Clinics in Obstetrics

Clinics in Obstetrics

Tania Gurdip Singh MS (Obstetrics and Gynecology)
Fellowship in Gynecological Endoscopy
Bodyline Trauma and Maternity Center
New Delhi, India

Foreword
Nutan Jain

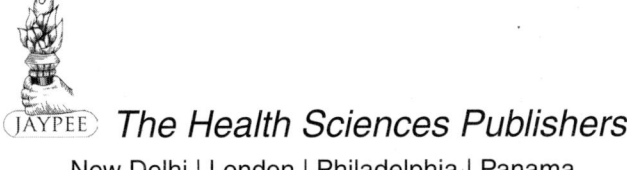

The Health Sciences Publishers
New Delhi | London | Philadelphia | Panama

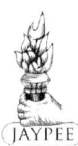

Jaypee Brothers Medical Publishers (P) Ltd.

Headquarters
Jaypee Brothers Medical Publishers (P) Ltd.
4838/24, Ansari Road, Daryaganj
New Delhi 110 002, India
Phone: +91-11-43574357
Fax: +91-11-43574314
E-mail: jaypee@jaypeebrothers.com

Overseas Offices

J.P. Medical Ltd.
83, Victoria Street, London
SW1H 0HW (UK)
Phone: +44-20 3170 8910
Fax: +44(0)20 3008 6180
E-mail: info@jpmedpub.com

Jaypee-Highlights Medical Publishers Inc.
City of Knowledge, Bld. 237, Clayton
Panama City, Panama
Phone: +1 507-301-0496
Fax: +1 507-301-0499
E-mail: cservice@jphmedical.com

Jaypee Medical Inc.
The Bourse
111, South Independence Mall East
Suite 835, Philadelphia, PA 19106, USA
Phone: +1 267-519-9789
E-mail: jpmed.us@gmail.com

Jaypee Brothers Medical Publishers (P) Ltd.
17/1-B, Babar Road, Block-B, Shaymali
Mohammadpur, Dhaka-1207
Bangladesh
Mobile: +08801912003485
E-mail: jaypeedhaka@gmail.com

Jaypee Brothers Medical Publishers (P) Ltd.
Bhotahity, Kathmandu, Nepal
Phone: +977-9741283608
E-mail: kathmandu@jaypeebrothers.com

Website: www.jaypeebrothers.com
Website: www.jaypeedigital.com

© 2015, Jaypee Brothers Medical Publishers

The views and opinions expressed in this book are solely those of the original contributor(s)/author(s) and do not necessarily represent those of editor(s) of the book.

All rights reserved. No part of this publication may be reproduced, stored or transmitted in any form or by any means, electronic, mechanical, photocopying, recording or otherwise, without the prior permission in writing of the publishers.

All brand names and product names used in this book are trade names, service marks, trademarks or registered trademarks of their respective owners. The publisher is not associated with any product or vendor mentioned in this book.

Medical knowledge and practice change constantly. This book is designed to provide accurate, authoritative information about the subject matter in question. However, readers are advised to check the most current information available on procedures included and check information from the manufacturer of each product to be administered, to verify the recommended dose, formula, method and duration of administration, adverse effects and contraindications. It is the responsibility of the practitioner to take all appropriate safety precautions. Neither the publisher nor the author(s)/editor(s) assume any liability for any injury and/or damage to persons or property arising from or related to use of material in this book.

This book is sold on the understanding that the publisher is not engaged in providing professional medical services. If such advice or services are required, the services of a competent medical professional should be sought.

Every effort has been made where necessary to contact holders of copyright to obtain permission to reproduce copyright material. If any have been inadvertently overlooked, the publisher will be pleased to make the necessary arrangements at the first opportunity.

Inquiries for bulk sales may be solicited at: jaypee@jaypeebrothers.com

Clinics in Obstetrics

First Edition: **2015**

ISBN: 978-93-5152-199-0

Printed at Rajkamal Electric Press, Plot No. 2, Phase-IV, Kundli, Haryana.

Dedicated to

*My great parents for their immense and constant support,
inspiration and faith in me.
My beloved husband for his extreme patience,
who, in his own way, tolerated and encouraged the demands of my career.
Together they have made this journey worth the effort.*

Foreword

Appearing for the examinations and viva voce remains a stressful task for most of the postgraduate students. After completing their medical schooling, they are at the doorsteps of venturing into life as independent experts in their respective fields. The challenges of clearing the examinations loom large on them. Even the finest of students find it difficult to revise the entire syllabus in a short time, close to their practicals. Addressing this universal problem, Dr Tania Gurdip Singh has come out with a unique book—*Clinics in Obstetrics*.

Obstetrics is ever-evolving. Hitech gadgets for monitoring and treating fetus as an individual have all brought about definite changes in the management protocols. Keeping the latest trends in view, all the chapters have been formulated. The book is basically meant for the preparation of practical and viva voce for both the postgraduate and undergraduate students. It covers history, examination and management of all the cases in obstetrics in complete detail. Each chapter is discussed with a hypothetical case, followed by stepwise discussion of each differential diagnosis and how to reach the final diagnosis. I feel this text will add a lot to the existing literature on obstetrics and will prove indispensable for the postgraduate students. It is need-based and well fulfills its purpose.

Dr Tania is a dedicated and hardworking individual, with a passion for excellence. I am sure her book is in accordance with her persona and will be a glittering gem in the array of existing literature in obstetrics.

A great academic achievement!

Nutan Jain MS (Obstetrics and Gynecology)
Vardhman Trauma and Laparoscopy Centre (P) Ltd
Muzaffarnagar, Uttar Pradesh, India
www.vardhmanhospital.com; www.drnutanjain.com

Preface

Obstetrics is a highly evolving field. The teaching and examination in obstetrics has become more practical-oriented. There is a tendency of the medical students to study the theory in depth, wherein the clinical aspect gets neglected, due to which there is a big fear when practicals and viva voce approach.

A very wrong belief among the students is that the questions will only be asked pertaining to the case and its final diagnosis, but, in reality, the case always goes on differential diagnosis because the examiner is aware of the fact that the students know the final diagnosis. In order to be confident in clinical cases, a proper approach to practical cases is a must.

The time duration between the theory and practical examinations is very less and most students are weak in case presentations, which makes them grumble before practicals and fumble in practicals. A student does not have time to look into different books in this short period of time. What he/she has to do is to just pick up this book, revise and go confidently to the examination hall. This book provides unique and recent information in the most original form, and that too in a stepwise manner.

The book is basically meant for the preparation of practical and viva voce for both the postgraduate as well as the undergraduate students. For the sake of simplicity, the book is divided into two sections: Section 1 for *Long Cases* and Section 2 for *Short Cases*. Each chapter contains important points in history, indicating where exactly to lay stress, explaining how history differs in each case (i.e. where the examiner can catch the student!). A hypothetical case is discussed, followed by stepwise discussion of each differential diagnosis and how to reach the final diagnosis. All the cases have been covered in full detail. Tests, which have lost their importance and are not implicated in routine practice, are not mentioned. It covers the management of all the cases in complete aspect.

The students may not know something in recent advances but will not be spared if it comes to basics, which might look very simple but are not recollected during examination. So, keeping this in mind, all the basic questions have been covered to refresh a student's knowledge.

Not only for the undergraduate and postgraduate students, this book will be highly beneficial for the clinicians also, who practice in the field of obstetrics. This book will prove to be useful for the nursing students as well. This is a very student-friendly or, rather I would say, an examination-friendly book, in a very comprehensive manner, with very original and authentic information, covering all the recent guidelines. It is a small effort on my part to reeve all the basic information and latest updates in a single thread.

Tania Gurdip Singh

Acknowledgments

I take this opportunity to thank all my teachers, friends and well-wishers, which is very much justified at this stage of the completion of my book, and even more so is a sense of gratitude.

It is my great privilege, though am finding words inadequate to express my indebtedness and deep gratitude to my respected teacher, Dr Nutan Jain. Her never-ending willingness to render help, loving guidance, coupled with her rich knowledge and keen interest, were a constant source of inspiration for me throughout.

I am deeply grateful to all my revered teachers Dr BR Desai, Dr BR Nilgar, Dr MK Swamy, Dr MB Bellad and Dr Kamal P Patil for their valuable guidance. I learnt from them that sincerity and hard work give a great pleasure at the end. I shall ever remain obliged to them.

I am very grateful to Shri Jitendar P Vij (Group Chairman) and Mr Ankit Vij (Group President) for showing trust in me and getting this book published. I sincerely thank Mr Tarun Duneja (Director-Publishing), Mr PS Ghuman (Assistant General Manager), Ms Samina Khan (Executive Assistant to Director-Publishing), Mr Rajesh Sharma, Mr Sunil Dogra and Mr Nilambar Pant (Production Coordinators), Mr Ashutosh Srivastava (Assistant Editor), Mr Chandra Dutt and Mr Hemant Kumar (DTP Operators), and Mr Pawan Kumar (Designer) of M/s Jaypee Brothers Medical Publishers (P) Ltd, New Delhi, India, who rendered great help in the completion of this project. I must acknowledge the tireless work of Mr Prashant Soni (Senior Proofreader) for excellent proofreading. The sincerity towards his work is outstanding. I am thankful for his productive suggestions and cooperation in completing this project.

I shall be failing in my duty if I do not acknowledge, with a deep sense of gratitude, all my patients, from whom I have learnt a lot.

"A mother is the truest friend we have. When trials, heavy and sudden, fall upon us, when adversity takes the place of prosperity, when friends who rejoice with us in our sunshine desert us, when trouble thickens around us, still will she cling to us, and endeavor by her kind percepts and counsels to dissipate the clouds of darkness and cause peace to return to our hearts."
—**Washington Irving**

I cannot express in words the indebtedness I owe to my dearest parents, who took pains for me and without whose inspiration and blessings, this work could not have been accomplished. Wholeheartedly, I am thankful to them for bringing me up in discipline. I must give full credit to them.

I owe my sincere admiration to my loveliest brother Gagandeep, who always nourished my ambitions and is behind every success of my life; my respected in-laws, who are always encouraging and supporting.

It is with a deep sense of gratitude that I take this opportunity to thank my beloved husband Earl Jaspal (Consultant Pediatrician and Head, Department of Neonatology, Government Hospital, Ambala, Haryana, India) for his constant encouragement and benevolent guidance. I am very much thankful to him for his important contributions for the following chapters in the book—Pain Abdomen during Pregnancy, Pyrexia in Pregnancy, Puerperium, Post-term Pregnancy,

Rh Negative Pregnancy, Jaundice in Pregnancy, HIV in Pregnancy and Thyroid Disorders in Pregnancy. As a truly caring person, he always had time to listen and also offered sincere advice with patience and understanding. His invaluable directions, vigilant supervision and constructive suggestions for improvement were the mainstreams to bring this work to the present shape. He is really a gem of a person. My daughter Aira is the ultimate source of motivation and is a real boost in whatever I do, including this work.

And, finally, I thank God for making all these wonderful people happen to me and pray for His continued blessings and success.

Contents

Section 1: Long Cases

1. **Antenatal Care** *Tania G Singh*	3
2. **Anemia in Pregnancy** *Tania G Singh*	48
3. **Recurrent Pregnancy Loss** *Tania G Singh*	102
4. **Antepartum Hemorrhage in Early Pregnancy** *Tania G Singh*	140
5. **Antepartum Hemorrhage in Late Gestation** *Tania G Singh*	183
6. **Uterine Size More than Expected** *Tania G Singh*	215
7. **Uterine Size Less than Expected** *Tania G Singh*	253
8. **Diabetes in Pregnancy** *Tania G Singh*	279
9. **Hypertensive Disorders in Pregnancy (HDP)** *Tania G Singh*	301
10. **Previous Cesarean Section** *Tania G Singh*	324
11. **Pain Abdomen during Pregnancy** *Tania G Singh, Earl Jaspal*	358
12. **Breech Presentation** *Tania G Singh*	403
13. **Cardiac Disease in Pregnancy (Part I)** *Tania G Singh*	421
14. **Cardiac Disease in Pregnancy (Part II)** *Tania G Singh*	445

15. **Pyrexia in Pregnancy** — 473
Tania G Singh, Earl Jaspal

16. **Postpartum Hemorrhage** — 518
Tania G Singh

17. **Puerperium** — 559
Tania G Singh, Earl Jaspal

Section 2: Short Cases

18. **Post-term Pregnancy** — 603
Tania G Singh, Earl Jaspal

19. **Convulsions in Pregnancy** — 622
Tania G Singh

20. **Rh Negative Pregnancy** — 652
Tania G Singh, Earl Jaspal

21. **Jaundice in Pregnancy** — 672
Tania G Singh, Earl Jaspal

22. **HIV in Pregnancy** — 698
Tania G Singh, Earl Jaspal

23. **Thyroid Disorders in Pregnancy** — 718
Tania G Singh, Earl Jaspal

Index — *743*

SECTION 1

Long Cases

SECTION OUTLINES

- **Antenatal Care**
  Tania G Singh
- **Anemia in Pregnancy**
  Tania G Singh
- **Recurrent Pregnancy Loss**
  Tania G Singh
- **Antepartum Hemorrhage in Early Pregnancy**
  Tania G Singh
- **Antepartum Hemorrhage in Late Gestation**
  Tania G Singh
- **Uterine Size More than Expected**
  Tania G Singh
- **Uterine Size Less than Expected**
  Tania G Singh
- **Diabetes in Pregnancy**
  Tania G Singh
- **Hypertensive Disorders in Pregnancy (HDP)**
  Tania G Singh
- **Previous Cesarean Section**
  Tania G Singh
- **Pain Abdomen during Pregnancy**
  Tania G Singh, Earl Jaspal
- **Breech Presentation**
  Tania G Singh
- **Cardiac Disease in Pregnancy (Part I)**
  Tania G Singh
- **Cardiac Disease in Pregnancy (Part II)**
  Tania G Singh
- **Pyrexia in Pregnancy**
  Tania G Singh, Earl Jaspal
- **Postpartum Hemorrhage**
  Tania G Singh
- **Puerperium**
  Tania G Singh, Earl Jaspal

CHAPTER 1

Antenatal Care

Tania G Singh

Obstetrics (in Latin 'obstare' means 'to stand by'): It is the branch of medicine that deals with the care of women during pregnancy, childbirth, and the recuperative period following delivery.

Awareness of all signs, symptoms and various examinations pertaining to a particular gestational age is immensely important (which forms the basis of 'Obstetrics').

A pregnant patient can approach a doctor at any period of gestation.

Before moving on to the history, a student should first be aware of what the patient will complain about, what he has to look for and which investigations are to be done and at which period of gestation.

Without the knowledge of all normal signs and symptoms of pregnancy, it is nearly very difficult to take history in a normal antenatal case.

First Trimester (First 12 Weeks of Pregnancy)

The first antenatal visit (between 6 and 10 weeks).

CLINICAL FEATURES

Symptoms

- *Amenorrhea*
- *Nausea and vomiting*
- *Frequency of micturition*
  - Due to congestion and pressure on the bladder
  - Appears from 8 to 12 weeks
  - Reappears again near the end of pregnancy when the fetal head descends into the maternal pelvis
- *Breast changes*
  - Discomfort
  - Enlargement
  - Pain/heaviness
- Fatigue/lassitude
- Change in appetite
  - Craving for certain foods, odors and particular objects
- Sleepiness
- Emotional changes/mood swings

Signs

Breast Signs

- Appear at 6 to 8 weeks
- Enlargement with vascular engorgement
- Discomfort—fullness, heaviness and pricking sensation
- Nipple and primary areola become more pigmented and sensitivity increases
- Montgomery's tubercles appear
- Expression of colostrum as early as 12th week
- More in primigravidae.

Pelvic Signs

Placental sign
Bleeding at the time of the next menstruation.

Hartman's sign
Implantation bleeding.

Ladin's sign
- A clinical sign of pregnancy in which there is softening in the midline of the uterus anteriorly at the junction of the uterus and cervix
- Occurs at about 6 weeks gestation.

Goodell's sign
- A significant softening of the vaginal portion of the cervix from increased vascularization of uterus in pregnancy
- Named after William Goodell
- Can be seen at 6th week.

Von Braun-Fernwald's sign
- A clinical sign in which there is an irregular softening and enlargement of the uterine fundus during early pregnancy
- Occurs at 5 to 8 weeks gestation
- Named after Karl von Braun-Fernwald.

Chadwick's sign
- Bluish discoloration of the cervix, vagina and labia resulting from increased blood flow
- Can be observed as early as 6 to 8 weeks after conception
- Discovered in 1836 by a French doctor, Étienne Joseph Jacquemin
- James Read Chadwick drew attention to it in 1886.

Piskaçek's sign
- Named after Ludwig Piskaçek and Kevin
- Can be observed at 7 to 8 weeks
- One half of uterus—more firm than other half (implantation site)
- Observing a soft palpable bulge at the uterine cornu.

Osiander's sign
Increased pulsations felt through lateral fornix by 8 weeks.

Hegar's sign
- Its absence does not exclude pregnancy
- Bimanual examination with two fingers in the anterior fornix and the fingers of the other hand on the abdomen behind the uterus
- The internal and external fingers can be approximated due to the fact that the lower segment is soft and empty and upper part of the body of the uterus is enlarged → fingers of both the hands can be approximated against the soft uterine isthmus
- Present from 6 weeks until the 12th week of pregnancy
- Difficult to recognize in multiparous women
- Described by Ernst Ludwig Alfred Hegar, a German gynecologist, in 1895.

Palmer's sign
- Regular and rhythmic contractions of the uterus in early pregnancy
- Pregnancy should be of at least 8 weeks duration
- Method:
  - Two fingers of gloved right hand are placed into the vagina and left hand palpates the lower abdomen from above
  - Wait for 2 to 3 minutes → uterus becomes firm and then ill-defined in accordance to its contraction and relaxation.

(In the presence of USG, Palmer's sign and Hegar's sign have lost their importance.)

Uterus

- Remains a pelvic organ until 12th week
- From 12 to 14 weeks, it can be felt as suprapubic bulge.

Vagina and Vulva

- Vagina and vulva are bluish/violet in color, particularly the vestibule
- Vagina becomes moist, warm and lax
- There is an increase in the amount and acidity of the vaginal discharge.

(None of the early clinical signs of pregnancy are reliable. Pregnancy needs to be confirmed by UPT and/or USG.)

LABORATORY TESTS

Immunological Tests for the Diagnosis of Pregnancy

Principle

Measurement of human chorionic gonadotropin (hCG) in maternal urine or serum with antibody, either polyclonal or monoclonal, available commercially.

Tests Used

Urine pregnancy tests
- Agglutination test: Latex particles or sheep erythrocyte (tube) coated with anti-hCG
- Agglutination inhibition tests
- Dip stick test
- Rapid and simple tests based on enzyme-labeled monoclonal antibodies assay.

Causes of false positive results
- Proteinuria
- Hematuria
- Done at the time of ovulation (cross-reaction with Luteinizing hormone)
- hCG injection for infertility treatment within the previous 30 days
- Thyrotoxicosis (high TSH)
- Early days after delivery or abortion
- Trophoblastic diseases
- hCG secreting tumours.
- Premature menopause (high LH and FSH)

Causes of false negative results
- Missed abortion
- Ectopic pregnancy
- Too early pregnancy
- Urine stored too long at room temperature
- Interfering medications.

Serum pregnancy tests
- Radioimmunoassay of β-subunit of hCG
- Radio receptor assay.

Test using both urine and serum
- Enzyme-linked immunosorbent assay (ELISA)

	Sensitivity	Time to complete	Postconception age when first positive	Gestational age when first positive
Radioimmunoassay	5 mIU/mL	4 hours	10–18 days	3–4 weeks
Immunoradiometric assay (more sensitive)	150 mIU/mL	30 minutes	18–22 days	4 weeks
Immunoradiometric assay (less sensitive)	1500 mIU/mL	2 minutes	25–28 days	5 weeks
Enzyme-linked immunosorbent assay (more sensitive)	25 mIU/mL	80 minutes	14–17 days	3.5 weeks
Enzyme-linked immunosorbent assay (less sensitive)	<50 mIU/mL	5–15 minutes	18–22 days	4 weeks
Fluoroimmunoassay	1 mIU/mL	2–3 hours	14–17 days	3.5 weeks

- hCG is detectable in the serum
  - In ≈ 5% of patients, 8 days after conception and
  - In > 98% of patients, by day 11.
- At 4 weeks' gestation (Day 18–22 postconception), the dimer and β-subunit of hCG doubling times are approximately 2.2 days (standard deviation ± 0.8 days)
- It falls to 3.5 days (standard deviation ± 1.2 d) by 9 weeks' gestation
- Levels peak at 10 to 12 weeks' gestation and then begin to decline rapidly until another, more gradual rise begins at 22 weeks' gestation, which continues until term.

The pregnancy test becomes negative about:
- 1 week after labor
- 2 weeks after abortion
- 4 weeks after evacuation of vesicular mole.

Progesterone

- Serum progesterone is a reflection of progesterone production by the corpus luteum, which is stimulated by a viable pregnancy
- Measured by radioimmunoassay and fluoroimmunoassay
- Results after 3 to 4 hours
- A dipstick ELISA that can determine a serum progesterone level of < 15 ng/mL is also available
- Serum progesterone
  - \> 25 ng/mL → viable intrauterine pregnancy (97.5% sensitivity)
  - < 5 ng/mL → a nonviable pregnancy (100% sensitivity)
  - 5 to 25 ng/mL → further testing using ultrasound, additional hormonal assays or serial examinations are warranted.

Early Pregnancy Factor

- Early pregnancy factor (EPF) assay may be useful in the future as an aid in diagnosing pregnancy *before implantation*
- It is a poorly defined immunosuppressive protein that is present in maternal serum shortly after conception
- The earliest available marker to indicate fertilization
- Detection:
  - Detectable in the serum 36–48 hours after fertilization
  - Peaks early in the first trimester
  - Almost undetectable at term
  - Also appears within 48 hours of successful IVF embryo transfers
  - Cannot be detected 24 hours after delivery or at the termination of an ectopic or intrauterine pregnancy
  - Also undetectable in many ectopic pregnancies and spontaneous abortions, indicating that if EPF is not identified, that pregnancy may represent a poor prognosis
- Today EPF has limited clinical application because the molecule is difficult to isolate
- Detection of EPF currently relies on a complex and unwieldy assay named the rosette inhibition test.

Home Pregnancy Tests

- These tests now use the modern immunometric assay
- Most of these tests claim '99% accuracy'
- The broad 99% accuracy statement is made for tests with sensitivities for hCG concentrations ranging from 25 mIU/mL (fairly sensitive) to tests with sensitivities of 100 mIU/mL (less sensitive)
- Home pregnancy tests are most commonly used in the week after the missed menstrual period (fourth completed gestational week)
- Urine hCG values are extremely variable at this time and can range from 12 mIU/mL to > 2500 mIU/mL
- This variability continues into the fifth week, when values have been shown to range from 13 mIU/mL to > 6000 mIU/mL
- Both weeks have a percentage of urine hCG values that is below the sensitivities of detection for common home pregnancy tests (range 25–100 mIU/mL)
- Therefore, during 4th and 5th weeks, they may not be highly accurate

- Collection of urine for the test:
  - Try to perform first thing in the morning, though this is not mandatory
  - Collect urine in a clean, dry, plastic container
  - Wash only with water
  - Ensure that there is no detergent residue in the container
  - Take out the strip from the pack and keep it on a flat surface
  - Put about 2 to 3 drops of urine on it with a dropper (provided in the kit)
  - Do not spill urine on the reading strip
  - Wait for 3 to 5 minutes (depending on manufacturer's instructions) and then read the test results
  - Trying to read the results before the stipulated time or waiting too long can both lead to inaccurate readings.

Reading the Test

- 'C' indicates a control (this band must always appear because this is the comparison band)
- 'T' indicates the test sample
- If only one red/pink/purple band appears in the region marked 'C', it means that the test is negative
- If two red/pink/purple bands appear, one in the 'C' region and the other in the region marked 'T', it means that the test is positive for pregnancy
- In case no bands appear or if a faint line appears in the 'T' region, then the test is invalid
- Repeat the test with a new pack after 72 hours.

Other Routine Blood Tests

- Hemogram
- Screening for hemoglobinopathies
- Complete urine analysis (to detect asymptomatic bacteriuria, if present)
- VDRL, HIV (after pretest counseling and written consent)
- ABO Rh. If rhesus negative, check husband's blood group
- HbsAg, Anti-HBC Ag
- Rubella susceptibility
- USG to confirm intrauterine gestation, cardiac activity, measure gestational age using CRL, to rule out multiple gestation and ectopic pregnancy
- Cervical cytology, if indicated
- A wet smear of any symptomatic vaginal discharge (i.e. itching, burning or offensive)
- Down's syndrome screening using:
  - 'Combined test' (nuchal translucency, β-hCG, pregnancy-associated plasma protein-A) at 10+0 to 13+6 weeks
  - Ultrasound for nuchal translucency between 10+0 and 14+0 weeks (CRL 36–84 mm).

Indications for Prenatal Counseling and Screening

Prepregnancy

- Maternal age ≥ 35 years
- Consanguinity, ethnicity, family history of genetic disorder
- History of recurrent spontaneous abortions, stillbirths, neonatal deaths and malformations in previous babies
- Family history of a known/suspected genetic disorder, e.g. thalassemia, muscular dystrophy, cystic fibrosis, Down's syndrome.

Antenatal
- Abnormal fetal USG
- Abnormal maternal serum screening
- Teratogen exposure
- Maternal infection.

Summary of prenatal genetic screening tests

Noninvasive tests

	Screen name	Markers	Possible timeframes	Best timeframes
1st trimester	USG	NT	11–13 wks 6d	12–13 wks 3d
	Combined screen	NT + PAPP A + hCG	10–13 wks 6d	10 wks 2d–11 wks 6d
2nd trimester	Triple test	MSAFP + uE3 + hCG	15–20 wks	
	Quadruple test	hCG + Inhibin A + MSAFP + uE3	15–20 wks 6d	15 wks 2d–17 wks
	USG	Anomaly scan	18–22 wks	
Combined 1st and 2nd trimesters	IPS (integrated prenatal screen)	PAPP + NT in 1st trimester and Quadruple in 2nd trimester	Reports given only after both the tests (by making single risk determination)	
	SIPS (serum integrated prenatal screen)	PAPP A + Quad test (w/o NT)		
	Stepwise sequential screening	PAPP A + NT with an age associated risk If at ↑ risk → 2 options Invasive testing in 1st trimester OR Triple or Quad test in 2nd trimester	1st trimester	

Interpretation of Various Markers

Maternal serum α fetoprotein (AFP)
- Oncofetal → produced by yolk sac initially and after its involution, by fetal liver (in early pregnancy)
- AFP is present in amniotic fluid initially through diffusion across immature skin and later through kidneys and fetal urination
- Amniotic fluid AFP is swallowed by fetus and recirculates with final degradation by fetal liver
- Very small amounts are present in maternal serum through diffusion across the placenta and amnion
- Levels:
  - Nonpregnancy levels → 1 µ/L
  - 16 to 18 weeks period of gestation → 18 to 40 µ/L
  - When fetal serum level is 2 µ/L and maternal serum level is 20 µ/L → amniotic fluid AFP will be 20,000 µ/L
- Fetal plasma and amniotic fluid AFP → peak in midtrimester of pregnancy
- Maternal serum AFP →↑ until 28 to 32 weeks of gestation

Elevated in
- Multiple gestation
- Fetal demise
- Fetomaternal hemorrhage
- Placental abnormalities
- Uterine abnormalities
- Maternal ovarian or hepatic tumour
- Fetal congenital defects
1. Neural tube defect
    i. Spina bifida
    ii. Anencephaly
    iii. Encephalocele
2. Open ventral wall defect
    i. Omphalocele
    ii. Gastroschisis
3. Congenital nephrosis (because of fetal proteinuria)
4. Triploidy
5. B/L renal agenesis
6. Congenital skin disorders
    i. Aplasia cutis
    ii. Epidemolysis bullosa
7. Autosomal recessive PCKD
8. Sacrococcygeal teratoma
9. Cystic adenomatoid malformation of lung
- Unexplained increase of maternal serum AFP
    - AFP>2.5 MOM in the absence of the above-mentioned causes
    - Associated with:
        - Chorionic villitis and placental vascular lesions
        - Maternal uterine malformation

Reduced in (<0.25 mm)
Spontaneous abortion
Preterm labor/delivery
Stillbirth
Infant death
Macrosomia
Obstetric complications (when ↑)
IUGR
APH
Preterm labor/delivery
Fetal death >24 weeks
Spontaneous abortion
Gestational hypertension and preeclampsia
Polyhydramnios
Low Apgar
Asphyxia
NICU admission

- Increase AFP in amniotic fluid and maternal serum → only when NTDs are open, i.e. when neural tissue is exposed or covered by only a thin membrane
- When NTDs are skin covered, AFP does not escape from fetal circulation and there is no increase of AFP in the mother
- AFP is an important screening test because 80% of infants with NTD are born into families with no prior history of disorder
- Optimal time for screening (for NTDs)
    - 16 to 18 weeks
    - When LMP is known, dating done is according to it
    - When LMP is not known, dating is done according to BPD in the 2nd trimester (at 14 weeks)
        - BPD is usually smaller in fetuses with spina bifida and maternal serum AFP will appear higher; therefore, improved detection rate
- Other factors which affect MSAFP
    - Maternal weight → obese females have ↓ levels (because larger size results in greater dilution of fetally derived AFP)
    - *Race:* Black and Asian females > nonblack race
    - IDDM → levels are lower
    - Multifetal reduction in 1st trimester →↑ levels in 2nd trimester

- Summary
  Increase in:
  - Neural tube defects
  - Trisomy 18

  Decrease in:
  - Down's syndrome.

Maternal serum hCG
- Secreted by syncytiotrophoblasts
- Elevated hCG
  - Cut-offs varying from > 2.0 MoM to > 4.0 MoM
  - *Causes:*
    - Fetal chromosomal abnormalities (Down's syndrome)
    - Placental anomalies (Molar pregnancy)
    - Multiple pregnancy
    - IUFD
    - Hypoxic cytotrophoblasts demonstrate increased proliferation and increased hCG production
    - Other placental abnormalities
      - Chorioangiosis of placenta (abnormal capillary proliferation associated with uterine hypoxia)
      - Placental mosaicism
- Obstetric complications with unexplained elevation:
  - IUGR
  - Hypertensive disorders of pregnancy
  - Preterm labor and preterm delivery
  - Stillbirth
  - Velamentous cord insertion
- Low hCG
  - Defined as a value < 0.5 MoM
  - *Unexplained low hCG:*
    - Normal fetal anatomy
    - Viable pregnancy
    - Normal fetal karyoptype
    - Pregnancy outcomes, when low hCG
    - In 1st trimester—miscarriage
    - In 2nd trimester—normal
- Summary
  Decrease in:
  - Trisomy 18

  No change in:
  - NTDs

Maternal serum unconjugated estriol (uE3)
- How and where is it produced?
  - Fetal adrenal glands produce DHEAS
  - Fetal liver converts DHEAS to 16 α OH-DHEAS
  - Inplacenta, 16 α OH-DHEAS is deconjugated by a sulfatase
  - Resulting molecule is aromatized to uE3

- Decrease in trisomy 21 and 18
- No change in open NTDs
- High levels are not associated with adverse perinatal outcomes
- Low levels (<0.75 MoM) are associated with:
  - Fetal chromosomal abnormalities
  - Fetal death
  - Fetal metabolic conditions
    - Steroid sulfatase deficiency
    - Congenital adrenal hypoplasia/Hypocortisolism
    - Smith-Lemli-Opitz syndrome
    - Placental aromatase deficiency
    - Kallman syndrome
- Complications (when low)
  - IUGR
  - Small for gestational age
  - IUFD
  - Oligohydramnios.

Maternal serum inhibin A

- Levels are much reduced in primary antiphospholipid antibody syndrome
- Levels are much increased in:
  - Triploidy
  - HELLP syndrome
  - Following loss of 1 twin in 1st trimester
- Obstetric complications (when levels are increased → ≥ 2 MoM)
  - IUGR
  - Preterm delivery
  - IUFD
  - Hypertensive disorders
- Summary
  Increase in:
  - Down's syndrome
  No change in:
  - Open NTDs
  - Trisomy 18.

Maternal serum pregnancy associated with plasma protein-A (PAPP-A)

- Produced by placenta and decidua
- Increases the bioavailability of IGF, which, in turn, mediates trophoblast invasion and modulates glucose and amino acid transport in the placenta
- *Levels increased*
  - No adverse outcome
- *Levels decreased*
  - Spontaneous abortions
  - IUGR
  - Preterm delivery
  - IUFD
  - Hypertensive disorders.

Recommendations
- *1st trimester:* Combined screening
- *2nd trimester:* Quadruple or triple test

ULTRASONOGRAPHY

Transvaginal

Period of gestation (weeks)	Ultrasound features

Week 4	**Gestational sac**
	• Gestational sac size = 3 to 6 mm
	• Grows at the rate of 1 mm/day through the 9th week
	• Sometimes may not appear by the end of the 5th week
	• Initially round, anechoic structure
	• Gestational age calculation
	  – When no structures are visible within the gestational sac:
	    - Mean sac diameter (MSD) in mm + 30 = Gestational age in days
	  – When embryo is seen inside it, MSD is no longer accurate

Week 5	**Gestational sac** • Size = 6–12 mm **Yolk sac** • Seen with TVS when mean sac diameter is ≈ 8 mm to 10 mm • Its presence confirms the diagnosis of an intrauterine pregnancy • By 5 weeks 4 days, it should definitely be present **Fetal pole** • Adjacent to yolk sac (near the wall) **Cardiac activity** • By the end of the 5th week • Normal heart rate at this time = 60–90 bpm (In early pregnancies, the actual cardiac rate is less important than its presence or absence) • Must be detected when embryo length is 5 mm **Lacunar structures** • Cavities or spaces at the site of implantation
Week 6	**Gestational sac** • Size = 14–25 mm **Crown rump length** • Gestational age in the 1st trimester is calculated from the fetal CRL (± 6 days) • This is the longest demonstrable length of the embryo or fetus, excluding the limbs and the yolk sac • Most accurate between 7 and 10 weeks of pregnancy • From 6 to 11 weeks, CRL grows at a rate of ≈ 1 mm/day • CRL = 4–7 mm **Fetal pole** • Length = 0.2–0.3 inches • Grows at the rate of about 1 mm/day, from 6th week **'Dating the fetus'** • Gestational age = 6 weeks plus (CRL in days) • *Example:* CRL 16 mm (2 wks 2 days) would have a gestational age of 8 wks and 2 days

Contd...

Contd...

Period of gestation (weeks)	Ultrasound features
Week 7	CRL (crown to rump length) • 5 mm to 12 mm Length • < 0.5 inch Weight • < 1 g Heart rate • Increases from 130–160 bpm *Other features:* • Heart is beating with one chamber • A dividing wall is formed in the heart • Arm and leg buds begin to grow • The lower jaw and the vocal cords are beginning to form • The mouth opening is formed • The inner ear is being created • The digestive tract is developing • The navel string is being created • The following organs are being formed: the lungs, the liver, the pancreas and the thyroid gland • Neural tube begins to fuse

Week 8	CRL
	• 16 mm to 20 mm
	
	Length
	• 0.6 to 0.9 inch
	
	Weight
	• Approximately 1 g
	
	Fetal structures (at the end of the 8th week):
	• Elbows
	• Feet buds
	• Hands bud
	• Even fingers are visible
	• Initiate minor movements
	• Stomach is being made from part of the gut
	• Face begins to take shape
	• Mouth and nostrils start developing
	• Teeth begin to develop under the gums
	• Eyes can now be seen as small hollows on each side of the head
	• Brain cavities—seen as large 'holes' in the embryonic head
	• Heart
	  – Rate—160 bpm
	  – Covers ≈ 50% of the chest area
	• Sometimes, it is possible to recognize the fluid-filled stomach below the heart

Contd...

Contd...

Period of gestation (weeks)	Ultrasound features
Week 9	CRL → 20–30 mm
	Length → 0.9 to 1.2 inch
	Weight → 2 g
	Other features: • Fingers and toes well defined • Cartilage and bones begin to form • Upper lip as well as the nose tip is being formed • Tongue begins to develop and the larynx is developing • Eyelids are developed, although they stay closed for several months • Main construction of the heart is complete • Heart rate reaches a maximum of about 175 bpm
Week 10	CRL → 31–41 mm (1.2 to 1.6 inches)
	Weight → 2–4 g
	Other features: • From this week until birth, the developing organism is called a fetus • Size of fetus → of a small strawberry • Feet are 2 mm long • Neck is beginning to take shape • Body muscles are almost developed • Fetus has begun movement, even shifts • Jaws are in place • Mouth cavity and the nose are joined • Ears and nose seen clearly • Fingerprints are already evident in the skin • Nipples and hair follicles begin to form
Week 11	CRL → 41–54 mm
	Length → 1.6 to 2 inches
	Weight → 7 g
	Other features: • Fingers and toes have completely separated • Taste buds start developing • Fetus has tooth buds, the beginning of the complete set of 20 milk teeth • Can swallow and stick out the tongue • Whole body except the tongue is sensitive to touch • Cartilage now calcifying to become bone
Week 12	Fetus is ≈ 6.5 cm long
	Weight → 14–20 g
	Other features: • Fetus starts moving spontaneously • Face is beginning to look like a baby's face • Fingernails and toenails appear • Fetus can suck the thumb and get hiccups Nuchal translucency and nasal bone (described henceforth)

Nuchal Translucency (NT)

- Single most powerful marker for Down's syndrome
- Refers to normal subcutaneous fluid-filled space between back of fetal neck and overlying skin
- Seen in all normal fetuses
- Called 'translucency' because, on ultrasound, this appears as a black space beneath the fetal skin
- Normally < 2.5 mm
- ≥ 2.5 mm → may indicate Down's syndrome or another chromosomal abnormality
- Time: 10 to 14 weeks (CRL 36–84 mm)
- Condition   NT
  Trisomy 21   ↑
  Trisomy 18   ↑
  Pregnancy loss <24 weeks   ↑
  Congenital heart defect   ↑

How to Measure?

- Midsagittal plane with fetal spine down
- Image—magnified. Only head, neck and upper thorax should be visible
- Neck—neutral (neither hyperflexed or hyperextended)
- Skin at fetal back clearly differentiated from underlying amniotic membrane
  How?
  a. Look for separate echogenic lines
  b. Note that skin line moves with fetus
- Calipers on inner border of echolucent space and perpendicular to long axis of fetus

Possible Causes for Increased Fluid-filled Space

- Cardiac failure 2° to structural malformation
- Abnormality in extracellular matrix
- Abnormal or delayed development of lymphatic system.

Septated cystic hygroma: When NT space is enlarged extending along entire length of fetus and in which septations are clearly visible.

Nasal Bone

- Clear association between absence of fetal nasal bone and Down's syndrome but absent Nasal Bone (NB) is not related to NT
- It is an independent marker
- Occasionally it may not be seen at 11 weeks.

How to Visualize?

- Midsagittal plane
- Spine position
- Slight neck flexion

- Two echogenic lines at fetal nose profile should be visualized
  Superficial: Nasal skin
  Deeper: Nasal bones (should be more echolucent at its distal end)
- USG beam should not be parallel to the plane of nasal bone because this will lead to error of ABSENT nasal bone.

Optimal Timing of USG for Fetal Anomalies

Anencephaly	10–12 weeks
Spina bifida	16–18 weeks
Limbs (all long bones should be measured)	16+ weeks (serial at 4 weeks interval)
Hydrocephalus/microcephaly	16+ weeks (serial at 4 weeks interval)
Renal (especially obstructive uropathy)	16+ weeks (serial at 4 weeks interval)
Face and mouth	18–22 weeks (preferably 3D or 4D)
Anterior abdominal wall	16–18 weeks

Following Important Points to be Explained at this Juncture

- Antenatal care should start at the time pregnancy is confirmed
- Booking visit should be as early as possible, preferably when the second menstrual period has been missed, i.e. at a gestational age (duration of pregnancy) of 8 weeks
- Ideally 8 to 10 antenatal appointments for nulliparous and 6 to 7 for parous women
- Basic investigations and appropriate screening tests must be done to identify high-risk patients
- Exercise (brisk walking) for 30 to 40 minutes 5 days/week seems to be appropriate
- Folic acid (400 micrograms/day, till 12 completed weeks to reduce the risk of neural tube defects) and vitamin D (10 micrograms/day) should be prescribed
- Vitamin A intake > 700 micrograms might be teratogenic and should, therefore, be avoided
- Diet, proper calorie intake and ideal weight gain should be explained at the beginning to avoid complications later in pregnancy.

PREGNANCY DIET AND WEIGHT GAIN

Types of Diet

Vegan: This diet includes fruits, vegetables, beans, grains, seeds and nuts. All animal sources of protein—including meat, poultry, fish, eggs, milk, cheese and other dairy products—are excluded from the diet.

Lacto-vegetarian: This diet includes dairy products in addition to the foods listed above in the vegan diet. Meat, poultry, fish and eggs are excluded from the diet.

Lacto-ovo-vegetarian: This diet includes dairy products and eggs in addition to the foods listed above in the vegan diet. Meat, poultry and fish are excluded from the diet

Pescatarian: This diet includes dairy products and eggs in addition to the foods listed above in the vegan diet. Meat and poultry are excluded from the diet, but fish is permitted, focusing on the fattier omega-3 rich varieties.

Mixed (nonveg): This diet includes vegies, dairy products, poultry, meat and fish.

General Principles

- In general, pregnant women need between 2,200 calories and 2,900 calories a day, which should be gradually increased with the growth of the fetus
  - 1st trimester → does not require any extra calories
  - 2nd trimester → additional 340 calories a day are recommended
  - 3rd trimester → recommendation is 450 calories more a day
- Add variety to your food
- Protein sources:
  - *For vegans:* Nuts, peanuts, butter, legumes, soy products, quinoa and tofu
  - *For nonvegans:* Meat, poultry, fish, eggs or dairy products
- Choose foods high in starch and fiber, such as whole-grain breads, cereals, pasta, rice, fruits and vegetables
- Eat and drink at least four servings of calcium-rich foods a day to help ensure that you are getting 1200 mg of calcium in your daily diet. Sources of calcium include dairy products, seafood, green-leafy vegetables, dried beans or peas, and tofu
- Vitamin D helps the body absorb calcium. Adequate amounts of vitamin D can be obtained through exposure to the sun and in fortified milk, eggs and fish. Vegans should receive 10 to 15 minutes of direct sunlight to the hands, face or arms three times per week or take a supplement
- Eat at least three servings of iron-rich foods per day to ensure getting 27 mg of iron in the daily diet. Sources of iron include enriched grain products (rice), eggs, green-leafy vegetables, broccoli, Brussels sprouts, sweet potatoes, dried beans and peas, raisins, prunes and peanuts
- Choose at least one source of vitamin C everyday. Sources of vitamin C include oranges, grapefruits, strawberries, honeydew, broccoli, cauliflower, Brussels sprouts, green peppers, tomatoes and mustard greens
- Choose at least one source of folic acid everyday. Sources of folic acid include dark, green-leafy vegetables, and legumes, such as lima beans, black beans, black-eyed peas and chickpeas
- Choose at least one source of vitamin A every alternate day. Sources of vitamin A include carrots, pumpkins, sweet potatoes, spinach, squash, turnip greens, beet greens, apricots and cantaloupe
- Choose at least one source of vitamin B_{12} a day. Vitamin B_{12} is found in animal products including fish and shellfish, eggs and dairy products. Vegans are at risk of not consuming enough vitamin B_{12}
- Avoid:
  - Leftover food
  - Frozen and deep-frozen food
  - Cold drinks
  - Tobacco
  - Alcohol
  - Smoking
- Liver and liver products may also contain high levels of vitamin A, and, therefore, consumption of these products should also be avoided
- Tea, coffee, chocolates and ice-cream can be taken only in moderation (only 2 cups of either tea or coffee permitted/day). Chocolate contains caffeine—the amount of caffeine in a chocolate bar is equal to 1/4th cup of coffee
- Those who suffer from constipation, gas and bloating must avoid peas and other 'heavy-to-digest' cereals and potatoes. They must take green gram as it is easy to digest and gives protein
- Butter, clarified butter, milk, honey, fennel seeds and sweets made from jaggery rather than white sugar can be taken in small quantity

- Items such as sandwich, bakery bread, bun, dhokla, pizza, khandvi, pancake, khaman dhokla, steamed rice cake, curd, tomato, tamarind and kadhi usually increase the swellings and acidity. So, try to avoid such items but if such problems do not exist, you can take in small quantity
- Most important, water intake should, by no means, be < 2.5 liters/day
- Limit fats and cholesterol
- DO NOT DIET or try to lose weight during pregnancy.

Calorie Chart for Basic Food Items

Fruits per 100 Grams

- Apple 56
- Avocado Pear 190
- Banana 95
- Chickoo 94
- Cherries 70
- Dates 281
- Grapes (Black) 45
- Guava 66
- Kiwi Fruit 45
- Lychees 61
- Mangoes 70
- Oranges 53
- Orange juice 100 mL 47
- Papaya 32
- Peach 50
- Pears 51
- Pineapple 46
- Plums 56
- Strawberries 77
- Watermelon 26
- Pomegranate 77

Vegetables per 100 Grams

- Broccoli 25
- Brinjal 24
- Cabbage 45
- Carrot 48
- Cauliflower 30
- Fenugreek (Methi) 49
- French beans 26
- Lettuce 21
- Mushroom 18
- Onion 50
- Peas 93
- Potato 97
- Spinach 23
- Tomato 21
- Tomato juice 100 mL 22

Cereals per 100 Grams

- Bajra 360
- Maize flour 355
- Rice 325
- Wheat flour 341

Indian Breads (Per Piece)

- 1 medium chapatti 119
- 1 slice white bread 60
- 1 paratha (no filling) 280

Milk and Milk Products (Per Cup)

- Butter 100 g 750
- Buttermilk 19
- Cheese 315
- Cream 100 g 210
- Ghee 100 g 910
- Milk (Buffalo) 115
- Milk (Cow) 100
- Milk (Skimmed) 45

Calories in Other Items

- Sugar 1 tbsp 48
- Honey 1 tbsp 90
- Coconut water 100 mL 25
- Coffee 40
- Tea 30

Weight Gain in Pregnancy

- **Underweight:** BMI below 18.5
- **Normal weight:** 18.5 to 24.9
- **Overweight:** 25.0 to 29.9
- **Obese:** 30.0 and above

Weeks	Weight gain (Pounds)	Weight gain (kg)
0–10 weeks	No weight gain	No weight gain
10–14 weeks	3–4 pounds	1.5 kg
14–20 weeks	4–6 pounds	2.5 kg
20–30 weeks	10–12 pounds	4.5 kg
30–36 weeks	6 pounds	2.7 kg
36–38 weeks	2 pounds	1.0 kg
38–40 weeks	Almost no weight gain	Almost no weight gain
Total	25–30 pounds	12–14 kg

Second Trimester (13–28 Weeks)

There should be a minimum of 3 visits in this trimester

CLINICAL FEATURES

Symptoms

- Amenorrhea
- Morning sickness and urinary symptoms decrease
- Progressive abdominal enlargement.

Signs

- Breasts become engorged
- Uterus feels soft and elastic, and becomes ovoid-shaped
- Braxton-Hicks contractions are evident.

Vaginal Examination

- Bluish discoloration of the vulva, vagina and cervix is much more evident
- Increased softening of the cervix
- Internal ballottement can be elicited between 16th–28th week. The fetus is too small before 16th week and too large to displace after 28th week.

14–16 Weeks

- Review, discuss and record the results of all the screening tests undertaken in the 1st trimester
- Colostrum becomes thick and yellowish by 16th week
- Injection tetanus toxoid 0.5 mL IM (1st dose) should be given
- Prescribe iron and calcium.

	WHO Tetanus toxoid immunization schedule		
Dose	When to give	Protection %	Duration of protection
TT-1	At first contact or as early as possible in pregnancy	Nil	None
TT-2	At least 4 weeks after TT-1	80	3 years
TT-3	At least 6 months after TT-2 or during subsequent pregnancy	95	5 years
TT-4	At least 1 year after TT-3 or during subsequent pregnancy	99	10 years
TT-5	At least 1 year after TT-4 or during subsequent pregnancy	99	Throughout childbearing

1. *Hemogram*
   - If hemoglobin level is <10 g/100 mL, investigate and consider additional iron supplementation
   - If MCH <27 picograms, offer HPLC (high performance liquid chromatography)
   - If woman is found to be carrier of a clinically significant hemoglobinopathy, father should also be screened without delay.

2. *Rhesus negative blood group*
   - If Rh negative blood group with husband rhesus positive, offer indirect coomb's test
   - If ICT is negative, repeat at 28 and then at 34 weeks
   - If positive, send for anti-D antibodies titer.
3. *VDRL positive*
   - If either the VDRL (Venereal Disease Research Laboratory) or the RPR (Rapid Plasmin Reagin) test is negative, then the patient does not have syphilis and no further tests for syphilis are needed
   - If the titer is ≥1:16, the patient has syphilis and must be treated
   - If the titer is ≤ 1:8, the laboratory should test the same blood sample by means of the TPHA (Treponema Pallidum Hemagglutin Assay) or FTA (Fluorescent Treponemal Antibody) test:
     i. If the TPHA (or FTA) test is also positive, the patient has syphilis and must be fully treated
     ii. If the TPHA (or FTA) is negative, then the patient does not have syphilis and, therefore, need not be treated
     iii. If a TPHA (or FTA) cannot be done, and the patient has not been fully treated for syphilis in the past 3 months, she must be given a full course of treatment.
4. *HIV positive*
   - Confirm by western blot or repeat ELISA.
5. *Screening for fetal anomalies*
   - For women who book later in pregnancy, serum screening test (triple or quadruple test) should be offered between 15+0 and 20+0 weeks
   - If the result is screen positive for Down's syndrome or any other abnormality, she should be given the option for amniocentesis or chorionic villus sampling.

18–20 Weeks

Symptoms and signs
- Breast → enlarged with prominent veins under the skin
- Quickening:
  - When movements made by the fetus are perceived for the first time by the mother
  - Occurs at 18–20 weeks in primigravida
  - At 16–18 weeks in multigravida
- At 20 weeks, the following can be usually observed:
  - Secondary areola
  - Prominent montgomery's tubercles extend to the secondary areola
  - Variable degree of striae (both pink and white) may be visible in lower abdomen
  - Linea nigra
  - Palpation of fetal parts
  - Active fetal movements
  - External ballottement (fetus is relatively smaller than the volume of the amniotic fluid)
  - Fetal heart sound detected with stethoscope
  - Two other sounds confused with FHS are:
  Uterine soufflé:
    - Soft blowing and systolic
    - Synchronous with maternal pulse
    - Due to increased blood flow through the dilated uterine vessels
  Funic or fetal soufflé:
    - Due to rush of blood through the umbilical arteries
    - A soft, blowing murmur
    - Synchronous with the FHS

Investigations
- Measure weight and blood pressure
- Detailed ultrasound level II (between 18 and 22 weeks)
- If any anamoly is detected, further decision accordingly
- If placenta is found extending to the internal os, repeat scan for placental localization should be offered at 32 weeks
- Continue iron and calcium
- Injection TT 0.5 mL IM (2nd dose).

24–25 Weeks

- Face—chloasma gravidarum may appear at 24th week
- Measure weight and blood pressure
- Plot symphysis—fundal height
- Test urine for proteinuria and rule out asymptomatic bacteriuria
- OGTT with 75 g glucose
- Fetal echocardiography, if mother has heart disease or any fetal cardiac abnormality detected at the time of anamoly scan.

Fundal height (McDonald's Rule)

Fundal height, or McDonald's rule, is a measure of the size of the uterus used to assess fetal growth and development during pregnancy. It is measured from the top of the mother's uterus to the top of the mother's pubic bone in centimeter.

Gestational age	Fundal height
40 weeks	1–2-finger width below subcostal arch
36 weeks	At costal arch
32 weeks	Between umbilicus and xiphoid process
28 weeks	3-finger width above umbilicus
24 weeks	At umbilicus
20 weeks	3-finger width below umbilicus
16 weeks	3-finger width above symphysis

Symphysis—Fundal Height (by Tape)

- To determine:
  - Period of gestation
  - Growth of the fetus
  - Multiple pregnancies
  - Complications of pregnancy, e.g. amniotic fluid disorders, hydatidiform mole and fetal growth disturbances
- Between 20 and 34 weeks gestation, the height of the uterus correlates closely with measurements in centimeter (except in obesity)

Step I
- Explain the procedure to the mother and gain verbal consent
- Wash hands
- Obtain a nonelastic measuring tape
- Ensure that the mother is comfortable in a supine position and extended legs, with an empty bladder
- Expose enough of the abdomen to allow a thorough examination.

Step II
- Ensure the abdomen is soft (not contracting)
- Perform abdominal palpation to enable accurate identification of the uterine fundus.

Step III
- Use the measuring tape with the centimeter on the underside to reduce bias
- Place the zero mark of the tape measure at the uppermost border of the symphysis pubis
- Measure from the top of symphysis pubis to the top of fundus
- The tape should stay in contact with the skin.

Step IV
- Measure along the longitudinal axis without correcting to the abdominal midline
- Do not hold the tape between the fingers
- Tape should then be turned so that the numbers are visible and the value can be recorded
- Measure only once
- Measurements should be in centimeter only.

Caution:
- If the bladder is full, it can increase the fundal height by 3 cm
- Supine position has the least variations in measurements
- After 34 weeks, it is not recommended as it may give erroneous readings due to descent of fetus into the pelvis
- A discrepancy of >2 cm should be reported.

ULTRASOUND

Level II Scan

- A scan is performed at 18 to 22 weeks when the fetus is large enough for an accurate survey of the fetal anatomy and when dates and growth can also be assessed
- Also known as—dating, anomaly or targeted scan
- Measurement of BP, FL, AC, HC, EFW is taken
- Localization of placenta and amount of liquor is determined
- Accurate dating can only be done as early in gestation as possible after 13 weeks, after which dating will not be that reliable
- Detailed Level II scan is beyond the scope of this book but few notable features are worth mentioning.

Period of gestation	Ultrasound features
Weeks 13–17	• Ribs appear • Nose and chin well-defined • Opening and closing of mouth • External genitalia almost defined • Ears fully developed • Cheek bones appear • First hair appears at 14 weeks • Fetus can make a fist at 15 weeks • Fat begins to form underneath the skin • Baby hears external voices, sleeps and dreams by 16 weeks • Umbilical cord grows thicker and stronger • Retina has become sensitive to light—week 17 • First stools (meconium) are now beginning to accumulate by week 17
Weeks 18–24	• Vernix starts forming • Genitals are distinct and recognizable by week 19 • Scalp hair has sprouted • Growth of hair on rest of the body • Regular sleeping and waking rhythm • Mother's movements can wake her baby • Eyebrows become visible by week 23 • Fetus weighs around 600 g and is about 30 cm long by week 24
Weeks 25–28	• Hands—fully developed • Brain is growing rapidly • Sexual organs are fully developed • Eyes begin to open, blink and close • Weight is 1000 g and length is almost 37.5 cm by week 28.

At this point, it is important to give a brief description of ultrasonographic changes in amniotic fluid and placenta in an uncomplicated pregnancy.

Amniotic Fluid

Appearance

- During the first two trimesters:
  - Clear and yellow
- During the third trimester:
  - Colorless
- Approximately from 33 to 34 weeks onwards:
  - Cloudiness and flocculation occur, at first very slowly, then after the 36th–37th week steadily and faster.
- At term:
  - Moderately cloudy and contains a moderate number of flakes of vernix
- The appearance of the amniotic fluid, depending on the degree of cloudiness and on the number of flakes, has been expressed by means of a score system, the so-called *'Macroscore.'*

Quantity and Constituents

- Completely surrounds the embryo after the 4th week of pregnancy

- Main constituents are:

1st trimester
- Water and electrolytes only

2nd trimester
- Water and electrolytes (99%)
- Glucose
- Lipids from the fetal lungs
- Proteins with bactericide properties
- Flaked-off fetal epithelium cells (they make a prenatal diagnosis of the infantile karyotype possible)
- Normally has a pH of 7.0 to 7.5.

Quantity Changes

- 20 mL in the 7th week
- 400 mL at 20th week
- 600 mL in the 25th week
- 800 mL at 28th week
- 1000 mL in the 30th to 34th weeks
- 800 mL at birth
- 400 mL in the 42nd week
- From the 5th month onwards, the fetus also begins to drink amniotic fluid (400 mL/day)
- Near to the end of pregnancy, the amniotic fluid is replaced every 3 hours.

Functions

- Amniotic fluid is 'inhaled' and 'exhaled' bythe fetus—essential for the development of lungs
- Swallowed amniotic fluid also forms urine and contributes to the formation of meconium
- Amniotic fluid protects the developing fetus by cushioning against blows to the mother's abdomen
- Allowing for easier fetal movements
- Promotes muscular and skeletal development.

Placenta

Placental grading refers to an ultrasound grading system of the placenta depending upon its maturity. This primarily portrays the extent of calcifications.

Grading system		
Grades	Period of gestation	Features
'0'	<18 weeks	Uniform echogenicity; Smooth chorionic plate
'I'	18–29 weeks	Occasional parenchymal calcification/hyperechoic areas
'II'	>30 weeks	Occasional basal calcification/hyperechoic areas; May also have comma-type densities at the chorionic plate
'III'	>39 weeks	Significant basal calcification; Chorionic plate interrupted by indentations; An early progression to grade III is a matter of concern and is sometimes associated with placental insufficiency

Third Trimester (29–40 Weeks)

Signs and Symptoms

- Amenorrhea continues
- As the fetus and uterus grow, the patient will complain of more and more discomfort
- Abdomen enlarges further
- There may be physiological edema of the feet
- Frequency of micturition again increases
- Fetal movements are more distinct
- Pigmentation and striae are more dark.

Examination

- Very important in this trimester is to distinguish lie, presentation, position and attitude of the fetus
- To know the Leopold maneuver
- To distinguish between physiological and pathological edema
- Pelvic examination
- Bishop's scoring system.

'Lie'

Relationship between the longitudinal axis of the fetus and mother.

Can be:
- Longitudinal (resulting in either cephalic or breech presentation)
- Oblique (unstable, will eventually become either longitudinal or transverse)
- Transverse (resulting in shoulder presentation).

'Presentation'

This refers to the leading anatomical part of the fetus, i.e. the one closest to the pelvic inlet of the birth canal.

The various presentations are:
1. Cephalic presentation (96.5%)
2. Breech presentation (3%)
3. Shoulder presentation (0.5%).

'Presenting Part'

The part which is usually felt first on per vaginal examination.
Depending on the degree of flexion, in a cephalic presentation, the presenting part can be:
- Vertex—the most common and associated with the fewest complications
- Sinciput
- Brow
- Face
- Chin.

'Attitude'

Relationship of fetal head to spine.

Can be:
- Flexed (this is the normal situation) → sinciput is higher than the occiput
- Neutral ('military') → deflexed state, when both sinciput and occiput are at the same level
- Extended.

'Denominator'

It is the bony point on the presenting part which comes in contact with the various quadrants of the maternal pelvis.

Presenting part	Denominator
Vertex	Occiput
Face	Mentum
Brow	Frontal eminence
Breech	Sacrum
Shoulder	Acromion

'Position'

Relationship of presenting part to maternal pelvis. Based on various presentations, the different positions can be as follows:
- Vertex presentation with longitudinal lie:
    - Left occipitoanterior (LOA)—the occiput is close to the vagina (hence known as vertex presentation). It faces anteriorly (forward with mother standing) and towards left. This is the most common position and lie
    - Right occipitoanterior (ROA)—the occiput faces anteriorly and towards right. Less common than LOA, but not associated withlabor complications
    - Left occipitoposterior (LOP)—the occiput faces posteriorly (behind) and towards left
    - Right occipitoposterior (ROP)—the occiput faces posteriorly and towards right
    - Occipitoanterior—the occiput faces anteriorly (absolutely straight without any turning to any of the sides)
    - Occipitoposterior—the occiput faces posteriorly (absolutely straight without any turning to any of the sides).
- Breech presentation with longitudinal lie:
    - Left sacrum anterior (LSA)—the buttocks, as against the occiput of the vertex presentation, lie close to the vagina (hence known as breech presentation), anteriorly and towards the left
    - Right sacrum anterior (RSA)—the buttocks face anteriorly and towards the right
    - Left sacrum posterior (LSP)—the buttocks face posteriorly and towards the left
    - Right sacrum posterior (RSP)—the buttocks face posteriorly and towards the right
    - Sacrum anterior (SA)—the buttocks face anteriorly
    - Sacrum posterior (SP)—the buttocks face posteriorly
- Shoulder presentation with transverse lie has the following different positions, based on the location of the scapula:
    - Left scapula-anterior (LSA)
    - Right scapula-anterior (RSA)
    - Left scapula-posterior (LSP)
    - Right scapula-posterior (RSP)

Edema

Causes (differential diagnosis):
1. Physiological
2. Preeclampsia
3. Anemia/hypoproteinemia
4. Cardiac failure
5. Chronic renal disease
6. DVT

Physiological Edema

Cause: Increased venous pressure of lower extremities by gravid uterus pressing on common iliac veins.

Features:
a. Slight degree (ankle edema) usually confined to 1 leg (right > left)
b. Unassociated with increase in BP or proteinuria
c. Disappears on rest alone

How and where to check?
- Over medial malleolus and anterior 1/3rd of tibia
- Press with thumb for 5 seconds

Approach to a Patient of Edema

Edema
↓
Localized? → Yes → Venous or lymph obstruction
↓
No
↓
Albumin < 2.5 g/dL → Yes → Severe malnutrition OR Chronic liver disease OR Nephrotic syndrome
↓
No
↓
↑ JVP or ↓ Cardiac output → Yes → Heart failure
↓
No
Azotemia or active urine sediment → Yes → Renal failure
↓
No
↓
Drug induced (steroids, estrogen, vasodilators)
Hypothyroidism

28–30 Weeks

- Measure blood pressure and weight
- Check edema (pedal)
- Check hemoglobin
- Offer anti-D prophylaxis to all rhesus-negative women
- Measure symphysis fundal height.

32–34 Weeks

- Measure weight, blood pressure and symphysis fundal height
- Ultrasound for fetal well-being, liquor, placental localization
- Urine routine to be done
- Repeat ICT at 34–36 weeks
- Some prefer to give anti-D again at 34 weeks (if dual dose regimen was adopted at 28 weeks) *(Refer to chapter on Rh-negative pregnancy)*
- Confirm the presenting part by Leopold's maneuvers.

Leopold's Maneuvers

- Named after the gynecologist Christian Gerhard Leopold
- Determines position and presentation of the fetus
- Difficult to perform on obese women and women who have polyhydramnios
- The maneuvers consist of four distinct actions
- The woman is relaxed and adequately positioned
- Bladder is emptied
- The woman should lie on her back with her shoulders raised slightly on a pillow and her knees flexed
- Abdomen uncovered
- Warm the hands by rubbing prior to palpation.

First Maneuver: Fundal Grip

- While facing the woman, palpate the woman's upper abdomen with both the hands
- Determine the size, consistency, shape and mobility of the form that is felt
- Fetal head is hard, firm, round, and moves independently of the trunk while the buttocks feel softer, are symmetric, and the shoulders and limbs have small bony processes; unlike the head, they move with the trunk.

Second Maneuver: Umbilical Grip or Lateral Grip

- Attempt to determine the location of the fetal back
- Still facing the woman, palpate the abdomen with gentle—but also deeppressure using the palm of the hands
- First the right hand remains steady on one side of the abdomen while the left hand explores the right side of the uterus
- This is then repeated using the opposite side and hands
- The fetal back will feel firm and smooth while fetal extremities (arms, legs, etc.) should feel like small irregularities and protrusions
- The fetal back, once determined, should be continuous with the part found at fundus and also to the one in the maternal inlet or lower abdomen.

Third Maneuver: First Pelvic Grip

- Face the woman's feet
- The fingers of both the hands are moved gently down the sides of the uterus towards the pubis
- The side, where the resistance to the descent of the fingers towards the pubis is greatest, is where the brow is located
- If the head of the fetus is well-flexed, it should be on the opposite side from the fetal back
- If the fetal head is extended and the occiput is felt instead → it is located on the same side as the back.

Fourth Maneuver: Pawlick's Grip (Second Pelvic Grip)

- In this maneuver, attempt to determine which fetal part is lying above the inlet, or lower abdomen
- First grasp the lower portion of the abdomen just above the pubic symphysis with the thumb and fingers of the right hand
- This maneuver should yield the opposite information and validate the findings of the first maneuver
- If it is the head and is not engaged, it may be gently pushed back and forth.

To Summarize

Examination	Determined by
Lie of fetus	Inspection → uterus appears longitudinal Fundal grip 1st pelvic grip
Presentation	1st pelvic grip
Attitude	1st pelvic grip Well flexed—sinciput higher than occiput Deflexed—both sinciput and occiput at the same level
Presenting part	1st pelvic grip Sinciput on same sides as limbs
Position	Inspection—convex uterine contour Lateral grip Auscultation
Engagement	1st pelvic grip—both poles not felt per abdomen Divergence of examining fingers If the fingers converge—head is not engaged

36–38 Weeks

- Measure weight and blood pressure
- Fetal presentation
- 'Lightening'—when the baby has dropped down in the pelvis and the diaphragm is relieved of pressure
- If it is a breech presentation, ECV can be offered after excluding contraindications to it
- Per vaginal examination for:
  - Adequacy of pelvis
  - Any cervical changes
  - And then mode of delivery is discussed with the patient

- Explain the patient about the labor process in brief
- The woman is made aware of signs of onset of true labor pains and that she should report if she has the following:
  - Pain in the abdomen which is radiating
  - Intermittent and increasing in frequency, duration and intensity
  - Per vaginal leak or blood-stained discharge
  - Decreased fetal movements
- If cesarean section is to be done, indication is discussed with the woman and appropriate gestational age for it is to be decided
- Women should be made aware of the advantages of breastfeeding.

Pelvic Assessment

In vertex presentation: Assessment is done at any time beyond 37th week but better at the beginning of labor because due to the softening of tissues, assessment can be done effectively during this time.
Empty bladder
Dorsolithotomy position
Aseptic precautions
Cover the abdomen.
NOTE: Sterilized gloved fingers once taken out should not be reintroduced.

Sacral Promontory

- Attempt should be made to tip the sacral promontory
- Try to establish the length of the diagonal conjugate
- Method:
  - Fingers are to follow anterior sacral curvature
  - In normal pelvis, it is difficult to feel sacral promontory (or felt with difficulty)
  - To reach it, elbow and wrist are to be depressed sufficiently and fingers are mobilized in an upward direction
  - Point at which bone recedes from fingers is sacral promontory
  - Fingers are then mobilized under symphysis pubis and a marking is placed over the gloved index finger by the index finger of the left hand
  - Internal fingers are removed
  - Distance between marking and tip of middle finger gives measurement of diagonal conjugate
  - Practically: If middle finger fails to reach promontory or touches it with difficulty→ conjugate is adequate for average size head to pass through
- If it is easily tipped, it should alert one to the possibility of a contracted pelvis.

Curvature of the Sacral Curve

- It is next assessed to see if it is flat or well-curved
- A well-curved sacrum allows for internal rotation of the fetal head.

Pelvic Side Walls

- Assessed next to see if they are parallel or convergent
- Normally not easily palpable.

Ischial Spines

- These are palpated to see if they are prominent and sticking in (that is, decreasing the space in midpelvis)
- Normally these are everted.

Sacrosciatic Notch

- Sufficiently wide to place 2 fingers over sacrospinous ligament covering the notch
- Gives information of the capacity of posterior segment and side walls of the lower pelvis.

Posterior Surface of Symphysis Pubis

- Smooth rounded curve
- Angulation/beaking → abnormal.

Pubic Arch

- Normally rounded
- Should accommodate palmar aspect of 2 fingers
- Configuration more important than pubic angle.

Subpubic Angle

- Before the fingers are removed from the vagina, the subpubic angle is assessed to see if it is acute or obtuse.

Now take out your fingers

Intertuberous Diameter

- Having removed the fingers, the intertuberous diameter is assessed to see if it accommodates more than four knuckles → if it does, it is adequate.

Conclusion

The most suitable pelvis for vaginal delivery is that of a gynecoid pelvis that has adequate dimensions.

Features of a gynecoid pelvis include:
- A wide diagonal conjugate
- A well-curved sacrum
- Parallel side walls
- Ischial spines that are not prominent
- A wide subpubic angle; and lastly
- A wide intertuberous diameter.

40–41 Weeks

- Measure blood pressure
- Height of uterus will be at 32 weeks due to engagement of fetal head; therefore, look at the flanks → if full, the duration of pregnancy is 40 weeks

34 **Section 1:** *Long Cases*

- Membrane sweeping is done followed by induction of labor, if labor pains do not start on their own
- Bishop score is calculated
- Discuss about the risks associated with prolonged pregnancy (decreased liquor, meconium aspiration, etc.).

Modified Bishop Score or Prelabor Scoring or Preinduction Score

- Bishop score is a prelabor scoring system to assist in predicting whether induction of labor will be required
- Components included to calculate the score are (original Bishop's score):
  - Cervical dilation
  - Cervical effacement
  - Cervical consistency
  - Cervical position
  - Fetal station
- According to the Modified Bishop's preinduction cervical scoring system, effacement has been replaced by cervical length in cm

Score	0	1	2	3
Dilatation	Closed	1–2	3–4	5
Length	>4	3–4	1–2	0
Consistency	Firm	Medium	Soft	–
Position	Posterior	Midline	Anterior	–
Station	–3	–2	–1/0	+1, +2

Interpretation

- Total score = 13
- Favorable score = 6–13
- Unfavorable score = 0–5
- A score of ≤ 5 suggests that labor is unlikely to start without induction
- A score of ≥ 9 indicates that labor will most likely commence spontaneously.

Another modification for the Bishop's score is the 'modifiers'. Points are added or subtracted according to the special circumstances as follows:
One point is added for:
- Existence of preeclampsia
- Every previous vaginal delivery.

One point is subtracted for:
- Postdated pregnancy
- Nulliparity (no previous vaginal deliveries)
- PPROM (Preterm premature rupture of membranes).

ULTRASOUND

Period of gestation	Ultrasound features
Week 29–34	• Wrinkled skin is becoming smoother now • In boys, the testicles have moved down to the groin by week 30 • Eyes open completely • Toenails and fingernails are completely formed • Eyes open when awake and close when sleeping • Excellent chance of survival outside the womb

Calculation of Gestational Age

Menstruation—Labor Interval (Naegele's Rule)

Expected date of delivery (EDD)
- 1st day of the last menstrual period + 7 days + 9 calendar months
  OR
- 1st day of LMP + 7 days − 3 calendar months + 1 year
  OR
- 1st day of LMP + 280 days (40 weeks).

A General History in Pregnancy

Chief complaints of the patient

Past Obstetric History (Gravida, Parity, Abortions, Ectopic, Twins, Death)

Importance
a. Married life (years). The woman may have conceived many years after her marriage
b. Consanguinity
c. Whether ANCs were taken in each previous pregnancy
d. Complications in previous antenatal periods (preeclampsia, preterm labor, gestational diabetes, antepartum hemorrhage, etc.)
e. Grand multiparity
f. Miscarriages (to rule out bad obstetric history and its causes, which are different for each trimester)
g. Ectopic pregnancy (whether managed medically or surgically; which surgery was done; was the tube saved; any blood transfusions were done; if medically treated, any reaction to the drug used, when was the treatment ended)
h. Any h/o molar pregnancy (ask patient to get previous records in the next visit; what treatment was given; histopathology report after D and C; was chemotherapy given and for how long)
i. Any h/o twin gestation (nonidentical twins tend to recur)
j. Any perinatal deaths [at what period of gestation, cause, how was it suspected or was it an incidental finding, delivery by induction or spontaneous, how was the appearance of the baby

(macerated, peeling of skin, skin color, any gross congenital anomalies seen, did the baby cry after birth, as the women sometimes are not able to distinguish intrauterine death or death immediately after birth); any histopathology sample of the baby was sent; if yes, ask for reports]
k. Mode of each delivery—vaginal or cesarean section; prolonged labor; birth weight of each baby; home or institutional delivery; gestational age at delivery; instrumental delivery; any complication after vaginal deliveries
l. If delivery was by cesarean section—cause, type of incision, any postoperative complications, history of blood transfusion
m. Was Anti-D taken in cases of Rh-negative pregnancy
n. Whether any baby was kept in NICU, why and for how long
o. Intervals between pregnancies
p. Whether all babies are alive and healthy
q. Whether breastfeeding done after each delivery and for how long.

Present Pregnancy

a. Type of conception (spontaneous or after-infertility treatment)
b. Any history of fever with or without rash, vaginal bleeding, burning micturition, etc.
c. Following minor symptoms should be enquired:
 - Nausea and vomiting
 - Heart burn
 - Constipation
 - Edema of the ankles and hands.

Menstrual History

Importance

a. Last menstrual period
b. Periods were regular or irregular
c. Whether the patient had any spotting after her last periods (may be implantation bleed)
d. Any history of oral or injectable contraception. These patients must have menstruated spontaneously after stopping contraception, otherwise the date of the last period should not be used to measure the duration of pregnancy.

Past Personal History/History of Medications, Surgeries, Allergies (Some medical conditions may become worse during pregnancy)

a. Hypertension
b. Diabetes mellitus
c. Rheumatic or other heart diseases
d. Epilepsy
e. Asthma
f. Tuberculosis
g. Psychiatric illness
h. Any other major illness or blood transfusions in the past
i. Any past medication can be a pointer of a specific illness. Certain drugs can be teratogenic to the fetus. So, they need to be changed or stopped at all.
j. Allergies to drugs need to be mentioned clearly on antenatal card
k. Any previous (major or minor) surgeries need to be enquired.

Family History

Parents and first-degree relatives with a condition such as diabetes, multiple pregnancy, bleeding tendencies or mental retardation have an increased risk of these conditions in the patient and the fetus. Some birth defects are inherited.

Of utmost importance are the risk factors for gestational diabetes:
a. Body mass index above 30 kg/m^2
b. Previous macrosomic baby weighing ≥ 4.5 kg
c. Previous gestational diabetes
d. Family history of diabetes (first-degree relative with diabetes)
e. Family origin with a high prevalence of diabetes:
   - South Asian (specifically women whose country of family origin is India, Pakistan or Bangladesh), black Caribbean Middle Eastern (specifically women whose country of family origin is Saudi Arabia, United Arab Emirates, Iraq, Jordan, Syria, Oman, Qatar, Kuwait, Lebanon or Egypt).

Social Circumstances of the Patient

a. Unemployment, poor housing (kutcha or pucca house, electricity) and overcrowding increase the risk of tuberculosis, malnutrition and intrauterine growth restriction. Patients living in poor social conditions need special support and help. Family income needs to be calculated according to Kuppuswamy scale
b. Daily calories of the patient need to be counted
c. Smoking/alcohol/tobacco consumption is enquired.

Kuppuswamy Scale (2012)

Kuppuswamy's socioeconomic status scale has been in use as an important aid to measure socioeconomic status of families in urban communities. The original version was given in 1976, which was later updated in 2003 by Mishra and Singh and again in 2007 by Kumar and colleagues. As changes in inflation rates change the monetary values of the monthly income range scores, Kuppuswamy scale has been again updated in 2012.

It includes education, occupation and family income per month

(A) Education:	Score
1. Profession or honours	7
2. Graduate or postgraduate	6
3. Intermediate or post-high-school diploma	5
4. High-school certificate	4
5. Middle-school certificate	3
6. Primary-school certificate	2
7. Illiterate	1

(B) Occupation:	Score
1. Profession	10
2. Semiprofession	6
3. Clerical, shop-owner, farmer	5
4. Skilled worker	4
5. Semiskilled worker	3
6. Unskilled worker	2
7. Unemployed	1

(C) Family income per month (2012):   Score
1. = 30375   12
2. 15188–30374   10
3. 11362–15187   6
4. 7594–11361   4
5. 4556–7593   3
6. 1521–4555   2
7. =1520   1

Total score   Socioeconomic status
1. 26–29   Upper (I)
2. 16–25 Middle   Upper middle (II)
3. 11–15   Lower middle (III)
4. 5–10 Lower   Upper lower (IV)
5. <5   Lower (V)

Physical Examination

General Appearance

a. Consciousness, orientation to time, place and person, occupation (to exclude occupational hazards or occupation as a cause of stress)
b. Built, sleep, nutrition, height, weight, BMI
c. Calories need to be calculated and proper diet needs to be explained
d. Face
   Chloasma uterinum (gravidarum)
   - Brownish pigmentation of the bridge of the nose and the maxillae, simulating a butterfly appearance
   - Occasionally, the pigmentation is more generalized, affecting the forehead and the cheeks
   Acromegalic features
   - More manifest in the 2nd half of pregnancy
   - Ascribed to the possible increase of the growth hormone of the anterior pituitary or placenta.

Systemic Examination

a. Pallor, icterus, cyanosis, clubbing, lymphadenopathy (neck, axillae, inguinalareas), edema (feet, hands, face)
b. Thyroid
   - A visibly enlarged thyroid gland, a single palpable nodule or a nodular goiter is abnormal and needs further investigation
   - A slightly, diffusely enlarged thyroid gland is normal in pregnancy
c. Breasts
   - Enlargement, warmth, tenderness—in which quadrant, is generalized or isolated
     – Early pregnancy: mostly manifest in the upper and outer quadrants
     – Late pregnancy: becomes more generalized and felt all over the breasts
   - Dilated veins under the skin
   - Nipple enlargement, pigmentation, more erectile or not
   - Discharge from nipples (color, consistency, amount)
   - Inverted or flat nipples

- Areola—size and pigmentation
- Montgomery's follicles—'glandular tubercles'
- Any breast lump
d. Spine (lordosis, kyphosis, scoliosis)
e. Respiratory system
   - Breath sounds, bilateral air entry, respiratory rate, dyspnea
f. Cardiovascular system
   - BP, PR
   - Functional murmurs (a soft, midsystolic, nonradiating, ejection murmur heard best over the mitral or aortic areas) are common in pregnancy.

Blood Pressure Recording in Pregnancy—Ideal Method
- First one should be familiar with the 5 phases of Korotkoff sounds
- Phase I: 1st appearance of sounds marking systolic pressure
- Phases II and III: Increasing loud sounds
- Phase IV: Muffling of sounds
- Phase V: Disappearance of sounds.

Position
- Rest—5 minutes
- Sitting with feet supported on flat surface (avoid supine position)
- Remove every tight clothing from the arm
- Arm well supported at the level of the heart (different arm positions can alter the BP significantly)
- Measure BP on both the arms at the first visit (this excludes rare vascular disorders)
- BP of the arm giving higher reading is to be taken
- In labor → left recumbent position.

Cuff
- Length—1.5 times the circumference of the arm
- Wide enough to cover at least 2/3rd of the upper arm
- Arm circumference >33 cm → use larger cuff
- Smaller cuff size will overestimate BP
- Larger cuff will underestimate BP
- Lower edge of the cuff should be 2–3 cm above the point of brachial artery pulsation (easy access to antecubital fossa)
- Application should be firm.

Measurement apparatus
- Mercury sphygmomanometer is still considered the best for measuring BP (especially in pre-eclamptic patients)
- Automated devices may underestimate BP by 10–15 mm Hg.

Measurement
- Do not kink or twist the tube on the cuff
- Inflated and deflated smoothly
- Korotkoff V is taken for diastolic BP
- Korotkoff IV only when sounds are audible as level approaches '0' mm Hg (due to hyperdynamic circulation of pregnancy).

g. Abdomen *(always warm your hands before abdominal palpation)*
   - Pigmentation "linea nigra"
   - Striae gravidarum (color, site)
   - Any scar (any previous surgery), its site (horizontal, vertical) and present condition
   - Fetal movements
   - Fetal parts
   - External ballottement
   - Contractions
   - Fundal height
   - Symphysis fundal height (with measuring tape)
   - Tenderness, any mass palpable, organomegaly
   - Leopold maneuvers
   - Fetal heart sound.
h. Both external and internal genitalia
   - Any ulcers, purulent or excessive discharge, enlarged inguinal lymph nodes should be looked for
   - Suspicious looking cervix (cervical smear must be taken) or any growth on the cervix
   - Bimanual examination (for size of uterus, if not palpable per abdomen), condition of the internal os
   - Any tenderness in the fornices
   - Pelvic assessment (if appropriate at that gestational age).

In the end, calculate period of gestation and write the provisional diagnosis

To Summarize

Calculation of period of gestation is by:
1. Last normal menstrual period (if dates are sure)
2. Size of the uterus on bimanual (up to 12 weeks) examination
3. Abdominal examination from 12–22 weeks, when fundal height is still below the umbilicus, is considered very accurate
4. SFH between 24 and 36 weeks
5. The size of the fetus (rule out IUGR/SGA or large for date fetus)
6. Ultrasound measurements:
   - If the ultrasound examination is done at ≤ 14 weeks, the error in determining the gestational age is only one week
   - If patient is >24 weeks pregnant, ultrasound cannot be used to determine the gestational age
   - If still not clear, look for serial growth after 3 weeks.

Uterus bigger than dates suggests:
- Error in calculating dates or wrong dates
- Multiple pregnancy
- Polyhydramnios
- Large for the gestational age
- Diabetes mellitus
- Complete molar pregnancy
- Hydrops
- Any mass (fibroid, ovarian tumour, etc.) with pregnancy
- Sometimes fetus in breech presentation looks bigger.

Uterus smaller than dates suggests:
- Error in calculating dates or wrong dates
- Intrauterine growth restriction
- Oligohydramnios
- Small for gestational age
- Transverse lie
- Fetal descent into the pelvis
- Intrauterine death
- Rupture of membranes.

Few Other Queries are Always in a Pregnant Woman's Mind

Lifestyle Considerations

Working during pregnancy is safe.

Food-acquired Infections

Pregnant women should be informed of primary prevention measures to avoid:

Toxoplasmosis infection
- Washing hands before handling food
- Thoroughly washing all fruits and vegetables, including ready prepared salads, before eating
- Thoroughly cooking raw meats (> 67°C/153°F)
- Wearing gloves and thoroughly washing hands after handling soil and gardening
- Avoiding cat feces in cat litter or in soil
- Freezing meat to at least –20°C/–4°F also kills T. gondii cysts
- Clean surfaces and utensils that have been in contact with raw meat
- Do not consume raw eggs or raw milk
- Do not drink water potentially contaminated with oocysts
- Be aware that:
  - The process of curing, smoking or drying meat does not necessarily result in a product free of parasite cysts
  - Refrigeration does not destroy the parasite (still viable after 68 days at +4°C)
  - Microwave oven cooking does not destroy parasites.

Infection by listeriosis
- Drinking only pasteurized or UHT milk
- Not eating ripened soft cheese (there is no risk with hard cheese, such as Cheddar, or cottage cheese and processed cheese)
- Not eating uncooked or undercooked ready-prepared meals.

Salmonella infection
- Avoiding raw or partially cooked eggs or food that may contain them (such as mayonnaise)
- Avoiding raw or partially cooked meat, especially poultry.

Medicines

- Few medicines have been established as safe to use in pregnancy
- To be taken under supervision.

Exercise in Pregnancy

- Beginning or continuing a moderate course of exercise during pregnancy is not associated with adverse outcomes
- Contact sports, high-impact sports and vigorous racquet sports that may involve the risk of abdominal trauma, falls or excessive joint stress, and scuba diving, which may result in fetal birth defects and fetal decompression disease are to be avoided in pregnancy.

Sexual Intercourse in Pregnancy

- Sexual intercourse in pregnancy is not known to be associated with any adverse outcomes.

Alcohol Consumption in Pregnancy

- Pregnant women and women planning a pregnancy should be advised to avoid drinking alcohol in the first 3 months of pregnancy if possible because it may be associated with an increased risk of miscarriage
- If women choose to drink alcohol during pregnancy, they should be advised to drink no more than one small (125 mL) glass of wine
- Although there is uncertainty regarding a safe level of alcohol consumption in pregnancy, at this low level, there is no evidence of harm to the unborn baby.

Smoking in Pregnancy

- Ask about active or even passive smoking (in case the husband is a smoker)
- Risks associated—low birth weight and preterm birth
- The benefits of quitting at any stage should be emphasized.

Air Travel during Pregnancy

- Pregnant women should be informed that long-haul air travel is associated with an increased risk of venous thrombosis, although the fact that whether or not there is additional risk during pregnancy is unclear
- Wearing correctly fitted compression stockings is effective at reducing the risk.

Car Travel during Pregnancy

- Correct use of seat belts (that is, three-point seat belts 'above and below the bump, not over it') should be explained.

Travelling Abroad during Pregnancy

- Pregnant women should be informed that if they are planning to travel abroad, they should discuss about considerations such as flying conditions, vaccinations and travel insurance.

Management of Common Symptoms of Pregnancy

Nausea and Vomiting in Early Pregnancy

- Women should be informed that most cases of nausea and vomiting in pregnancy will resolve spontaneously within 16 to 20 weeks and that nausea and vomiting are not usually associated with a poor pregnancy outcome

- The following interventions appear to be effective in reducing symptoms:
  - *Nonpharmacological:* ginger, P6 (wrist) acupressure
  - *Pharmacological:* antihistamines.

Heartburn

- Lifestyle and diet modification
- Antacids may be offered to women whose heartburn remains troublesome despite lifestyle and diet modification.

Constipation

- Diet modification, such as bran or wheat fiber supplementation
- Increase water intake.

Hemorrhoids

- Diet modification
- If clinical symptoms remain troublesome, standard hemorrhoid creams should be considered.

Varicose Veins

- Varicose veins are a common symptom of pregnancy that will not cause harm
- Compression stockings can improve the symptoms but will not prevent varicose veins from emerging.

Leg Cramps

- Administration of adequate calcium and vitamin D3
- Gentle massage of the legs
- Local application of topical analgesics.

Vaginal Discharge

- Increase in vaginal discharge is a common physiological change that occurs during pregnancy
- If it is associated with itch, soreness, offensive smell or pain on passing urine, there may be an infective cause and so investigation should be considered
- A 1-week course of a topical imidazole is an effective treatment and should be considered for vaginal candidiasis infections in pregnant women
- The effectiveness and safety of oral treatments for vaginal candidiasis in pregnancy are uncertain and these treatments should not be offered.

Backache

- Women should be informed that exercising in water, massage therapy and group or individual back care classes might help to ease backache during pregnancy.

Breast Care

- Maintain cleanliness
- Massage the breasts
- Try to express the discharge (colostrum).

Prediction, Detection and Initial Management of Mental Disorders

Topics to be discussed during health education sessions

1. Healthy eating
2. Danger symptoms and signs
3. Dangerous habits, e.g. smoking or drinking alcohol
4. Description of the onset and process of labor must be included, especially when the patient is a primigravida
5. HIV counseling of both the partners
6. Breastfeeding
7. Care of the newborn infant
8. Family planning.

Preconception History and Counseling

HISTORY

Genetic History

Risk Factors

1. *Risk factors for numerical chromosomal abnormalities and new mutations*
   - Maternal age
   - Paternal age ($\geq$ 40 years, r/o child having new gene mutations)
   - Radiation/chemicals/drugs
2. *Risk factors for inherited mutations*
   - Presence of such an illness in either parent, in his or her family or in a previous child
   - Couple's ethnic background:
     - Cystic fibrosis in Europe, the Mediterranean region and Middle East
     - Sickle cell anemia and thalassemia (where prevalence of malaria is ↑)
     - Tay-Sachs disease and several other rare disorders in Ashkenazi Jewish background
     - Neural tube defects
   - Consanguinity—risk of autosomal recessive disorders increases.

Family History

Construct three-generation pedigree, which includes the following:

Genetic Disorders in the Family

- Muscular dystrophy
- Hemophilia
- Cystic fibrosis
- Fragile X syndrome
- Congenital heart disease
- Phenyl ketonuria
- Dwarfism
- Sickle cell anemia
- Tay-Sachs disease.

Multifactorial Congenital Malformations

- Spina bifida
- Anencephaly
- Cleft palate and cleft lip
- Hypospadias
- Congenital heart disease.

Familial Diseases with a Major Genetic Component

- Developmental disability
- Premature atherosclerosis
- Diabetes mellitus
- Psychosis
- Epileptic disorders
- Hypertension
- Rheumatoid arthritis
- Deafness
- Severe refractive disorders of the eye.

Age

- Women < 20 or > 35 years carry increased risks.

Health History

Chronic Conditions

- Diabetes mellitus
- Anemia
- Thyroid disorders
- Gynecological disorders
- Asthma
- STDs
- Heart disease
- Hypertension
- Deep venous thrombosis
- Kidney disease
- SLE
- Epilepsy
- Hemoglobinopathies
- Cancer
- Seizure disorders
- Tuberculosis
- Rheumatoid arthritis
- Mental health/psychiatric disorders.

Infectious Conditions

- Rubella or varicella susceptible—offer vaccination if not vaccinated
- Hepatitis B and C—routine preconception testing is not currently recommended

- Routine serologic testing for toxoplasmosis is not recommended
- Evaluate (woman and her partner) for sexually transmitted disease (e.g. Chlamydia, HIV, gonorrhea, syphilis)
- Periodontal screening
- *Nonpregnant women immunized with a live or live-attenuated vaccine should be counseled to delay pregnancy by at least four weeks.*

Reproductive History

- Menstrual history (regularity, duration and amount of flow, length of cycle, clots, dysmenorrhea)
- Contraceptive
- Sexual history
- Infertility
- Abnormal Pap smear
- In utero exposure to diethylstilbestrol
- Past obstetric history
  - Early/late miscarriages/stillbirths
  - Number of pregnancies and live issues
  - Mode of previous deliveries
  - Length/course of labor
  - Complications (preterm labor or delivery, gestational diabetes mellitus, hypertension in pregnancy, postpartum depression).

Lifestyle Assessment

- BMI
- Nutrition
- Physical activity
- Sufficient sleep
- Minimum stress
- Prescription and over-the-counter drug use
- Other substance abuse
- Environmental exposures (current and past).

COUNSELING

1. Ideal BMI—19.6–26.0 kg/mt^2
2. Laboratory testing:
   - CBC
   - Urinalysis
   - ABO Rh
   - VDRL
   - HIV
   - HbsAg
   - Rubella antibody titer
   - FBS/OGTT ⎤
   - TFT   ⎬ when indicated
   - TORCH   ⎦

3. Folic acid or folate (vitamin B_9)
   The recommended strategy(ies) for primary prevention or to decrease the incidence of fetal congenital anomalies include(s) various options:
   Option A:
   Patients with no personal health risks, planned pregnancy and good compliance require:
   - Folate-rich foods—fortified grains, spinach, lentils, chickpeas, asparagus, broccoli, peas, Brussels sprouts, corn and oranges
   - A multivitamin with folic acid (0.4–1.0 mg) × 2–3 months before conception and throughout pregnancy and postpartum period (4–6 weeks and as long as breastfeeding continues).

   Option B:
   Patients with health risks (previous child with neural tube defects, epilepsy, Type I DM, use of folate antagonists, obesity with BMI >35 kg/m^2, family history of neural tube defects, belonging to a high-risk ethnic group, e.g. Sikhs) require:
   - Increased dietary intake of folate-rich foods
   - A multivitamin with 5 mg folic acid, beginning at least three months before conception and continuing until 10 to 12 weeks postconception. From 12 weeks postconception and continuing throughout pregnancy and the postpartum period (4–6 weeks or as long as breastfeeding continues), supplementation should consist of a multivitamin with folic acid (0.4–1.0 mg).
4. Vitamin D intake of minimum 5 μg/day for nonpregnant women with limited exposure to sunlight (i.e. those whose hands and face are exposed to the open air for < 15 minutes/day) and 10 μg/day for pregnant women
5. Avoid exposure to cat feces, raw/undercooked meats and unpasteurized milk
6. Smoking and alcohol cessation
7. Consumption of vitamin A to < 3000 μg/day
8. Polytherapy changed to monotherapy in case of epilepsy with prior consultation with a neurologist
9. Adequate glycemic control in a patient of pregestational diabetes
10. Consultation with cardiologist if having cardiac disease
11. ACE inhibitors should be changed to a different drug.

SUGGESTED READING

1. Antenatal care: NICE clinical guideline; 62. June 2010.
2. BCPHP obstetric guideline 19, Maternity care pathway. Feb 2010.
3. Belizan J, Villar J, et al. Diagnosis of intrauterine growth retardation by a simple clinical method: Measurement of uterine height. Am J Obstet Gynecol. 1978;131:6:643-64.
4. Kuppuswamy's socioeconomic scale: Updating income ranges for the year 2012. Indian Journal of Public Health. January-March, 2012;Volume 56: Issue 1.
5. Measuring fundal height with a tape measure: Clinical Guidelines. OGCCU King Edward Memorial Hospital, Perth, Western Australia. September 2012.

CHAPTER 2

Anemia in Pregnancy

Tania G Singh

HISTORY IN A CASE OF ANEMIA AND SIGNIFICANCE OF EACH CONTENT

General Information

- Name
- Age → <17 years, additional demand ≈ 270 mg during the course of pregnancy
- Address → resident of endemic or tropic areas
- Marital status
- Education level
- Economic resources (Income and category according to Kuppu Swamy Scale)
- Employment (type of work and position of the patient) → if agriculture → ↑ sweat → iron loss 15 µg/month
- Housing (type, size, number of occupants, electricity, cooking facilities) → unemployment, poor housing and overcrowding ↑the risk of TB, malnutrition and IUGR.

HISTORY OF PRESENT ILLNESS (HOPI)

- Asymptomatic — iron deficiency in the absence of anemia. It can manifest as:
    - Mild anemia (hemoglobin > 10 g/dL)
    - Gradual onset of anemia
    - In active, well-conditioned persons
- Excessive vomiting, nausea, loss of appetite
- Leg cramps, which occur on climbing stairs, also are common in patients deficient in iron.

Nonspecific Symptoms

- Fatigue
- Generalized weakness
- Lassitude
- Dyspnea on exertion
- Light-headedness, giddiness
- Palpitations
- Pruritus (Iron deficiency anemia).

Dietary/Personal History

- Diet (veg/nonveg/mixed)
- *Inadequate iron or protein intake:* Iron deficiency

- *Strict vegetarian:* Vitamin B_{12} deficiency
- *Diet lacking in fruits and vegetables:* folate deficiency
- Dysphagia or loss of appetite
- Calculate kcal/day
- Smoking — IUGR
- Alcohol — IUGR
- Malabsorption with hypochlorhydria → ↓ absorption
- A fundamental concept is that after age of 1 year, dietary deficiency alone is not sufficient to cause clinically significant iron deficiency, so a source of blood loss should always be sought
- Pica — compulsive eating of nonfood substances
  - Pica is not a cause of iron deficiency anemia; it is a symptom of iron deficiency anemia
  - It is the link between iron deficiency anemia and lead poisoning, which is why iron deficiency anemia should always be sought when a child is diagnosed with lead poisoning. Both substances decrease the absorption of dietary iron
  - Pagophagia (ice eating) — most common form of pica in patients with iron deficiency anemia
  - Usually, they crave for ice to suck or chew
  - Occasionally, patients are seen who prefer cold celery or other cold vegetables in lieu of ice
  - Clay and dirt eating (geophagia) also occurs
  - Starch (amylophagia)
  - Hair (trichophagia).
- Sleep
- *Bladder:* UTI/dysuria
- *Bowel habits:* Constipation/diarrhea/dysentery/hemorrhoids.

History of Hemorrhage

- Two-thirds of body iron is present in circulating red blood cells as hemoglobin
- Each gram of hemoglobin contains 3.47 mg of iron; thus, each mL of blood lost from the body (hemoglobin 15 g/dL) results in a loss of 0.5 mg of iron
- Causes:
  - Bleeding is the most common cause of iron deficiency from:
    - History of passing worms in stools
      - Blood depletion (0.5–2 mg daily)
      - Each worm extracts ≈ 0.05 mL/day
      - There is intestinal hurry → ↓ iron absorption
  - With hematuria, hematemesis, hemoptysis, patients will present before they develop chronic iron deficiency anemia
  - But GI bleed (e.g. melena) may go unnoticed: *Blood must remain in GI tract for at least 14 hours before melena develops*
  - Increased menstrual bleed. Ask the patient about history of passage of clots, number of days of bleeding, use of multiple pads
  - IUCD in situ just prior to index pregnancy (IUCD users tend to bleed more)
  - Any obstetric hemorrhage in present pregnancy.

Obstetric History

- Repeated pregnancy at short intervals with prolonged lactation (≈ 2 years are required to replenish ≈ 1000 mg iron lost in pregnancy in healthy females with adequate diet)

- Pregnancy interferes with maternal erythropoiesis by competing for folic acid, vitamin B, proteins, iron → hence explains polymorphism of anemia in pregnancy.

Past History

- Blood transfusion
- Allergy to medication or food
- Current use of any medications:
  - Antacids or any other medications which need to be changed or interfere with iron absorption
  - Oxidant medications provoke G6PD.

Family History

- Hereditary spherocytosis
- Sickle cell anemia (Black patients)
- Thalassemia (Asian, Black or Mediterranean patients)
- Other hemoglobinopathies
- Glucose-6-phosphate dehydrogenase deficiency (G6PD).

History of Chronic Illness (Anemia of Chronic Disease)

- Chronic infection
- Collagen vascular disease
- Malignancy
- Hypothyroidism
- Hypoadrenalism
- Renal disease
- Hypopituitarism
- History of gastrectomy or malabsorption (e.g. diarrhea)
  - Vitamin B_{12} deficiency
  - Iron deficiency anemia
  - Folate deficiency anemia
- Recent infection (Infection↑↑ interference with erythropoiesis)
  - Urinary tract (UTI, asymptomatic bacteriuria, pyelonephritis)
  - Malaria ⎱ recently or in
  - Tuberculosis ⎰ index pregnancy
  - Unexplained fever
  - *Parvovirus:* Erythroblastopenia
  - *Hepatitis:* Aplastic anemia
- Abdominal pain
  - Peptic ulcer disease
  - Lead toxicity
  - Porphyria

General/Local Examination

- Built
- PICCLE (pallor, icterus, cyanosis, clubbing, lymphadenopathy, edema)

Chapter 2: *Anemia in Pregnancy* **51**

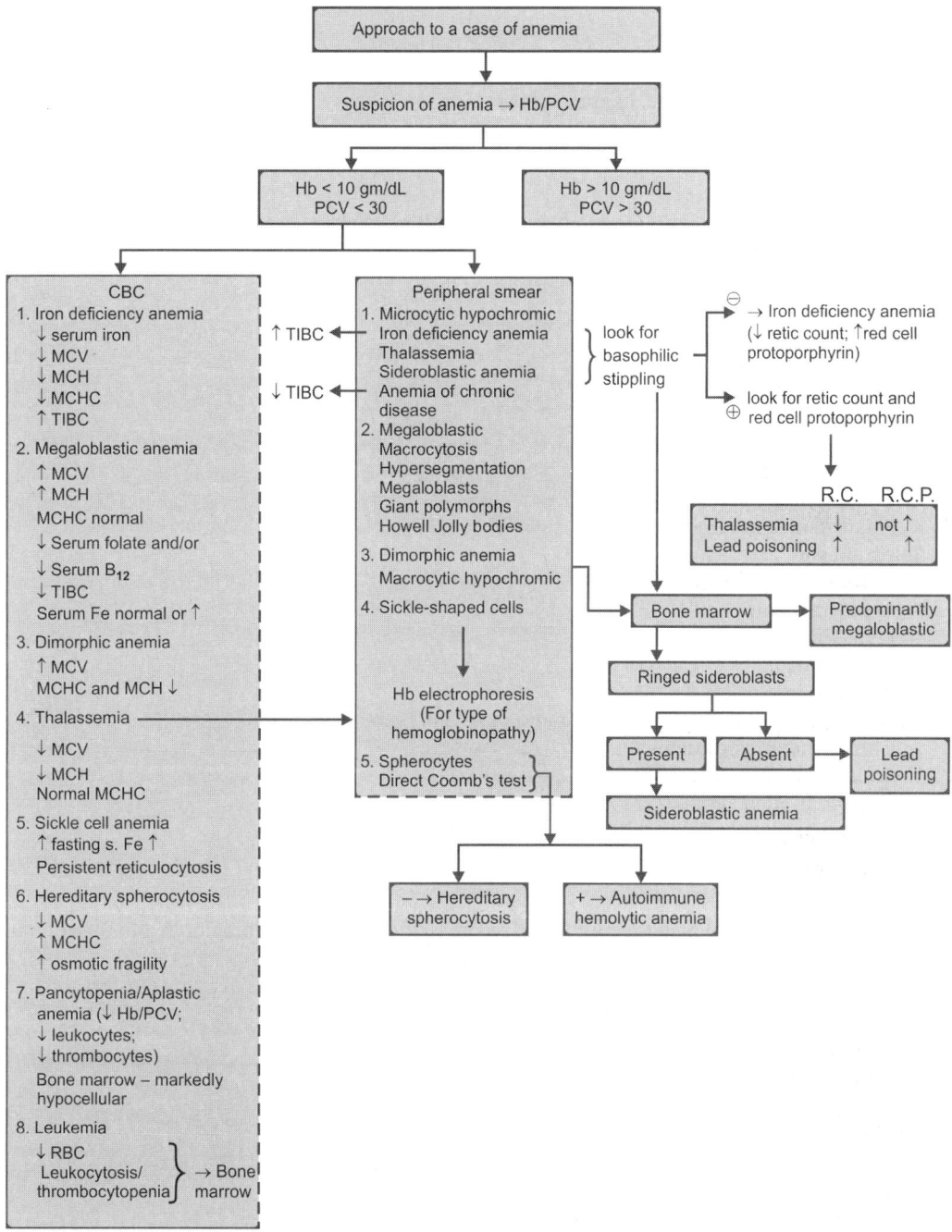

- PR
- BP
- RR (look for dyspnea)
- Lymph nodes in neck, axillae, inguinal areas
- Ankle swelling or swelling of legs.

RS, CVS, CNS

Weight, Height, BMI

Thyroid, Breasts

Signs (Clinical Clues)

- Pallor in severe anemia (hematocrit<25%, hemoglobin<7 g/dL)
  - Pale conjunctiva or mucous membranes
  - Pallor at the nail beds or palmar creases
- Jaundice
  - Hemolytic anemia
  - Hepatitis
- Angular cheilitis
  - Iron deficiency anemia
- Glossitis
  - Iron deficiency anemia
  - Vitamin B_{12} deficiency
  - Folate deficiency anemia
- Splenomegaly
  - Chronic hemolytic anemia
  - Acute infection
  - Leukemia
  - Lymphoma
  - Portal hypertension
- Frontal bossing with prominent malar and maxillary bone
  - Chronic hemolytic anemia
- Neurologic changes (dementia, ataxia, paresthesia)
  - Vitamin B_{12} deficiency
- Symphysis fundal height – to look for IUGR secondary to anemia.

1. **Define anemia**

   Definition
   - Any condition in which the number of red cells, the amount of hemoglobin and the volume of packed red blood cells per unit volume is less than normal
   - A pathophysiological condition in which the body cannot meet its demands for oxygen.

   WHO
   - No anemia ≥ 11 g/dL
   - Mild 10–10.9 g/dL
   - Moderate 7–9.9 g/dL
   - Severe 4–6.9 g/dL
   - Very severe < 4 g/dL

   CDC
   - Hb <11 g/dL in 1st and 3rd trimesters
   - Hb <10.5 g/dL in 2nd trimester (Packed cell volume ≈ 32%)

   Pregnancy
   - For practical purposes, Hb <10 g/dL at any time during pregnancy is considered anemia, as plasma volume expands resulting in Hb dilution
   - Hb ≤ 9 g/dL → need to investigate.

Prevalence
- High prevalence ≥ 40%
- Medium prevalence 15–39%
- Low prevalence 5–14.9%
- Not a problem <5%.

Global scenario
- India has the highest prevalence of iron deficiency anemia among women in the world, including adolescents: 60-70% of Indian adolescent girls are anemic (2010)
- Worldwide—2 billion people affected (25% of the population)
- Out of this 40-75% are in developing world
- 58% of pregnant women in India are anemic } Guidelines for control of IDA,
- Maternal mortality because of anemia — 20-40% (in India) } NRHM, 2013

2. **RBC 'Rule of 3'**

For normal erythrocytes:
- Hemoglobin (g/dL) ≈ 3 × RBC count (millions)
- Hematocrit (%) ≈ 3 × hemoglobin (g/dL) ± 3%.
Failure to obey this rule suggests an abnormality in erythrocytes (e.g. sickle cells, etc.)

3. **Iron distribution in the body**

Distribution

Total quantity of iron in the body ≈ 4 g. Out of this,
- 65% — present as hemoglobin
- 15-30% — mainly in RES and liver parenchymal cells in the form of ferritin (iron stores)
- 4% — myoglobin
- 1% — various heme compounds that promote intracellular oxidation
- 0.1% — combined with protein transferrin in blood plasma.

Absorption of 1.4 mg/day is required from the diet in women to maintain hemostasis.
To maintain adequate supplies of iron for heme synthesis, 20 mg of iron is recycled daily, going from senescent red cells that are removed from the circulation to new cells in the bone marrow.

Transport and Metabolism

Three stages-

1. Secretion

Liver → secretes apotransferrin into bile $\xrightarrow{through}$ bile duct is absorbed in small intestine.

2. Absorption

In duodenum (2nd part) and jejunum → apotransferrin + iron → transferrin (loosely bound, can be released to any tissue cell at any point in the body) → stimulates receptor on enterocytes → enters it and is released as plasma transferrin.

3. Actual metabolism

Fe^{3+} (in food) $\xrightarrow{\text{Fe reductase present in luminal border of enterocytes}}$ Fe^{2+} (from duodenal lumen to inside erythrocyte)

$\xrightarrow{\text{DCT 1 (Transporter protein)}}$ Fe^{2+} enters in enterocyte where it is stimulated by ferroxidase and is converted into Fe^{3+}.

This ferric iron has three forms:
1. Within the enterocyte, it forms a complex with ferritin → when intestinal epithelial cells are shed, ferritin is also shed with it.

2. In plasma, combines with transferrin → this will be excreted.
3. It is stored in combined form with apoferritin.

Tissues → free iron is stored as ferritin and hemosiderin.

Ferritin
- Storage form
- Deposited especially in reticuloendothelial cells and liver hepatocytes
- Apoferritin + Fe → ferritin (in cell cytoplasm).

Hemosiderin
- Small quantities are stored as this
- Extremely insoluble
- When total quantity of iron in body is more than apoferritin storage pool

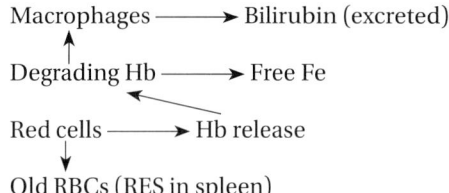

- Fe excreted — 0.6 mg daily
- Fe lost in menses — 0.7 mg/day

4. **Components of blood**
   Red blood cells
   - Shape
     - Biconcave disc
   - Size
     - Diameter
       - 7.5 µm
     - Thickness
       - Center →<1 µm
       - Periphery - 2.5 µm
   - Average life span → 120 days
   - Concentration in blood → 4.7–5.0 mill/cmm in women
   - Daily RBC production requires ≈ 30–35 mg of iron/day (from recycling of storage pool iron)
   - Production (Erythropoiesis → "erythro" — red and "poiesis" — to make)
     - Embryonic life
       - From stem cells in yolk sac
     - Fetal life
       - RBCs in liver, spleen and bone marrow
     - Newborn — childhood
       - Bone marrow of all bones and liver
     - Adult life
       - Bone marrow present in vertebra, sternum, ribs, iliac crest and proximal ends of long bones

Differentiation of Erythrocyte

Hemocytoblast (a multipotent hematopoietic stem cell) → Common Myeloid Progenitor (a multipotent stem cell) → Unipotent Stem Cell → Proerythroblasts → Basophil erythroblast → Polychromatophilic erythroblast → Orthochromatic erythroblast → Reticulocyte → Erythrocyte.

These different appearances can be seen under light microscope after staining with James Homer Wright stain.

Regulatory Factors

- Erythropoietin
  - Produced by renal tubules (90%) and liver (10%)
  - Secretion stimulated by:
    - Decrease in tissue oxygenation
      - Low blood volume
      - Anemia
      - Low hemoglobin
      - Poor blood flow
      - Chronic lung disease
      - High altitudes
    - Placental lactogen
    - Progesterone
  - Stimulates stem cells in marrow → increases red cell production
  - Molecular weight: 55,000 kD
- Hepcidin **(recent advances)**
  - Peptide hormone
  - Composed of 25 amino acids
  - Synthesized in the liver and detectable in blood and urine
  - Plays a role in the regulation of hemoglobin production and thus affects erythropoiesis.

Role of Hepcidin in Iron Deficiency Anemia

- It acts as a coordination between use and storage of iron in the body
- It acts on the inhibition of intestinal iron absorption and iron release by macrophages and enterocytes and is a mediator in the cycle of iron absorption between the liver and intestine
- Measurement of hepcidin concentrations can be used for different diagnoses of anemia, such as iron deficiency anemia, which is characterized by low levels of this hormone
- Iron homeostasis is regulated by two main mechanisms:
  1. An intracellular mechanism, dependent on the amount of iron available for the cell
  2. A systemic mechanism, in which hepcidin plays a crucial role
- Inadequate oxygen (blood loss/hypoxia) →↑ production of erythrocytes →↓ Hepcidin and its inhibitory effects → more iron is made available from diet and from storage pool in macrophages and hepatocytes
- Hepcidin binds to ferroportin (protein required for ferrous transport into plasma) → regulates iron export into plasma
  - ↓ hepcidin → ferroportin exports iron → iron released in bloodstream
  - ↑ hepcidin → internalization and degradation of ferroportin molecules → iron release decreases progressively →↓ iron absorption in enterocytes

- Hepcidin ↑ in anemia of chronic disease but the classic iron deficiency anemia in humans is associated with low hepcidin expression, which makes this hormone a potential marker for detection of iron deficiency anemia coexisting with anemia of chronic disease
- Diagnosis and therapy for anemia based on hepcidin may provide a more effective approach to prevent toxicity associated with iron overload.

Maturation

Vitamins

- RNA → vitamin B12 (early stages)
- DNA → folic acid (late stage)
- Folic acid requires vitamin C for folinic acid synthesis
- Deficiency of vitamin B_{12} → defective synthesis of both RNA and DNA } Maturation failure
- Deficiency of folic acid → defective synthesis of DNA only } of RBCs

Result in megaloblast production having very little O_2 carrying capacity and have short life span

Minerals

- Iron (mainly)
- Traces of copper and cobalt } Hemoglobin synthesis

Proteins

- Supply amino acid for synthesis of globin moiety
- *In nonpregnant state, iron flows mainly towards cells in marrow*
- *In pregnancy, iron flows towards trophoblastic cells of placenta and delivered to fetus*

Hemoglobin

- Globular proteins, comprising 1/3rd of the weight of red cell
- Molecular weight 68000
- Concentration in whole blood
  - Females — 13.5–14 gm% per mL
  - Each gram of hemoglobin can combine with 1.3 mL of O_2
- Consists of heme and globin
- Each red cell contains ≈ 640 million Hb molecules
- Synthesis
  - 65% in erythroblasts
  - 35% in reticulocyte stage
  - Heme synthesis occurs in mitochondria
  - Globin synthesis occurs in polyribosome
- It has eight functional globin chains
- Globin synthesis is first detected in primitive erythroid precursors of yolk sac at ≈ 3 weeks gestation
- Embryonic
  - Hb Gower I
  - Hb Portland
  - Hb Gower II

- Fetal
  - HbF ($\alpha_2 \gamma_2$)
  - HbA ($\alpha_2 \beta_2$)

  change from fetal to adult hemoglobin occurs at 3–6 months after birth
- Adult
  - HbA ($\alpha_2 \beta_2$) → > 95%, consists of 4 polypeptide chains, each with its own heme group
  - HbA2 ($\alpha_2 \delta_2$) → 1.5–3.2%
  - HbF ($\alpha_2 \gamma_2$) → 0.5–0.8% (<1%)

Classification of Anemia

Can be classified as:
- Physiological
- Pathological
  - Acquired
  - Inherited

Acquired

- Deficiency anemia
  - Iron deficiency
  - Folic acid deficiency
  - Vitamin B_{12} deficiency
  - Protein deficiency
- Hemorrhagic
  - Acute
    - Antepartum hemorrhage
  - Chronic
    - Hookworm infestation
    - Bleeding piles
- Bone marrow insufficiency
  - Hypoplasia or aplasia due to radiation, drugs (aspirin, indomethacin)
- Anemia of infection
  - Malaria, tuberculosis
- Anemia due to chronic disease
  - Renal disease or neoplasm.

Inherited

- Thalassemia
- Hereditary hemolytic anemia (RBC membrane defects, spherocytosis)
- Sickle cell hemoglobinopathy.

Concept of Physiological Anemia in Pregnancy

- RBC increases by (350 mL) 20–30%
- Plasma volume increases by (250 mL) 40–50%
- Erythrocyte dilution by 5–15%
- Decrease in hemoglobin concentration by ≈ 2 g/dL
- Total blood volume, increases by (1500 mL) 30–40%

- Because of hemodilution → physiological anemia occurs → hemoglobin is brought down to 11 g%
- Blood picture of physiological anemia in pregnancy: normocytic, normochromic.

Benefits

- Decreases blood viscosity → decreases load on heart
- Facilitates blood flow through placenta
- Increases blood volume → acts as protective barrier against blood loss in third stage of labor.

Harmful Effects

- In case of cardiac disease, the increased circulatory burden can be dangerous, especially in the presence of anemia and fetus may be less efficiently oxygenated because of decreased oxygen carrying capacity of diluted blood.

Daily Intake of Dietary Iron

- 15 mg can replenish daily loss of 1.5 mg of iron
- Absorption rate → 10%.

Factors Leading to Anemia during Pregnancy

- *Increased demand*
  - Increased absorption by presence of HCl in stomach
  - Multiparity (increased iron demand by 2-folds)
  - Women with rapidly occurring pregnancy within 2 years following last delivery
  - Teenage pregnancy (e.g. at the age of 17, additional demand is ≈ 270 mg during pregnancy) → becomes nil by age 21
  - Parturition
  - Lactation
    - Adequate balanced diet → 18–20 mg of iron
    - Absorption rate increased by 20%, therefore, demand is hardly fulfilled.

- *Diminished intake of iron*
  - Low socioeconomic status
  - Vegetarian diet
  - Lack of balanced diet or poor intake (e.g. diet rich only in carbohydrates)
  - Alcoholism
  - High-risk ethnic groups
  - Drugs — alphadopa/levodopa/ciprofloxacin/cimetidine → interfere with iron absorption
  - Achlorhydria and copious intake of antacids decreases absorption
  - Loss of appetite and vomiting
  - Indian tradition — housewife eats last, after all male members and children have eaten and, in many families, the women eat only the leftovers. Hence, even though the food prepared for the family is the same, women are more prone to develop IDA than other members of the family.

- *Disturbed metabolism: presence of infection*
  - Asymptomatic bacteriuria
  - Chronic and latent pyelonephritis
  - UTI

  Therefore, antibacterial therapy is necessary before response to hematinics is expected.

- *Decreased absorption*
  - Dietary factors (tannins, phytates in fiber, calcium in milk, tea, coffee, carbonated drinks)
  - Upper GI pathology
    - Chronic gastritis
    - Chronic diarrhea
    - Gastric lymphoma
    - Celiac disease
    - Crohn's disease
  - Medications that decrease gastric acidity or bind iron
  - Gastrectomy or intestinal bypass
  - Duodenal pathology
  - Chronic renal failure patients.
- *Iron loss*
  - Loss by sweat ≈ 15 mg/month
  - Repeated pregnancy at short intervals (along with prolonged lactation)
    - It requires ≈ 2 years to replenish ≈ 1000 mg of iron lost during delivery and lactation
  - Increased blood loss during menstruation
  - Hookworm infestation
    - 0.5–2 mg of iron daily (each worm extracts up to 0.05 mL of blood/day)
    - A hookworm burden of 40–160 worms (depending on the iron status of the host) is associated with iron deficiency anemia
  - Malaria (falciparum and vivax), chronic blood loss due to bleeding piles/dysentery
  - Sickle cell anemia and thalassemia
    - About 10% of the world's thalassemia patients belong to the Indian subcontinent and 3.4% of them are carriers
    - In India, about 32,400 infants are born with hemoglobinopathies every year
  - GI bleeding
  - Regular blood donors
  - Hematuria
  - Intravascular hemolysis: hemoglobinuria
  - Extreme physical exercise (endurance athletes)
  - Pathological (hemolytic)
- *Prepregnancy health status: anemic or inadequate state of stored iron*
- *Polymorphism*
  - Another important problem posed by anemia in pregnancy is its polymorphism. Pregnancy interferes with maternal erythropoiesis by competing for available raw materials.

5. How does *H. pylori* infection lead to iron deficiency anemia?

Iron deficiency occurs due to the following:
- *H. pylori* infection is intraluminal in proximal part of small intestine where iron absorption takes place and any disruption in metabolism and absorption would lead to iron deficiency anemia
- *H. pylori* infection may be caused via the decreased expression of DMT1 (divalent metal ion transporter 1)
- Ferric iron must be reduced to ferrous iron before absorption. Gastric acid and low gastric juice pH are needed for this reduction. Atrophic gastritis caused by *H. pylori* infection can decrease the excretion of gastric acid, which can decrease the absorption of iron

- Increased iron uptake by *H. pylori* is another mechanism for iron deficiency caused by *H. pylori* infection
- *H. pylori* may compete with the host for the availability of food iron
- Iron inside the enterocyte is stored as ferritin and is lost with the enterocytes sloughed at the villus tip. *H. pylori* infection can cause duodenal diseases including duodenal ulcer, which may increase the slough of enterocytes. This may be responsible for ID development to some extent.

6. **Why is iron not prescribed in first trimester?**
   - Absorption of exogenous iron is regulated by state of body store
   - Females generally have adequate iron stores when they enter pregnancy, leading to its little absorption in the 1st trimester
   - Later in gestation, there is increased demands → depletion of stores and accordingly iron absorption is increased from 7% in 1st trimester to 66% in 3rd trimester.

7. **What are the iron requirements/day in different trimesters?**
   - Normal iron requirement in pregnancy is roughly 4.0 mg/day, i.e. ≈ 120–150 mg/month

   In pregnancy
   - *Early:* 2.5 mg/day
   - *20–32 weeks:* 5.5 mg/day (1.9 mg/1000 kcal in 2nd trimester)
   - *>32 weeks:* 6–8 mg/day (2.7 mg/1000 kcal in 3rd trimester).

   Lactation
   2.4 mg/day

8. **Effects of anemia on mother and fetus**
   Mother

   During pregnancy
   - Abortions
   - *Preeclampsia:* Because of malnutrition and hypoproteinemia
   - Intercurrent infection:
     - A diminished resistance to infection
     - Flares up pre-existing lesion
     - Infection itself impairs erythropoiesis by bone marrow depression
   - Heart failure at 30–32 weeks
   - Preterm labor
   - IUD (24% at term)

   During labor:
   - Uterine inertia
   - Postpartum hemorrhage
   - Cardiac failure:
     - Due to accelerated cardiac output which occurs during labor or immediately after delivery
     - As the blood in uterine circulation is squeezed in general circulation, it puts undue strain on weak heart already compromised by hypoxia
   - Shock

   Puerperium
   - Puerperal sepsis
   - Subinvolution

- Failing lactation
- Puerperal venous thrombosis
- Pulmonary embolism

Risk periods
- At approximately 30-32 weeks of pregnancy
- During labor
- Immediately following delivery
- Any time in puerperium especially 7-10 days after delivery due to pulmonary embolism

Fetus
Usually remains unaffected even if mother suffers from iron deficiency anemia

Risks include:
- Preterm
- IUGR
- IUD

Baby:
- Low Apgar score
- Developmental delay
- Iron deficiency in infancy.

9. **Stages of iron deficiency anemia (IDA)**
   There are three stages–

   Depletion of iron stores
   - Signifies that iron supply to bone marrow and other tissues is marginally inadequate but there is still no anemia
   - Diagnosis:
     - Ferritin <15 ng/mL
     - Normal hemoglobin/hematocrit
     - Normal RBC indices
   - Ferritin ⟶ molecular weight 4,50,000 kDA ⟶ marker of storage iron
   - It is a stable glycoprotein which accurately reflects iron stores in the absence of inflammatory change
   - 1st lab test to become abnormal
   - Not affected by recent iron ingestion
   - Initially rises, then falls by the end of the 2nd trimester to 50% of prepregnancy levels, reflecting hemodilution of pregnancy → again slightly ↑ after 32 weeks
   - 1 ng/mL of serum ferritin = 8 mg of storage iron
   - Measured by ELISA
   - Normal value: 50-150 ng/mL
   - Treatment to be considered when levels fall to <30 ng/mL

Different categories of IDA	*Hemoglobin*	*s. ferritin*
Iron deficiency but not anemic	>11 gm/dL	<15 ng/mL
Iron deficiency anemia	<11 gm/dL	<15 ng/mL
Anemia not due to iron deficiency	<11 gm/dL	>15 ng/mL

   Iron-deficient erythropoiesis (IDE)
   Peripheral smear → Normocytic cells
   Serum transferrin saturation(%) → Serum iron: TIBC

Normal values:
- Serum iron 60–120 µg/dL (decreases in later part of the day and with infection)
- TIBC 325–400 µg/dL
- Transferrin saturation 20–50%
- *In iron deficiency anemia: iron/TIBC × 100 → % saturation*
- *60/400 × 100 → 15% → transferrin saturation (%)*

Erythrocyte zinc protoporphyrin concentration (ZPP):
- Represents substrate used for heme synthesis
- ZPP increases when iron availability decreases, as zinc, rather than iron, is incorporated into the protoporphyrin ring → gives an indication of availability of iron to tissues
- Not influenced by plasma dilution
- Levels rise in 3rd trimester
- Mild IDE–ZPP ratios between 40 and 70 µmol/mol. heme
- More advanced IDE–ZPP > 70 micromol/mol. heme
- Though rarely performed, has greater sensitivity and specificity for iron depletion

Serum transferrin receptor (Tfr) measurements:
- Transmembrane protein which transports iron into cell
- There is little change in the early stages of iron store depletion, but once iron deficiency is established, the serum Tfr concentration increases in direct proportion to total transferrin receptor concentration
- Measured by ELISA → to assess cellular Fe status
- Consists of a single protein of 85 kD
- Expensive test
- Little data on its use in pregnancy.

Frank iron deficiency anemia
- Tfr concentration ≈ 8.8 mg/L
    - Normal baseline average ≈ 5.3 mg/L → 3-fold increase (this precedes decrease in MCV or increase in FEP)
- Serum Tfr: serum ferritin
    - <100 (when adequate stores are present)
    - >2000 (significant functional iron depletion)
    - 500 (at the point of storage depletion)

10. **How will you differentiate between iron deficiency anemia and thalassemia?**
    - Cells are smaller and along with that are of unequal sizes and staining, i.e. anisocytosis and polychromasia in thalassemia
    - This variation in red cell distribution width → important feature to differentiate iron deficiency anemia and thalassemia.

\multicolumn{2}{c}{Features pointing towards etiology of anemia}
Features	*Etiology*
Presence of jaundice	Hemolytic
Leg ulcer	Sickle cell anemia
Spotted nails and koilonychia	Iron deficiency anemia
Neurological deficit	Megaloblastic anemia
Cold intolerance, reduced resistance to infection	Iron deficiency anemia
Hepatosplenomegaly	Hemolytic anemia
Malignancy and parasitic infestation	Thalassemia
Frontal bossing	Thalassemia
Lymphadenopathy or sternal tenderness	Blood dyscrasias and metastasis
Scleral icterus	Hemolytic
Restless leg syndrome	Iron deficiency anemia
Glossitis	Pernicious anemia/folic acid or vitamin B_{12} deficiency
Tongue fiery red	Vitamin B deficiency
Pale tongue	Pernicious anemia
Fatigue, leg cramps on climbing stairs, craving ice or cold vegetables	Iron deficiency anemia
Petechiae	Thrombocytopenia from a bone marrow disorder
Glossy tongue, with atrophy of the lingual papillae	Iron deficiency anemia
Ecchymosis, purpura, lymphadenopathy, splenomegaly	Hemolytic malignancy
Melena, hematochezia, hematuria, hematemesis	Iron deficiency anemia secondary to bleeding
Cheilitis, glossitis, decreased proprioception and vibratory sensation	Vitamin B_{12} deficiency
Dermatitis herpetiformis (DH) or Duhring's disease	Iron deficiency anemia secondary to malabsorption
Dysphagia with solid foods together with esophageal web (dysphagia results from weakened esophageal muscle contractions)	Plummer-Vinson syndrome
Pseudotumour cerebri	Iron deficiency anemia (a rare finding in severe cases)

11. **What is koilonychia and angular cheilitis?**

Koilonychia
- Nail disease
- Sign of iron-deficiency anemia
- Literal meaning—"spoon nails"
- Refers to nails (usually of the hand) which have lost their convexity, becoming flat or even concave in shape
- Koilonychia is the opposite of nail clubbing
- Process of change is: brittle nails → straight nails → spoon-shaped nails

Angular cheilitis (cheilosis or angular stomatitis)
- Fissures at the corners of the mouth (angular stomatitis)
- An inflammatory lesion at the labial commissure, or corner of the mouth
- Often occurs bilaterally
- Manifests as deep cracks or splits
- In severe cases, the splits can bleed when the mouth is opened and shallow ulcers or a crust may form.

MANANGEMENT OF IRON DEFICIENCY ANEMIA

I. *Iron demand in pregnancy*
II. *Determine the cause of anemia (discussed above)*
III. *Preventive measures*
- Dietary diversification
- Diet fortification
- Micronutrient deficiencies: Awareness of risk factors and health consequences
- WHO prophylaxis (National program)
- FANC (including intervention strategies to prevent iron deficiency in the newborns)
- Control of parasitic infections
- General measures (improvement in sanitation and safe drinking water).

IV. *Treatment proper*

I. Iron demand in pregnancy

- Total 900 mg (range 700–1400 mg)
- Out of 900 mg
  - 500–600 mg → goes to uterus and its contents
  - 150–200 mg → average blood loss at delivery
  - 150–200 mg → required in lactation
  - 500 mg → consumed by increased maternal Hb mass (but this is returned to stores after delivery)
- Total increase in red cell volume ≈ 350 mL and 1 mL contains 1.1 mg of iron
- On the credit side:
  - Savings of ≈ 225 mg (because of anemia of pregnancy)
  - Total → 900–225 = 600–700 mg → *likely iron deficit*

III. Preventive measures

Dietary diversification:
- Indian diet contains ≈ 15 mg of iron/day, out of which ≈ 10% is available for absorption
- There should be a critical balance between enhancers and inhibitors of iron absorption

- Enhancers:
  - Heme iron (absorbed 2-3-fold readily than nonheme iron), present in meat, liver, poultry, fish, other seafood
  - Ascorbic acid or vitamin C, present in fruits, juices, potatoes and some other tubers, and other vegetables such as green leaves, cauliflower and cabbage
  - Fermentation or germination of cereals or legumes (as it increases the bioavailability by reducing the content of phytate)
- Inhibitors:
  - Phytates in cereal bran, cereal grains, high-extraction flour, legumes, nuts and seeds
  - Tannins in tea and coffee, cocoa, herbal infusions in general, certain spices (e.g. oregano)
  - Calcium, particularly from milk and milk products
- Foods rich in iron:
  - *Nonheme iron:* Jaggery, amla, chick pea (chana sag), spinach, amaranth, onion stalks, mustard leaves, fenugreek leaves, mint, colocasia leaves, lentil (dal), kala chana, soyabean, til, red gram and black gram, watermelon, pumpkin, cabbage, drumsticks, coriander leaves
- Foods rich in folic acid:
  - Green vegetables (spinach, methi, broccoli), fruits, liver, kidney
- Foods rich in vitamin B_{12}:
  - Meat, fish, eggs, milk
- Foods rich in vitamin C (conversion of ferric into ferrous salts):
  - Citrus fruits, amla (Indian gooseberry), fresh vegetables
- Certain household practices should be improved:
  - Avoid prolonged cooking
  - Recommend that vegetables rich in vitamin C, folate and other water-soluble or heat-labile vitamins be minimally cooked in small amounts of water
  - Encourage the consumption of tea, coffee, chocolate, or herbal teas at times other than with meals
  - Staple Indian diet consists of cereals and cereals contain phytic acid. Phytate reduces iron absorption
  - Medications that raise the gastric pH (e.g. antacids, proton pump inhibitors, histamine H_2 blockers) should be avoided while on iron therapy
- Heme iron is absorbed very efficiently by the body whereas only 1 to 7% of nonheme iron is absorbed
- Because nonheme iron is present mainly as ferric iron in food, it must be reduced to the ferrous and divalent form (Fe^{2+}) prior to uptake by intestinal enterocytes
- Around 1-2 mg/day of additional diet is needed to balance losses in the urine, sweat and stools.

Controversy: whether iron and vitamin B_{12} supplementation to be offered routinely to all pregnant females?
- Increased Hb and ferritin levels are associated with increased risk of IUGR, preterm labor and preeclampsia
  - Studies have shown that there is possible iron overload of gut mucosa and oxidative damage to tissues following daily iron intake
  - Excessive iron is highly toxic as it generates free radicals
- Vitamin B_{12} prophylaxis
  - Not required routinely except in strict vegetarians, who will not take animal products
  - Dose: 3-10 mcg/day.

Micronutrient Deficiencies: Risk Factors and Health Consequences

Iron

Risk factors
- Low intakes of meat, fish, poultry and high intakes of cereals and legumes
- Preterm delivery or low birth weight
- Pregnancy and adolescence
- Heavy menstrual losses
- Parasitic infections (i.e. hookworm, schistosomiasis, ascaris) which cause heavy blood losses
- Malaria (causes anemia, not iron deficiency anemia)
- Low intakes of vitamin C (ascorbic acid)
- Allergy to cow's milk.

Health consequences
- Reduced cognitive performance
- Lower work performance and endurance
- Impaired iodine and vitamin A metabolism
- Anemia
- Increased risk of maternal mortality and child mortality (with more severe anemia).

Folate (Vitamin B_9)

Risk factors
- Low intakes of fruits and vegetables, legumes and dairy products
- Malabsorption and intestinal parasitic infections (e.g. Giardia lamblia)
- Genetic disorder of folic acid metabolism.

Health consequences
- Megaloblastic anemia.

Risk factor for–
- Neural tube defects and other birth defects (orofacial clefts, heart defects) and adverse pregnancy outcomes
- Elevated plasma homocysteine
- Heart disease and stroke
- Impaired cognitive function
- Depression.

Vitamin B_{12} (Cobalamin)

Risk factors
- Low intakes of animal products
- Malabsorption from food due to gastric atrophy induced by *H. pylori* or bacterial overgrowth
- Genetic disorder of vitamin B_{12} metabolism.

Health consequences
- Megaloblastic anemia
- Severe deficiency can cause developmental delays, poor neurobehavioral performance and growth in infants and children, nerve demyelination and neurological dysfunction.

Risk factor for
- Neural tube defects
- Elevated plasma homocysteine
- Impaired cognitive function.

Calcium

Risk factors
- Low intakes of dairy products.

Health consequences
- Decreased bone mineralization
- Increased risk of osteoporosis in adults
- Increased risk of rickets in children.

Vitamin D

Risk factors
- Low exposure to ultraviolet radiation from the sun
- Wearing excess clothes
- Having darkly pigmented skin.

Health consequences
Severe forms result in rickets in children and osteomalacia in adults.

National Anemia Prophylaxis Program

Overview:
- Launched in 1970
- Aim: To prevent nutritional anemia in mothers and children
- A part of RCH program
- Program also includes health and nutrition education
- Based on clinical assessment of anemia, target group includes–
  - Children 6–60 months
  - School children 6–10 years
  - Adolescents 11–18 years of age
    Dosage:
    - 100 mg elemental iron + 500 µgm folic acid for 100 days (girls to be given greater priority)
    - The following intervention is proposed for women in reproductive age-group:
      - IFA supplementation (100 mg elemental iron and 500 mcg of folic acid) throughout the calendar year, i.e. 52 weeks each year
      - Albendazole (400 mg) tablets for biannual deworming for helminthic control
      - IFA supplements to women in reproductive age-group during doorstep distribution of contraceptives
  - Pregnant woman
    Dosage:
    - 1 tab of 100 mg elemental iron + 500 µgm folic acid prophylactically daily
    - If clinically anemic, 2 such tablets to be given daily × 100 days

- Nursing mothers
  Dosage:
  - 1 tablet containing 100 µgm elemental iron + 500 µgm folic acid daily × 100 days

WHO Recommendations

- 60 mg of elemental iron + 400 mcg of folic acid × 6 months (where prevalence of anemia is <40%)
- This dose is to be supplemented for 3 months postpartum where prevalence is >40%
- Weekly supplementation of 200 mg of elemental iron seems to be equally efficacious as daily dose of 100 mg in nonanemic pregnant females
- Advantages:
  - Less side effects
  - ↓ noncompliance

Food Fortification
- Worldwide ≈ 2 billion people are affected by 'Hidden Hunger' which is defined as:
  - "Deficiencies in **essential micronutrients** (vitamins and minerals) in individuals or populations negatively affecting health, cognition, function, survival and economic development"
  - Micronutrients (vitamins and minerals), which are required in very small amounts are not produced by the body but are essential for:
    - Good health
    - Normal brain growth
    - Healthy aging
    - Good performance
    - Healthy babies
    - Strengthening immune system
    - Normal growth

Fortification/Enrichment
Addition of one or more essential nutrients to a food whether or not it is normally contained in the food, for the purpose of preventing or correcting a demonstrated deficiency of one or more nutrients.

Three types:
1. Conventional fortification
   - Staple foods (flour, sugar, milk, oil, rice)
   - Dairy (milk, yoghurt)
   - Spreads (margarine)
   - Condiments (salt)
2. Home fortification
   - Crushable/soluble tablets
   - Powders
   - Spreads
3. Biofortification
   - Agricultural products (rice, maize, sweet potato)

Also can be classified as follows:
- Mass fortification — foods that are consumed by general population
- Targeted fortification — to fortify foods designed for specific population subgroups, such as complementary foods for young children or rations for displaced populations

- Market-driven fortification — to allow food manufacturers to voluntarily fortify foods available in the market.

The most difficult challenge is to find which particular iron compound is to be fortified and with which food item.

Focused Antenatal Care (FANC) by WHO

- Focused antenatal care (FANC) comprises four visits rather than the older schedule of monthly visits
- The aim is to distribute:
  - Iron and folic acid to all women
  - Mebendazole for the presumptive treatment of hookworms starting from the 2nd trimester
- Advantages:
  - Fewer visits reduce the burden on the pregnant female
  - Quality of services improves
  - Motivation of women to adhere to iron supplementation increases.

Intervention Strategies which Help Provide the Neonate with Adequate Iron Reserve

Amount of iron at birth plays a very important role in sustaining adequate iron status of the infant in the first 6 months and even beyond because breast milk is physiologically low in iron.

Intervention strategies: Three intervention strategies help provide the neonate with adequate iron reserve.

First: Prevention of low birth weight:
- Iron is directly proportional to the lean tissue mass and blood volume of the baby, both functions of its intrauterine growth
- Low birth weight babies are, therefore, most vulnerable to early iron depletion postnatally.

Second: Prevention of maternal iron deficiency anemia:
- Earlier it was thought that fetus acts as a parasite and obtains enough iron, irrespective of the status of the mother
- However, recent evidence suggests that maternal iron deficiency during pregnancy compromises the status of the neonate.

Third: Delayed clamping of the umbilical cord after birth:
A short delay of 2–3 minutes allows a small but important amount of blood to continue to flow to the fetus from the placenta, increasing the red cell mass and, therefore, the iron endowment of the neonate.

Prevention of Parasitic Infections

- *Ankylostomiasis or hookworm infection:* Tab. mebendazole 100 mg bid × 3 days (always keep a watch for reinfection)
- *Malaria:* Weekly 2 tablets of chloroquine (300 mg base) from the 2nd trimester onwards in the endemic areas.

IV. Treatment Proper

Points to be remembered before starting the therapy:
- Oral route is the first choice to replenish iron stores unless indicated otherwise
  - Oral therapy takes about 6-10 weeks for Hb to return to normal level
  - In iron deficiency anemia, stores are exhausted and need to be replenished, which begins only after Hb returns to normal
  - Therefore, stopping iron soon after Hb is normal—means inadequate therapy and predisposes to recurrence
- Absorption of iron diminishes after Hb has returned to normal and, therefore, replenishment of stores is a very slow process, taking about 3-4 months
  - Thus iron therapy should be continued for 5-6 months
  - The best absorption occurs during the first few weeks of treatment
  - A positive response to treatment can be defined as a daily increase in hemoglobin concentration of 0.1 g/dL from the 4th day onwards
- Start iron tablet with 1 tablet/day, increase gradually till full dose is reached and well tolerated
- If the patient complains of side effects, try a low-dose preparation with an iron enhancer like ascorbic acid or try alternative salts with less gastric intolerance
- > 2 tablets/day → not recommended and not favored
- Side effects are directly related to the amount of elemental iron and the actual compound and not to the brand used
- Ferrous salts → 3 times readily absorbed than ferric forms
- Ideally iron should be taken on an empty stomach but it ↑ side effects. Therefore, it can be taken in between meals. If taken after meals, absorption is ↓ to 5%
- Tea, coffee, antacids, calcium salts (other than calcium carbonate and citrate) should be avoided for at least 2-3 hours after iron intake
- Vitamin C is an enhancer, so it can be taken with iron
- Liquid preparations:
  - Expensive
  - Deteriorate on storage
  - Metallic taste
  - Make feces black
  - Cause temporary discoloration of teeth (due to formation of iron sulfide), therefore:
    - Take with straw OR
    - Mix with water or fruit juice OR
    - Use a dropper to the back of the mouth and then rinse the mouth thoroughly
- There is no significant difference in absorption when a ferrous salt is given in the form of sulfate, gluconate, lactate, fumarate or succinate but absorption is poor
  - When given as carbonate, citrate and pyrophosphate
  - In ferric forms
  - Colloidal iron preparations
  - Iron carbohydrate complexes
- Cheapest and well-absorbed form — ferrous sulfate
- Most commonly used salt in commercial preparations - ferrous fumarate
- Response to oral therapy
  - Usually begins 1 week after starting treatment and thereafter hemoglobin increases at the rate of 0.8 g/dL/week
  - Retic count ↑ by 7-10 days

- Side effects:
  - *Upper GIT:* Nausea, gastric discomfort, loss of appetite, staining of teeth with liquid preparations
  - *Lower GIT:* Constipation, diarrhea, flatulence
- Enteric coated or sustained release oral iron preparations are generally not recommended as majority of the iron is carried past the duodenum, resulting in poor absorption
- Colloidal ferric hydroxide has high elemental iron (52.26%) → gets reduced to ferrous state easily by action of gastric juices → assuring its greatest and better absorption with minimal gastric irritation
- Daily versus weekly iron supplementations — studies have shown that weekly supplementation is simple, economical, with less side effects and equally efficacious when compared to daily doses.

Various oral iron preparations		
Preparation	*Iron compound (mg/tab)*	*Elemental iron [mg/tab (%)]*
Ferrous sulfate (hydrous)	300	60 (20%)
Ferrous sulfate (dried)	200	65 (32.5%)
Ferrous gluconate	300	36 (12%)
Ferrous fumarate	200	66 (33%)
Ferrous succinate	100	35 (35%)
Ferric ammonium citrate	125	25 (17-22%)
Carbonyl iron	100	90 (90%)
Iron polymaltose complex	100 mg/50 mg	-
Ferrous ascorbate		100
Ferrous fructose		25%
Ferrous lactate		19%
Ferrous carbonate		16%
Ferrous glycine citrate		23%
Iron choline		12%

Newer Oral Iron Preparations

Iron III Hydroxide Polymaltose Complex (Mumfer)

Advantages:
- Less side effects (nonionic)
- Can be used in those who cannot tolerate other oral preparations
- Does not stain teeth
- Can be taken at any time irrespective of meals
- No metallic taste.

Disadvantages:
- Recently therapeutic efficacy of IPC is questioned
- Comparatively costlier as compared to other preparations
- Ferric iron preparation
- Very poor bioavailability.

Iron Bisglycinate

- Glycine (smallest of all amino acids) on reacting with ferrous iron, forms a more stable compound, bisglycinate chelate with least GI symptoms
- It protects the iron from harmful chemical reaction in stomach and duodenum. Therefore, phytates will not reduce its absorption
- Different studies have shown this compound to be very efficacious in restoring Hb levels in shorter duration of time with low doses.

Disadvantage:
- High cost.

Carbonyl Iron

- "Carbonyl"—refers to a manufacturing process
- Iron is obtained by controlled heating of vaporized iron pentacarbonyl → leading to the deposition of unchanged elemental iron (purity >98%) as microscopic spheres of diameter < 5μ → which then becomes soluble in gastric juices
- The gastric juices solubilize this iron, consuming H+ ions → increasing its pH → for much slower but complete absorption
- ↓↓ toxicity (no risk of iron poisoning even if taken by children by mistake)
- Has high bioavailability and less side effects than other preparations.

Na Feredetate

- Newer formulation, chelate form of iron
- Does not dissociate in stomach, thereby producing minimal gastric irritation
- Bioavailability is 2.5 to 10 times of ferrous sulfate and carbonyl iron respectively
- Produces faster rise in hemoglobin as compared to conventional and carbonyl iron
- Absorption → unaffected by phytates and oxalates
- Available as Tabs and solution
- Tablet provides:
  - 231 mg of sodium feredetate equivalent to 33 mg of elemental iron
  - 1.5 mg of folic acid
  - 15 mcg of vitamin B_{12}
- Each 5 mL of solution contains
  - 231 mg of sodium feredetate equivalent to 33 mg of elemental iron
  - Available in lemon orange flavor.

Gastric Delivery Systems

- Bioadhesive polymer (cross-linked polyacrylic acid)
- It adheres to the gastric mucosa or epithelium and floats there
- Releases iron slowly (over 5–12 hours) but continuously in stomach, reducing the dosage to once daily
- Eliminates GI side effects
- Absorption ↑↑
- Very costly.

Short Gun Therapy of Anemia

- Contains different vitamins and trace elements
- An added advantage
- High cost
- Technical Advisory Board (India) has recommended that B complex, other vitamins and zinc should not be included in iron and folic acid containing hematinics.

Iron poisoning:
- Second most common cause of poisoning among children after aspirin
- Children get tempted by the sugar coating on the tablets
- 1 g of drug is quite enough to cause poisoning.

Parenteral Administration

- *Caution before use:* Iron deficiency should be confirmed by ferritin levels before use of parenteral preparations as free iron may lead to the production of hydroxyl radicals with potential toxicity to tissues
- Rate of response → same as oral therapy
- Oral iron to be discontinued when IM or IV iron is given, otherwise receptor sites get choked → ↑ toxicity from free circulating iron (especially 48 hours before, in case of iron sorbitol).

Indications for Parenteral Therapy

- Demonstrated intolerance to oral iron
- Disorder of GIT (Inflammatory bowel disease) — poor absorption
- Along with erythropoietin
- Noncompliance/Nonadherence → patient is not taking it at all (color of stools to be asked)
- Late in pregnancy
- Poor response to oral therapy (≈ after 4 weeks in a confirmed case of iron deficiency anemia)
- Chronic uncorrectable bleeding
- Hemoglobin < 6 g/dL (60 g per L) with signs of poor perfusion, in patients who would otherwise receive transfusion.

Contraindications

- History of anaphylaxis or reactions to parenteral iron therapy
- First trimester of pregnancy
- Active, acute or chronic infection
- Chronic liver disease.

Preparations

Iron Carbohydrate Complexes
- Iron dextran (Imferon)
- Iron sorbitol (Iron sorbitol citric acid complex—Jectofer)
- Iron sucrose (Orofer S).

Routes

Intramuscular

- **Technique:** Test dose 0.5 mL (at same site where full dose is to be given)
- After 1 hour, give full dose
- Give only into muscle mass of upper outer quadrant of buttock in a Z track technique (before injection, skin is laterally displaced so as to avoid staining in case it leaks into subcutaneous tissues)
- Do not rub the injection site
- **Recommended dosage:** 1.5 mg/kg/day or on alternate days
- **Formula:** [(normal Hb—patient's Hb) × wt (kg) × 2.21] + 1000
- It takes ≈ 200 mg of elemental iron to raise Hb by 1 gm/dL of blood
- Anaphylaxis is less with IM than IV preparations
- Side effects:
  - Pain
  - Discoloration at injection site
  - Injection abscess
  - Sarcomatous change (rare).

Iron dextran	Iron sorbitol citric acid complex
IM and IV preparation both	IM only
High molecular weight	Low molecular weight and high transferrin saturation capacity; therefore, it cannot be given as high IV bolus or infusion
Available as 2 mL (IM) and 10 mL (IV)	Available as 1.5 mL ampule
Elemental iron — 50 mg/mL	Elemental iron — 50 mg/mL
50–90% absorbed	Absorbed completely
Slow absorption	Absorption rapid
Not excreted in urine	30% excreted in urine; therefore, treatment is comparatively costlier
Molecule — large as compared to sorbitol	Small molecule as compared to dextran
Takes 3–4 weeks for complete absorption	≈ 2/3rd of the dose is absorbed from local site in 3 hours and little or no residue remains at injection site after 10 days
Side effects: • Joint pain (swelling in joints) in 20% • Fever in 5% of cases	Pain at injection site

Intravenous

- Advantages over IM therapy
  - Less painful
  - Better compliance — complete treatment ensured
  - Less hospital stay
- Dose calculation: $\dfrac{\text{Hb deficit (g/dL)} \times \text{blood volume (65 mL)/kg body weight} \times 3.4}{100}$
- Where 3.4 is → mg iron/gm Hb

- Total dose is diluted in 0.9% NS
- 5% dextrose → ↑ incidence of local pain and phlebitis
- *Test dose:* 0.5 mL (25 mg) diluted in 50 mL IV over 10–15 min
  ↓ After 1 hour
- Give total dose (to be completed within 30 minutes).

Iron sucrose
- Polynuclear ferric hydroxide
- Molecular weight 34000–60000 daltons
- Can be given only by intravenous route
- Each 2.5 mL/5 mL ampule contains 50 mg and 100 mg elemental iron respectively, i.e. each mL contains 20 mg of iron
- Plasma $t_{1/2}$ ≈ 6 hours
- After IV administration, it dissociates into iron and sucrose
- Peak levels reach in 10 minutes
- Does not oversaturate transferrin
- Dose calculation: The cumulative dose depends on total iron deficit
  Total iron (mg) = [2.4 × wt.(kg) × Hb deficit (gm)] + 1000 mg (for pregnancy)
- Administration: as slow IV injection or infusion
  - *Slow IV injection*: 100 mg injected IV over 2–5 minutes
  - *IV infusion*: 5 mL iron sucrose is usually diluted in 100 mL of 0.9% NaCl, immediately prior to infusion and infused IV at the rate of 100 mg of iron over a period of at least 15 minutes
  - Unused diluted solution must be discarded
  - Each dose of 100 mg IV may be repeated up to 3 times per week → max. of 200 mg/sitting
- Advantages:
  - More safe
  - Effective
  - Well-tolerated
  - Very rare anaphylactic reaction
- Disadvantage: high cost
- Caution:
  - The whole infusion should get over in 20–30 minutes (and not 4–5 hours)
  - Most cases of anaphylactoid reaction (recently observed) occurs in the last half hour of the slow infusions, due to the release of free iron radicals with delayed infusions and not due to compound
- Contraindications:
  - In patients with evidence of iron overload
  - In patients with known hypersensitivity to formulation
  - In patients with anemia not caused by iron deficiency
- Side effects (though uncommon)—keep the patient in hospital for minimum 2 hours for observation:
  - Hypotension
  - Chest pain
  - Hypertension
  - Hypervolemia
  - CHF
  - Cramps
  - Musculoskeletal pain
  - Diarrhea

- Nausea/vomiting
- Abdominal pain
- Elevated liver enzymes
- Skin irritation
- Pruritus
- Application site reaction
- Dizziness
- Dyspnea
- Headache
- Fever
- Asthenia/malaise
  - Response to treatment
    - Reticulocyte count >12%
    - Rate of rise in Hb in pregnancy is 0.8 g/dL/week and in nonpregnant women 1.0–1.2 g/dL/week
    - Maximum Hb response does not appear till 4–9 weeks; therefore, if Rx is not started until last month of pregnancy → insufficient time to increase Hb till delivery
  - *Absence of response:* complete investigation including bone marrow biopsy.

Severe Anemia in Late Pregnancy and Labor

Late Pregnancy

- Blood transfusion — life-saving in the last 4 weeks of pregnancy
- Packed cells are to be transfused slowly instead of whole blood
- Diuretics (frusemide) — simultaneously administered
- Propped up position
- O_2 inhalation
- Vitals charting
- Intermittent chest auscultation
- Keep a check on uterine contractions (may go into preterm labor).

Labor/Delivery

- Propped up position
- O_2 inhalation
- Strict watch on volume of fluids
- Intermittent chest auscultation
- Partograph (do not allow prolonged labor)
- Blood cross-matched and saved—more prone to PPH
- Antibiotics cover
- Active management of 3rd stage of labor
- Avoid IV ergometrine
- Keep other oxytocics ready
- If possible, delay blood transfusion till delivery
- Digitalization and cardiac support in cardiac failure.

Postpartum

- Breastfeeding
- Treatment of infections

- Contraception for at least 2 years
- Continue iron and folic acid for minimum 3 months postpartum.

Failure of Treatment in Case of Iron Deficiency Anemia

Causes

- Noncompliance
- Continuous blood loss through hookworm infestation or bleeding piles
- Coexisting infection
- Faulty iron absorption
- Folic acid deficiency
- Noniron deficiency microcytic anemia
  - Thalassemia
  - Pyridoxine deficiency
  - Lead poisoning.

Place of Blood Transfusion in Case of Iron Deficiency Anemia

- Hemoglobin<5 gm/dL → at any gestational age
- After 36 weeks of pregnancy
- Nonresponders → to oral or parenteral therapy
- PPH.

Place of Exchange Transfusion

- Rare
- Indicated in very severe cases in cardiac failure.

Role of Erythropoietin in Anemia

Indications

- Pregnancy with renal insufficiency
- Refractory anemia
- Severe anemia in late pregnancy
- Member of Jehovah's witnesses.

Product Detail (In India)

Available as:
- Vials containing 1000, 2000 and 4000 IU
- Prefilled erythropoietin syringe for subcutaneous use.

Safety:
- Seems to be safe for the fetus: It does not cross the placental barrier and, therefore, lacks any direct fetal effect
- Also safe for the mother.

Prerequisite for successful treatment:
- Adequate iron supplementation.

Contraindications:
- Uncontrolled hypertension
- Hypersensitivity to the drug.

Side effects (uncommon):
- High blood pressure
- Muscle and joint pain
- Flu-like syndrome (headache, dizziness, insomnia, pyrexia, cough, URTI)
- Pruritus, rashes, urticaria
- Nausea, vomiting, stomatitis, dysphagia
- Injection site pain and irritation.

Route:
- For subcutaneous or IV administration only
- Not for intradermal, intramuscular or intra-arterial administration
- IV route recommended for patients on hemodialysis.

Precautions:
- Do not shake or vigorously agitate vial → prolonged, vigorous shaking may denature the glycoprotein, rendering it biologically inactive
- Rotate subcutaneous injection sites
- Single-dose vials contain no preservative
- Use only 1 dose/vial
- Do not re-enter the vial
- Discard any unused portion
- Do not combine unused portions or save unused portions for later use
- Do not administer in conjunction with other drug solutions. However, at the time of subcutaneous administration, single-use vials may be admixed in a syringe with bacteriostatic sodium chloride 0.9% and benzyl alcohol 0.9% in a 1:1 ratio
- Multidose vials contain benzyl alcohol and admixing is not necessary
- Individualize dosing and use the lowest dose sufficient to reduce the need for blood transfusions.

Drug Administration

Two methods exist:

Method 1
Erythropoietin + iron sucrose in the same sitting
   200 mg iron sucrose diluted in 100 mL 0.9% NS infused over 15–20 minutes → flush cannula with 5 mL saline solution → inject erythropoietin (1 mL) bolus.

Method 2
Erythropoietin s/c with oral iron therapy
   150 IU/kg × 3 times/week for a total of 4 weeks
- When adjusting therapy, consider hemoglobin rate of rise, rate of decline and hemoglobin variability
- A single hemoglobin excursion may not require a dosing change
- Evaluate the iron status in all patients before and during treatment and maintain iron repletion.

NRHM (NATIONAL RURAL HEALTH MISSION) RECOMMENDATIONS, 2013

- As anemia is very common among pregnant women in India and majority of anemia-related complications occur at low resource settings, utmost importance should be given to treatment of anemia at subcenter/outreach/PHC/CHC levels
- Screening — by Sahli's hemoglobinometer or by Standard Hemoglobin Color Scale.

Antepartum

Hb between 9 and 11 g/dL

- 2 IFA tablets/day × minimum 100 days
- Reassess Hb after a month → if normal → stop treatment
- If not → refer to higher center.

Hb between 8 and 9 g/dL

- Investigate for the cause
- Rest same as above.

Hb between 7 and 8 g/dL

- Investigate for the cause
- If iron deficiency → IM iron therapy in divided doses + folic acid (if no other obstetric or systemic complications)
- Repeat Hb after 8 weeks
- If she is in her 3rd trimester → refer to higher center
- Multiple dose regimen
  - Intramuscular (IM) — Test dose of 0.5 mL given deep IM and woman observed for 1 hour
  - Iron dextran or iron sorbitol citrate complex given as 100 mg (2 mL) deep IM in gluteal region daily
  - Recommended dose is 1500–2000 mg (IM in divided doses) depending upon the body weight and Hb level.

Hb between 5 and 7 g/dL

- Refer to higher center.

Hb <5 g/dL

- Immediate hospitalization in tertiary care.

Postpartum

- Hemoglobin checked within first 48 hours after delivery
- If woman is nonanemic, prophylactic regime should be given (1 tab daily × 100 days)
- If Hb < 10 gm/dL (WHO) → treat.

IMPORTANT POINTS

12. Causes of microcytic hypochromic anemia
Microcytic hypochromic anemia is found in:
- Iron deficiency anemia
- Thalassemia
- Sideroblastic anemia: Lead poisoning

Lead causes inhibition of several enzymes involved in heme synthesis including ALA synthetase and it leads to sideroblastic anemia with microcytic hypochromic picture.

Characteristic hematological features of lead poisoning:
- Sideroblastic anemia
- Hemolysis
- Punctate basophilia

Condition	Iron deficiency	Thalassemia	Sideroblastic anemia	Anemia of chronic disease
Smear	Microcytic hypochromic	Microcytic hypochromic	Micro hypo or dimorphic picture	Normocytic normochromic > microcytic hypochromic
Serum iron	Low	Normal or ↑	Normal or ↑	↓
TIBC	↑	N	N or ↑	↓
% saturation	<10 (↓)	N or ↑	N or ↑	↓
Ferritin (μg/L)	<15	↑	↑	N or ↑
Hb pattern	N	Abnormal	N	N

Hemochromatosis:

- Disorder of iron storage in which there is an inappropriate ↑ in intestinal iron absorption → deposition of ↑ amounts of iron in parenchymal cells with eventual tissue damage and impaired function of organs
- None of the conditions other than hemochromatosis present with ↑ serum iron with ↑ serum ferritin and ↑ % saturation of transferrin.

13. Name the conditions where iron overload occurs.

Iron loading anemia
- Thalassemia major
- Sideroblastic anemia
- Chronic hemolytic anemia
- Transfusional and parenteral iron overload.

Chronic liver disease
- Hepatitis C
- Alcoholic cirrhosis (advanced)
- Nonalcoholic steatohepatitis
- Porphyria cutanea tarda
- Postportocaval shunting.

Hereditary hemochromatosis

Dietary iron overload
- ↑ erythropoietin →↑ hematopoiesis and ↑ demand for iron, producing state of iron deficiency
- Polycythemia vera being a state of ↑ erythropoietin → there is iron deficiency rather than iron overload.

14. **How has anemia of chronic disease normal ferritin levels but reduced iron?**
    - Anemia of chronic disease is characterized by block in delivery of iron from RES to erythroid progenitors
    - Therefore, patients have normal/↑ iron stores in marrow and N/↑ ferritin level
    - Because of block in delivery, serum iron levels fall and so does TIBC and transferrin saturation.

SIDEROBLASTIC ANEMIA

- Uncommon form
- Presence of ↑↑ number of sideroblasts in bone marrow
- *Sideroblasts:* Erythroid precursors with demonstrable cytoplasmic iron
- Ring sideroblasts are normoblasts in which amount of iron is so greatly ↑ that it appears as cytoplasmic granules arranged in a complete ring around the nucleus
- *Defect:* In incorporating iron into Hb molecule within the erythrocyte.

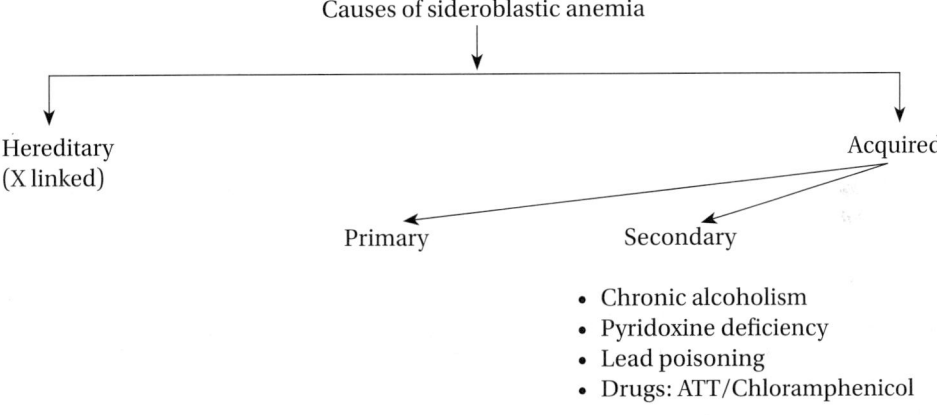

PORPHYRIA

- Inherited or acquired disturbances in heme biosynthesis
- Manifests as:
  - CNS dysfunction
  - Sensitivity of skin to sunlight
- Types:
  - Hepatic porphyria
  - Erythropoietic porphyria.

HEMOGLOBINOPATHY

Thalassemia

Case: A 24-year old lady came for regular antenatal check-up, a known case of thalassemia minor with 30 weeks period of gestation. Husband's reports are normal. She does not have any complaint. Abdominal height is corresponding to the period of gestation.

How will you make out that patient has thalassemia minor?

In general,
- Hemoglobin and PCV → for severity of disease
- RBC indices → type of anemia
- Hb electrophoresis → Hemoglobinopathies (Thalassemia and sickle cell disease)
- Peripheral smear (stained with Giemsa stain) → diagnosis of anemia.

Step I: RBC Indices

- MCV and MCH → low
- MCHC → Normal
- Serum iron and TIBC → normal or ↑

Step II: Confirm by Electrophoresis

- ↑HbA$_2$ ($\alpha_2\delta_2$) → >3.5% with or without ↑ HbF

Step III: Investigations of the Partner

Send Hb electrophoresis

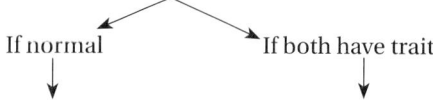

If normal   If both have trait

Nothing is to be done   Offer prenatal diagnosis (there is 25% chance that the fetus will have thalassemia major)

If yes, terminate pregnancy

15. **How will you counsel this patient?**
    - There is seldom any degree of hemochromatosis, if usual iron and folate supplements are taken
    - Do not ever receive parenteral preparations, carrying a risk of hemochromatosis
    - Has a good maternal and fetal outcome
    - Blood transfusions are rarely required.

16. **How will you explain Hb electrophoresis to the patient?**

    Hb electrophoresis
    - For routine Hb analysis
    - Quantification and identification of various hemoglobins
    - Best technique for diagnosis of thalassemia syndromes
    - *Thalassemia syndromes*
        - These are a heterogeneous group of inherited anemias characterized by reduced or absent synthesis of either α or β globin chains of HbA
        - Most common single gene disorder.

Explanation
- Hemoglobin is a conjugated protein
- Molecular weight → 68000
- It has four heme molecules
- On the other hand, globin has four possible chains

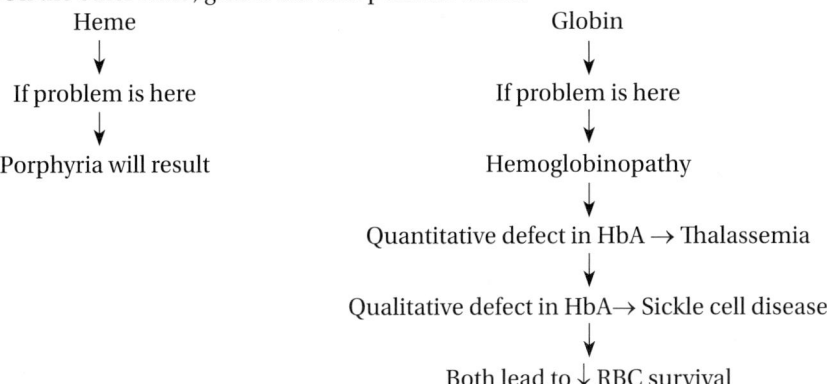

Possible chains of Globin
I. HbA ($\alpha_2\beta_2$)
   - A pair of alpha and a pair of beta chain
   - It is > 95% in normal adult blood
II. HbA$_2$ ($\alpha_2\delta_2$)
   - Approximately 1–3%
III. HbF ($\alpha_2\gamma_2$)
   - Fetal hemoglobin
   - 80% of Hb in cord blood at term
   - Falls to 25% by 1st month of life
   - Almost completely changed to HbA in 1st year of life
   - Constitutes < 1% of adult blood.

Classification
When synthesis of alpha chain is suppressed:
- Level of all the three is reduced, i.e.
  - HbA ($\alpha_2\beta_2$)
  - HbA$_2$ ($\alpha_2\delta_2$)   } Leading to Alpha thalassemia
  - HbF ($\alpha_2\gamma_2$)

When synthesis of beta chain is suppressed:
- Adult Hb is reduced → leading to Beta thalassemia

Inheritance
Autosomal recessive.

Beta Thalassemia

- Results from point mutations of the 2 genes responsible for beta chain that are located on chromosome 11
- Characterized by total or near total absence of β chains resulting in marked decrease in HbA
- Result:
  - Compensatory increase in other chains:
    - γ chain synthesis persists in adult life (↑ HbF)
    - δ chain synthesis is also increased (↑ HbA$_2$)

- Precipitation of excess unpaired α chains
  - Excess of α chains precipitate in cytoplasm of affected RBC → destruction of RBC → anemia
- β⁺ thal → reduced synthesis of β globin chain; heterozygous
- β⁰ thal → absent synthesis of β globin chain; homozygous.

		Beta thalassemia		
Classification	β globin genes	HbA	HbA$_2$	HbF
Normal	Homozygous β	97–99%	1–3%	<1%
Thal major	Homozygous β⁰	0%	4–10%	90–96%
Thal major	Heterozygous β⁺	0–10%	4–10%	90–96%
Thal intermedia	Homozygous β⁺	0–30%	0–10%	60–100%
Thal minor	Heterozygous β⁰	80–95%	4–8%	1–5%
Thal minor	Heterozygous β⁺	80–95%	4–8%	1–5%

Alpha Thalassemia

- Results from gene deletions of the 4 genes responsible for alpha chains that are located on chromosome 16
- Result:

Mutation of 1 gene
- "Silent" carrier
- No clinical or laboratory abnormality

Mutation of 2 genes
- Alpha thalassemia "Minor"
- It goes unrecognized
- Pregnancy well tolerated

Mutation of 3 genes
- "Hb H disease" (Hb H Ds) or "Intermediate"
- Hb Bart (4 γ chains) → present at birth
- Gradually replaced by HbH (4 β chains) → 5–30%
- These women suffer from hemolytic anemia
- During pregnancy → anemia worsens

Mutation of 4 genes (Bart's Hydrops Fetalis Syndrome)
- Most severe form → "α Thalassemia major"
- Incompatible with life
- They have no functioning alpha chain genes (--/--)
- Mother may develop mirror syndrome
  - Hydramnios
  - Edema
  - Preeclampsia
- Neonate born with hydrops fetalis
- Hepatosplenomegaly and cardiomegaly present
- Predominant hemoglobin is Hemoglobin Bart, along with Hemoglobin Portland and traces of Hemoglobin H
- Bart's hemoglobin has high oxygen affinity so cannot carry oxygen to tissues
- Fetus dies *in utero* or shortly after birth
- At birth, has severe hypochromic, microcytic anemia
- Pregnancy → dangerous to mother
- Increased risk of severe preeclampsia and postpartum hemorrhage.

Pathophysiology of the Disease

- Lack of adequate HbA → anemia → ↑ tissue hypoxia → ↑ EPO production → ↑ erythropoiesis in the marrow and at times extramedullary also → expansion of medullary cavities of various bones
- Liver/spleen enlarges → extramedullary hematopoiesis.

Manifestations:

Marrow expansion
- Hemolytic facies with frontoparietal, occipital bossing
- Malar prominence
- Malocclusion of teeth
- Distortion of ribs and vertebrae
- Pathological fractures of long bones due to cortical thinning
- Sinus and middle ear infection due to ineffective drainage
- Folate deficiency
- Increased absorption of iron from intestine
- Hypermetabolic state → fever, wastage, leg ulcers.

Hepatomegaly
- Iron released from breakdown of endogenous or transfused RBCs cannot be utilized for hemoglobin synthesis → hemosiderosis
- Hemochromatosis
- Infections (transfusion related) → Hepatitis B, Hepatitis C, HIV
- Chronic hepatitis
- Jaundice—obstructive (due to gallstones).

Splenomegaly
- Work atrophy due to constant hemolysis
- Hypersplenism
- Jaundice-unconjugated hyperbilirubinemia.

17. **Which is more common of the two?**
    - Beta thalassemia (Cooley's Anemia) is more common of the two
    - Alpha thalassemia is rare.

    Clinical spectrum of β thalassemia
    Thalassemia major
    - Serious homozygous form
    - Severe microcytic hypochromic anemia
    - Detected early in childhood
    - Present in early infancy with:
        - Progressive pallor
        - Hepatosplenomegaly
        - Bony changes
    - Fatal during first few years of life if left untreated
    - Hemoglobin level between 4 and 8 g/dL
    - Peripheral blood shows:
        - Markedly hypochromic, microcytic erythrocytes
        - Extreme poikilocytosis, target cells, teardrop cells and elliptocytes
        - Marked basophilic stippling

- Repeated blood transfusions required
- Physical growth and development delayed.

Thalassemia minor
- Heterozygous form
- Presents late and patient can lead a normal life except for persistent mild hemolytic anemia
- Compatible with normal life
- They have one normal beta gene and one mutated β gene
- Hemoglobin level in 10–13 g/dL range, with normal or slightly elevated RBC count
- Anemia usually hypochromic and microcytic
- Rarely seen hepatomegaly or splenomegaly
- Make sure that these are not diagnosed with iron deficiency anemia.

Thalassemia intermedia
- Patients are able to maintain minimum hemoglobin (7 g/dL or greater) without transfusions
- They are also homozygous
- Patient presents somewhere between two extremes with variable clinical manifestations
  - Progressive pallor
  - Hepatosplenomegaly
  - Bony changes
  - Significant increase in bilirubin
- Life is fairly comfortable
- Not dependent on blood transfusions
- Anemia usually becomes worse with infections, pregnancy, or folic acid deficiencies
- Tend to develop iron overloads as a result of increased gastrointestinal absorption.

Management of β Thalassemia major in pregnancy

Where's the problem?

These patients have iron overload

Iron deposition in various organs

- Brain (hypothalamus and pituitary) → Endocrine abnormalities → Hypogonadotrophic hypogonadism.
  Manifests as:
  - Primary or secondary amenorrhea
  - Chronic anovulation
  - Decreased estradiol levels
- Hypothyroidism
- Diabetes mellitus
- Direct ovarian damage due to iron deposition and redox-active iron in follicular fluid.

Preconception period (very important)
- Need to investigate the following:
  - Maternal cardiac status
  - Thyroid function tests
  - FBS/PPBS/HbA$_1$C
  - Serum ferritin
  - Blood group and type
  - Screening for blood group antibodies (anti-Kell and Duffy) should be performed → If not available → ICT
  - Hepatitis B, C, HIV
  - Partner's electrophoresis

- Chelation therapy
  - With desferrioxamine + vitamin C
  - Aim → serum ferritin level of 1000–2000 ng/mL
- Start folic acid.

Antenatal management
- Investigations mentioned above
- Discontinue:
  Desferrioxamine
  - Harmful effects on fetus
  - Risk of iron deficiency in neonates
  Vitamin C
  - It increases dietary absorption of iron
- Iron supplements should not be given
- These fetuses are at increased risk of:
  - Anemia →↑ blood transfusions (continue folic acid throughout pregnancy)
  - Increased risk of IUGR (frequent fetal growth monitoring and biophysical profile)
  - Increased risk of pregnancy loss
  - Cardiac failure due to overload of pregnancy
  - Increased chances of undergoing cesarean section.

Intrapartum management
- IV line
- Propped up position
- O_2 inhalation
- Maintain partograph → prolonged and obstructed labor in no way is accepted
- Do not increase total blood volume; this can precipitate cardiac failure and pulmonary edema
- Oxytocics and cross-matched blood to be kept ready
- Active management of 3rd stage of labor
- Avoid IV ergometrine.

Puerperium
- Continue breastfeeding
- Desferrioxamine restarted within a week in the postpartum period
- Contraceptive counseling
- OCPs avoided because of the risk of thrombosis especially if splenectomy done.

Management of α thalassemia

Diagnosis by CVS or amniocentesis

When there is mutation of 1 or 2 genes
- Iron and folate therapy
- Never to be given parenteral therapy
- Pregnancy → well tolerated.

HbH disease
- 5 mg folate/day
- Offspring will either be a silent carrier or will carry "trait".

α Thalassemia major
- Incompatible with life and pregnancy
- Vaginal delivery is complicated due to large placenta and fetus.

SICKLE CELL DISEASE (SCD)

Definition

- Sickle cell anemia, an inherited autosomal recessive blood disorder, is the prototype of structural hemoglobinopathies characterized by production of structurally abnormal hemoglobin chain.

Also known as:
- "HbSS"
- "SS disease"
- "Hemoglobin S"
- Drepanocytosis.

It was thought to have originated in areas of the world where malaria was common, since people with sickle trait do not get malaria.

Epidemiology

- SCD is the most common inherited condition worldwide
- Sickle cell disease is prevalent in many parts of India, where the prevalence has ranged from 9.4 to 22.2% in endemic areas.

Pathology

Understanding the Disease

Normal hemoglobin cells are smooth, round, flexible and quite elastic, like the letter "O", which enables them to deform to pass through the vasculature easily

↓

Sickle cell hemoglobin cells are stiff, rigid, sticky, lose their elasticity and form into the shape of a sickle, or the letter "C," promoted by low oxygen tension

↓

These cells fail to return to normal shape when normal oxygen tension is restored. As a consequence, these rigid blood cells are unable to deform as they pass through narrow capillaries, leading to vessel occlusion and ischemia

↓

Due to the decreased number of hemoglobin cells circulating in the body, a person with sickle cell disease is chronically anemic

↓

Although the bone marrow attempts to compensate by creating new red blood cells, it does not match the rate of destruction

↓

Healthy red blood cells typically live 90–120 days, but sickle cells only survive 10–20 days and are destroyed by spleen

↓

In this process, spleen is also damaged → ischemia and infarction occurs → hyposplenism → auto splenectomy

Cause

- Caused by a point mutation in the β-globin chain of hemoglobin, causing the hydrophilic amino acid glutamic acid to be replaced with the hydrophobic amino acid valine at the sixth position
- The β-globin gene is found on chromosome 11
- The association of two wild-type α-globin subunits with two mutant β-globin subunits forms hemoglobin S (HbS)
- Under low-oxygen conditions (being at high altitude, for example), the absence of a polar amino acid at position six of the β-globin chain promotes the non-covalent polymerization (aggregation) of hemoglobin, which distorts red blood cells into a sickle shape and decreases their elasticity
- The loss of red blood cell elasticity is central to the pathophysiology of sickle-cell disease
- *HbA is $\alpha_2\beta_2$:* It thus needs to have both α and β chains. β chains are defective in sickle cell disease such that:
    - In heterozygotes or sickle cell trait: 40% chains are defective
    - In homozygotes or sickle cell disease: 100% chains are defective
    - Therefore, there are no β chains in sickle cell anemia (homozygous) and, therefore, no HbA
    - HbA2 is $\alpha_2\delta_2$ ⎱ There is no underlying defect in δ chains
    - HbF is $\alpha_2\gamma_2$ ⎰ or γ chains in sickle cell disease and, hence, HbF and HbA$_2$ may well be seen
- Most important factor which affects rate and degree of sickling (polymerization) is amount of HbS and its interactions with other Hb chains
- Affected newborn seldom exhibits clinical features of sickle cell disease. Anemia develops over the first 2–4 months paralleling replacement of much of fetal Hb by HbS
- Clinical manifestations are uncommon before 5–6 months of age.

Sickle cell trait patients do not have manifestations as that of sickle cell disease because HbS is <50% and HbA has low affinity for HbS.

Sickle cell trait patients have:
- 40% Hb in form of HbS
- 60% Hb in form of HbA → interferes with HbS only when deoxygenated
- Both low concentration of HbS and presence of interfering HbA act to prevent effective HbS aggregation and polymerization and, therefore, red cells in sickle cell trait (heterozygotes) do not sickle
- Other, rarer forms of sickle-cell disease are compound heterozygous states in which the person has only one copy of the mutation that causes HbS and one copy of another abnormal hemoglobin allele
- They include sickle-hemoglobin C disease (HbSC), sickle beta-plus-thalassemia (HbS/β$^+$) and sickle beta-zero-thalassemia (HbS/β^0).

Sickle cell anemia is characterized by hyposplenism/autosplenectomy. Repeated episodes of splenic infarction cause the spleen to be reduced to small calcified remnant—'Autosplenectomy'.

Clinical Manifestations

Chronic Manifestation

- **Sickle red cells**
    - ↑ mechanical fragility
    - ↑ blood viscosity—'seeding in microvasculature'

- Hemolysis:
  - Anemia
  - Icterus
  - Gallstones—Cholelithiasis and cholecystitis may result from excessive bilirubin production and precipitation due to prolonged hemolysis.
- ***Chronic pain***: Even in the absence of acute vaso-occlusive pain, many patients have chronic pain that is not reported
- ***Chronic renal failure*** due to sickle cell nephropathy—manifests itself with hypertension, proteinuria, hematuria and worsened anemia. If it progresses to end-stage renal failure, it carries a poor prognosis.

Acute Manifestation

- ***Infarctive or painful crisis***
  - Severe skeletal pain but no change in Hb%.
- ***Sequestration crisis:***
  - Sudden massive pooling of red cells in spleen with an acute fall in Hb concentration with the potential for hypovolemic shock
  - Because of its narrow vessels and function in clearing defective red blood cells, the spleen is frequently affected → infarction of spleen
  - This autosplenectomy increases the risk of infection from encapsulated organisms.
- ***Hemolytic crisis:***
  - Uncommon
  - Acute accelerated ↓ in Hb concentration with ↑↑ in jaundice
  - This is particularly common in patients with co-existent G6PD deficiency.
- ***Vaso-occlusive crisis***
  - ↑ blood viscosity → ischemia, pain and infarction
  - Following organs are affected:
    - Lung – Pulmonary hypertension due to vaso-occlusive disease in lung vessels—leading to strain on the right ventricle and a risk of heart failure; typical symptoms are shortness of breath, decreased exercise tolerance and episodes of syncope
    - Bone – Osteomyelitis
    - The most common cause of osteomyelitis in sickle cell disease is Salmonella (especially the non-typical serotypes, *Salmonella typhimurium, Salmonella enteritidis, Salmonella choleraesuis* and *Salmonella paratyphi B*), followed by Staphylococcus aureus and Gram-negative enteric bacilli perhaps because intravascular sickling of the bowel leads to patchy ischemic infarction
    - Avascular necrosis (aseptic bone necrosis) of the hip and other major joints, which may occur as a result of ischemia
    - Spleen – hyposplenism; autosplenectomy
    - Priapism
    - Kidney – Acute papillary necrosis
    - Eye – Background retinopathy, proliferative retinopathy, vitreous hemorrhages and retinal detachments, resulting in blindness
    - Stroke, which can result from a progressive narrowing of blood vessels, preventing oxygen from reaching the brain. Cerebral infarction and cerebral hemorrhage in adults
    - Silent stroke is a stroke that causes no immediate symptoms but is associated with damage to the brain. Silent stroke is probably five times as common as symptomatic stroke, predominating in the younger patient.

- **Aplastic crisis**
  - This is an acute worsening of the patient's baseline anemia, producing pallor, tachycardia, and fatigue
  - This crisis is normally triggered by parvovirus B19, directly affecting erythropoiesis by invading the red cell precursors and eventually leading to their destruction
  - Parvovirus infection nearly completely prevents red blood cell production for two to three days, which in normal individuals, is of little consequence, but the shortened red cell life of sickle-cell patients results in an abrupt, life-threatening situation
  - Reticulocyte counts drop dramatically during the disease, and the rapid turnover of red cells leads to the drop in hemoglobin
  - This crisis takes four days to one week to disappear
  - Overwhelming post-(auto) splenectomy infection (OPSI), which is due to functional asplenia, caused by encapsulated organisms such as *Streptococcus pneumoniae* and *Haemophilus influenzae*.

  Most episodes of sickle cell crises last between five and seven days.

Consequences of Anemia

- Cardiomegaly: Heart failure
- Hepatomegaly
- Reactive bone marrow hyperplasia
  - Stunted growth
  - Bossing skull
  - Fish mouth vertebra
- Chronic leg ulcers

Granulocytosis (leukocytosis) and not leukopenia (WBC ↑ 12000-15000/μL)
- Most common acute presentation of sickle cell anemia is: Bone pain (recurrent episodes) → produced as a result of intermittent episodes of vaso-occlusion in connective tissue and musculoskeletal structures → painful ischemia.

Management

Preconceptional Counseling

- These women should ideally be reviewed annually from adolescence
- Patient should be made aware of the factors favoring sickling/polymerization
  - *Hypoxia:* (2,3 diphosphoglycerate ↑ polymerization)
  - Dehydration
  - Stress/overexertion
  - *Acidosis:* (↓ pH enhances polymerization)
  - *Hb concentration:* Higher concentration →↑ polymerization
  - Combination of HbS with other Hbs → It depends upon extent of homology with other Hbs

Descending order of ability to copolymerization are HbS, C, D, O, Arab, A, J and F (Least with HbF)
- Any urinary infection, if present should be treated before pregnancy
- Patient should be made aware of the increased risk of:
  - Worsening anemia
  - Sickling crises and acute chest syndrome
  - Urinary tract infection during pregnancy

- Recommend pregnancy keeping in mind any previous damage due to serious complications and their screening in advance
  - Echocardiography—to screen for pulmonary hypertension
  - Blood pressure and urine analysis—to rule out hypertension and/or proteinuria
  - RFT/LFT
  - Ophthalmic examination
  - Screening for iron overload (if undergone multiple transfusions or who have high ferritin levels)
  - Screening for red cell antibodies
- Partner's Hb electrophoresis
- Prenatal diagnosis
- Folic acid 5 mg daily
- Patients taking hydroxy urea (to decrease the incidence of crisis and acute chest syndrome) should be counseled regarding the associated congenital defects in the fetus and the drug should be stopped at least 3 months prior to conception
- Angiotensin-converting enzyme inhibitors and angiotensin receptor blockers should be stopped before conception
- Penicillin prophylaxis and vaccinations (Hep B, influenza, pneumococcal vaccine, etc.) should be considered especially in those who are hyposplenic
- Effects of pregnancy on the disease and how the disease affects pregnancy, should be discussed in detail.

Effect of Pregnancy on Sickle Cell Disease

- In some, pregnancy may go uneventful
- In others, there may be worsening of the disease
- Sickle cell crises may still occur in pregnancy and can be managed conservatively
- Pre-existing kidney disease and congestive heart failure may worsen during pregnancy, even with proper treatment and care.

Effect of Sickle Cell Disease on Pregnancy

The risks for pregnancy depend on whether the mother has sickle cell disease or sickle cell trait.

Mother

Sickle cell trait
- Not much affected
- There is an increased incidence of:
  - Painful crises during pregnancy
  - IUGR
  - Antepartum hospital admission
  - Postpartum infection
  - UTI.

Sickle cell disease
- Encounter frequent urinary tract infections
- Lung infection
- They can have iron-deficient anemia while pregnant woman requiring iron supplementation
- Gallstones

- Acute painful crisis
- Antenatal hospitalization
- Maternal mortality
- Delivery by cesarean section
- Infection
- Thromboembolic events
- Antepartum hemorrhage
- Hypertensive disorders of pregnancy
- Cardiac enlargement and heart failure from anemia.

Fetus
- Miscarriage
- Intrauterine growth restriction
- Preterm birth
- Low birth weight
- Stillbirth and neonatal death.

Antepartum Management

Sickle cell trait
- Folic acid 5 mg daily
- Mother not at higher risk
- But baby may be affected if the father also carries the trait
- Investigate the husband at the 1st visit, if not done preconceptionally
- If the baby's father has sickle cell trait, amniocentesis or other methods of prenatal diagnosis may be offered to help determine if the fetus has the trait or the disease.

Sickle cell disease
Care of the mother
- She should see both obstetrician and the hematologist
- Early and regular prenatal care is very important
- Folic acid 5 mg daily
- Avoid excessive nausea and vomiting to prevent dehydration
- More frequent prenatal visits allow for close monitoring of the disease and for fetal well-being
- Healthy diet, prenatal vitamins, folic acid prevent exertion and extreme temperatures
- Blood pressure (often have a low BP) and urine analysis at each visit
- Urine culture—performed monthly
- Serial ultrasounds and Doppler studies (in case of IUGR fetus)
- Though pregnancy is not contraindicated while patient is on hydroxyurea, but stop the drug as soon as pregnancy is diagnosed and ultrasound should be done to rule out any defects
- Live attenuated vaccines should be deferred in pregnancy
- Iron supplementation only if there is documented iron deficiency
- Low dose aspirin 75 mg daily from 2nd trimester onwards, to minimize the risk of preeclampsia is advisable and is stopped at 34 weeks
- If admitted to hospital, LMWH should be considered
- No recommendation for prophylactic blood transfusions
- Blood transfusions to replace the sickled cells if acute emergency arises. This is to be continued several times in pregnancy

- There is no recommendation as to when to start the transfusion but Hb < 6 gm% or a fall in Hb of ≥ 2 gm% any time in pregnancy is an indication for blood transfusion
- Such women are to be screened for antibodies that may be transferred from transfused blood
- The most common antibodies are to the Rh factor
- Exchange transfusion in case of acute chest syndrome or acute stroke.

Investigations
- CBC
- Blood group and type
- Antibody screen
- HIV
- HbsAg
- Anti HCV
- LFT/KFT
- Viral screen
- Urine routine and culture
- Partner screening (as soon as pregnancy is diagnosed).

Care of the fetus
- Started in the 2nd trimester
- TAS (level II scan)
- Nonstress test (after 32 weeks)
- Biophysical profile
- Doppler flow studies (if IUGR).

Place of blood transfusion
- Only when there are concomitant serious complications
- From 26 weeks onwards
- Exchange transfusion (2 units removed for every 3-4 units transfused).

Intrapartum Care

- Delivery should be in a tertiary care center
- If growth is normal, induction of labor is offered at 37 completed weeks
- Blood should be promptly available in case of emergency
- Keep the woman warm
- IV fluids—to prevent dehydration
- O_2 through mask
- Pulse oximeter—to detect early hypoxia
- If oxygen saturation is ≤ 94% → ABG analysis
- Maternal vitals and FHR monitoring meticulously
- Avoid repeated vaginal examinations—to minimize risk of infection
- Left lateral position
- Avoid prolonged and obstructed labor (avoid maternal exertion and exhaustion)
- Vaginal delivery allowed
- Cesarean section for other indications
- Avoid general anesthesia
- Regional anesthesia is recommended.

Postpartum Care

- Antibiotics
- Thromboprophylaxis (Low-molecular-weight heparin)
  - Should be administered:
    - While in hospital
    - 7 days postdischarge following vaginal delivery or
    - For a period of 6 weeks following cesarean section
- Antithrombotic stockings
- Family planning:
  - Permanent sterilization
  - Progesterone only pills
  - Injectable progesterone (Depo provera)
  - LNG IUD
  - Estrogen containing contraceptives can also be used
  - Avoid OCPs and IUCD.

Complications

Painful Crisis

- Most frequent complication during pregnancy
- Incidence ranges from 27 to 50%
- Most frequent cause of hospital admission
- Avoidance of precipitants such as a cold environment, excessive exercise, dehydration and stress is important
- Pain management:
  - Mild pain—paracetamol
  - Mild-to-moderate pain—NSAIDs (only in 2nd trimester)
  - Moderate pain—Weak opioids
  - Severe pain—Stronger opiates (morphine) by oral, subcutaneous, IM or IV route
  - Pethidine to be avoided.

Acute Chest Syndrome

- Second most common complication
- Reported in 7–20% of pregnancies
- Respiratory symptoms—tachypnea, chest pain, cough, dyspnea
- Management:
  - IV antibiotics
  - Hydration
  - Oxygen
  - Blood transfusion
  - Ventilatory support → if severe hypoxia.

Acute Stroke

- It is an emergency
- Urgent exchange transfusion.

Acute Anemia

- Isolate the woman (may be attributed to erythrovirus)
- It may be due to malaria or splenic sequestration
- Reticulocyte count
- Blood transfusion
- With erythrovirus, there is a risk of vertical transmission to the fetus, leading to hydrops. Therefore, careful fetal monitoring is necessary.

18. **Mother has sickle cell disease. Father is normal. Chances of children having disease and trait are 0 and 100% respectively. How?**
    - Sickle cell disease is the homozygous state of HbS (SS) where 'S' stands for gene coding HbS
    - Sickle cell trait is the heterozygous state of HbS (SA), where A stands for absent gene
    - The individual has no gene for HbS (AA)
    - If mother is SS and father AA → offsprings → SA (sickle cell trait)
    - Therefore,
        - SCD → will be 0%
        - SCT → will be 100%.

Prognosis

- About 90% of patients survive upto age 20, and close to 50% survive beyond the fifth decade
- Acute splenic sequestration has a peak incidence between 6 months and 3 years and can be rapid in onset → death
- Most common cause of mortality → sepsis and acute chest syndrome
- Chronic transfusion therapy (repeated BT) required in severely ill patients.

MEGALOBLASTIC ANEMIA

Osler (1919) was the first to describe megaloblastic anemia in pregnancy.

Case: A 30-year-old G2P1L1 with 26 weeks 1 day period of gestation, a strict vegan, has come with occasional vomitings and mouth ulcers, feeling very weak since morning, having a fever upto 99°F. She has been taking iron routinely since 2nd trimester. Her investigations show the following results:

Hb 10 gm%
PCV 30%
MCV 105 µm³
MCH 37 pg
MCHC 33%

How will you interpret this report. What is your provisional diagnosis?

Probable diagnosis: **Megaloblastic anemia (resistant to iron therapy)**

Interpretation:
Hb ↓; PCV↓; MCH ↑; MCV ↑; MCHC is normal

What is Megaloblastic Anemia?

Deficiency of folic acid and/or vitamin B_{12}
↓
Inhibition of DNA synthesis during red blood cell production
↓
Cell cycle cannot progress from the G2 growth stage to the mitosis (M) stage
↓
Cell growth continues without division → presents as Macrocytosis
↓
Slower onset, especially when compared to other types of anemia

Mechanism

- Vitamin B_{12} deficiency alone will not cause the syndrome in the presence of sufficient folate
- The actual mechanism is loss of B_{12}-dependent folate recycling, followed by folate deficiency → which, in turn, will affect the nucleic acid synthesis (specifically thymine) → leading to defects in DNA synthesis
- Folic acid supplementation in the absence of vitamin B_{12} prevents this type of anemia (although other vitamin B_{12}-specific pathologies continue).

Why is There Impaired DNA Synthesis or Abnormal Maturation?

- For maturation, the following are required:
  - Vitamin B_{12} → In synthesis of RNA
  - Folic acid → In synthesis of DNA
  - Vitamin C → For conversion of folic acid to folinic acid
- Therefore, if there is inadequate vitamin B_{12} → Defective synthesis of DNA and RNA
- If folic acid is not adequate → Defective synthesis of DNA only
- Folic acid is required for conversion of uridine to thymidine in nucleic acid synthesis.

Folic Acid (An Overview)

- Also known as folate, vitamin M, vitamin B_9, vitamin Bc or folacin; pteroyl-L-glutamic acid and pteroyl-L-glutamate are forms of the water-soluble vitamin B_9
- Composed of the aromatic pteridine ring linked to para-aminobenzoic acid and one or more glutamate residues
- Folic acid is itself not biologically active, but its biological importance is due to tetrahydrofolate and other derivatives after its conversion to dihydrofolic acid in the liver
- Humans cannot synthesize folate *de novo*; therefore, folate has to be supplied through the diet to meet their daily requirements
- Functions:
  - Synthesizes DNA
  - Repairs DNA
  - Methylates DNA
  - Acts as a cofactor in certain biological reactions
  - Aids in rapid cell division and growth
- Derived its name from the Latin word '*folium*' (which means '*leaf*'); therefore, leafy vegetables are principal sources of folic acid
- Folate in body stores: 500–20,000 µg
- A complete lack of dietary folate takes months before deficiency develops
- Common symptoms of folate deficiency include:
  - Diarrhea
  - Macrocytic anemia with weakness or shortness of breath
  - Nerve damage with weakness and limb numbness (peripheral neuropathy)
  - Pregnancy complications
  - Mental confusion, forgetfulness or other cognitive declines, mental depression
  - Sore or swollen tongue
  - Peptic or mouth ulcers
  - Headaches
  - Palpitations

- Irritability and behavioral disorders
- Low levels of folate can also lead to homocysteine accumulation
- DNA synthesis and repair are impaired and this could lead to cancer development
- Folate requirement of newborn → 20–50 µ/day.

Incidence

- 0.2–5%
- Deficiency of folic acid → very common
- Deficiency of vitamin B_{12} → rare.

Why is Vitamin B_{12} Deficiency Rare?

- Very long storage life
- Stores usually not depleted by pregnancy
- Absorption usually normal in pregnancy
- Vitamin B_{12} binds to intrinsic factor (secreted by gastric parietal cells) → absorbed in distal ileum
- Pre-existing vitamin B_{12} deficiency is often associated with infertility
- Intake (animal products):
  - In nonpregnant females → 2 µg/day
  - In pregnancy → 3 µg/day
- Only strict vegans have a problem → may require supplementation in pregnancy.

Causes of Megaloblastic Anemia in Pregnancy

It is mainly because of folic acid deficiency:
- Deficient supply (poor nutrition)
- Decreased intake because of hyperemesis
- Defective absorption (e.g. in tropical sprue)
- Alcohol consumption (interferes with folate metabolism)
- Smoking (↓ availability)
- Frequent child birth and multiple gestation (increased demands)
- Hemolytic factors:
  - Congenital → sickle cell disease
  - Parasitic → e.g. malaria
  - Hemorrhagic states:
    - Peptic ulcer
    - Hookworms
    - Hemorrhoids
- Infection decreases life span of RBCs → folic acid is required to make more RBCs
- Increased demand (in pregnancy → minimum 400 µg/day)
- Female on anticonvulsant drugs (in epilepsy) → rapid decrease in RBC folate
- Intestinal malabsorption syndrome → recurrence in subsequent pregnancies
- Woman on OCPs → why?
  - Because they have reduced cobalamin levels, which may exaggerate a pre-existing cobalamin deficiency
- Hepatic disorders (↓storage)
- Vitamin C deficiency
- Excessive cooking destroys much of folate.

Other Investigations which can Confirm Diagnosis of Megaloblastic Anemia

Hemogram

- Hb ≤ 10 gm%
- MCV >100 μm^3
- MCH >33 pg
- MCHC normal
- The reticulocyte count is decreased due to destruction of fragile and abnormal megaloblastic erythroid precursor
- Leukopenia/Thrombocytopenia
- Serum iron → normal or ↑
- Total iron binding capacity →↓

Peripheral Smear

Presence of any two of the following:
- Hyper-/multisegmented neutrophils (≥ 5 lobes) → *'Senile neutrophil'*
  - This is thought to be due to decreased production and a compensatory prolonged lifespan for circulating neutrophils, which increase number of nuclear segments with age
- Anisocytosis (increased variation in RBC size) and poikilocytosis (abnormally shaped RBCs)
- Macrocytosis (larger than normal RBCs) and Giant polymorphs
- Megaloblasts
- Ovalocytes present
- Howell-Jolly bodies (chromosomal remnant).

Other Findings

- Increased LDH level (The isozyme is LDH-2 which is typical of the serum and hematopoietic cells)
- Increased homocysteine and methylmalonic acid in Vitamin B_{12} deficiency
- Increased homocysteine in folate deficiency
- Normal levels of both methylmalonic acid and total homocysteine rule out clinically significant cobalamin deficiency.

Diagnostic (Definitive)

- Serum folate (fasting) < 3 ng/mL (6.68 mmol/L) → Diagnostic
- Erythrocyte folate activity < 20 ng/mL (50 mmol/L) → indicates folic acid deficiency
- Serum B_{12} < 90 pg/mL
- Normal levels of vitamin B_{12}:
  - Nonpregnant levels (279–966 pg/mL)
  - 1st trimester (118–438 pg/mL)
  - 2nd trimester (130–656 pg/mL)
  - 3rd trimester (99–526 pg/mL).

Rarely Done

- Serum bilirubin → may be increased
- Bone marrow → megaloblastic erythropoiesis.

Which is more Dangerous. Iron Deficiency Anemia or Megaloblastic Anemia?

- Full blown megaloblastic anemia can kill a patient far more readily than iron deficiency anemia. Therefore, treatment should be energetic.

How would You Treat this Patient?

- Deworm the patient
- Iron supplementation → is a MUST with folic acid
- Folic acid 5 mg starting atleast 3 months before conception → throughout pregnancy → up to 4 weeks postpartum
- Injection Vitamin B_{12} 100 µg daily or on alternate days or Inj. Methylcobalamin
  - Methylcobalamin → It is a kind of endogenous coenzyme B_{12}
  - It has an important role in transmethylation as a coenzyme in synthesis of methionine from homocysteine
  - Promotes nucleic acid and protein synthesis
  - 1 mL of injection contains 500 µg vitamin B_{12}
- Vitamin C 100 mg three times a day should be included
- Transfusion → Antepartum hemorrhage is the main indication (but before that take blood sample for peripheral smear) → it will unmask folate deficiency
- *Established anemia:* Start an additional tablet of 5 mg folic acid, especially in the last month of pregnancy, along with
  - Parenteral iron (while waiting for investigations)
  - In multiple gestation (risk of preterm labor)

Once megaloblastic hemopoiesis is established, treatment of folic acid deficiency becomes more difficult, due to megaloblastic changes in GIT, resulting in impaired absorption. It becomes normal in 5 weeks with oral treatment → if ineffective, parenteral treatment.

Conditions where Folate Requirement is increased even in Nonpregnant State

- Hemolytic anemia
- Patients on treatment for the following disorders:
  - Type 2 diabetes
  - Epilepsy
  - Rheumatoid arthritis
  - Lupus
  - Psoriasis
  - Asthma
  - Inflammatory bowel disease
- Women on OCPs
- Associated chronic infection or disease
- Previous child with NTDs
- Liver disease
- Sickle cell disease
- Celiac disease
- Consumption of more than one alcoholic drink a day
- With kidney disease and in patients on dialysis.

Maternal and Fetal Complications

- Abortion
- Dysmaturity
- Prematurity (fetus at risk of megaloblastic anemia because preterm infant in folate-deficient mother is in severe negative folate balance because of high growth rate)
- Abruptio
- Fetal malformation (cleft palate, NTDs).

SUGGESTED READING

1. Auerbach1 M, Ballard H. Clinical use of intravenous iron: administration, efficacy, and safety. Hematology 2010.
2. Bencaiova G, Krafft A, Burkhardt T, et al. Variable efficacy of recombinant human erythropoietin in anemic pregnant women with different forms of heterozygous hemoglobinopathy. Acta Haematol. 2006;116:259-65.
3. Divakar H. *Iron-deficiency Anemia in Pregnant Women:* What is preventing the practitioners from using IV iron sucrose? Int J Inft Fet Med. 2012;3(1).
4. Focusing on anemia. World Health Organization, 2004.
5. Guidelines for control of iron deficiency anemia. Adolescent Division, Ministry of Health and Family Welfare, Government of India. 2013.
6. Guidelines on food fortification with micronutrients. World Health Organization (WHO).
7. Iron Deficiency—investigation and Management. Guidelines and Protocols Advisory Committee, British Columbia Medical Association. June 15, 2010.
8. Kalaivani K. Prevalence and consequences of anemia in pregnancy. Indian J Med Res 2009;130:627-33.
9. Kalaivani. Use of intravenous iron sucrose for treatment of anemia in pregnancy. Indian J Med Res 2013; 138:16-7.
10. Killip S, Bennett JM, Chambers MD. Iron Deficiency Anemia. Am Fam Physician 2007;75:671-8.
11. Krafft A, Bencaiova G, Breymann C. Selective use of recombinant human erythropoietin in pregnant patients with severe anemia or nonresponsive to iron sucrose alone. Fetal Diagn Ther. 2009;25:239-45.
12. Lemos AR, Ismael LAS, Boato CCM, et al. Hepcidin as a biochemical parameter for the assessment of iron deficiency anemia. Rev Assoc Med Bras. 2010;56(5):596-9.
13. Lynch S Iron. Am J Clin Nutr. 2011;94(suppl):673S-8S.
14. Management of Sickle Cell Disease in Pregnancy. RCOG Green-top Guideline No. 61. July 2011.
15. Patil SS, Khanwelkar CC, Patil SK. Conventional and newer oral iron preparations. Int J Med Pharm Sci. 2012;2(3).
16. Pavord S, Myers B, Robinson S, et al. UK guidelines on the management of iron deficiency in pregnancy. British Committee for Standards in Haematology. July 2011.
17. Santiago P. Ferrous versus ferric oral iron formulations for the treatment ofiron deficiency: a clinical overview. The Scientific World Journal. 2012.
18. Stoltzfus RJ. Iron interventions for women and children in low-income countries. J Nutr. 2011;141:756S-62S.
19. Zhang Zhi-feng, Yang Ning, Zhao Gang, Zhu Lei, et al. Effect of Helicobacter pylori eradication on iron deficiency. Chin Med J. 2010;123(14):1924-30.

CHAPTER 3

Recurrent Pregnancy Loss

Tania G Singh

Case: An unbooked patient, $G_4P_0L_0A_3$ with 5 months amenorrhea presented in emergency at around 13 o'clock with chief complaints of leaking per vaginum since morning followed by pain in the abdomen, which started only 1 hour back. On revealing history, first two abortions occurred in 1st trimester and third abortion in 2nd trimester. On examination, vitals were stable and fundal height was corresponding to the period of gestation. On palpation, she was getting 3 to 4 contractions lasting for 35 to 40 seconds in 10 minutes. On per vaginal examination, cervix was 4 to 5 cm dilated, soft globular presenting part felt with absent membranes. Only laboratory reports available with the patient were haemoglobin—10 g% and B +ve blood group.

What is your provisional diagnosis? What important and relevant points would you like to include in the history to reach the diagnosis? How will you investigate the case?

Provisional diagnosis: G_4A_3 with 5 months amenorrhea with bad obstetric history (recurrent pregnancy loss) with preterm premature rupture of membranes (PPROM) in active labor.

IMPORTANT POINTS IN HISTORY

Age of Both Partners

- Risk ↑↑ if female >35 years and male >40 years.

Obstetrics History

- Consanguinity
- Gestational age at the time of pregnancy loss (by LMP/USG)
- Whether spontaneous or induced
- History of curettage done after abortion
- Histopathological documentation/karyotype report available
- History of live births/stillbirths
- Was the fetus malformed?
- History of high BP/IUGR (in case of losses after 20 weeks).

Menstrual History

- Length and regularity of menstrual cycles (to look for oligo-ovulation, PCOS, dys-synchronous fertilization).

Past History

- For how long has the couple been attempting conception? (It may indicate subclinical/preimplantation pregnancy loss)

- History of thyroid disorder (lassitude, weakness, extreme changes in weight, diet, hyperactivity)/DM/TB/syphilis/chronic illness
- History of PCOS
- Personal thrombotic history or ever VDRL was +ve? (VDRL +ve in APLA, syphilis, febrile illness, IV drugs abuse, immunization, laboratory error)
- Other autoimmune disorders (SLE, etc.)
- Alcohol, cigarette smoking, caffeine
- History of drugs, radiation, toxins, any treatment taken earlier?
- History of any surgical procedure on cervix (midtrimester) → conization, forcible dilatation of cervix.

Family History

History of
- Thrombosis (indicates inherited thrombophilias)/stroke
- Recurrent pregnancy loss
- Stillbirths
- Birth defects
- Uterine anomalies.

General Physical Examination

- Built (height, weight, BMI) indicates DM/thyroid disorder/obesity
- Nutrition
- Hirsutism, acanthosis, skin texture (features of hyperandrogenism)
- Thyroid exam/breast exam (galactorrhea)
- PR, BP, temperature, pedal edema (for thyroid disorder, hypertension).

P/A

- Fundal height, contractions, any previous scars, any other mass felt.

P/S

- Vaginal/cervical anatomy (torn cervix or grossly short cervix/septum)
- Signs of infection
- Previous trauma
- Masculinization.

P/V

- Uterine size and shape
- Any gross uterine anomaly
- Any other mass palpable.

Special Investigations

- Thyroid function tests/thyroid autoantibodies
- HbA_1C/GTT

- APLA (LA, aCL, anti-β2GP1 antibodies)
- Thrombophilia testing (factor V leiden, antithrombin 3, protein C and S, prothrombin gene, fasting homocysteine)
- Platelets/PT/aPTT
- Urine culture and sensitivity, cervical swab, HVS
- Karyotype of both partners (and of abortus, if possible)
- USG (congenital anomalies, fibroids, features of PCOS, cervical length).

QUESTIONS LIKELY TO BE ASKED

1. **Define early pregnancy loss, biochemical pregnancy loss, primary, secondary and tertiary loss.**

    Early pregnancy loss: Confirmed empty sac or sac with fetus but no fetal cardiac activity <12 weeks.

    Biochemical pregnancy loss: Pregnancy not located on scanning.

    Primary RPL: ≥3 losses with no pregnancy progressing beyond 20 weeks.

    Secondary RPL: ≥3 losses after a pregnancy that has progressed beyond 20 weeks which might have ended in a live or stillbirth.

    Tertiary RPL: At least 3 miscarriages that are not consecutive but are interspersed with pregnancies that have progressed beyond 20 weeks gestation and might have ended in live birth, stillbirth or neonatal death.

    Definition by Percy Malpas in 1938.

    Seconded by Eastman in 1946.

2. **What is the incidence and what are the two most important covariates?**
    - Incidence: 0.34% of women who become pregnant experience RPL.
    - Approximately 15% of all clinically recognizable pregnancies end in pregnancy loss, with three or more losses affecting 1–2% of women of reproductive age and two or more losses affecting around 5%.
    - Up to 15 to 20% of women with recurrent pregnancy loss have antiphospholipid antibodies (APLA).
    - Two most important covariates:
        – Number of successive losses:
            - After 1 loss—risk is 21%
            - After 2 losses—29%
            - After 3 losses—31%
        – Maternal age >35 years

    NOTE: Investigations may be started after 2 consecutive miscarriages.

3. **Recurrent pregnancy loss causes:**

Etiology	Incidence
(a) Genetic causes (1st trimester)	3.5 to 5%
• Chromosomal	
• Single gene defects	
• Multifactorial	

(b) Anatomic causes (2nd trimester) 12 to 16%

Congenital
- Incomplete Mullerian fusion or septum resorption
- Diethylstilbestrol exposure
- Uterine anomalies
- Cervix incompetence (rare).

Acquired
- Cervical incompetence
- Synechiae
- Leiomyoma
- Adenomyosis.

(c) Endocrine and metabolic causes 17 to 20%
- Luteal phase insufficiency
- PCOS (including insulin resistance and hyperandrogenism)
- Other androgen disorders
- Diabetes mellitus
- Thyroid disorders
- Prolactin disorders.

(d) Infectious disorders (1st trimester) 0.5 to 5%
- Bacteria, viruses, parasites, zoonotic, fungal.

(e) Immunological causes (1st trimester) 20 to 50%

Cellular mechanisms
- Suppressor cell or factor deficiency
- Alterations in MHC antigen expression
- Alterations in cellular immune regulation
  - Th_1 immune responses to reproductive antigens (embryo or trophoblast)
  - Th_2 cytokine or growth factor deficiency
  - Hormonal—progesterone, estrogen, prolactin, androgen alterations
  - Tryptophan metabolism.

Humoral mechanisms
- Antiphospholipid antibody syndrome
- Antithyroid antibodies
- Antisperm antibodies
- Antitrophoblast antibodies
- Blocking antibody deficiency.

(f) Thrombotic factors (1st trimester)
- Inherited thrombophilias
- Acquired.

(g) Other factors 10%
- Altered uterine receptivity (integrins, adhesion molecule)
- Environmental (toxins, illicit drugs, cigarettes, caffeine)
- Placental abnormalities (circumvallate, marginate)
- Medical illness (cardiac, renal)
- Male factors
- Exercise.

(h) Unexplained causes 35 to 50%

4. **Elaborate various genetic factors**
   Account for 50 to 60% of losses in the 1st trimester (chromosomal abnormalities)
   Abnormality may be in: 1. Total number; and 2. Structure.

Total Number

Trisomy   *(50%)*

- Trisomy 16   (31%)
- Trisomy 22   (11.4%)
- Trisomy 21   (10.5%)
- Found in 60% of blighted ova
- Reason for such anomaly—nondisjunction (Twice more at meiosis)
- Common in females than males
- Risk of miscarriage → 15%.

Monosomy X   *(20%)*

- Karyotype 45 XO
- *Cause:* It may be due to loss of X chromosome at the time of fertilization or due to nondisjunction during meiosis
- Permits viable offspring.

Triploidy   *(15%)*

- Mean chromosome number is 69
- Most common cause—double fertilization of single ova
- There may be empty sac or obvious fetal anomalies like omphalocele, cleft lip and palate.

Tetraploidy   *(5%)*

- Mean chromosome number is 92
- Due to failure of corresponding cytoplasmic division after chromosome division.

Structure

Translocations → Balanced (most common) and unbalanced
- Balanced
  - Reciprocal (5%):
    - Occurs between 2 heterologous chromosomes and results in balanced carriers
    - Twice more common in females than males
    - Risk of miscarriage is 15%.
  - Robertsonian:
    - Occurs between 2 homologous chromosomes and results in either a carrier state, abortion or a normal fetus
    - Occurs between acrocenter chromosome no. 13, 14, 15, 21 and 22
    - Risk of miscarriage is low
    - Risk more in female carriers than male carriers.
- Unbalanced
  - Here total chromosome number is altered, resulting in lethal monosomies or trisomies.

Inversions (0.3%)/Intrachromosomal Rearrangements

Paracentric
- Involve only 1 arm
- Harmless.

Pericentric
- Involve both arms
- 1 in 1000 couples with RPL
- Overall risk → 0.3.

Recent Advances
- Neither family history nor a history of prior preterm births is sufficient to rule out a potential parental chromosomal abnormality.
- As number of miscarriages increases, prevalence of chromosomal abnormality decreases and chance of recurring maternal cause increases.
- If karyotype of miscarried pregnancy is abnormal, there is a better prognosis in the next pregnancy.

5. **Elaborate thrombophilias (inherited)**
   Thrombophilia
   - Defined as a tendency to thrombosis (arterial and venous) → abnormal placental vascularization → placental thrombosis (cause 50% of VTE in pregnancy).

   Inherited thrombophilias:
   - Most commonly linked with RPL
   - 3- to 8-fold increase in fetal loss:
     - Antithrombin 3 deficiency: Late losses (more than all other factors except protein S deficiency which causes the highest) >> early losses
     - Protein C deficiency: Both early and late losses
     - Protein S deficiency: Highest for late losses
     - Activated protein C resistance: 3- to 4-fold increase in 1st trimester losses
     - Prothrombin gene mutation: 2- to 3-fold increase in early and late losses
     - Hyperhomocysteinemia: Point mutations are common in MTHFR (methylene tetrahydrofolate reductase) → hyperhomocysteinemia and thrombosis → causing neural tube defects
     - MTHFR gene defect
     - Factor V Leiden defect → Both early and late pregnancy losses, recurrent pregnancy losses.
   - Cause is unclear → maternal thrombophilia could interfere with implantation and initial development of uteroplacental circulation.
   - Adverse fetal outcomes:
     - Isolated and recurrent early and late spontaneous pregnancy losses
     - Intrauterine growth restriction
     - Intrauterine fetal death
     - Placental abruption
     - Preeclampsia
     - Cause (in almost all cases)—venous and arterial thrombosis → ↓ placental circulation → impaired development and function of placenta

- Explanation:

Before 10 weeks	After 10 weeks
Transfer of nutrients from mother to fetus through transudation (through uterine vasculature)	Establishment of intervillous circulation→ maternal blood directly flows into intervillous spaces

↓

Therefore, it causes early and late pregnancy losses and all adverse fetal outcomes mentioned above.

Pregnancy is a state of compensated DIC. Clot formation can be initiated through 2 pathways → extrinsic and intrinsic. Both respond to blood vessel damage and subsequently release of tissue factor.

Tissue Factor (TF)
- Glycoprotein
- Present on surface of cells surrounding blood vessels
- Not expressed on endothelium of blood vessel itself
- Therefore, exposure of blood to TF is an indicator of vessel damage
  TF + Factor VII → stimulates extrinsic pathway

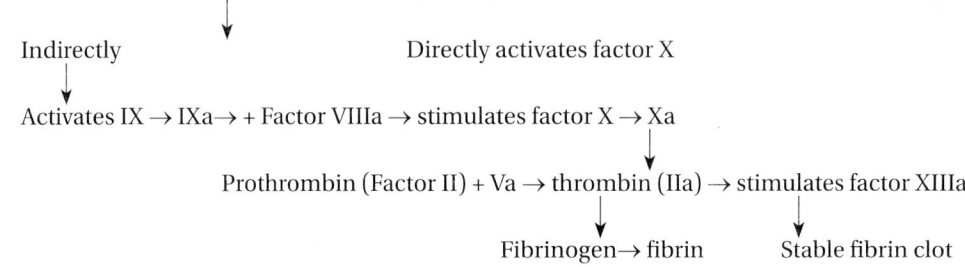

Indirectly ↓ Directly activates factor X

Activates IX → IXa→ + Factor VIIIa → stimulates factor X → Xa

Prothrombin (Factor II) + Va → thrombin (IIa) → stimulates factor XIIIa

Fibrinogen→ fibrin   Stable fibrin clot

To avoid uncontrolled thrombosis
- Thrombomodulin and thrombin at the sites of endothelial damage → stimulates proteins C and S → inhibits Va and VIIIa
- Antithrombin:
  - Binds to IXa/Xa/XIa/XIIa → accelerates dissociation of VIIa + TF complex
  - Binds to and inhibits thrombin.
- Plasminogen activator inhibitor → acts on plasmin → breakdown of fibrin clot (fibrinolysis) → release of fibrin degradation products
- Pregnancy is a hypercoagulable state. All prothrombotic changes in pregnancy can be detected from 3rd month. They all reverse 4 to 6 weeks following delivery:
  - Fibrinogen–300 to 600 mg% (↑ by 50%)
  - Factor VII–↑ 10 times by term
  - Factor VIII–↑ 2 times by term
  - Factors IX and X–increase in pregnancy
  - Factor XI–↓ by 60%
  - Factor XIII–↓ by 50%
  - *Platelets:* Width and volume increase but concentration decreases due to hemodilution. There is an increase in number of younger and larger platelets
  - Clotting time—no change
  - Fibrinolytic system—depressed till 60 minutes after delivery of placenta

- Vascular damage associated with delivery is an additional significant risk factor for thrombosis, making immediate postpartum period an important continuation of prothrombotic state associated with pregnancy.

6. **Elaborate immunological causes (cellular immune mechanisms)**

   Immune cells in endometrium and maternofetal interface consists mainly of 3 cell types:
   - T-cells
   - Macrophages
   - Uterine natural killer cells (uNK cells).

   T-cells
   - Constitute 45% of leukocytes in proliferative endometrium
   - Absolute number remains constant throughout the cycle and in early pregnancy
   - Relative number decreases as proportion of uNK cells increases.

   Macrophages
   - Constitute 15–20% of endometrial leukocytes
   - Number significantly increases during secretory phase and in early pregnancy.

   Uterine natural killer cells
   - Also called large granular lymphocytes
   - Differ from NK cells found in peripheral blood
   - Peripheral blood NK cells express CD3, CD4, CD8, CD16, CD57 cells and show minimum expression of CD56+ cells
   - uNK cells mainly express CD56+, CD3+, CD38
   - *CD56+ uNK cells show most dramatic menstrual cycle changes*
     - During proliferative phase, constitute 40%
     - In midsecretory phase, comprise 70% of endometrial leukocytes
     - Number increases further during early pregnancy
     - CD56+ cells undergo apoptosis few days prior to menses, but are maintained if pregnancy occurs.

   Differences in immune cell population in Recurrent Pregnancy Loss patients
   - Both number and activity of CD56+ NK cells increase in 1st trimester in peripheral blood in patients with RPL
   - There is decrease of CD56+ NK cells in deciduas but increase in endometrium in patients with RPL
   - There is no change in CD3+ T-cells, both in peripheral blood and maternofetal interface in patients with RPL
   - Number of macrophages remains the same in deciduas of early pregnancy but increase is seen in endometrium
   - Ratio of CD4+/CD8+ in endometrium increases in women with RPL.

   Major Histocompatibility Complex Molecules-Human Leukocyte Antigen Expression
   - Cytotrophoblast cells do not express classical MHC molecules HLA-A and HLA-B
   - They express nonclassical HLA-G and HLA-E molecules
   - Role of HLA-G:
     - Attachment of blastocyst to endometrium
     - Control of trophoblast invasion
     - Protects from NK cells
   - In patients with RPL → there is decreased expression of HLA-G molecules in extravillous and endovascular cytotrophoblasts.

Role of cytokines

Proinflammatory cytokines (type I)	Anti-inflammatory cytokines (type II)
• INFγ, TNFβ, IL-2, TNFα	IL4, IL6, IL10, IL13
• Down regulated in pregnancy normally but increase in patients with RPL	Upregulated at the time of implantation

Q. Do abnormal sperms cause RPL?

- Paternal genes (androgenomes) have positive effect on growth of placenta
- Maternal genes (gynogenomes) promote growth of embryo
- Sperm DNA damage causes:
  - Decondensation
  - Increased fragmentation
  - Sperm chromosomal aneuploidy
- All these lead to:
  - Poor semen quality
  - Low fertilization rates
  - Impaired preimplantation development
  - Increase in miscarriages
  - Increase in incidence of disease in offspring (including childhood carcinoma)
- Cause of DNA damage → oxidative stress and aberrant apoptosis
- Abnormal sperms, if unchecked, manifest clinically as unexplained RPL.

7. **Elaborate humoral immune mechanisms**

   Antiphospholipid antibody syndrome (APAS)
   - Also known as "HUGHES SYNDROME"
   - ***Definition:*** Disorder of coagulation, which causes blood clots (thrombosis) in both arteries and veins as well as pregnancy-related complications, i.e. miscarriages, preterm delivery, severe preeclampsia
   - ***Classification***
     - Primary: > 50% of all patients
     - Secondary: associated with other autoimmune disorders (SLE, Rheumatoid arthritis, etc.).
   - ***Incidence***
     - 15–20% in RPL
     - In low-risk obstetrics history < 2%
     - Fetal loss rate → 50–75%
     - Live birth rate with no interventions → 10%
     - Can occur in any trimester, but commonest in 1st trimester
     - The best predictor of pregnancy outcome in women with APAS is past obstetric history
     - The clinical phenotype of APAS varies widely, suggesting that different women have different types and quantities of antiphospholipid antibodies (APLA).
   - ***Patient suspected to have APAS***
     - RPL
     - Unexplained 2nd/3rd trimester loss
     - Early onset of severe preeclampsia
     - Venous or arterial thrombosis
     - Unexplained IUGR
     - False +ve serological marker of syphilis
     - SLE/other connective tissue disorders.

- *Pathophysiology*
  - APLA → endothelial cell →↓ Prostaglandin I_2 and Thrombaxane A_2
  - Inhibition of $\beta_2 GP_1$ (natural anticoagulant) which again inhibits platelet prothrombinase and ADP. This, in turn, inhibits platelet aggregation
  - Annexin V: soluble, hydrophilic protein produced by villous trophoblast
    Annexin V + phospholipid → anticoagulant in intervillous spaces
    APLA inhibits Annexin V by competitive inhibition
    APLA inhibits activation of Protein C and S pathway.
- *Causes of RPL:*

  On implantation
  - Cytotrophoblast cells express phosphotidylserine on their surface
  - Binding of APLA to them causes direct cellular injury and inhibition of syncytia formation

  On postimplantation
  - Thrombogenic action →↓ placental perfusion
  - Annexin V →↓ in APAS → placental insufficiency and fetal loss
- Nonthrombotic pathogenesis of APLA → Trophoblast invasion impairment
- APLA: Family of antibodies that binds to negatively charged phospholipids, phospholipid-binding proteins or a combination of the two
- Antibodies:
  - LA-IgG and IgM
  - aCL-IgG, IgM, IgA
  - anti-β2 glycoprotein 1
  - Others:
    - Phosphatidylserine
    - Phosphotidylethalomine
    - Phosphatidylinositol
    - Phosphotidylglycerol
    - Phosphotidylcholine

I. Lupus anticoagulant (LA):
   - Misnomer
   - 1st association between LA and pregnancy loss → 1975
   - Antibody directed against prothrombin or annexin V
   - Causes prolonged APTT (abnormally)
   - Requires prothrombin to exert their action

II. Anticardiolipin antibodies (aCL):
   - 1st association between aCL and pregnancy loss → 1985
   - Not all are pathogenic → IgM aCL MAY NOT BE PATHOGENIC
   - Detected after:

     Viral infections
     - Syphilis
     - Adenovirus
     - Chickenpox
     - Mumps
     - Q-fever
     - TB
     - Parvovirus

- HIV
- CMV

Drugs
- Procainamide
- Chlorpromazine
- Sodium valproate
- aCL require β-GP1 to exert their action

III. Anti-$β_2$ glycoprotein-1:
- β GP1 → a phospholipid-binding protein which inhibits prothrombinase activity
- New addition to diagnostic criteria
- $β_2$GP1 is an apolipoprotein and a member of the complement control protein family; it binds to cell surface receptors and negatively charged surfaces
- Anti-$β_2$ G1 are those that bind specifically to a limited epitope on domain 1 of the protein (Gly40-Arg43) that is most strongly associated with thrombosis.

- **Complications of APAS**

Obstetric
1. Thrombotic complications—70% in venous system.
   Venous thrombosis in APAS is most commonly lower limb deep vein thrombosis (DVT) and/or pulmonary embolism (PE) but any part of the venous system may be involved, including superficial, portal, renal, mesenteric and intracranial veins.
2. Gestational hypertension/preeclampsia
   - Severe early onset
   - In 32%
3. IUGR/Preterm
   - Uteroplacental insufficiency
   - More likely, exhibit nonreassuring NST
4. RPL
   - APAS → causes 15% of RPL
   - 40% in fetal period (hypercoagulability → uteroplacental insufficiency →↓ intervillous blood flow)
5. IUD
6. Chorea gravidarum
7. Neonatal thrombosis

General/Others (nonobstetric)
1. CVS:
   - MI/Angina. Myocardial infarction is less common, although subclinical myocardial ischemia may be under-recognized
   - Premature atherosclerosis
   - Thrombocytopenia, valvular lesions (which are most commonly occult)
2. Dermatologic:
   - Livedo reticularis/racemosa
   - Sphincter hemorrhages
   - Skin infarcts
   - Leg ulcers
   - Superficial thrombophlebitis

3. Musculoskeletal:
   - DVT
   - AVN
   - Transverse myelopathy (occurs in SLE)
4. Neurologic:
   - Cerebrovascular accidents
     - The most frequent site of arterial thrombosis in APAS is in the cerebral vasculature resulting in transient cerebral ischemia (TIA)/stroke
   - Migraines
   - Multi-infarct dementia
   - Pseudotumour cerebri
   - Seizures
   - Peripheral neuropathy
5. GI:
   - Hepatic infarction
   - Budd Chiari syndrome
6. Pulmonary:
   - Pulmonary embolus
   - Nonthromboembolic pulmonary hypertension
7. Endocrine:
   - Adrenal insufficiency
8. Renal:
   - Renal arterial/venous thrombosis
   - Hypertension
   - Glomerular thrombosis
   - Renal insufficiency

- ***Catastrophic Antiphospholipid Syndrome***
  - Microvascular thrombosis in APAS
  - Least common but may manifest as the potentially lethal 'catastrophic antiphospholipid syndrome' (CAPS)
  - Multiple simultaneously occurring vascular occlusions in body → death (50%)
  - Diagnosis: at least 3 organ system involvement
  - Manifestation:
    - Renal failure (78%)
    - ARDS (66%)
    - Cerebral microthrombi (50%)
    - Dermatological abnormalities (50%)
    - DIC (25%)
  - Precipitating factors:
    - Infection
    - Surgery
    - Discontinuation of anticoagulants
  - Treatment:
    - Prompt use of anticoagulation (in the absence of concurrent hemorrhage) and identification and treatment of possible underlying infection remains the cornerstone of treatment
    - Glucocorticoids, in the absence of infection

- Intravenous immunoglobulin and/or plasma exchange
- If there is lupus flare, cyclophosphamide should be considered
- Though recurrences are rare, still patients should be left on long-term anticoagulation.

8. **Elaborate the anatomical factors**

Anatomic abnormalities of both uterine cervix and uterine body have been associated with RPL
- Congenital:
  - Müllerian anomalies
- Acquired:
  - Cervical incompetence
  - Leiomyomas
  - Intrauterine adhesions

Acquired causes:

I. Cervical incompetence:
- Associated with rapid, painless passage of conceptus without associated bleeding
- Classically 2nd trimester abortions (after 12–13 weeks). Why?
  - When decidua vera and decidua capsularis fuse and weight of conceptus gets directly transmitted to an incompetent os, it gives way
- Occurs in 0.5–1% of pregnancies (due to structural or functional deficiency of cervix → congenital or acquired)
- Congenital → rare
- Acquired (iatrogenic) → common, after:
  - D and C
  - Induced abortion by D and E (10%)
  - Vaginal operative delivery through undilated cervix
  - Amputation of cervix or cone biopsy
  - Laceration/tears

USG evaluation of cervix → Which route?
1. TAU
2. TLU (translabial/transperineal)
3. TVS → preferred

Why not TAU and TLU?

TAU:
- Full bladder is required to obtain a good image but it results in elongation of cervix and mask funneling of internal os
- Fetal parts can obscure the cervix, especially after 20 weeks
- Distance from probe to cervix → degraded image quality.

TLU:
- Patient lies on table with hips and knees flexed
- Gloved transducer in sagittal orientation on perineum between labia majora
- Main drawback: gas in rectum can impede visualization of cervix, especially external os.

TVS:

Technique

Empty bladder
- Transvaginal probe covered by condom
- Insert probe (in anterior fornix of vagina)

- Sagittal long-axis view obtained of endocervical canal, along its entire length
- Distance from surface of posterior lip to cervical canal should be equal to distance from surface of anterior lip to cervical canal
- There should be no increased echogenicity (suggestive of increased pressure)
- Enlarge image, so that cervix occupies at least 2/3rd of image
- Measure cervical length from internal os to external os along the endocervical canal
- Ideally, obtain 3 measurements and record the SHORTEST best measurement in mm
- Apply transfundal pressure for 15 seconds and record cervical length again.

Limitations and pitfalls:
- Full bladder→ pressure on cervix→ mask funneling or opening of internal os
- Too much pressure→ mask funneling or opening of internal os and elongates the cervix
- Contraction → may mimic appearance of funneling of internal cervical os.

When to consider lower uterine segment (LUS) contraction?
  - When cervical length measures >50 mm
  - Cervical canal assumes 'S'-shape
  - LUS (either anteriorly or posteriorly or both) is thickened and asymmetric
- Underdeveloped LUS → often before 14 weeks, LUS is difficult to distinguish from endocervical canal because gestation sac has not reached a sufficient size to completely expand lower part of uterus. Therefore, measurement of true CL is very difficult before 14 weeks.

Digital examination—why not to use?
- It is subjective (interobserver variability of 52%)
- Not accurate for evaluating internal os (whole upper half of cervix is not measureable by this method)
- Nonspecific
- USG CL measurements, on an average, are 11 mm longer than manual estimations

What to measure?
- Cervical length
  and
- Funneling

Cervical length
- From internal os to external os along the endocervical canal
- Short CL is usually straight
- Curved cervix→ CL > 25 mm (reassuring finding)
- If AB is >5 mm, then cervical canal is to be measured in 2 steps or else measure as straight line
- Total CL: funnel length + functional CL
- Functional CL: sonographic CL (which we usually take) → if funneling is present, record SHAPE

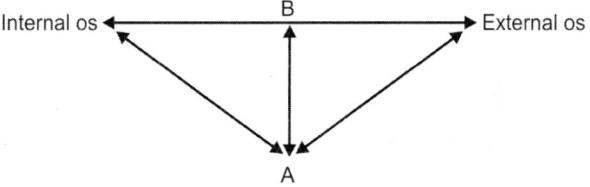

Funneling

4 different shapes of funnel:
- "T"-shaped
  - Closed normal cervix

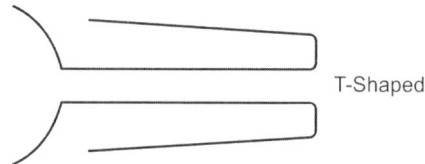

- "Y"-shaped
  - Small funnel (< 25%)
  - Cervical length ≥ 25 mm
  - May not be clinically significant

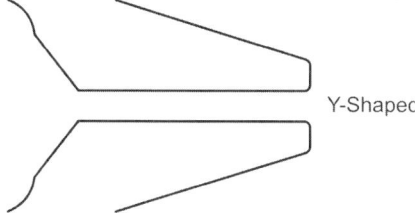

- "V"-shaped
  - More significant funnel
  - Closer to external os

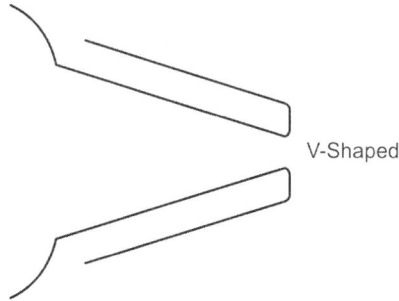

- "U"-shaped
  - FUNNEL OF MOST CONCERN
  - Clinical situation in which more often the cervix can be dilated by manual examination
    a. Minimum (< 25% funneling)
       - Common finding
       - Not associated with increase in preterm labor
    b. Moderate (25–50%)
       - Almost always CL is short (25 mm)
    c. Severe (>50%)
       - Risk of preterm labor is increased if both short CL and funneling are present, rather than short CL alone

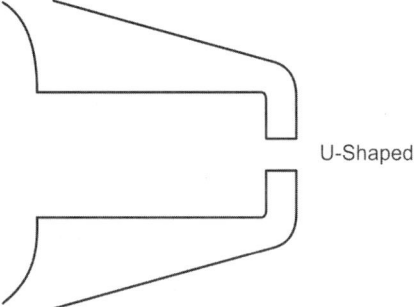
U-Shaped

- Normal CL: a normal CL is 25–50 mm (lower 10 centile and upper 10 centile) at 14–30 weeks
- Short CL: < 25 mm at these gestational ages
- CL >50 mm is also normal but often reflects a measurement that includes LUS (especially before 16 weeks)
- Best time for measurement of, or development of, short cervix or funneling is 18–22 weeks. WHY??
    - Between 10 and 14 weeks:
        - Prediction of preterm birth is very low because most females destined to deliver preterm have cervical shortening usually detected at ≥16 weeks
        - LUS is difficult to distinguish from true cervix (in late 1st and early 2nd trimester)
    - After 30 weeks:
        - CL progressively shortens in preparation for term labor, so that CL<25 mm (15–24 mm) after 30 weeks can be physiologic and not associated with preterm birth
- In case of RPL—determine between 14 and 18 weeks (for early intervention)
- Best measure at 14–18 weeks (1st) followed by a measurement between 18 and 22 weeks (2nd)
- Twins: CL≤25 mm at 24 weeks gestation → best of all predictors of preterm birth in twins (various studies have shown and concluded)
- Cerclage: The higher (closer to internal os) the cerclage sutured, the most effective is the prevention of preterm birth. How does it help?
    - CL usually INCREASES postcerclage → this increase is associated with increased chance of term delivery
- **Recent advances:** almost NO woman, even the most high-risk, has a short CL in 1st trimester; therefore, the pressure the growing gestational sac exerts on cervix will be unlikely to open up even the weakest of cervices.
- More appropriate nomenclature based on indication for cervical suture is now recommended and is mentioned below.

Recent terminologies
History-indicated cerclage
- Prophylactic cerclage inserted at 12–14 weeks in an asymptomatic woman on the basis of an indication provided in her history
- Indicated in women with ≥ 3 previous 2nd trimester losses or ≥ 3 preterm births.

Ultrasound-indicated cerclage
- Therapeutic cerclage inserted on the basis of short cervical length obtained on ultrasonography, usually performed between 14 and 24 weeks
- Placed if the diagnosed ultrasound cervical length is ≤ 25 mm and period of gestation is not > 24 weeks
- Funneling alone is not an indication to apply this cerclage.

Rescue cerclage
- Salvage cerclage inserted in cases of premature cervical dilatation (detected either on ultrasound or on per speculum examination) and/or with fetal membranes extending beyond the external os
- Cervical dilatation should not be >4 cm.

Transvaginal cerclage (McDonald)
- A transvaginal purse-string suture placed at the cervicovaginal junction, without bladder mobilization.

High transvaginal cerclage (Shirodkar)
- A transvaginal purse-string suture placed following bladder mobilization, to allow insertion above the level of the cardinal ligaments.

Transabdominal cerclage
- Cerclage at the cervicoisthmic junction placed via laparotomy
- Sole indication—previous failed transvaginal cerclage
- Can be inserted preconceptionally or in early pregnancy but there is increased maternal morbidity. So, rarely performed.

Occlusion cerclage
- Occlusion of the external os by placement of continuous nonabsorbable suture in order to retain the mucus plug.

Contraindications to cervical cerclage insertion
- Active preterm labor (≥ 4 cm cervical dilatation)
- Clinical evidence of chorioamnionitis
- Continuing vaginal bleeding
- PPROM
- Evidence of fetal compromise
- Gross congenital anamolies
- IUD.

Risks
- Bleeding during insertion
- Rupture of membranes
- Premature contractions
- Use of anesthesia during removal of cerclage inserted by Shirodkar's technique
- Bucket handle tear if labor sets in, with suture in place.

Recent advances/Recommendations
- An ultrasound examination for cardiac activity and to rule out gross congenital anomalies should be performed before placing cerclage
- Prophylactic perioperative tocolysis and antibiotics should be offered to women undergoing cervical cerclage, though NOT recommended in routine practice
- Abstinence should not be routinely recommended
- Serial ultrasound monitoring of cervical length postcerclage is useful for administration of steroids
- Progesterone is not routinely recommended after cerclage
- Usually removed at 36^{+1}–37^{+0} weeks
- Removed at the time of operation in cases of elective cesarean section
- Removed earlier in cases of established preterm labor.

II. Intrauterine adhesions (Asherman syndrome or Fritsch syndrome)
- JG Asherman described the syndrome in 1948
- Defined as presence of scar tissue, adhesions and/or fibrosis within endometrial cavity
- *Other terms* used to describe the condition are as follows:
  - Injurious intrauterine adhesions
  - Uterine/cervical atresia
  - Traumatic uterine atrophy
  - Sclerotic endometrium
  - Endometrial sclerosis
  - Intrauterine synechiae
- Causes:
  - Curettage (providing trauma to the basal layer → development of intrauterine scars resulting in adhesions that can obliterate the cavity to varying degrees → failure of endometrium to respond to estrogen)
    - After spontaneous, incomplete or elective abortion or after vaginal delivery (to remove the placental bits)
    - For PPH
    - After cesarean section
  - Removal of fibroid tumours (myomectomy)
  - Use of intrauterine devices
  - Pelvic irradiation
  - Schistosomiasis
  - Genital tuberculosis
  - Chronic endometritis from genital tuberculosis is a significant cause of severe IUA in the developing world, often resulting in total obliteration of the uterine cavity which is difficult to treat
- Classification: Many classifications have been proposed:

Valle and Sciarra's 1988 classification
- *Mild*: Filmy adhesions composed of basal endometrium producing partial or complete uterine cavity occlusion
- *Moderate*: Fibromuscular adhesions that are characteristically thick, still covered by endometrium that may bleed on division, partially or totally occluding the uterine cavity
- *Severe*: Composed of connective tissue with no endometrial lining and likely to bleed upon division, partially or totally occluding the uterine cavity.

Society for Hysteroscopy, 1989
I—Thin or filmy adhesions easily ruptured by hysteroscope sheath alone, cornual areas normal
II—Singular firm adhesions connecting separate parts of the uterine cavity, visualization of both tubal ostia possible, cannot be ruptured by hysteroscope sheath alone
IIa—Occluding adhesions only in the region of the internal cervical os. Upper uterine cavity normal
III—Multiple firm adhesions connecting separate parts of the uterine cavity, unilateral obliteration of ostial areas of the tubes
IIIa—Extensive scarring of the uterine cavity wall with amenorrhea or hypomenorrhea
IIIb—Combination of III and IIIa
IV—Extensive firm adhesions with agglutination of the uterine walls. Both tubal ostial areas occluded.

Donnez and Nisolle 1994 classification
A—Central adhesions
  a. Thin flimsy adhesions (endometrial adhesions)
  b. Myofibrous (connective adhesions)
B—Marginal adhesions (always myofibrous or connective)
  a. Wedge-like projection
  b. Obliteration of one horn
C—Uterine cavity absent on HSG
  a. Occlusion of the internal os (upper cavity normal)
  b. Extensive agglutination of uterine walls (absence of uterine cavity—true Asherman's).

Classification by March and Israel (depending upon occlusion of uterine cavity)
A—< 1/4 of uterine cavity involved
- Thin flimsy adhesions
- Ostia/fundus minimally involved or clear

B—1/4–3/4 of uterine cavity involved
- No agglutination of walls
- Ostia/upper fundus only partially involved

C—> 3/4 of uterine cavity involved
- Agglutination of walls/thick bands present
- Ostia/upper cavity occluded.

Classification system of Nasr, et al. also includes obstetric history
- Cause of RPL:
  - Constrictions of the uterine cavity by adhesions
  - Lack of adequate functional endometrium to support implantation
  - Defective vascularization of the residual endometrial tissue due to fibrosis
- Risks and complications:
  - Infertility
  - Endometriosis
  - Placental abnormalities
  - Miscarriages
  - Cervical incompetence
  - IUGR
  - Premature birth
  - Uterine rupture.

III. Leiomyoma
- Submucous fibroid: Disturb endometrial function→ compromise normal implantation
- Pedunculated fibroid (polyp) and large intramural fibroid (>3 cm): Hyperirritability of myometrium → abortions
- Do leiomyomas affect fertility? Actually no problem in conception but possible effects are:
  - Alter uterine contractility→ affect sperm transport
  - Obstruct uterine cavity/tubal ostia→ affect sperm transport
  - Distort uterine cavity→ affect sperm transport and embryo transport
  - Alter position of cervix→ compromise exposure to semen
  - Associated endometrial thinning/infection/altered vascularity→ affect implantation/embryo growth.

Congenital causes:
- Result from the abnormal formation, fusion or resorption of Müllerian ducts during fetal life

- Present in:
  - 1–10% of the unselected population
  - 2–8% of infertile women
  - 5–30% of women with a history of miscarriage.

Uterine development
Formed at around 8–16 weeks of fetal life from the development of the two paired paramesonephric ducts called Müllerian ducts.

The process involves three main stages:
i. Organogenesis: The development of both Müllerian ducts
ii. Fusion: The lower Müllerian ducts fuse to form the upper vagina, cervix and uterus. This is termed as 'lateral fusion'. The upper cranial part of the Müllerian ducts will remain unfused and form the Fallopian tubes.
iii. Septal absorption: After the lower Müllerian ducts fuse, a central septum is left, which starts to resorb at ≈ 9 weeks, eventually leaving a single uterine cavity and cervix. Wolffian ducts are a precursor and inducer of female reproductive tract development and play a crucial role in renal development. In addition, they act along with the Müllerian tubercle to form part of the vagina. As a result, abnormalities originating from mesonephric maldevelopment may also have an effect on genital tract and uterine formation (e.g. renal anomalies with unicornuate uterus).

Classification of uterine anomalies
- First proposed by Buttram and Gibbons in 1979 based on the degree of failure of the Müllerian ducts to develop normally and divided them into groups with similar clinical manifestations, treatments and prognosis
- Revised and modified first in 1983 and then in 1988 by the American Society of Reproductive Medicine (formerly known as the American Fertility Society) to provide a classification which is now most widely accepted and used worldwide (Letterie, 1998)
- This consists of seven groups, some with further subdivisions.

Classification   *Anomaly*
Class I (Agenesis/hypoplasia)   Vaginal, Cervical, Fundal, Tubal, Combined
- Well-formed uterus is rarely associated with absence of fallopian tubes
- Age 15–18 years
- Primary amenorrhea present
- Rectoabdominal examination—uterus absent
- Renal anomalies—very common
- Chromosomal analysis not required
- MRI → Ideal method for demonstrating uterine malformation

Class II (Unicornuate)   Communicating, Noncommunicating, No horn, No cavity
- Absence or incomplete development of 1 müllerian duct → unicornuate uterus with only 1 fallopian tube
- Cervix and vagina normal in appearance and function (may be) → but they strictly represent only one half of fully developed organ
- Symptoms—few, if dysmenorrhea present → pain limited to one side on which horn is present
- Association with adverse pregnancy outcomes:
  - Favors abortion but more of preterm delivery
  - Breech presentation
  - Fundal insertion of placenta
  - Uterus usually contracts significantly in all stages of labor

Class III (Didelphys)   Didelphys
- Cause: Imperfect fusion of mullerian ducts
- When 2 mullerian ducts remain separate, 2 halves of uterus remain distinct and each has its own cervix

Class IV (Bicornuate)   Complete, Partial
- Only lower parts of ducts fuse, leaving cornua separate
- Cervix and vagina may be single or double

Class V (Septate)   Complete, Partial
- From outside → uterus appears normal
- Contains complete or incomplete septum (which reflects a failure in breakdown of walls between 2 ducts)
- Cervical canal may be single or double
- Vagina—whole or septate
- Tends to miscarry more in 1st trimester
- **Septate and subseptate vagina:**
    - Sagittal septum with cresenteric lower edge → in upper vagina or throughout its length
    - Can occur alone or in conjunction with septate or bicornuate uterus → may have 1 or 2 cervices
    - This is because of late fusion of mullerian ducts → giving rise to 2 mullerian tubercles OR because of canalization of 2 sinovaginal bulbs

Class VI (Arcuate)   Arcuate
- Flat topped uterus
- Fundal bulge has not developed after fusion of ducts
- If only external part of uterus is affected, fundal myometrium is abnormally thin
- Tends to miscarry more in 2nd trimester

Class VII (DES related)   DES related
- Benign vaginal adenosis/cervical hoods
- Septa/collars/T-shaped uteri/wide lower segment
- Constriction bands
- Perifimbrial paratubal cysts
- Vaginal clear cell adenocarcinoma (very rare)
- But NOT associated with renal anomalies.

Limitations of the classification
1. It does not specify the diagnostic methods or criteria that should be used in order to diagnose the anomalies and, as a result, this is solely based on the subjective impression of the clinician performing the test
2. The classification is by no means comprehensive
3. Rarer anomalies, such as a hypoplastic noncavitated uterus with two rudimentary horns, an uterus with a vaginal anastomosis and cervical atresia, a septate uterus with cervical duplication and a longitudinal vaginal septum and a normal uterus with a double cervix and vagina, and a blind cervical pouch are not included.

Symptoms associated with congenital anomalies
- *Mostly recognized at the time of pregnancy or as a result of pregnancy mishap*
- *Menstrual cycle*
    - Usually normal
    - Menorrhagia can occur because of increased bleeding surface in cases of two well-developed horns

- Dysmenorrhea:
  - Unusual arrangement of musculature
  - Abnormal contractions
  - Unequal development of 2 horns → one-sided dysmenorrhea
- Failure to contain flow by single intravaginal tampon → clearly shows:
  - Septate vagina and uterus didelphys
- *Coitus*
  - Dyspareunia
  - Bleeding (from vessel in lower edge of septum)
- *Obstetric*
  - Infertility
  - Only deformity, which significantly disturbs it, is fully septate vagina because may be coitus is taking place in the half, which is not communicating with the cervix
  - Cornual pregnancy
  - Sacculation of uterus → presents as either organic or functional abnormality during pregnancy
  - Abortions and preterm labor → due to:
    - Abnormal contractions
    - Inadequate stretching and hypertrophy to accommodate pregnancy
    - Poor implantation
    - Placentation on septum
  - Malpresentation:
    - Subseptate/bicornuate deformity—transverse lie
    - Didelphys/unicornuate—breech presentation
  - Inefficient uterine action:
    - Usually in 3rd stage of labor
  - Manual removal of placenta (may lead to PPH):
    - May be necessary in bicornuate/subseptate uterus
  - High vaginal septum:
    - Prevent cervix from dilating
  - Obstructed labor:
    - Nonpregnant horn of uterus didelphys enlarges during pregnancy because it has been subjected to same hormone influence as pregnant horn
    - Sometimes it remains low in pelvis and constitutes a tumour which obstructs delivery
    - Labor is also obstructed by vaginal septum (CLASSICAL SITUATION WHEN BREECH PRESENTATION ASTRIDES THE SEPTUM)
  - Recurrent pregnancy loss:
    - Septate uterus (most common)
  - Preterm delivery:
    - Unicornuate and bicornuate.

Effect of malformation on pregnancy
Clinical pregnancy rates
- Arcuate uteri → no difference as compared to normal uterus
- Canalization defects (septate and subseptate) → significant reduction in pregnancy rates
- Unification defects (unicornuate, bicornuate, didelphys) → no difference

1st trimester abortions
- Arcuate uterus → no difference
- Canalization defects → significant increase in abortions
- Bicornuate and unicornuate uteri show a slightly increased risk of abortions

2nd trimester abortions (mainly from 13 to 23 weeks)
- Arcuate uterus → significant increase
- Canalization defects → insignificant except for septate uterus which shows a slightly higher risk
- Unification defects
- Bicornuate → has double the risk
- Unicornuate and didelphys → slightly increased risk

Preterm birth rate
- Arcuate uteri → no increase
- Canalization defects → septate and subseptate uteri have increased risk
- Unification defects → significant association

Fetal malpresentation
- Arcuate uteri → statistically significant increase
- Canalization defects → increased rate
- Unification defects → significant and consistent increase (present in each type of unification defect).

9. **Explain the various endocrine abnormalities accounting for RPL**
   Corpus luteum insufficiency
   Normally:
- From ovulation till 7-9 weeks of gestation → progesterone production by corpus luteum maintains pregnancy
- 7-9 weeks → luteal placental shift → developing trophoblastic cells take over progesterone production.
   ### *Luteal phase defect*
- Characterized by inadequately or improperly timed endometrial development at potential sites, resulting from a qualitative or quantitative disorder in corpus luteum function
- Progesterone is the only steroid necessary to induce complete decidualization
- Under continued influence of progesterone, secretory endometrium produces a number of specific proteins crucial for implantation
- Progesterone may also inhibit uterine prostaglandin production and prevent embryo rejection by maternal immune system
- Causes of LPD (many and not well understood).
   Hypersecretion of Luteinizing Hormone (not completely understood)
   – May have direct effect on:
   - The developing oocyte (premature aging)
   - Endometrium (dyssynchronous maturation)
   - Or both
   – Many patients have features of PCOS.

   Hyperprolactinemia
   – Deficient LH levels
   – Accelerated luteolysis
   – Intrinsic cellular defects of CL
   – Inadequate endometrial progesterone receptors.

   Androgen overproduction
   Endometriosis
   – Endometrial implants may cause:
   - Deterioration of corpus luteum
   - ↑ PGF_2 interferes with corpus luteal function

- In endometrium, intraperitoneal chronic inflammatory changes leading to ↑ IL and TNF in peritoneal fluid → abortion.

PCOS
- ↑ LH levels and hyperandrogenism (implicated in RPL) may lead to:
  - ↑ LH in follicular phase of conception cycle → abortion
  - Adverse effect on oocyte maturation
  - More associated in infertility patients of PCOS when they conceive
  - Obese PCOS patients have more chances of RPL.

Hyperinsulinemia
- Independent risk factor for early pregnancy loss in PCOS
- ↓ levels of glycodelin and insulin-like growth factor 1 (IGFBP1)

Declining ovarian function
- High D3 FSH>20
- Low D3 inhibin B < 0.6 U/mL
- Low D3 estradiol < 20 ng/mL
- Low antral follicle count on USG <5
- Low antimullerian hormone <15 picomol/L.

Thyroid dysfunction
- Thyroid autoimmunity (TAI) reported first by Stagnaro—Green et al.
- Defined as the presence of autoantibodies against thyroid peroxidase (TPOab) and/or thyroglobulin (TGab)
- Their presence reflects a generalized activation of the immune system and a highly reactive immune system against the fetoplacental unit
- Prevalence of thyroid dysfunction during pregnancy is ≈ 2-3% and is mainly caused by chronic autoimmune thyroiditis
- Thyroid autoantibodies are found in 5-15% of women of reproductive age but are not necessarily accompanied by thyroid dysfunction
- Recurrent pregnancy loss occurs in 1-3% of all couples with either thyroid dysfunction or autoimmunity
- Studies have shown that presence of thyroid autoantibodies in euthyroid women can be associated with a subtle deficiency in thyroid hormone concentrations or a lower capacity of the thyroid gland to adequately adapt to the demands of pregnancy. They may have a lower thyroidal reserve during pregnancy when a greater amount of thyroid hormones is demanded.
- Complications:

  Subclinical hypothyroidism
  - Preeclampsia
  - Increased perinatal mortality

  Thyroid autoantibodies
  - Increased risk of subfertility
  - Miscarriage (occurs mainly within the 1st trimester of gestation, when the fetus is critically dependent on maternal thyroid hormones)
  - Recurrent miscarriage
  - Preterm birth
  - Placental abruption
  - Postpartum thyroid disease
  - Presence of thyroid autoantibodies before conception carries a significantly increased risk of miscarriage.

Diabetes Mellitus
- Poorly controlled DM → 3-fold increased risk of miscarriage
- No evidence to support an association between well-controlled DM and RPL
- OGTT and HbA$_1$C recommended → if ↑ in 1st trimester →↑ risk of spontaneous abortion.

Hyperprolactinemia
- Not clear
- Insufficient evidence to assess effect of hyperprolactinemia as risk factor for RPL.

10. **Role of infection in RPL**

    Role of infection in RPL is unclear:
    - Any severe infection that leads to bacteremia or viremia can cause sporadic miscarriage
    - For an infective agent to cause RPL, it must be capable of persisting in genital tract and avoiding detection or must cause insufficient symptoms to disturb the woman
    - Routine TORCH should be abandoned
    - Agents implicated in spontaneous abortion:

    HSV/CMV
    - Directly infect placenta and fetus
    - Resulting villitis and tissue destruction → pregnancy disruption

    Bacterial vaginosis
    - Can lead to 2nd trimester loss
    - Linked to PPROM/chorioamnionitis/preterm labor/LBW infants/postpartum endometritis

    Others
    - Varicella, parvovirus, rubella, toxoplasmosis, HSV, chlamydia, monocytogenes → cause immunologic activation.

11. **Mention the miscellaneous factors implicated in RPL**

    Exposure to medications
    - Antiprogestogens
    - Antineoplastic
    - Inhalation anesthetics
    - Folic acid antagonists.

    Exposure to ionizing radiation
    - Prolonged exposure to organic solvents
    - Environmental toxins (heavy metals) → have both endocrine and immune effects → poor placentation → pregnancy loss.

    Alcohol
    - 3–5 drinks/week →↑ risk by 1.5–2 fold.

    Cigarette smoking

    Coffee and caffeinated beverages → adverse pregnancy outcome.

    Obesity/stress/NSAIDs (during early pregnancy) → isolated spontaneous pregnancy loss.

    Factors **NOT** implicated in recurrent pregnancy loss:
    - Moderate exercise
    - Coitus in the absence of cervical incompetence
    - Video display terminals, microwave ovens, high altitudes (flight attendants).

DIAGNOSIS OF RPL

Genetic Causes

- Karyotype of both partners
- Karyotype of abortus.

Immunological Causes (Cellular Immune)

- Immunological laboratory tests used earlier → of no value
- Neither transfusion of paternal leukocytes prior to conception nor IV immunoglobulins improve live birth rate in a woman with RPL
- Use of 3rd party donor white cells or trophoblast membrane transfusion—abandoned
- Alloimmunization has potential risks of:
  - Transfusion reaction
  - Graft versus host reaction
  - Transmission of infections like Hepatitis B/HIV.

Humoral Immune Mechanisms

Lupus Anticoagulant

- Tests:
  - aPTT
  - Dilute Russel viper venom test
  - Kaolin clotting time
- Results as –ve or +ve
- Two test systems of different principles should be employed to ensure the detection of weak LA and to improve specificity. Clinical evidence based on associations with thrombosis suggests that DRVVT has good utility and should be one of these tests
- The other tests will usually be:
  - An aPTT using a reagent with proven LA sensitivity
  - A modified aPTT OR
  - A dilute prothrombin time
- If the aPTT is suggestive of LA but the DRVVT is negative, a confirmatory step (e.g. using a high phospholipid concentration, platelet neutralizing reagent or LA-insensitive reagent) is needed to fulfil the criteria for LA
  - When LA testing is required for patients receiving oral anticoagulants, LA testing is better done with taipan snake venom time as the utility of the DRVVT is disputed. The taipan snake venom time has high specificity for LA
  - When testing for APAS is indicated, testing for:
    - LA
      and
    - IgG antibodies to β2 GP1 (either by an IgG aCL ELISA or an IgG anti-β2 GP1 ELISA) should be performed.

Anticardiolipin (aCL) antibodies: IgG and IgM (sensitivity 80–90%) → ELISA

- Results → negative/low/medium/high
- Expressed as GPL/MPL (1 unit represents binding activity of 1 mcg/mL of affinity-purified aCL antibody)

- GPL → IgG } (values of > 40, > 40 MPL and
- MPL → IgM } >99%tile of normal are +ve).

Anti-β2 GP1 antibodies

- aCL ELISA typically detects antibodies to β2 GP1
- LA tests are sensitive to anti-β2 GP1 and also antibodies to prothrombin
- Included in 2006 consensus
- Considered more specific
- IgG/IgM titers are detected.

Diagnostic Criteria/Sapporo's Revised Criteria, 2006

Clinical criteria:
- ≥1 episodes of vascular thrombosis (arterial, venous or small vessel thrombosis) in any organ
- Pregnancy morbidity:
  - ≥1 unexplained death of morphologically normal fetus ≥10 weeks of gestation
  - ≥1 premature births < 34 weeks because of eclampsia, preeclampsia or placental insufficiency
  - ≥3 unexplained consecutive spontaneous abortions < 10 weeks period of gestation with maternal anatomic, hormonal and paternal karyotype abnormality excluded.

Laboratory Criteria:
- LA present in serum/plasma on ≥2 occasions atleast 12 weeks apart
- aCL antibodies of IgG and/or IgM isotype in serum/plasma present in medium or high titer (i.e. > 40 GPL or MPL or > 99%tile) on ≥2 occasions at least 12 weeks apart, measured by standard ELISA
- Anti β2 GP1 antibody of IgG and/or IgM isotype in serum/plasma in titer >99% tile present on ≥2 occasions at least 12 weeks apart, measured by standard ELISA.

NOTE:
- APAS diagnosed when at least 1 of the clinical and 1 laboratory criteria are met (1+1)
- Significance of isolated +ve aCL IgM antibodies, although regarded as APLA is also debated.

Three Prominent Features of the Updated APAS Classification

- Incorporation of the beta 2-glycoprotein 1 enzyme-linked immunosorbent assay (ELISA) as a diagnostic test in addition to the cardiolipin ELISA (CL-ELISA) and the lupus anticoagulant (LA) assay(s)
- Recommendation that classification of APAS requires the persistence of antibodies for at least 12 weeks; and
- Setting of definitive cut off values for the CL-ELISA and the beta 2-GP1-ELISA.

Risk of Pregnancy Loss with APAS

- RPL<13 weeks   RPL<24 weeks   Late Loss
  IgG aCL > anti-β2 GP1   Highest with LA   Highest with aCL (medium and high titers)

APAS and Thrombosis

Association with DVT

Risk factors:
- LA
- Anti-β2GP1

- Anti-prothrombin antibodies
  - IgG anti-β2 GP1 is associated with thrombosis whereas IgM anti-β2 GP1 and aCL (IgG/IgM) are not
  - Anti-β2 GP1 replaces aCL measurement and only the IgG isotype should be tested for.

Association with Arterial Thrombosis

- Both LA and IgG aCL are associated with arterial thrombosis but that IgM aCL are not
- Anti-β2 GP1 is not associated
- β2GP1-dependent LA has been shown to be associated with arterial thrombosis.

Tests to be Done

- LA → most predictive test for thrombosis
- Presence of IgG aCL or IgG anti-β2 GP1 in those who are LA positive increases the specificity
- Measuring IgM antibodies in patients with thrombosis does not add any useful information
- Tests should be repeated after an interval of 12 weeks to demonstrate persistence.

APAS and Pregnancy

- LA has a stronger association with pregnancy loss than the other anti-phospholipid antibodies
- Association of anti-β2 GP1 and pregnancy loss is uncertain
- Both IgG and IgM aCL are associated with recurrent fetal loss
- Testing for aCL IgA antibodies is not recommended.

INHERITED THROMBOPHILIAS

Hyperhomocysteinemia

- Inherited and acquired → causes neural tube defects
- Common in India (north 3.9/1000, south 11.9/1000)
- Raw vegetables → missing from diet
- We routinely do not test for homocysteine
- We should supplement folic acid + vitamin B_6 + vitamin B_2 to prevent or in hyperhomocysteinemia
- Levels can be measured after 12 hours of fasting:
  - Normal range is 5–15 µmol/L
  - Moderate rise 16–30 µmol/L ⎫ causes genetic defects or
  - Intermediate rise 31–100 µmol/L ⎭ dietary deficiency
  - Severe > 100 µmol/L → coronary artery thrombosis at an early age.

ANATOMIC CAUSES

Congenital Malformations

Diagnostic Signs

Class II
- Uterus which leans well to one side of the pelvis and which cannot easily be straightened → strong suspicion of unicornuate uterus
- HSG → helps to identify but not always

Classes III-VII: Imperfect fusion of Mullerian ducts:
- Per vaginal examination: septate vagina and two cervices may be obvious
- On bimanual examination: 2 separate uterine horns or depression in fundus may be felt → if both fail → an impression that the uterus is unusually wide from side to side (very suggestive sign)
- Septate uterus cannot be diagnosed on bimanual exam but may be recognized by passing a sound
- Diagnosis best made by:
  - Hysteroscopy or HSG
  - MRI—excellent modality for accurate diagnosis (but expensive)
- Clinical diagnosis of septate vagina and uterus didelphys is difficult when:
  - Unequal development of 2 sides
  - Septum is displaced
- During pregnancy, diagnosis of uterine bicornis or didelphys:
  - By feeling the nonpregnant horn lying to one side and a little in front of or behind the main horn
  - Frequently mistaken for subserous leiomyoma or ovarian cyst
  - Can be avoided by careful palpation, which reveals varying shape and consistency due to intermittent contractions in case of uterine horn
  - Shape of pregnant horn and lie of fetus → may guide
  - During manual removal of placenta (MRP) or curettage for abortion→ cavity of uterus to be explored by hand, finger, sound, curette to exclude septum or bicornuate deformity.

Diagnostic Procedures

HSG
- HSG, first performed by Rindfleisch in 1910
- It provides valuable information regarding the interior cavity of the uterus
- When it shows an unicornuate uterus, however, a second cervical opening must be considered; if it is found, further injection of contrast into the cervix may lead to the diagnosis of an uterine didelphys or a complete septate uterus
- In assessing an unicornuate uterus with HSG, blocked or noncommunicating rudimentary horns will not appear on film
- HSG does not evaluate the external contour of the uterus and, therefore, it cannot reliably differentiate between a septate and a bicornuate uterus. Some authors suggest that an angle of <75° between the uterine horns is suggestive of a septate uterus and an angle of >105° indicates a bicornuate uterus
- Small septal defects can also be missed with HSG.
- Considered accurate in diagnosing most DES-linked uterine anomalies.

Sonohysterography
- Also known as hysterosonography or saline-infused sonography
- It uses the introduction of fluid into the uterine cavity to enhance ultrasound imaging. It, therefore, improves the internal delineation of the uterine contour
- It is a safe procedure and not particularly painful for the patient
- Highly accurate in both diagnosing and categorizing congenital uterine anomalies
- Sensitivity and specificity → 93% and 99% respectively.

3D USG
- Noninvasive
- Very high accuracy rate in diagnosing congenital uterine anomalies
- Also accurate in classifying the anomalies.

Hysteroscopy
- Allows direct visualization of the intrauterine cavity and ostia
- Very accurate in identifying congenital uterine anomalies after an abnormal HSG finding
- Evaluation of the external contour of the uterus is not possible and is, therefore, inadequate in differentiating between different anomaly types.

Hysterolaparoscopy
- Gold standard (both diagnostic and therapeutic)
- Complications may arise in the hands of an inexperienced surgeon.

MRI
- Noninvasive approach of assessing the internal and external contour of the uterus
- Criteria used to distinguish bicornuate from septate uteri:
  - A 10 mm threshold of fundal indentation
  - An intracornual distance of >4 cm OR
  - An angle between the two indenting medial margins of the fundus of >60°.

ENDOCRINE ABNORMALITY

Luteal Phase Defect
- Low D_{21} progesterone <10 ng/mL
- Day 5, 7, 9 progesterone postovulation (as progesterone levels fluctuate) <13 ng/mL
- USG → lack of echogenic area coupled with either absent corpus luteum or ↓ blood flow through corpus luteum
- Short luteal phase <13 days → diagnostic
- Low levels of progesterone-blocking factor in endometrium
- Endometrial biopsy lag > 2 days → invasive, not preferred.

Thyroid Disorders
- Hormone replacement therapy in pregnant women with subclinical hypothyroidism even in case of only marginally increased thyroid-stimulating hormone (TSH) is recommended
- Therapy has also been recommended in euthyroid women with circulating antibodies against thyroperoxidase (TPO-Ab) and/or thyroglobulin (Tg-Ab)
- In early gestation, measure:
  - Serum TSH
  - Free T4
  - Thyroid autoantibodies
- If serum TSH ↑ or free T4 is below normal → LT4 is administered
- Presence of thyroid autoantibodies and serum TSH < 2 mU/L → LT4 treatment is not warranted. Serum TSH and free T4 should be measured later in gestation, preferably at the end of the 2nd trimester
- For women with thyroid autoantibodies and TSH between 2 and 4 mU/L in early gestation, treatment with LT4 should be considered.

TREATMENT OF RPL

Therapeutic Options

- Use of donor oocyte/sperms
- PGD or PIGD (Preimplantation genetic diagnosis)
- Antithrombotic interventions
- Repair of anatomic abnormalities
- Correction of endocrine abnormalities
- Treatment of infection
- Immunological interventions and drugs
- Psychological counseling and support.

Genetic Abnormality

3 Alternatives

- Antithrombotic therapy
- PGD: identifies embryo (affected)→removes single cell from each embryo matured by IVF→ performs genetic testing on this cell to rule out chromosomal abnormality or presence of specific genetic diseases (cystic fibrosis)→ normal embryos replaced in uterine cavity
- Patients with Robertsonian translocations involving homologous chromosomes (because their genetic anomaly always results in embryonic aneuploidy) → use of donor oocyte/sperm, depending on the affected partner, is recommended.

Anatomic Abnormality

Inherited Causes

Class I
Agenesis
Hypoplasia of uterus (mainly)

Hypoplasia: ESSENTIAL CRITERIA (**all must be present**)
- Subnormal menstrual cycle
- Uterine cavity of ≤ 6 cm
- Endometrium which appears unstimulated on microscopy.

Clinical Features

- 1° amenorrhea
- Late menarche ⎫
- Infrequent menstruation ⎬ underlying ovarian inactivity
- Infertility ⎭
- On per vaginal exam:
  - Uterus small in overall length and width
  - Cervix relatively long
- USG → endometrium thin.

Treatment

- If hypoplasia is there because the uterus is unresponsive to ovaries, estrogens have no effect on it
- If hypoplasia is the result of inadequate ovarian stimulus, then estrogens will promote full development of uterus but the effect is temporary and unless ovarian function becomes normal in the meantime, uterus returns to its former state when treatment is suspended.

Class II
Unicornuate uterus
- If true—no treatment
- Rudimentary horn of apparent unicornuate uterus—excise if communicating with the main cavity.

Class IV
Bicornuate uterus
- Incision is made over uterus and the two horns are sutured together to form a single cavity
- Scars heal well
- Intraoperatively, it is hardly seen
- Pregnancy and labor possible
- Some prefer elective cesarean section.

Class V
Septate uterus

Older methods are now replaced by hysteroscopic procedures

Give GnRH × 2 months → endometrial atrophy (OPTIONAL)

↓

Cut septum with scissors, resectoscope (most preferred) or laser (argon, KTP or Nd-YAG)

↓

Septum is avascular, but myometrium may bleed

↓

Resectoscope → coagulates the bleeders (simultaneously)

Use laparoscope together with hysteroscopy to:
- Confirm septate uterus
- Determine end-point of resection—myometrial fibers can be seen hysteroscopically and the light can be seen transmitted through fundus uniformly

Main complications: uterine perforation and fluid overload

↓

Healing (of septal area) occurs in 2 months and is covered by endometrium

↓

No prophylaxis for intrauterine adhesions (estrogen/IUCD not required).

Acquired Causes

Uterine synechiae

Hysteroscopic resection followed by:
- Estrogen therapy ⎫ ─────→ for endometrial formation
  and   ⎬ × 2 months
- Insertion of IUCD ⎭ ─────→ to prevent scar formation and recurrence of adhesions

Submucous leiomyoma
- Myomectomy ⟶ hysteroscopic resection

Cervical tear ⟶ trachelorrhaphy

Incompetent cervix
Abdominal approach
- Rarely required
- Mainly for congenitally short cervix or amputated cervix
- Abdominal cervical cerclage is successfully being performed nowadays laparoscopically.

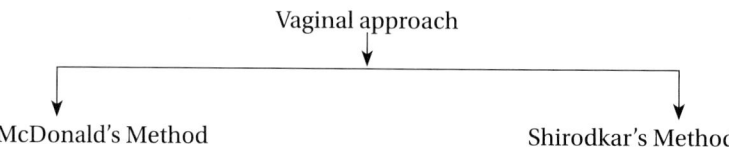

McDonald's Method	Shirodkar's Method
Purse string suture with braided silk or mersiline is placed. Suture is passed through outer half of cervical thickness starting at 12 o'clock position. Suture is passed at junction of portiovaginalis and vaginal vault taking 4 bites. Knot is kept anterior.	An encircling suture is placed around internal os after dissection of bladder. Nonabsorbable suture like silk or nylon or mersiline is used and placed below mucosa by a special curved needle. More physiological as it is exactly at internal os.

Complications
1. Hemorrhage
2. Onset of threatened abortion
3. Infection
4. Bucket handle tear of cervix, if uterine contractions begin
5. Ischemic necrosis of cervix (rarely).

Endocrine Abnormality

LPD

- Progesterone supplementation 250–500 mg IM weekly or Inj. hCG 5000 IU weekly till functional uteroplacental shift occurs
- Natural progesterone 200 mg daily (as vaginal pessary or orally)
- While giving hCG and/or progesterone, USG is performed every 2 weeks for:
  – Fetal viability
  – Congenital malformation
  – Fetal growth.

Hyperinsulinemia

- Metformin (category B drug)
  – Decreased risk of early pregnancy loss from 41.9% to 8.8%
  – Increased follicular and luteal phase serum glycodelin and IGFBP-1 →↑ vascularity and blood flow
- Progesterone support.

DM/Hypothyroidism/Hyperprolactinemia →*Treat accordingly*

Immunological causes (cellular mechanisms)

Progesterone
- Favors development of human T-cells producing T-Helper 2 cells
- Blocks production of T-Helper 1 cytokines
- Dydrogesterone:
  - High bioavailability
  - Molecular structure and pharmacological effects similar to endogenous progesterone
  - High affinity for progesterone receptor.

Tests for abnormal sperms
- Sperm DNA decondensation test
- Sperm DNA fragmentation assay.

Humoral Cell Mechanisms

APAS

Low-dose Aspirin (75–80 mg)
- Mechanism of action: selectively inhibit thrombaxane A_2 without affecting prostacyclin production
- Started as soon as UPT comes positive
- Success rate (with aspirin alone): 40%
- Stopped at 34 weeks: why?
  - Closure of ductus arteriosus when used near term
  - Oligohydramnios
  - Neonates: hemolysis, increased blood transfusion, metabolic acidosis
- Side effects
  - Increased bleeding during surgery
  - Fetal gastroschisis.

Heparin (1st Line Therapy)
- Unfractionated heparin (UFH) 5000 IU s/c BD
- Formation of irreversible complexes between antithrombin III and coagulation factors complex
- Started when cardiac activity is seen on USG
- aPTT done weekly and dose adjusted until anticoagulation achieved (it inactivates factors IIa and Xa and affects aPTT, a measure of thrombin activity)
- Platelet count—1 week after starting and monthly thereafter

Regimens	Prophylactic	Anticoagulation
1st trimester (T1)	7500–10,000 IU every 12 hourly	Every 8–12 hours maintaining levels
T2 and T3	10,000 IU every 12 hourly	

Monitoring
- Maintain aPTT values between 1.5–2 times control
- aPTT not used in case of LA positive patients
- Success rate (aspirin + UFH) → 70%

Complications:
1. Osteopenia:
   - Reversible on stopping therapy
   - In 1-2% of cases
   - Advice: calcium, vitamin B, weight-bearing exercises, graduated elastic compression stockings
2. Symptomatic vertebral fracture in 2.2-3% patients
3. Heparin-induced thrombocytopenia (HIT):
   - In 0.5% of cases
   - Manifests between 3 and 21 days
   - If severe, can cause limb ischemia, cerebrovascular accidents and myocardial infarction
   - Uncommon with prophylactic dose

   HIT type I (nonimmune):
   - Mild and reversible
   - Occurs within 1st few days of treatment
   - Common after high-dose UFH
   - Patients do not exhibit symptoms, recover over the following 3-4 days

   HIT type II (immune):
   - Rapid drop of platelet count
   - Occurs between 6 and 10 days of treatment
   - Formation of heparin-dependent antibodies can result in platelet activation.

Low Molecular Weight Heparin

- Enoxaparin 20-40 mg/day s/c
- Advantages:
  - Once daily administration
  - Less laboratory monitoring → response much more predictable
  - Increased bioavailability because it binds less to plasma proteins
  - Lesser degree of osteopenia and bleeding
  - Decreased risk of heparin-induced thrombocytopenia because of lower affinity to platelets and vWF
  - Derived from depolymerization of standard heparin → yields fragments ≈ 1/3rd the size of UFH
  - It inhibits factor Xa and augments tissue factor pathway inhibitor
  - Has minimal effect on thrombin (factor IIa)
  - Therefore, monitoring requires anti-Xa assay and not aPTT
  - Metabolized in liver by heparinase
  - Fragments excreted in urine
  - $t_{1/2}$ is increased in cirrhotic and renal failure cases.

Unfractionated heparin	LMWH
Molecular weight 5000-35,000 daltons	2000-8000 daltons
Single chain 40-50 saccharide units	13-22 saccharide units
Ratio of anti-Xa:IIa—1:1	Varies between 2:1 and 4:1
Strong inhibition of platelet adhesion to vascular wall	Moderate inhibition
Augments microvascular bleeding	Minimum alteration in microvascular bleeding
Bioavailability 30% after s/c use	70% after s/c use
Short t½, doses every 8-12 hours	Longer t½, can be given as OD dose

LMWH

Regimens
Enoxaparin
Dalteparin

Prophylactic
40 mg OD (20 mg if body wt<50 kg)
5000 IU OD

Anticoagulant
1 mg/kg BD
20 U/kg BD

Intermediate dose
Enoxaparin   40 mg OD   } until 16 weeks
Dalteparin   5000 IU OD   } followed by 12 hourly

- Monitoring:
  - Anti-factor Xa.

SCHEME OF MANAGEMENT IN CASE OF APLA POSITIVE

With Previous History of Thrombosis

- Anticoagulation (in therapeutic doses) throughout pregnancy and 6 weeks postpartum.

With Previous Pregnancy Mishap

- Aspirin + Heparin (standard treatment)
- aPTT and factor Xa levels weekly (till adjustment of dose)
- Platelet count 1–2 weeks after initiating therapy
- Routine monitoring with aPTT or serum Xa levels is NOT required
- Antenatal visits:
  - Up to 20 weeks → every 2–4 weeks
  - Thereafter 1–2 weeks
  - Serial USG 3–4 weeks after 20 weeks (for IUGR and oligohydramnios)
  - 2nd trimester: uterine artery velocity waveform on USG (for predicting adverse fetal and neonatal outcomes)
- Close maternal and fetal surveillance due to increased risk of preeclampsia, IUGR, abruption
- At 32 weeks → fetal kick count, weekly NST and BPP
- Induction at 38–39 weeks (warfarin stopped; start heparin 7–10 days earlier)
- Heparin discontinued any time with:
  - Uterine contractions
  - Elective induction is planned
- No specific neonatal complications per se because of APAS (only secondary to IUGR or IUD)
- Postpartum period:
  - Heparin × 6 weeks
  - Warfarin after 2–3 days and heparin discontinued once adequate INR is achieved
- OCPs contraindicated (risk of thrombosis).

Warfarin

- Patient with history of recurrent thrombosis or cerebral thrombotic events
- Can be given between 13 and 36 weeks
- MOA: interfering with synthesis of vitamin K-dependent clotting factors in the liver
- Anticoagulant effect develops within 1–3 days
- Secreted in milk. However, quantity of active form is insufficient to affect the suckling infant
- $t_{1/2}$ is 36–48 hours, thus single dose 3–5 mg OD

- Start of therapy:
  Warfarin + Heparin → INR done after 2 days of initiating the therapy → repeat daily → INR >2 (2 continuous days) → stop Heparin
- INR values maintained between 1.5 and 2.5
- Started on postnatal day 2.

Glucocorticoids

- Generally used in secondary APAS
- Prednisone 40 mg/day
- Successful pregnancy rate 60–70%
- Side effects:
  - Osteopenia/Osteoporosis/Pathological fractures
  - Delayed wound healing
  - Overt/Gestational DM
  - Preterm delivery/PROM
  - Cushinoid features
  - Vertebral body collapse
  - Significant infection.

Intravenous Immunoglobulins

- Used when 1st line of management fails
- In cases of HIT
- Doses:
  - 0.4 g/kg IV × 5 days monthly OR 1 g/kg IV monthly
  - 0.3 g/kg every 4 weekly till 32 weeks
- Associated with anaphylactic reaction
- Inhibits APLA themselves and decreases their further production
- Helps mainly in refractory cases, i.e. pregnancy failure despite heparin use
- Disadvantages → high cost
- Side effects → anaphylaxis (particularly in patients with IgA deficiency)
- No added benefit if added to heparin treatment
- Decrease in number of IUGR babies.

Hydroxychloroquine

- Decreases thrombogenic activity of APLA
- Still no trials to prove its efficacy.

Infection

- In selected cases
- Appropriate antibiotics to both the partners
- Post-treatment culture (to verify eradication) before attempting conception.

Unexplained RPL

Even if no cause is found, still 65% couples will have a successful subsequent pregnancy. Therefore, reassurance, support and positive counseling are very essential.

SUGGESTED READING

1. Antiphospholipid syndrome: ACOG. January 2011.
2. Berghella V, Keeler SM, MS, et al: Effectiveness of cerclage according to severity of cervical length shortening: a meta-analysis, Ultrasound Obstet Gynecol. 2010;35:468-73.
3. Bill Giannakopoulos, Steven A Krilis. How I treat the antiphospholipid syndrome: Blood, Volume 114, Number 10, 2009.
4. Cervical Cerclage: Royal College of Obstetricians and Gynaecologists, RCOG Green-top Guideline No. 60, May 2011.
5. Chan YY, Jayaprakasan K, Tan A, et al: Reproductive outcomes in women with congenital uterine anomalies: a systematic review, Ultrasound Obstet Gynecol. 2011;38:371-82.
6. Chan YY, Jayaprakasan K, Zamora J, et al: The prevalence of congenital uterine anomalies in unselected and high-risk populations: a systematic review, Human Reproduction Update. 2011;17(6):761-71.
7. David Keeling, Ian Mackie, Gary W Moore: Guidelines on the investigation and management of antiphospholipid syndrome, British Journal of Haematology. 2012;157:47-58.
8. Emmyvan den Boogaard, Rosa Vissenberg, Jolande A. Land et al: Significance of (sub)clinical thyroid dysfunction and thyroid autoimmunity before conception and in early pregnancy: a systematic review, Human Reproduction Update. 2011;17(5):605-19.
9. Henriette Svarre Nielsen. Secondary recurrent miscarriage and H-Y immunity, Human Reproduction Update. 2011;17(4):558-74.
10. Konstantinos A Toulis, Dimitrios G Goulis, Christos A Venetis, et al: Risk of spontaneous miscarriage in euthyroid women with thyroid autoimmunity undergoing IVF: a meta-analysis, European Journal of Endocrinology. 2010;162:643-52.
11. Mei-Tsz Su, Sheng-Hsiang Lin, Yi-Chi Chen. Genetic association studies of angiogenesis and vasoconstriction-related genes in women with recurrent pregnancy loss: a systematic review and meta-analysis, Human Reproduction Update. 2011;17(6):803-12.
12. Mette Dahl, Thomas Vauvert F Hviid. Human leukocyte antigen class Ib molecules in pregnancy success and early pregnancy loss, Human Reproduction Update. 2012;18(1):92-109.
13. Saskia Middeldorp. Is Thrombophilia Testing Useful? American Society of Hematology. 2011;150-55.
14. Shannon M Bates. Consultative Hematology: The Pregnant Patient Pregnancy Loss, American Society of Hematology. 2010;166-72.
15. Shyi-Jou Chen, Yung-Liang Liu, Huey-Kang Sytwu. Immunologic Regulation in Pregnancy: From Mechanism to Therapeutic Strategy for Immunomodulation, Clinical and Developmental Immunology 2012.
16. Sotirios H Saravelos, Karen A Cocksedge, Tin-Chiu Li. Prevalence and diagnosis of congenital uterine anomalies in women with reproductive failure: a critical appraisal, Human Reproduction Update. 2008;14(5):415-29.
17. Tang AW, Alfirevic Z, Quenby S. Natural killer cells and pregnancy outcomes in women with recurrent miscarriage and infertility: a systematic review, Human Reproduction Update. 2011;26(8):1971-80.
18. The Use of Antithrombotics in the Prevention of Recurrent Pregnancy Loss. Royal College of Obstetricians and Gynaecologists, Scientific Impact Paper 26, June 2011.
19. Warning JC, McCracken SA, Morris JM. A balancing act: mechanisms by which the fetus avoids rejection by the maternal immune system, Reproduction. 2011;141:715-24.

CHAPTER 4

Antepartum Hemorrhage in Early Pregnancy

Tania G Singh

Case: A 28 years old woman approaches the emergency department with complaints of severe pain in lower abdomen on right side since the past 2 hours. She gives a history of irregular periods, which come every 2–3 months, so is not sure whether she is pregnant or not. She also complains of slight vaginal bleeding since the past 1 hour. On examination:
- PR: 110/min   Pallor ++
- BP 96/60 mmHg   Per-abdomen: tenderness present in right iliac region
- Pervaginal examination: uterus normal size, internal os closed, cervical motion tenderness present.

What is your likely diagnosis? What are the other conditions in which patient can become unstable?

Likely diagnosis: **Pregnancy of unknown location**
Step I → Complete history/calculate period of gestation/physical examination
Step II → Check vitals

Patient *remains* stable in–
- Threatened abortion
- Inevitable abortion
- Missed abortion (when comes with minimal spotting or brownish discharge)
- Unruptured ectopic.

Patient *becomes* unstable in–
- Ruptured ectopic
- Profuse bleeding due to incomplete abortion
- Profuse bleeding due to molar pregnancy.

Patient *can be* stable in–
- Mild to moderate bleeding due to incomplete abortion or molar pregnancy

Stable
Situation 1
Bleeding minimal → internal os closed

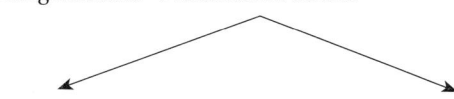

Pain absent
Uterine size corresponding to POG
↓
Threatened abortion/
Implantation bleeding/
Subchorionic hemorrhage/
Idiopathic bleeding in a viable pregnancy.

Pain present
Normal uterine size
↓
Ectopic

Situation 2
Bleeding moderate
a. Uterine size corresponds to POG → internal os open → inevitable abortion
b. Uterine size ≤ POG → internal os closed or may be slightly opened → partial mole
c. Uterine size >>POG → internal os closed or may be slightly opened → complete mole.

Unstable
Situation 1
Bleeding profuse
a. Uterine size <POG → internal os open → incomplete abortion
b. Uterine size ≤ POG → internal os closed or may be slightly opened → partial mole
c. Uterine size >> POG → internal os closed or may be slightly opened → complete mole.

Situation 2
Minimal to moderate bleeding
a. Adnexal/abdominal or uterine tenderness → internal os closed with normal uterine size → ruptured ectopic

Step III → Bleeding present due to nonobstetric cause → diagnose and treat as indicated

Diagnosis can be:
a. Cervical abnormalities (e.g., excessive friability, polyps, trauma, malignancy)
b. Infection of the vagina or cervix
c. Vaginal trauma.

CERTAIN IMPORTANT THINGS NEED TO BE DISCUSSED BEFORE PROCEEDING TO THE ACTUAL TOPIC

Normal Early Intrauterine Pregnancy

Causes of pain
- Can be due to ligamentous laxity, or
- Due to a growing hemorrhagic corpus luteum cyst
- Can be a spontaneous abortion in progress.

Sonographic findings

Intradecidual sign
- Earliest sonographic finding of an intrauterine pregnancy (IUP)
- Visualized at about 4.5 menstrual weeks
- It is a small fluid collection surrounded by an echogenic ring that is eccentrically located within the endometrium, just beneath the endometrial stripe
- Important thing is that-
  - Firstly, it should be visualized in two planes and not have a changing appearance
  - Secondly, the echogenic (hyperechoic) ring around the sac, differentiating it from thin walled decidual cysts (found at the junction of endometrium and myometrium),which are common in ectopic pregnancy but may also be found in normal early IUP
  - Therefore, in such a case, it is prudent to measure serum β hCG levels.

Double decidual sac
- Visualized at ≈ 5 weeks
- It is caused by the inner rim of chorionic villi surrounded by a thin crescent of fluid in the endometrial cavity, which in turn, is surrounded by the outer echogenic rim of the decidua vera (i.e. two concentric hyperechoic rings that surround an anechoic gestational sac). This sign is highly reliable for the diagnosis of an intrauterine gestational sac
- However, there is only a short window of time between visualization of the intradecidual sign and visualization of a yolk sac (a definitive sign of IUP), so the double decidual sac sign has limited value.

Yolk sac
- Visualized at ≈ 5.5 weeks, within the gestational sac (when it reaches 10 mm).

Cardiac activity
- Visualized at ≈ 5–6 weeks, when the gestational sac measures > 18 mm or when the embryonic pole measures ≥ 5 mm.

Note:
- If a patient presents with amenorrhea and bleeding and any of the above signs of early IUP are seen on USG → follow her with serum β hCG test and sonography until cardiac activity is seen
- Although the presence of an intrauterine gestational sac dramatically decreases the likelihood of an ectopic pregnancy, it is still important to perform a careful assessment of the adnexa, since heterotopic pregnancies can occur, especially in IVF patients.

Abnormal Early Intrauterine Pregnancy

Abortion can present as any of the following:
- Amenorrhea and pain

OR
- Amenorrhea and bleeding

OR
- Amenorrhea, pain and bleeding

TVS thresholds for definitive diagnosis of nonviable pregnancy
1. Nonvisualization of a yolk sac by the time the mean sac diameter is 8–13 mm
2. Nonvisualization of an embryo by the time the mean sac diameter is 16–18 mm
3. Nonvisualization of cardiac activity by the time the embryo is 5 mm in length

Most important point at this juncture is:
What is pseudosac? How will you distinguish between abnormal IUP and pseudosac of ectopic pregnancy?
- Collection of fluid within the endometrial cavity
- Represents a thick decidual reaction surrounding intrauterine fluid
- Absence of double decidual sac sign helps distinguish a pseudo-gestational sac from a true viable gestational sac
- Pseudosac is located centrally within the endometrial canal, whereas a normal gestational sac is located eccentrically within the canal (a viable gestational sac also exhibits low-resistance arterial flow on color Doppler flow images)
- Has a heterogeneous appearance due to presence of blood and debris
- At times, it can be seen moving.

But it is NOT diagnostic of ectopic (present in only 20% of ectopic pregnancies)

Presence of a gestational sac of 13 mm without a yolk sac with β hCG levels not rising normally points towards performing a D and C
If chorionic villi are present → abnormal IUP
If absent → ectopic.

Molar Pregnancy

- Classical appearance is not of pain, which usually occurs secondary to the enlarging uterus and ovarian theca lutein cysts late in 1st trimester
- A βhCG >100,000 mIU/mL with a heterogeneous appearance of the endometrium with multiple small cystic spaces is suspicious for molar pregnancy.

Corpus Luteal Cyst

Corpus luteum
- Normal structure in intrauterine pregnancy with varied appearances
- Located within the ovary or exophytic from the ovary, whereas ectopic pregnancies are most commonly located within the tube
- Even a complex cyst within the ovary has a very high possibility of being a corpus luteum as ovarian ectopics are quite rare
- Its wall is generally more hypoechoic than the wall of an ectopic pregnancy
- Corpus luteum moves with the ovary rather than separately from it (as would be expected from a tubal ectopic pregnancy).

Presence of free fluid – significance!
Most dependent location where fluid accumulates → cul-de-sac
Pregnancy and hemoperitoneum–2 possibilities
I. Ectopic pregnancy
II. Ruptured hemorrhagic corpus luteum cyst
- If the patient is unstable, do not waste time in performing the whole scan to rule out ectopic as management for both situations is same → laparotomy
- If the patient is stable – complete scan and β hCG can be performed.

PUL (Pregnancy of Unknown Location) or Negative Pelvic Sonogram

- A positive pregnancy test with no evidence of either an intrauterine pregnancy or an ectopic on TVS

- Differential diagnosis in such a case would be:
  - Normal early pregnancy (with intrauterine gestational sac), OR
  - Ectopic, OR
  - Spontaneous abortion
- Follow up with β hCG and TVS is mandatory in such cases - why?
  - Normal pregnancy
    - Intrauterine gestational sac grows at a rate of 0.8 mm/day; therefore, follow-up sonography in 2-3 days will demonstrate growth in normal pregnancy
  - Ectopic → 3 possibilities
    - ≈ 15-35% of ectopic pregnancies will not demonstrate an identifiable extrauterine mass at TVS OR
    - Resolved without intervention OR
    - A probability of ectopic pregnancy, found as either:
      - An extrauterine inhomogeneous mass *(Blob sign)*
      OR
      - An extrauterine empty gestational sac *(Bagel sign)*
  - Spontaneous abortion
    - Complete abortion where serum β hCG has resolved without intervention.

ECTOPIC PREGNANCY

An Overview

- Any pregnancy implanted outside the uterine cavity
- Fertilization of ovum occurs in the fallopian tube. As the zygote divides, it first becomes a morula and then a blastocyst, normally arriving in the uterine cavity and beginning implantation on day 6 after fertilization
- Anything that delays or impedes tubal transport may allow implantation to begin while the blastocyst is still in the tube.

Prevalence

- Accounts for ≈ 10-15% of all maternal deaths
- Incidence is 1.5-2% of all pregnancies among general population
- Prevalence among those presenting to an emergency department with 1st trimester bleeding or pain or both≈ 6-16%
- Risk of heterotopic pregnancy ranges between 1 in 10000 to 1 in 30000 in cases of spontaneous conception but is as high as 1 to 3% in women on ovulation induction owing to tubal damage in patients undergoing IVF.

Implantation Sites

- 95% of ectopic pregnancies are tubal in location
- Commoner on right side
- They can be:

Extrauterine (98%)

- Tubal (>95%)
  - Ampullary (75-80%)
  - Isthmic (10-12%)

- Interstitial/cornual (4-5%)
- Fimbrial end (5%)
- Ovarian (0.5%)
- Abdominal (1.0%)
  - Primary (rare)
  - Secondary
    - Intraperitoneal (common)
    - Extraperitoneal (rare)

Intrauterine (1.5-2%)

- Cervical (<1%)
- Angular.

Tubal Ectopic Pregnancy

- Usually becomes symptomatic at 5-6 weeks.

Etiology

- Previous ectopic pregnancy (7-15% risk)
- Preexisting tubal damage
  - Prior pelvic infection
    - Chlamydia (most common)
    - Gonorrhea
    - Other STDs
    - Salpingitis isthmica nodosa
  - Tubal disease occurring secondary to
    - Endometriosis
    - Appendicitis
    - Previous pelvic surgery
    - Current use of IUCD (it prevents implantation inside the uterus)
    - Use of POPs
    - Exposure to diethylstilbestrol (DES)
  - Prior tubal surgery
    - Tubal ligation
    - Reversal of ligation
- Infertility treatment/drugs
- History of placenta previa
- Congenital uterine anomalies
- Cigarette smoking
- No apparent cause

Serum or UPT (ELISA) are sensitive to β hCG levels of 10-20 mIU/mL and are positive in 99% of ectopic pregnancies.

Risk Factors

High-risk factors
1. Previous tubal surgery (reconstructive)
2. History of tubal ligation

3. Previous ectopic pregnancy
   - Previous 2 ectopics → overall increased risk by 16%
4. In utero DES exposure
   - 9-fold increased risk of ectopic pregnancy
5. Current use of intrauterine device
6. Documented tubal pathology.

Moderate risk factors
1. History of PID (gonorrhea/Chlamydia)
2. History of infertility
3. Multiple sexual partners.

Weak or almost no association
1. Outpatient treatment of chlamydia/gonorrhea
2. Smoking
3. Coitus before 18 years
4. Past use of intrauterine device
5. History of threatened abortion
6. Non-tubal surgery (previous pelvic or abdominal surgery)
7. Previous cesarean section
8. Vaginal douching.

Tubal surgery
- Reconstructive tubal surgery for tubal damage caused by a previous ectopic pregnancy or PID
- Patients with a history of tubal occlusion by cautery are at higher risk than those who had reversals after noncautery methods.

Tubal ligation failure
- Risk is highest in patients who had a tubal ligation using bipolar cautery and in women who underwent sterilization before 30 years of age
- The increased risk with bipolar cautery is most likely associated with fistula formation of the fallopian tube leading to subsequent failure
- There is currently no data on risk of ectopic pregnancy after hysteroscopic sterilization.

Presentation

- Most common gestational age → 6–10 weeks
- Classic triad of ectopic
  - Abdominal pain
  - Vaginal bleeding } Present in only 45% of patients
  - Adnexal mass

Note:
- 25–30% patients will not have vaginal bleeding
- 10% will have palpable adnexal mass
- ≈ 10% have negative pelvic examination
- Profuse vaginal bleeding is suggestive of incomplete abortion rather than ectopic
- Abdominal pain + vaginal bleeding → 39%
- Abdominal pain + vaginal bleeding + other risk factors → 54%.

Physical examination
- Abdominal tenderness (97.3%)
- Adnexal tenderness (98%)
- Amenorrhea with vaginal spotting/bleeding (60–80%)

- Tachycardia or orthostatic changes
- Cervical motion tenderness → in 3/4th of patients but may be present prior to rupture
- Uterine tenderness (from blood irritating the peritoneal surfaces)
- A palpable mass
- Rebound tenderness or peritoneal signs
- Pallor
- Abdominal distension
- Enlarged uterus
- Shock/collapse.

Other reported symptoms
- Breast tenderness
- Gastrointestinal symptoms
- Dizziness, fainting or syncope
- Shoulder tip pain (secondary to diaphragmatic irritation)
- Urinary symptoms
- Passage of tissue
- Rectal pressure or pain on defecation.

Even if the classic triad is present, still rule out the following possibilities:
- Implantation bleeding
- Acute appendicitis
- Miscarriage
- Ovarian torsion
- PID
- Ruptured corpus luteal cyst or follicle or chocolate cyst
- Tubo-ovarian abscess
- Urinary calculi.

Diagnosis

I. Ultrasonography

Transabdominal (TAS)
- Identification of products of conception in fallopian tubes is difficult
- Intrauterine pregnancy not recognized until 5–6 menstrual weeks or 28 days after timed ovulation
- Corpus luteum cysts and matted bowel can mimic tubal pregnancy

Indeterminate sac
- <1 cm → TAS
- 0.6 cm → TVS (sensitivity 20–80%).

Transvaginal (TVS)
Look for the following:
i. 1st USG sign of intrauterine pregnancy → gestation sac "double decidual sign" (double echogenic rings around the sac → eccentrically placed in uterus ≥ 1–3 mm in size) at 4.5–5 weeks
ii. Intrauterine gestation at 5.5 menstrual weeks → 1 week after missed periods → 100% accuracy
iii. Yolk sac → at 5–6 weeks and remain until about 10 weeks
iv. Embryo (fetal pole) and cardiac activity → 5.5–6 weeks

The presence for above features still does not rule out ectopic pregnancy
- Also look for:
  - Tubes and adnexa (separate from ovary) to evaluate for heterotopic pregnancy as it is common after IVF

- Fluid in cul-de-sac
- Adnexal masses—cannot be seen when they are small or when obscured by bowel.

II. βhCG (Human Chorionic Gonadotropin)
- A glycoprotein hormone that contains both an alpha and a beta subunit
- Levels begin to ascend in a curvilinear fashion early in pregnancy and continue until they reach plateau at ≈ 9–11 weeks
- The plateau lasts for only a few days and thereafter β-hCG levels begin to decline at 20 weeks
- In the absence of a reliable LMP, hCG level is instrumental
- Ideally β hCG levels should increase by 53–63% within 48 hours in normal pregnancy
- If β-hCG levels increase by <53% during a 48-hour period, there is almost always a nonviable pregnancy associated, be it intra- or extrauterine

What is Discriminatory Zone (DZ)?
Discriminatory zone is defined as the level of β hCG at which an intrauterine pregnancy should be visualized
- With TAS → 6500 mIU/mL ⎫ Above these levels, if it is not visualized, it is either
- With TVS → 1500 – 2500 mIU/mL ⎭ an ectopic or an intrauterine nonviable pregnancy.

Following possible situations:
i. β hCG level has reached DZ and no intrauterine pregnancy
   - Highly suspicious of ectopic → (exception: multiple gestation)
   - The lower limit of a normal rise of β hCG in a normal pregnancy is 66% in 48 hours and 114% rise in 72 hours (Mean Doubling Time)
   - Rise lower than this → suggestive of abnormal pregnancy
   - Normal rising β hCG levels → DOES NOT RULE OUT ECTOPIC PREGNANCY.
ii. β hCG > DZ and no definite USG diagnosis
   It can be either dead fetus or ectopic
   Uterine evacuation indicated (D and C) → to differentiate between an early pregnancy loss and an ectopic

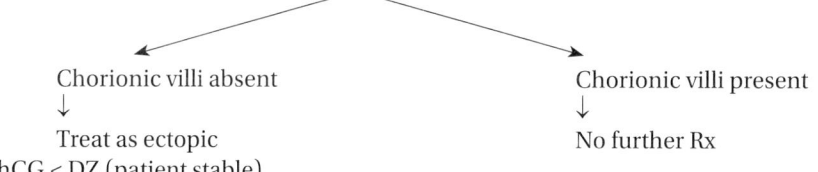

Chorionic villi absent → Treat as ectopic

Chorionic villi present → No further Rx

iii. β hCG < DZ (patient stable)
   Serial β hCG + repeat TVS (at 2–3 days interval)

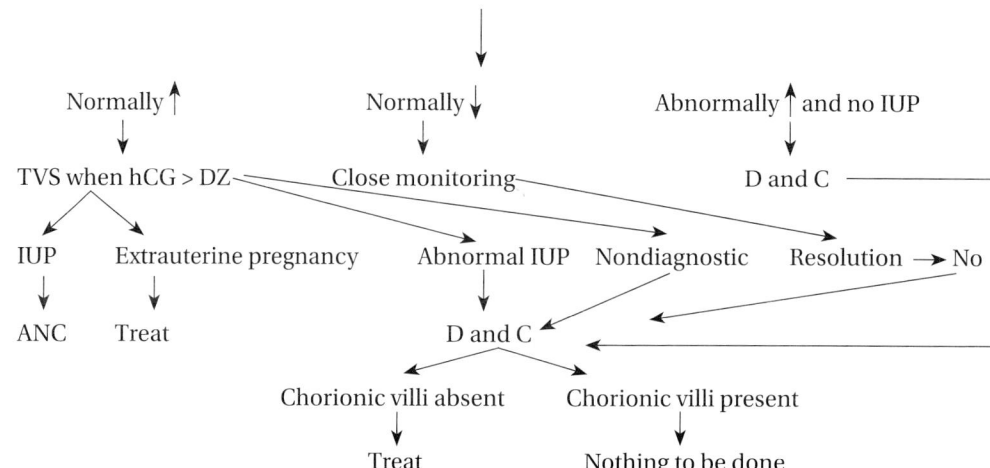

What is 'Phantom hCG'?
- It is a positive blood pregnancy test without being pregnant
- Patients will have a persistently but not significantly rising positive blood pregnancy test but the urine test is negative
- Reason—false positive reactivity to some substrate in the blood hCG test, displaying a consistently low positive hCG titer even though they are not pregnant
- It may lead to serious misdiagnosis and interventions, but can be detected with serial dilutions or by doing a UPT.

Causes of false-positive hCG measurements
a. Measurement of pituitary hCG-like substance
b. Production of free hCG β-subunit
c. Interference by non-hCG substances, including hLH or hLH β-subunit, both species-specific and heterophilic anti-animal immunoglobulin antibodies; rheumatoid factor; anti-hCG antibodies; and nonspecific serum factors
d. Assay issues such as carryover by positive displacement pipettes and contaminants that affect label detection (radioactive iodine or fluorophoresis).

Characteristics of false-positive hCG measurements include:
a. Low-level positive result (generally <1,000 mIU/mL and usually < 150 mIU/mL)
b. Positive serum but negative urine test
c. Serial dilutions of serum that are not parallel to the hCG standard and yield higher or lower levels of hCG when multiplied by dilution factor
d. Positive hCG results that are not consistent with clinical or surgical findings
e. No substantial changes in levels that were measured in serial blood samples, even after therapeutic procedures
f. Negative results in a different type of quantitative hCG assay.

Following steps are recommended when phantom hCG is found:
a. Measure urinary hCG
b. Re-measure the hCG concentration using a different method
c. Add normal mouse serum or other animal serum to the assay, test for anti-hCG antibodies
d. Measure hCG concentrations after several days or weeks.

III. Serum progesterone
Role and importance
- Usefulness of single progesterone level to diagnose ectopic is controversial
- During 1st 8–10 weeks, progesterone is produced by corpus luteum and remains relatively stable
- Progesterone > 25 ng/mL → consistent with normal pregnancy, if conceived spontaneously (97.5% sensitivity)
- But after ART →↑↑progesterone
- Progesterone < 5 ng/mL → 99% specific for abnormal pregnancy
  There are 2 possibilities–
  – Intrauterine pregnancy with dead fetus
  – Ectopic pregnancy
- <5 ng/mL occurs in 0.3% of normal pregnancies
- But this lower limit cannot differentiate between an early pregnancy failure and an ectopic pregnancy.

IV. Role of culdocentesis
- Performed only rarely
- Primarily when USG is not available

- Four possibilities
  i. Nonclotting bloody fluid OR fluid with fragments of old clots → bleeding ectopic
  ii. Yellow or straw colored fluid → ruptured ovarian cyst
  iii. If fluid does not clot → may have been obtained from adjacent blood vessel rather than from bleeding ectopic
      - Used to identify hemoperitoneum
      - Cervix is pulled towards symphysis with a tenaculum and a long 16 or 18 gauge needle is inserted through posterior fornix into cul-de-sac
  iv. If present, fluid is aspirated
- If no fluid is aspirated (unsatisfactory entry into cul-de-sac), it does not rule out ectopic.

To summarize:
- Two most vital diagnostic tests → TVS and β hCG
- Sensitivity and specificity on combining these two → 95–100%.

Treatment

Options available:
1. Surgery (salpingectomy, salpingostomy or salpingotomy either by laparoscopy or by open approach)
2. Medical/conservative –
   - Systemic route → Methotrexate (preferred route and drug)

   OR

   - Local route (administration of various drugs like methotrexate, prostaglandins or hyperosmolar glucose directly into the gestational sac transvaginally under sonographic or laparoscopic guidance)
3. Expectant management.

Surgical Route

Surgery can be offered as the 1st line of management in the following cases:
- Ectopic pregnancy with significant pain
- Ectopic pregnancy with adnexal mass of ≥ 35 mm
- Ectopic pregnancy with cardiac activity
- Ectopic pregnancy with serum hCG ≥ 5000 mIU/mL
- When patient is hemodynamically unstable
- When patient is not compliant
- When patient is breastfeeding
- Heterotopic pregnancy ⎫
- Tubal rupture   ⎬ In hemodynamically stable patient
- Imminent risk of rupture ⎭
- No desire for or an inability to comply with medical management
- Contraindication to methotrexate
- Failure of medical management such as tubal pregnancy > 5 cm or fetal cardiac activity seen on TVS.

There are two options – Laparotomy and laparoscopic surgery

Laparotomy
- If patient is unstable → Laparotomy (preferred and is an absolute indication)
- Also indicated when location is other than tubal pregnancy (ovarian, cervical, interstitial pregnancy).

Laparoscopic approach
- Usually employed in hemodynamically (with obvious abdominal hemorrhage that requires definitive treatment) stable patient
- In unruptured ectopic (cases where medical management is either not possible or not opted)
- Advantages:
  - Faster recovery
  - Shorter hospitalization
  - Reduced overall costs
  - Less pain, bleeding and adhesion formation
  - Lower analgesic requirements.

Laparoscopy *versus* Open approach
- No difference in overall tubal patency rates
- No difference in subsequent intrauterine pregnancy rates
- But there is a trend towards lower repeat ectopic pregnancy rates with laparoscopy.

Surgery can be:

Conservative
- Salpingostomy
- Salpingotomy
- Fimbrial expression of ectopic pregnancy.

Radical
- Salpingectomy.

Salpingectomy
- Segmental or entire removal of fallopian tube
- Indications:
  - Recurrent ectopic pregnancy in the same tube
  - Severely damaged tube
  - Uncontrolled bleeding (before or after salpingostomy) both for ruptured or unruptured ectopics
  - Heterotopic pregnancy
  - Lack of desire to bear more children
- Partial salpingectomy can be performed when ectopic pregnancy is small and fimbriae appear healthy.

Note: When removing the oviduct, it is advisable to excise a wedge of the outer 1/3rd or less of interstitial portion of the tube. This so called *corneal resection* is done in an effort to minimize the rare recurrence of pregnancy in tubal stump. Even with this future ectopic cannot be prevented.

Salpingostomy
- Method of choice in women of reproductive age who wish to preserve their fertility
- For removing pregnancy <2 cm in length and located in distal 1/3rd of fallopian tube
- Typically performed by making a linear incision ($\approx$ 10-15 mm) on the antimesenteric border of the fallopian tube at the point of maximal distention (i.e. over the ectopic)
- Removing the POCs by hydrodissection is recommended, avoiding-
  - Excessive handling of the tube
  - Excessive cautery to prevent further damage to the fallopian tube
- Incision left unsutured to heal by 2° intention
- Rate of intrauterine pregnancy is improved in patients having linear salpingostomy but recurrent ectopic rate is also higher

- Readily performed through laparoscope
- Drawback: risk of persistent trophoblast (incomplete removal of trophoblastic tissue, resulting in rising or plateauing serum β hCG postoperatively) and repeat ectopic pregnancy.

Salpingotomy

- Same procedure as salpingostomy except that incision is closed with 7-0 vicryl or similar suture.

Recent advances

- In the presence of a healthy contralateral tube, there is no clear evidence that salpingostomy should be used in preference to salpingectomy
- Laparoscopic salpingostomy should be considered as primary treatment when managing tubal pregnancy in the presence of contralateral tubal disease and the desire for future fertility
- In cases of salpingectomy, perform UPT after 3 weeks
- In cases of salpingotomy, perform serum β hCG after 1 week and then weekly until the results are negative.

Persistent Ectopic

- Defined as failure of s. β hCG levels to fall as expected after initial treatment. It is the result of incomplete removal of trophoblast
- Normally hCG is 10% of preoperative value by Day 12   OR
- Postoperative Day 1 hCG is < 50% of preoperative value (s. hCG may fall to normal → these cases present as "delayed hemorrhage")
- A well-recognized hazard after salpingostomy, systemic methotrexate treatment and expectant management
- Leads to recurrence of clinical symptoms
- Is an indication for additional treatment
- Precautions which can be taken–
  - Serial hCG monitoring till the levels become undetectable
  - Prophylactic single dose of MTX even after salpingostomy
- Risk of persistent ectopic increases:
  - In very early gestations and commencement of therapy before 42 menstrual days
  - Those measuring < 2 cm in diameter
  - With relatively higher initial β hCG values (>3000 IU/lit)
  - Rapid preoperative rise in s. hCG
  - Presence of active tubal bleeding
  - Implantation medial to salpingostomy site.

Risk is

- 2–11% with laparotomy
- 5–20% with laparoscopy (average ≈8%)
- 3.9–4.1% after salpingostomy
- 5–10% initially treated medically.

Treatment

- Serial hCG measurements after treatment
- Methotrexate 50 mg/m² (SINGLE DOSE).

Medical Management

Methotrexate (MTX)
- First case report of methotrexate for treatment of ectopic pregnancy appeared in 1982
- Medical treatment of choice currently
- It destroys the ectopic pregnancy tissue and allows the body to reabsorb the latter
- It was proposed for the treatment of ectopic, after observation that actively replicating trophoblasts in gestational trophoblastic disease were successfully treated with methotrexate
- Immunosuppressive drug (folinic acid antagonist)
- Metabolism:

Pathway 1

Binds to the catalytic site of enzyme dihydrofolate reductase
(enzyme used to reduce folic acid to tetrahydrofolate)
↓
Inhibits synthesis of purines and pyrimidines (thymidylate, serine and methionine)
↓
Disrupting synthesis of DNA, RNA and cell replication
↓
Leading to cell death

Pathway 2

Metabolized to methotrexate polyglutamates (which are long-lived metabolites)
↓
Inhibiting other folate-dependent enzymes

- Uses (treatment of):
  - Extrauterine pregnancy (EUP)
  - 1st trimester terminations
  - Gestational trophoblastic disease
  - Cancers
  - Psoriasis
  - Rheumatic diseases
- A low-dose MTX treatment protocol introduced by Stovall et al, 20 years ago is to date the treatment of choice for EUP when possible
- Most widely used → single dose (50 mg/m^2)
- For most women, it is between 75–90 mg/m^2
- S. β hCG levels checked on day 4 and 7
- Further dose given if hCG levels fail to fall by > 15% between day 4 and 7
- Most suitable for MTX are those with s.hCG < 3000 IU/lit and minimal symptoms
- Can be given as outpatient therapy → cost saving
- Failure:
  - When β hCG levels plateaus OR
  - Level increases OR
  - There is tubal rupture (which can even occur in face of declining β hCG levels).

Patient selection:
1. No significant pain
2. Unruptured ectopic with no cardiac activity
3. Adnexal mass < 35 mm

4. β hCG levels <1500 mIU/mL (even women upto 5000 IU /lit can be offered MTX therapy, if all other criterias are fulfilled)
5. No intrauterine pregnancy (confirmed on ultrasound)
6. Candidate reliable and willing for follow up
7. ABO Rh should be checked
8. Other important investigations to be done before.

Not candidates for MTX

- Liver disease: transaminase level > 2 times normal
- Renal disease: creatinine >1.5 gm/dl (133 µmol/L)
- Immune compromise:
  - WBCs <1500/mm^3 (1.5 × 10^9/lit)
  - Platelets < 1 lakh/mm^3
- Significant pulmonary disease (CXR should be done because of the risk of interstitial pneumonitis in these patients).

Contraindications

Absolute
- Active intra-abdominal hemorrhage
- Breastfeeding
- Immunodeficiency
- Liver/renal/severe pulmonary disease
- Alcoholism
- Pre-existing blood dyscrasias
- Peptic ulcer disease
- Known sensitivity to methotrexate.

Relative
- Gestational sac > 3.5–4 cm
- High initial hCG > 5000 mIU/mL
- Presence of cardiac activity.

Indications

Absolute
- Hemodynamically stable without active bleeding or signs of hemoperitoneum
- Patient desires future fertility
- Nonlaparoscopic diagnosis
- Patient compliant/reliable
- Administration of general anesthesia poses risk
- Patient has no contraindication to methotrexate.

Relative
- Period of gestation < 6 weeks
- Unruptured mass ≤ 3.5 cm at the greatest dimension
- No fetal cardiac activity
- β hCG limit does not exceed a predetermined value, i.e. β hCG < 15000 mIU/mL.

Methotrexate Therapy

Protocols

- Originally MTX *multidose* therapy was described in 1976 by Goldstein and again in 1989 by Bagshawe for treatment of GTD
- Later in 1989, Stovall introduced the *single* dose regimen to reduce drug related toxicity, patient compliance and deduction in costs.

Single Dose (Without Folinic Acid)

The term 'single dose' is actually a misnomer. While the term single describes the number of MTX injections, the regimen includes provision for additional doses when response is inadequate.

Candidates
- Women with serum β hCG concentrations < 1500 mIU/mL, a single-dose MTX regimen (50 mg/m² or 1 mg/kg IM) can be considered.

Dose
- 50 mg/sq. mt of body surface methotrexate IM on Day 1.

Lab values
- LFT/CBC/RFT (mainly creatinine) on Day 0
- β hCG on Day 0, 1, 4 and 7.

Repeat medication
- Repeat dose on Day 7, if β hCG does not decrease by 15% between day 4 and 7.

Follow up
- β hCG level weekly and continue regimen until no longer detected
- If difference is between day 4 and 7 is ≥ 15% → repeat weekly until undetectable
- If difference is < 15% → repeat methotrexate dose and begin new Day 1
- If cardiac activity is present by Day 7 → repeat methotrexate dose, begin new Day 1
- If β hCG levels are not decreased and fetal cardiac activity persists after 3 doses of methotrexate → surgical management.

Fixed Multiple Dose (Alternated with Folinic Acid – Leucovorin)

Candidates
- Hemodynamically stable
- Unruptured tubal ectopic
- No signs of active bleeding
- Serum β hCG concentrations < 3000 mIU/mL.

Dose
- Alternate every other day:
  1 mg/kg methotrexate IM (Day 1, 3, 5, 7)
  and
  0.1 mg/kg leucovorin IM (Day 2, 4, 6 and 8).

Note: Leucovorin is an antagonist to MTX that can help to reduce other prohibitive side effects, particularly when higher doses of MTX are used.

Lab values
- LFT/CBC/RFT on Day 0
- β hCG on Day 0,1, 3, 5 and 7 (i.e. every 48 hours) until levels decrease by 15%.

Repeat medication
- Repeat regimen (for up to 4 doses of each), if β hCG level does not decrease by 15% with each measurement (in 48 hours).

Follow up
- β hCG level weekly and continue regimen until no longer detected
- Mean time to resolution of ectopic pregnancy is 2–3 weeks after MTX therapy but can take 6–8 weeks, especially if pretreatment β hCG levels were high.

Note:
- In both treatment protocols, once hCG levels have met the criteria for initial decline, hCG levels are followed serially at weekly intervals to ensure that concentrations decline steadily and become undetectable
- hCG levels should decline to <5 mIU/mL before stopping treatment.

Effects Related to Drug

- Liver involvement (12%)
- Nausea, vomiting
- Conjunctivitis
- Stomatitis
- Gastric distress (gastroenteritis 1%)
- Dizziness/fever
- Pneumonitis (drug induced)
- Reversible alopecia (rare)
- Severe neutropenia (rare)
- Photosensitivity
- Bone marrow depression
- A proportion of women need to be admitted for observation and assessment by TVS – why?
  - Differentiating so called *'separation pain'* due to tubal abortion from pain due to tubal rupture
  - Separation pain usually develops between day 3 and 7 after treatment begins and subsides within 4–12 hours after onset
  - In 65–75% cases, increasing pain begins several days after therapy
  - Relieved by non-narcotic analgesics
  - If not relieved → check vitals and hematocrit and if ruptured, surgery becomes mandatory.

Effects Related to Treatment

- Increased abdominal pain
- Increase in β hCG levels from day 1 to day 4
- Increase in abdominal girth
- Vaginal bleeding or spotting (rare, due to thrombocytopenia, occurring within 2 weeks of injection).

Advice to Patients on Methotrexate Therapy

Prohibition during treatment
- Sexual intercourse
- Alcohol

- Folic acid
- Vitamins
- NSAIDs ⎫
- Aspirin ⎭ Lethal interactions

Maintain ample fluid intake
- Limit sun exposure during treatment, as methotrexate can cause sensitivity to sunlight and sunburn or dermatitis may occur
- Reliable contraception for 3–6 months after MTX because of possible teratogenic risk (minimum 3 months)
- Avoid gas forming foods as they may cause pain
- Avoid pelvic examinations and ultrasound during surveillance of MTX therapy
- Pregnancy occurring before 3 months is not an indication for termination unless USG indicates birth defects
- Although half-life of MTX is 8 to 15 hours, its presence in the liver has been reported to last up to 116 days after exposure
- Rh negative women with confirmed or suspected ectopic should receive anti D.

Congenital Anomalies Associated with MTX

I. CNS abnormalities
- Spina bifida
- Hydrocephaly
- Anencephaly
- Mental retardation

II. Skeletal abnormalities
- Synostosis of lambdoid sutures
- Partial or absent ossification of bones
- Micrognathia
- Cleft lip or palate
- Broad depressed nasal bone
- Hypertelorism
- Short limbs
- Syndactyly
- Absent digits
- Clubfoot.

III. Dextrocardia

IV. IUGR

Predictors of MTX Treatment Failure

- Presence of fetal cardiac activity
- Gestational mass > 4 cm
- hCG > 5000 mIU/mL
- Free blood in peritoneal cavity
- Rapidly increasing hCG concentrations before initiation of MTX treatment (> 50% rise in 48 hours)
- Continued rapid increase in hCG levels during treatment

Future Fertility and Risk of Recurrence

- ≈ 30% will have difficulty conceiving
- ≈ 77% → overall conception rate regardless of mode of management
- 5–20% → risk of recurrence
- 32% → risk with 2 consecutive ectopic pregnancies.

Note:
- Medical treatment fails in ≈ 5–10% of cases and rate is higher in pregnancy > 6 weeks gestation and tubal mass > 4 cm in diameter
- Failure of medical therapy requires retreatment, either medically or elective surgery
- If tubal rupture occurs (5–10% cases) → emergency surgery
- If patient is treated as outpatient, rapid transportation must be readily available
- Gastrointestinal symptoms associated with MTX therapy may mimic a ruptured ectopic, therefore, abdominal and pleuritic pain, weakness, dizziness or syncope together with hemorrhage must be reported promptly to rule out ruptured ectopic due to treatment failure.

Expectant Management

Based on the fact that the natural course of many early ectopic pregnancies is a self-limiting process, ultimately resulting in tubal abortion or reabsorption

Can be employed, if
- Clinically stable patient
- Pregnancy < 6 weeks
- Declining or stable β hCG levels
- Patient bleeding but not in pain
- Lower β hCG levels associated with best outcome (< 200 mIU/mL)
- Adnexal mass < 3.5–4 cm
- Patient returning for β hCG measurements and sonography at repeated intervals.

Heterotopic Pregnancy

- ≈1% of pregnancies resulting from assisted reproduction are heterotopic
- Of them, ≈ 50% present with acute rupture
- Suspect heterotopic pregnancy, if a patient underwent an abortion of an intrauterine pregnancy and still experiences persistent adnexal pain with abnormal β-hCG levels
- Treatment
  - Ultrasound guided ablation or laparoscopic removal of the extrauterine fetus
  - Intrauterine pregnancy to continue normally
  - MTX is contraindicated in them.

Interstitial Pregnancy

- Accounts for ≈ 2–4% of all ectopics
- Occurs when the gestational sac implants in the intramyometrial segment of the fallopian tube
- Risk factors
  - Prior salpingectomy
  - Pregnancy after IVF
- Highly morbid
  - Can lead to life-threatening hemorrhage because of the proximity of the uterine artery to the fallopian tube
  - Late presentation (as surrounding myometrium allows it to enlarge painlessly)

- Because this segment of the tube is highly distensible, interstitial pregnancies usually manifest at 8–10 weeks but may be seen as late as the 16th week of gestation
- Associated with very high serum β hCG levels
- If cardiac activity is present, direct injection of potassium chloride into the embryo along with systemic MTX is suggested
- USG features:
  - An eccentrically located gestational sac surrounded by myometrium either partially or by a thin layer measuring < 5 mm
  - Interstitial line sign, which represents "an echogenic line that extends into the upper regions of the uterine horn and borders the margin of the intramural gestational sac".

Cornual Pregnancy

- Refers to the implantation of a blastocyst within the cornua of a bicornuate or septate uterus
- Rare entity (< 1% of all ectopic pregnancies)
- Its rupture leads to massive bleeding
- USG features:
  - Gestational sac is surrounded by a thin rim (< 5 mm) of myometrium
  - The sac is in an eccentric position and is > 1 cm from the lateral wall of the endometrial cavity.

Cervical Pregnancy

- Occurs when implantation takes place within the endocervical canal, at times extending into lower uterine segment
- Rare (<1% of all ectopics)
- Etiology:
  - In vitro fertilization
  - History of prior curettage
- USG features:
  - Uterus may be shaped like an hourglass or a figure eight (8), as the fetus expands within the cervix
  - Cardiac activity below the internal os - highly suggestive of a cervical pregnancy
  - Normal endometrial stripe
- Differential diagnosis – inevitable abortion
  - Gentle manipulation of the gestational sac will differentiate a cervical pregnancy from an abortion in progress
  - If the sliding sign is seen (transducer probe can manipulate the gestational sac), this confirms that the gestational sac is not adherent to the cervix (excluding cervical pregnancy) and that the patient is aborting
  - Presence of cardiac activity excludes abortion in progress
  - In case of spontaneous abortion, sac shape and location should change on repeat scans
  - Doppler shows a hypervascular trophoblastic ring in cases of live cervical pregnancies
- Management:
  Tends to bleed profusely if surgical procedure is performed because of the large amount of fibrous tissue in the cervix. Therefore, three possible treatment modalities:
  - Direct percutaneous injection of potassium chloride under USG guidance (1–3 mL of 2 mEq/mL [2 mmol/lit]) OR
  - MTX systemic or local, when cardiac activity is present OR
  - Preoperative uterine artery embolization before D and E.

Hoffman Criteria for Cervical Pregnancy

- Echo free uterine cavity or presence of false gestational sac
- Decidual transformation of endometrium with dense echo structure
- Diffuse uterine wall structure
- Hourglass uterine shape
- Ballooned cervical canal
- Gestation sac in endocervix
- Placental tissue in cervical canal
- Closed internal os.

Ovarian Pregnancy

- Occurs when an ovum is fertilized and is retained within the ovary
- Account for 3% of ectopic pregnancies
- Strongly associated with the use of intrauterine devices
- Often manifest at the same time as tubal pregnancies
- The presence of:
  - Gestational sac
  - Chorionic villi, or
  - An atypical cyst with a hyperechoic ring within the ovary
  - Along with the normal fallopian tubes, is suggestive of an ovarian pregnancy
- First line management is surgery.

Scar (Cesarean) Pregnancy

- Prevalence – <1% of all pregnancies
- Implantation takes place within the scar of a prior cesarean section (most common site)
- Blastocyst is surrounded by myometrium and fibrous tissue
- Can be present in any uterine scar
- Symptoms:
  - Vaginal bleeding as early as 5–6 weeks and as late as 16 weeks
  - These pregnancies may also rupture, resulting in severe hemorrhage and collapse
- USG features:
  - An empty uterus
  - Empty cervical canal
  - Development of the sac in the anterior part of the lower uterine segment
  - Absence of myometrium between the bladder wall and the gestational sac.

Intra-abdominal Pregnancy

- Intraperitoneal implantation, typically in ligaments of ovary, obtaining blood supply from omentum and abdominal organs
- Seen separately from uterus, adnexa and ovaries
- Rare -1.4% of all ectopic pregnancies
- Catastrophic hemorrhage occurs, leading to almost 8 times higher maternal mortality when compared to ectopics in other locations
- May continue till term
- Treatment is surgical—laparotomy or laparoscopy.

ABORTION

Expulsion of the fetus from uterus either spontaneously or by induction before the period of viability, i.e. 22 weeks.

Types

i. Missed abortion
ii. Threatened abortion
iii. Inevitable abortion
iv. Incomplete abortion
v. Complete abortion.

} Spectrum of the same process

Missed Abortion

- Embryonic or fetal demise
- Products of conception are dead and retained inside uterine cavity
- Also called 'silent miscarriage'
- No signs and symptoms of abortion
- Vitals stable
- Usually in 1st trimester, sometimes missed abortion proceeds to form a blood mole where the fetus and placenta are surrounded by clotted blood within the capsular decidua. If a blood mole is retained in the uterus for some months, the fluid becomes absorbed and the fleshy hard mass which remains is called a 'carneous mole'.

History

- History of amenorrhea
- Brownish vaginal discharge
- Regressing symptoms of pregnancy:
  - Nausea/vomiting
  - Breast changes.

Diagnosis

- Vitals stable
- Uterine size (↓) → after considerable time has elapsed (minimum 2 weeks)
- FHS absent when supposed to be heard
- Cervix – uneffaced, os closed; feels firm
- No bleeding.

USG

- Embryonic pole ≥ 5 mm without fetal cardiac activity, or
- Embryonic pole < 5 mm and no interval growth over one week.

Whatever be the measurements, it is preferable to do a repeat scan before labeling it as missed abortion.

Note:
- For cardiac activity you can wait till 10 weeks provided CRL is increasing
- CRL 10 mm but no cardiac activity → missed abortion.

UPT
- Becomes absent.

Complications (though rare)
- DIC → they are autolyzed → thromboplastin released → initiate the coagulation mechanism
- Infection → any dead tissue is a nidus for infection → sepsis.

Management
- Admission
- Investigations
  - Hemoglobin
  - Urine routine
  - Blood group
  - Coagulation profile
- Termination
  - 1st trimester
    - Surgical (suction evacuation or D and C)
    - Medical – 800 mcg misoprostol single dose per vaginally preferably (NICE 2012)
    - Can be given orally if patient hesitant for vaginal route
    - If bleeding does not start after 24 hours-report back
    - Do not give mifepristone
  - 2nd trimester → medical, using prostaglandins
- Investigate the cause of abortion.

Threatened Abortion
- 'Warning signal'
- History of amenorrhea (<20 weeks)
- Vaginal bleeding → minimal/moderate
- Pain abdomen/backache → mild pain/cramping.

Diagnosis
- Vitals stable
- Per-speculum: minimal bleeding/spotting through os present
- Uterine size corresponds to period of gestation
- Cervix uneffaced
- Internal os closed.

USG
- Cardiac activity present
- Subchorionic hemorrhage may be present.

Management
- Admission/ambulatory care
- Investigations
  - Hemoglobin
  - Urine routine-very important
  - Blood group.

Advice on Discharge

- Bed rest
- Coitus contraindicated
- Progesterone supplements → natural micronized progesterone
- Investigate and treat the cause
- May or may not miscarry
- **Only abortion which has expectant line of management.**

Inevitable Abortion

- History of amenorrhea
- Vaginal bleeding – moderate → becomes severe at the time of expulsion
- Pain in abdomen- moderate/severe.

Diagnosis

- Vitals stable
- General condition proportionate to visible blood loss
- P/S: bleeding through os present
- P/V:
  - Uterine size corresponds to period of gestation
  - Uterus tender, firm
  - Cervix- effaced
  - Internal os open
  - Products of conception → felt at os
- Miscarriage unavoidable.

USG

- Products of conception visible
- Fetal cardiac activity may or may not be present.

Management

- Admission
- Investigations
  - Hemoglobin
  - Urine routine
  - Blood group and type
- Expedite the process of abortion
  - 1st trimester: surgical
  - 2nd trimester: medical
- Investigate the cause.

Incomplete Abortion

- Very important where we can lose the mother
- Commonest type
- History of amenorrhea
- Vaginal bleeding—moderate/severe

- Pain abdomen – moderate/severe
- History of having passed products of conception but not complete.

Diagnosis

- Vitals may be stable or patient is in hypovolemic shock
- P/S: profuse bleeding through os present
- P/V
  - Uterine size < period of gestation
  - Uterus tender, firm
  - Cervix – effaced; internal os partly closed
  - Products of conception felt at os
- Most likely to occur in 2nd trimester.

USG

- Irregular, heterogeneous and/or echogenic material along endometrial stripe or in cervical canal suggestive of retained products.

Management

- Admission
- Investigations
  - Hemoglobin
  - Blood group and type
- Resuscitation
- Investigate the cause
- Complete the process of abortion as fast as possible
- Can be managed surgically or medically
- Medical Rx:
  600 µg misoprostol per vaginally (single dose)
  Repeat UPT after 3 weeks

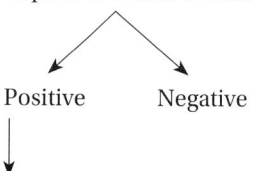

Positive   Negative

Report to exclude molar pregnancy or ectopic
- Surgical Rx:
  If gestational age ≤ 13 weeks

- Vacuum aspiration (misoprostol 400 µg sublingually or 600 µg orally can be given before evacuation to speed up the process).

Complete Abortion

History

- Amenorrhea (usually within first 8 weeks)
- Vaginal bleeding (moderate/severe)

- Pain in abdomen (cramps)
- Expulsion of a fleshy mass/POCs
- On examination:
  - Patient stable
  - Abdominal pain absent
  - Minimal spotting or no bleeding
  - Uterine size smaller than period of gestation
  - Feel of uterus-firm
  - Internal os closed.

USG

- Uterus empty
- Endometrial lining may be thickened
- Rule out any remaining bits (though rare).

Management

- No further treatment required.

Anembryonic Gestation

Definition

- Pregnancy in which a gestational sac develops without development of any embryonic structures; previously referred to as an "empty sac" or "blighted ovum".

USG

- Gestational sac > 13 mm without yolk sac, OR
- 18 mm without embryonic pole, OR
- Empty sac beyond 38 days' gestation and no interval growth over one week

Note: Anti-D to be given in all cases where deemed necessary.

MEDICAL TERMINATION OF PREGNANCY

Can be given at all periods of gestation with different doses and regimens.

Regimen I

First 7 weeks (49 days)
Mifepristone 200 mg orally

↓

After 24–48 hours

↓

Misoprostol (400 µg orally OR 800 µg sublingually OR 800 µg vaginally OR 800 µg by buccal route)

From 7–9 weeks (49–63 days)
Same as above except that oral route of misoprostol is contraindicated.

From 9-12 weeks (63-84 days)
Mifepristone 200 mg orally

↓

After 36-48 hours

↓

Misoprostol (800 µg vaginally) followed by

↓

200 µg misoprostol either vaginally or sublingually every 3 hours (a total of 4 doses).

From 12-24 weeks
Mifepristone 200 mg orally

↓

After 36-48 hours

↓

Misoprostol (800 µg vaginally OR 400 µg orally) followed by

↓

400 µg misoprostol either vaginally or sublingually every 3 hours (a total of 4 doses).

From 24 weeks onwards
Dose of misoprostol should be reduced as the gestation advances, as the uterus becomes more and more responsive even to minor doses.

Regimen II

Till 12 weeks
800 µg misoprostol vaginally OR sublingually followed by

↓

800 µg misoprostol every 3 hourly (a total of 4 doses, i.e. for a total duration of 12 hours).

From 12-24 weeks
Misoprostol 400 µg vaginally OR sublingually every 3 hourly (a total of 5 doses).

From 24 weeks onwards
Same as above.

SURGICAL TERMINATION OF PREGNANCY

Up to 12 weeks
- Vacuum aspiration
- Should not be followed by sharp curettage or D and C
- No need for cervical preparation but can be done as per the situation

From 12–24 weeks
- Dilatation and evacuation – safest and most effective
- Cervical preparation becomes obligatory
  - Misoprostol 400 µg sublingually or vaginally 2–3 hours prior to the procedure.

GESTATIONAL TROPHOBLASTIC DISEASE (GTD)

Broad term encompassing both benign and malignant growths arising from products of conception in the uterus.

Classification

Hydatidiform mole (HM)
- Complete HM
- Partial HM.

Gestational trophoblastic tumours
- Invasive mole
- Choriocarcinoma
- Placental-site trophoblastic tumour (very rare)
- Epithelioid trophoblastic tumour (even more rare).

Note:
Gestational trophoblastic neoplasia (can progress, invade, metastasize, and lead to death if left untreated).

Incidence and Risk Factors

- Varies worldwide, from a low of 23 per 100,000 pregnancies (Paraguay) to a high of 1,299 per 100,000 pregnancies (Indonesia).

Two factors have consistently been associated with an increased risk of GTD:
- Maternal age
- Prior history of H. mole
  - With previously diagnosed 1 H. mole, risk in subsequent pregnancy is 1%
  - Risk is 25% if > 1 prior HM
  - Age < 21 years and > 35 years
- Another reported obstetric risk factor for both complete and partial moles is a **history of spontaneous abortion**, increasing the risk to 2- to 3-fold
- Only consistent environmental association with an inverse relationship is between β carotene and animal fat dietary intake with the incidence of molar pregnancy
- Ovulation induction is also linked to have increased risk of molar pregnancy
- Risk factors for choriocarcinoma:
  - Prior complete hydatidiform mole (1000 times more likely when compared with normal pregnancy)
  - Ethnicity (increased in women of Asian and American Indian descent as well as African Americans)
  - Advanced maternal age (particularly for mothers > 45 years)
  - Long-term oral contraceptive use
  - Blood group A.

Hydatidiform Mole

- Refers to an abnormal pregnancy characterized by varying degrees of trophoblastic proliferation (both cytotrophoblast and syncytiotrophoblast) and gross vesicular swellings of chorionic villi associated with an absent or an abnormal fetus/embryo
- The etymology is derived from hydatisia (Greek "a drop of water"), referring to the watery contents of the cysts, and mole (from Latin mola – "millstone/false conception"). The term, however, comes from the similar appearance of the cyst to a hydatid cyst in an echinococcosis
- There is disintegration and loss of blood vessels in the villous core.

Complete Hydatidiform Mole

- Occurs when an ovum *that has extruded* its maternal nucleus (i.e. empty ovum) is fertilized by either
  - A single sperm (75–80%), with subsequent chromosome duplication, always yielding a mole with karyotype of 46 XX (since at least one X chromosome is required for viability and a karyotype of 46 YY is rapidly lethal to the ovum)
  OR
  - Two sperms (20–25%) yielding either a karyotype of 46 XX or 46 XY
- Androgenic in origin
- Always results in either case, a diploid karyotype
- **Rarely** reveals a fetus or amniotic fluid
- Diffuse swelling of villi
- Diffuse trophoblastic hyperplasia with varying degrees of atypia
- hCG often > 100,000 mIU/mL
- Absent scalloping of chorionic villi
- Absent trophoblastic stromal inclusions
- Gestational age at presentation is 6–16 weeks (mostly)
- USG: Characteristic vesicular pattern consisting of multiples echoes (holes) within the placental mass and usually no fetus
- Risk of developing into an invasive mole is 15–25%
- Need for chemotherapy is in 15% of cases
- Other obstetric and medical complications:
  - Vaginal bleeding in 80–90%
  - Undue enlargement of uterus in ≈ 28%
  - Anemia in ≈ 5%
- Preeclampsia (H. mole to be considered when PE develops in 1st and 2nd trimester) in 1%
- Hyperemesis (8%)
- Hyperthyroidism
  - Secondary to the homology between the beta-subunits of hCG and TSH, which causes hCG to have weak TSH-like activity
  - After evacuation TFT returns to normal
- Theca lutein ovarian cysts
  - ≈6 cm in diameter
  - In 15–50% cases
  - Abdominal distension/pelvic pressure
- Rarer symptoms
  - Thyroid storm (anesthesia and surgery may precipitate it)
    - Hyperthermia
    - Delirium
    - Convulsions

- Trophoblastic embolization
    - Chest pain
    - Dyspnea
    - Tachypnea
    - Tachycardia
    - Severe respiratory distress
    - Diffuse rales on auscultation
    - Bilateral pulmonary infiltrates on CXR
- Neurologic symptoms
    - Resulting from brain metastases, such as seizures in a female within the reproductive age group.

Partial Hydatidiform Mole

- Occurs when the ovum *retains its nucleus* but is fertilized by either–
    - Two sperms (90%) and the resulting triploid karyotypes are 69 XXY, 69 XXX, or 69 XYY
    OR
    - By a single sperm, with subsequent chromosome duplication (10% cases)
- Chromosomes of a partial mole are only 2/3rd paternal in origin
- 10% of partial moles represent tetraploid or mosaic conceptions
- Gestational age at presentation ≈ 24–26 weeks
- Uterus size corresponds to POG or smaller than that (SGA or IUGR)
- Chorionic villi with focal edema that vary in size and shape and scalloping
- Focal trophoblastic hyperplasia with mild atypia only
- hCG usually <100,000 mIU/mL
- Prominent trophoblastic stromal inclusions present
- Functioning villous circulation
- They have signs and symptoms of *incomplete or missed abortion*
- Main presenting symptom is vaginal bleeding, which occurs in ≈ 75% of patients
- Medical complications - rare
- USG
    - Usually shows a fetus, which may even be viable and amniotic fluid is visible
    - Cystic spaces in the placenta and a ratio of transverse to anteroposterior dimension of the gestation sac of >1.5, is required for the reliable diagnosis of a partial molar pregnancy
- Transformation to malignancy is rare (<5%)
- Merely, 0.5% require chemotherapy.

Suspicion of Persistent Disease

- Persistent GTN should always be suspected when a patient has continued or irregular vaginal bleeding (most common symptom) in the post-delivery period, although most commonly it follows a molar pregnancy but can follow a normal pregnancy, ectopic pregnancy, or abortion
→ *perform UPT after 3 weeks*
- As persistent trophoblastic neoplasia may develop after any pregnancy, it is recommended to have histological examination in cases of *all failed pregnancies (where USG could not recognize fetal parts or was not done or there was a difficulty in making a diagnosis of molar pregnancy) and repeat D and Cs*
- GTD should be considered whenever a premenopausal woman presents with:
    - Rapidly enlarging uterus
    - Irregular vaginal bleeding
- The most common antecedent pregnancy in GTD is that of an H. mole.

Management

Patient has come with bleeding per vaginam. How will you suspect it to be a molar pregnancy??

Step I → Complete history/ physical examination/check vitals
Step II → Send basic investigations (CBC, urine routine, ABO Rh, HIV, UPT and most important β hCG)
Step III → Perform USG
Step IV → Review all reports
Step V → GTD confirmed → Send additional investigations

- LFT, RFT, Thyroid function tests
- CXR (lungs are a primary site of metastasis for malignant trophoblastic tumours)
- ECG, if appropriate
- Head CT/MRI (in case of choriocarcinoma or central nervous system signs)
- ECHO, only in suspected cases of acute left ventricular failure due to anemia, thyrotoxicosis, pulmonary embolization, etc.

Step VII → Ask the patient whether she desires future fertility
Step VIIa → Yes → Evacuate the uterus (if hemodynamically stable)
Step VIIb → No → Can proceed with hysterectomy.

Blood availability should be confirmed prior to evacuation (especially when uterine size is > 16 weeks).

Evacuation of Molar Pregnancy

Suction curettage – irrespective of the uterine size except when fetal parts are large enough (as in case of partial mole) making suction evacuation impossible, then medical evacuation is done (v. rarely)

↓

Anesthesia

↓

Cervical preparation ***immediately*** before the procedure

↓

12–14 mm suction cannula passes into lower uterine segment → rotated → contents sucked

↓

Gentle sharp curettage

↓

Oxytocin infusion (saline drip with 30 units of syntocinon running at 30 drops/min) at the onset of evacuation, continued for several hours after

↓

Reassuring signs:
Prompt uterine involution
Cessation of bleeding
Ovarian cyst regression

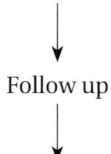

Follow up

Repeat hCG after 1–2 weeks of evacuation (within 6–8 weeks) to see for regression, till 3 consecutive tests show normal levels
[to detect trophoblastic sequelae (invasive mole or choriocarcinoma)]

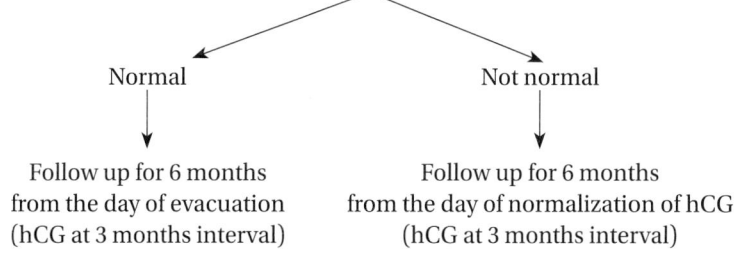

Normal	Not normal
Follow up for 6 months from the day of evacuation (hCG at 3 months interval)	Follow up for 6 months from the day of normalization of hCG (hCG at 3 months interval)

Hysterectomy

- Alternative to suction evacuation, if family completed
- The adnexa may be left intact even in the presence of prominent theca lutein cysts
- Advantages:
  - Evacuates molar pregnancy
  - Provides permanent sterilization
  - Eliminates the risk of local myometrial invasion as a cause of persistent disease

Is the patient free from metastasis after hysterectomy?
No, it has the potential to metastasize even after hysterectomy in ≈ 3–5% of cases, therefore, follow with serial β hCG and subsequent chemotherapy, if required.

Anesthesia during Evacuation

- Hemodynamically stable patient → spinal anesthesia (preferable)
- Advantages over general anesthesia include:
  - Ease of technique
  - Favorable effects on the pulmonary system
  - Safety in patients with hyperthyroidism and non-tocolytic pharmacological properties
  - Additionally, by maintaining patient's consciousness one can diagnose the complications like uterine perforation, cardiopulmonary distress and thyroid storm at an earlier stage than when the patient is sedated or is under general anesthesia
- Hemodynamically unstable or have a coagulation defect → general anesthesia.

Note:
- >50% patients will show regression within 2 months of evacuation
- There is **no** need to send the POCs for **histological examination** in confirmed cases of molar pregnancy

- Effective contraception is important
  - **During the follow-up period** (to avoid confusion occurring with a rising β hCG as a result of pregnancy)
    - OCPs and barrier methods during entire hormonal follow up period
    - IUCD should not be used until hCG levels are normal to reduce the risk of uterine perforation
    - Advantages of using OCPs:
      - They suppress endogenous luteinizing hormone, which may interfere with measurement of hCG at low levels
      - They do not increase the risk of postmolar trophoblastic neoplasia
  - **Further continuation** of contraception should be for 6 months after the first normal hCG
- **Prophylactic administration** of single chemotherapeutic agent at the time of evacuation or immediately after, reduces the risk of postmolar GTN from 15–20% to 3–8%
  Various agents and doses:
  - Methotrexate 50 mg IV drip lasting for 3–4 hours during evacuation
  - Actinomycin D IV 12 µg/kg daily (3 days prior and 2 days after)
  - Methotrexate 15 mg orally daily (3 days prior and 2 days after).

1. **Why complete molar pregnancy is not terminated by medical management?**
   Reasons:
   1. Oxytocic agents → contraction of the myometrium → embolization and dissemination of trophoblastic tissue through the venous system → profound deterioration of the patient → embolism and metastasis occurring in the lung
   2. Also these patients may be at increased risk for requiring treatment for persistent trophoblastic disease
   3. There can be increased blood loss
   4. Incomplete evacuation requiring dilatation and curettage is followed by cesarean section in subsequent pregnancies
   5. Evacuation of complete molar pregnancies with mifepristone and misoprostol should be avoided since it increases the sensitivity of the uterus to prostaglandins.

2. **Is prophylaxis with anti-D required?**
   Since there is poor vascularization of chorionic villi and absence of the anti-D antigen in complete moles, anti-D prophylaxis is not required but is very much required in partial moles.

3. **What is the fate of a twin pregnancy occurring with a mole?**
   Occurs once in every 22,000–100,000 pregnancies
   Twin gestation, a normal fetus and a complete mole, can have the following outcomes:
   a. 25% chance of live birth ⎫ if allowed to
   b. 36% risk of preterm labor and delivery ⎭ continue
   c. Risks
      - 40% chance of early fetal loss
      - 20% chance of preeclampsia
      - Increased risk of hemorrhage
      - Development of persistent GTN
   d. In many cases, it is not clear whether the pregnancy is a complete mole with a coexisting normal twin or a partial mole → ultrasound and prenatal fetal karyotype helps in such cases to differentiate between chromosomally normal, potentially viable fetuses and triploid nonviable fetuses
   e. Management by suction evacuation and curettage.

4. **Are there any factors, which can increase the likelihood of persistence of the disease?**
   In women with complete mole, risk of persistence or neoplastic transformation is approximately doubled in the setting of certain characteristics, which include the following:
   - Age > 35 years or age < 20 years
   - Pre-evacuation serum β hCG >100,000 mIU/mL
   - Large-for-date uterus
   - Large uterine molar mass
   - Large (>6 cm) ovarian cysts
   - Preeclampsia
   - Hyperthyroidism
   - Hyperemesis of pregnancy
   - Trophoblastic embolization
   - Disseminated intravascular coagulation.

5. **When will you suspect a persistent disease (GTN-invasive mole or choriocarcinoma)?**
   Components needed to diagnose post-molar GTN:
   - A rising β hCG titer of > 20% for 2 consecutive weeks (3 titers)
   - A tissue diagnosis of choriocarcinoma
   - A plateau of the β hCG (decrease of ≤ 10%) for 4 consecutive values over a period of 3 weeks
   - Persistence of detectable β hCG 6 months after mole evacuation
   - Metastatic disease
   - An elevation in β hCG after a normal value
   - Postevacuation hemorrhage not caused by retained tissues.

   GTN suspected/established → further metastatic workup and evaluation of risk factors
   1. Complete history and physical examination
   2. CBC including platelets
   3. Coagulation studies
   4. RFT/LFT
   5. ABO Rh
   6. Quantitative s. β hCG
   7. Pelvic ultrasound
   8. CXR → if chest X-ray is negative → CT scan of the chest
   9. CT scans of the abdomen and pelvis
   10. CT scan or MRI of the brain.

6. **Repeat curettage—Is there a role?**
   - Generally not recommended unless there is excessive uterine bleeding and evidence of intracavitary molar tissue exists on scan because it does not often induce remission or influence treatment and it may result in uterine perforation and hemorrhage.

7. **Now these patients are candidates for chemotherapy. What to give?**
   - Given the extremely good therapeutic outcomes of most of these tumours, an important goal is to distinguish patients who need less intensive therapies from those who require more intensive regimens to achieve a cure
   - Therefore, before chemotherapy, assess the woman with modified WHO and FIGO scoring system.

FIGO ANATOMICAL STAGING

Stage I: Disease confined to the uterus
Stage II: GTN extends outside of the uterus, but is limited to the genital structures (adnexa, vagina, broad ligament)

Stage III: GTN extends to the lungs, with or without known genital tract involvement
Stage IV: All other metastatic sites.

Modified WHO Prognostic Scoring System				
Scores	0	1	2	4
Age	<40	≥ 40	-	-
Antecedent pregnancy	Mole	Abortion	Term	-
Interval months from index pregnancy	<4	4-6	7-12	>12
Pretreatment s.hCG (IU/L)	$<10^3$	10^3-10^4	10^4-10^5	$> 10^5$
Largest tumour size (including uterus)	<3	3-4 cm	≥ 5 cm	-
Site of metastasis	Lung	Spleen, kidney	Gastrointestinal	Liver, brain
Number of metastasis	-	1-4	5-8	>8
Previous failed chemotherapy	-	-	Single drug	More drugs

Nonmetastatic stage I and low-risk metastatic (stage II, III and score 0-6) GTN
- Treated with single agent
- 3 protocols most popularly used
  - The 8-day Charing Cross regimen
    Methotrexate 50 mg IM (or 1 mg/kg) on days 1, 3, 5, and 7
    and
    Folinic acid 7.5 mg orally (or 0.1 mg/kg IM) on days 2, 4, 6, and 8 followed by Rest for 6 days
  - MTX 0.4 mg/kg (maximum 25 mg) per day IV or IM for 5 d; repeat every 14 days
  - Methotrexate can also be given as a weekly regimen, 30–50 mg/m² IM
- Cure rate ≈ 100%
- Multi-agent chemotherapy to be started, if
  - Significant elevation in hCG level
  - Development of metastases
  - Resistance to sequential single-agent chemotherapy
- Regardless of the treatment protocol used, chemotherapy is continued until hCG values have returned to normal and at least 1 course has been administered after the first normal hCG level.

High-risk metastatic GTN (FIGO stage IV and stages II-III score ≥ 7)
- Score ≥ 7 → treated with multiple agent therapy (EMA-CO)
- Cure rate ≈ 95%
- Cycles are repeated every 2 weeks (on days 15, 16, and 22) until any metastases present at diagnosis disappear and serum β hCG has normalized, then the treatment is usually continued for an additional 3–4 cycles.

EMA-CO REGIMEN

Day 1
- Etoposide 100 mg/m² IV for 30 min
- Dactinomycin 0.5 mg IV push
- Methotrexate 300 mg/m² IV for 12 h (100 mg/m² IV push, then 200 mg/m² in 500 mL 5% D).

Day 2
- Etoposide 100 mg/m² IV for 30 min
- Dactinomycin 0.5 mg IV push
- Folinic acid 15 mg IM or PO every 12 h × 4 doses, beginning 24 h after the start of methotrexate.

Day 8
- Cyclophosphamide 600 mg/m² IV infusion
- Vincristine 0.8–1.0 mg/m² IV push (maximum dose 2 mg).

When brain metastases are present, 2 options:

Option I
- Whole brain irradiation (3000 cGy in 200-cGy fractions) OR ⎱ Together with
- Surgical excision with stereotactic irradiation in selected patients ⎰ chemotherapy
- Changes in chemotherapy
    - Methotrexate infusion dose in the EMA-CO protocol is increased to 1 g/m²
    - Folinic acid 30 mg every 12 hours for 3 days starting 32 hours after the infusion begins.

Option II
- Intrathecal as well as high-dose IV methotrexate
- Overall cure rates with brain metastases are 50–80%.

The EMA-EP regimen
- Substitutes etoposide and cisplatin for cyclophosphamide and vincristine in the EMA-CO protocol
- Considered the most appropriate therapy for patients who have responded to EMA-CO but have plateauing low β hCG levels or who have developed re-elevation of β hCG levels after a complete response to EMA-CO.

Chances of Cure with GTD

- Prognosis is good even when the disease has spread to distant organs, *especially* when *only* the lungs are involved
- The probability of cure depends on the following:
    - Histologic type (invasive mole or choriocarcinoma)
    - Extent of spread of the disease/largest tumour size
    - Level of s. β hCG
    - Duration of disease from the initial pregnancy event to start of treatment
    - Number and specific sites of metastases
    - Nature of antecedent pregnancy
    - Extent of prior treatment.

Future Conception

- No conception until follow up is complete
- Those who received chemotherapy should not conceive for 1 year after completion of treatment
- Risks, if conception occurs before this:
    - Increased risk of miscarriage/stillbirth
    - Congenital anomalies (1.8% risk)
- Recommendation for all future pregnancies
    - Histopathologic examination of placenta and other products of conception
    - Determination of a 6-week postpartum β hCG level.

Long-term Outcome

- Earlier menopause in those who received chemotherapy
  - With single agent, it's advanced by 1 year
  - With multiple drug used, advanced by 3 years
- High-risk patients may be at increased risk of secondary cancers (with the use of etoposide), if treatment was extended to > 6 months
- Secondary cancers include:
  - Acute myeloid leukemia
  - Colon cancer
  - Melanoma
  - Breast cancer.

GESTATIONAL TROPHOBLASTIC NEOPLASIA

Overview

- ***Postmolar*** GTN (invasive mole or choriocarcinoma) most commonly presents as—
  - Irregular bleeding (most common) following evacuation of a hydatidiform mole
  - An enlarged, irregular uterus
  - Persistent bilateral ovarian enlargement
  - Occasionally, a metastatic vaginal lesion may be noted on evacuation, disruption of which may cause uncontrolled bleeding
- Choriocarcinoma associated with ***nonmolar*** gestation
  - Has no characteristic symptoms or signs, which are mostly related to invasion of tumour in the uterus or at metastatic sites
- In patients with postpartum uterine bleeding and subinvolution, GTN should be considered along with other possible causes
- Other symptoms:

  Bleeding as a result of uterine perforation or metastatic lesions
  - Abdominal pain
  - Hemoptysis
  - Melena

  Increased intracranial pressure from intracerebral hemorrhage
  - Headaches
  - Seizures
  - Hemiplegia

  Pulmonary symptoms
  - Dyspnea
  - Cough
  - Chest pain, caused by extensive lung metastases
- PSTTs and ETTs
  - Almost always cause irregular uterine bleeding often distant from a preceding nonmolar gestation, and rarely virilization or nephrotic syndrome
  - The uterus is usually symmetrically enlarged and serum hCG levels are only slightly elevated.

Invasive Mole (Chorioadenoma Destruens)

- Locally invasive, benign in nature
- Rarely metastatic

- May be preceded by either complete or partial molar pregnancy (in 10–17% of cases)
- Usually diploid in karyotype, but may have aneuploidy
- Microscopically, they show:
  - Trophoblastic invasion of the myometrium via direct extension through tissue or venous channels
  - Identifiable villous structures
  - Hyperplasia of cytotrophoblastic and syncytial elements
  - May resemble choriocarcinoma in histologic appearance
- Have more aggressive behavior than either complete or partial HMs
- Most often diagnosed clinically (without a histopathologic diagnosis), based on persistent hCG elevation after molar evacuation
- Mode of treatment—chemotherapy
- Have potential to regress spontaneously
- 15% metastatic → lung/vagina.

Choriocarcinoma

- Malignant tumour of the trophoblastic epithelium, characterized by:
  - Abnormal trophoblastic hyperplasia and anaplasia
  - Absence of chorionic villi
  - Hemorrhage
  - Necrosis
  - Direct invasion into myometrium
  - Vascular invasion resulting in spread to distant sites:
    - Lungs
    - Brain
    - Liver
    - Pelvis
    - Vagina
    - Spleen
    - Intestines
    - Kidney
- Aneuploid karyotype (mostly) and 3/4th of them contain a Y chromosome
- Occurs:
  - After a molar pregnancy in 50% of cases
  - After spontaneous abortion or ectopic pregnancy in 25% of cases
  - After full-term or preterm pregnancy in 25%
- ***Nearly all GTDs that are preceded by nonmolar pregnancies are choriocarcinomas***; the rare exceptions generally are PSTTs.

Treatment

- Treatment (chemotherapy) of invasive mole and choriocarcinoma depends on the risk category determined by the Modified WHO Prognostic Scoring System as adapted by FIGO
- Prompt institution of therapy and continuing follow-up at very close intervals until normal β hCG titers are obtained is the cornerstone of management.

Placental Site Trophoblastic Tumour (PSTT)

- A very rare tumour arising from the placental implantation site and resembles an exaggerated form of syncytial endometritis

- Consists predominantly of mononuclear intermediate trophoblasts without chorionic villi
- Trophoblastic cells infiltrate the myometrium
- Vascular invasion, hemorrhage and necrosis are much less as compared to choriocarcinoma
- Has propensity for lymphatic metastasis
- Human placental lactogen is present in the tumour cells, whereas immunoperoxidase staining for β hCG is positive in only scattered cells
- Elevations in serum β hCG are relatively low, therefore, is not considered a reliable tumour marker
- Much lower growth rates than choriocarcinoma
- More often diploid than aneuploid
- Most of them follow nonmolar gestations. Presentation after a full-term pregnancy is often delayed by months or years
- Resistant to chemotherapy, making hysterectomy the standard primary treatment when the tumour is confined to the uterus
- About 35% of PSTTs have distant metastases at diagnosis. Common sites include:
  - Lungs
  - Pelvis
  - Lymph nodes
- Less common sites:
  - Central nervous system
  - Kidneys
  - Liver metastases.

Management

Resistant to Chemotherapy

Treatment options:

Tumours confined to the uterus (FIGO Stage I)
- Hysterectomy is the treatment of choice.

Tumours with extrauterine spread to genital structures (FIGO stage II)
- Complete resection with or without adjuvant multi-agent chemotherapy.

Metastatic tumours (FIGO stages III and IV)
- Polyagent chemotherapy. Regimens include:
  - EMA/CO: Etoposide, methotrexate with folinic acid rescue, dactinomycin, cyclophosphamide, and vincristine. This appears to be the most commonly used regimen
  - EP/EMA: Etoposide and cisplatin with etoposide, methotrexate, and dactomycin
  - MAE: Methotrexate with folinic acid rescue, dactinomycin, and etoposide.

Note: Chemotherapy is also used in nonmetastatic tumours in the following cases:
a. Interval from last known pregnancy to diagnosis is >2 years
b. Deep myometrial invasion
c. Tumour necrosis
d. Mitotic count > 6/10 high power fields.

Survival Rate

- Nonmetastatic disease ≈ 100%
- Metastatic disease ≈ 50–60%.

Epithelioid Trophoblastic Tumour (ETT)

- An extremely rare variant of PSTT that simulates carcinoma
- Although originally termed atypical choriocarcinoma, it appears to be less aggressive than choriocarcinoma and is now regarded as a distinct entity
- Pathologically, it has a monomorphic cellular pattern of epithelioid cells and may resemble squamous cell carcinoma of the cervix when arising in the cervical canal
- Clinically resembles PSTT more than choriocarcinoma
- Most ETTs present many years after a full-term delivery
- It has a spectrum of clinical behavior from benign to malignant
- About 1/3rd of patients present with metastases, usually in the lungs.

Management

- Exceedingly rare
- Their behavior and prognosis is similar to placental-site trophoblastic tumours, so it is reasonable to manage them similarly.

Follow-up after Treatment for GTN

- After completion of chemotherapy:
  - Serum quantitative β hCG levels should be obtained at 1-month intervals for 12 months
  - Physical examinations are performed at intervals of 6–12 months
  - X rays or scans → rarely indicated
- Risk of relapse is ≈ 3% in the first year after completing therapy, but is exceedingly low after that
- Resumption of normal ovarian function
- Fertility is not decreased and pregnancy goes uneventful
- Contraception should be maintained during treatment and for 1 year after completion of chemotherapy, preferably using oral contraceptives to allow for:
  - Uninterrupted hCG follow-up, and
  - The elimination of mature ova that may have been damaged by exposure to cytotoxic drugs
- Future pregnancies (1-2% risk of a second GTD):
  - TVS in 1st trimester of subsequent pregnancy
  - Serum quantitative β hCG should be determined 6 weeks after any pregnancy
- There is no evidence of reactivation of disease after subsequent pregnancies.

Management

Recurrent or Chemoresistant Gestational Trophoblastic Neoplasia

- Recurrent disease indicates failure of prior chemotherapy unless initial therapy was surgery alone
- Nearly all recurrences occur within 3 years of remission (85% before 18 months)
- A patient whose disease progresses after primary surgical therapy, is generally treated with single-agent chemotherapy unless one of the poor prognostic factors that requires combination chemotherapy supervenes
- Relapse after prior chemotherapy failure automatically places the patient into the high-risk category. These patients should be treated with aggressive combination chemotherapy

- Long-term disease-free survival, in > 50%, is achievable with combination drug regimens using the following drugs:
  - Cisplatin
  - Etoposide
  - Bleomycin
  - Paclitaxel
  - 5-fluorouracil
  - Floxuridine
- Patients with chemotherapy-resistant and clinically detectable gestational trophoblastic neoplasia may benefit from salvage surgery.

Quiescent Gestational Trophoblastic Disease

- A term applied to a presumed inactive form of GTN
- Characterized by persistent, unchanging low levels (< 200 mIU/mL) of "real" hCG for at least 3 months, associated with a history of GTD or spontaneous abortion, but without clinically detectable disease
- hCG levels do not change with chemotherapy or surgery
- Subanalysis of hCG reveals no hyperglycosylated hCG, which is associated with cytotrophoblastic invasion
- Follow-up reveals subsequent development of active GTN in about one-quarter, which is heralded by an increase in both hyperglycosylated hCG and total hCG
- Management:
  - False-positive β hCG resulting from heterophile antibodies or LH interference should be excluded
  - Patient should be thoroughly investigated for evidence of disease
  - Immediate chemotherapy or surgery should be avoided
  - Patient should be monitored long term with periodic hCG testing
  - Pregnancy avoided
  - Treatment should be undertaken only when there is a sustained rise in hCG or the appearance of overt clinical disease.

Ultrasound Features of Molar Pregnancies

Complete Hydatidiform Mole

- Echogenic mass with multiple, diffusely distributed, small (1–30 mm) vesicles, in an enlarged uterus → the characteristic "cluster of grapes" or "snowstorm" or "honeycomb" appearance
- Absent fetus, except in rare case of coexistent diploid twin pregnancy. The latter could be differentiated from a partial mole by identifying a separate normal placenta
- Theca lutein cysts: Bilateral, multilocular ovarian cysts, some of which may occasionally be complicated by hemorrhage or rupture.

Partial Molar Pregnancy

- An enlarged placenta with nonuniformly distributed cystic spaces (very small in 1st trimester, so may not be apparent)
- A deformed gestational sac
- Fetus—may be alive or dead

- The fetus may be anomalous and demonstrate triploid features, such as growth restriction, hydrocephalus, cleft lip or syndactyly
- Rarely, molar pregnancy may occur in an ectopic location.

Persistent Trophoblastic Neoplasia

- The various types of PTN may appear similar on TVS, focal myometrial mass being the most common, which may be either uniformly echogenic or hypoechoic, or complex and multicystic
- Anechoic spaces within the mass may be due to hemorrhagic or necrotic tissue, cysts, or vascular spaces
- More extensive disease may appear as:
  - A lobulated and heterogeneously enlarged uterus that may be seen extending to adjacent structures, OR
  - A large, undifferentiated pelvic mass
- On Doppler ultrasound:
  - Extreme vascularity secondary to the contained arteriovenous shunts
  - There is loss of vessel discreteness
  - Trophoblastic vessels demonstrate a high-velocity, low-resistance waveform (but these are not specific to GTT).

Placental Site Trophoblastic Tumour

- May occur in either a hypovascular or a hypervascular form
- Hypovascular form is not associated with prominent vascularity on Doppler ultrasound.

SUGGESTED READING

1. Andrew McRae, Marcia Edmonds, Heather Murray. Diagnostic accuracy and clinical utility of emergency department targeted ultrasonography in the evaluation of first-trimester pelvic pain and bleeding: a systematic review. CJEM 2009;11(4):355-64.
2. Andrew W Horne, W Colin Duncan, Hilary OD Critchley. The need for serum biomarker development for diagnosing and excluding tubal ectopic pregnancy. Acta Obstet Gynecol Scand. 2010;89(3):299-301.
3. Clinical Policy: Critical Issues in the Initial Evaluation and Management of Patients Presenting to the Emergency Department in Early Pregnancy. Ann Emerg Med. 2003;41:123-33.
4. Deborah Levine. Ectopic Pregnancy. Radiology: Volume 245: Number 2—November 2007.
5. Diagnosis and treatment of gestational trophoblastic disease. ACOG, 2004, Jun 13.
6. Ectopic pregnancy and miscarriage. NICE clinical guideline 154, December 2012.
7. Ectopic pregnancy and miscarriage: diagnosis and initial management in early pregnancy of ectopic pregnancy and miscarriage, NICE, Dec 2012.
8. Ectopic pregnancy. A Guide for Patients. American Society for Reproductive Medicine.
9. Edward P Lin, Shweta Bhatt Vikram S Dogra. Diagnostic Clues to Ectopic Pregnancy. Radiographics 2008;28:1661-71.
10. Gerulath AH. Gestational trophoblastic disease. SJOGC 2 May 2002.
11. Ghansham Biyani, Sadik Mohammed, Pradeep Bhatia. Anaesthetic Challenges in Molar Pregnancy. The Indian Anaesthetists' Forum. June 2013;14(8):1-9.
12. Hajenius PJ, Mol F, Mol BWJ, Bossuyt PMM, Ankum WM, Van der Veen F. Interventions for tubal ectopic pregnancy (Review), 2009,The Cochrane Collaboration.
13. Jeremy K Brown, Andrew W Horne. Laboratory models for studying ectopic pregnancy. Curr Opin Obstet Gynecol. 2011;23(4):221-6.
14. John R Lurain. Gestational trophoblastic disease I: epidemiology, pathology, clinical presentation and diagnosis of gestational trophoblastic disease and management of hydatidiform mole. American Journal of Obstetrics and Gynecology, Dec 2010.

15. John R Lurain. Gestational trophoblastic disease II: classification and management of gestational trophoblastic neoplasia. American Journal of Obstetrics and Gynecology, Jan 2011.
16. Julie LV Shaw, Andrew W. Horne. The Paracrinology of Tubal Ectopic Pregnancy. Mol Cell Endocrinol. 2012;358(2):216-22.
17. Kimia Khalatbari Kani, Jean H Lee, Manjiri Dighe, Mariam Moshiri, et al. Gestational Trophoblastic Disease: Multimodality Imaging Assessment with Special Emphasis on Spectrum of Abnormalities and Value of Imaging in Staging and Management of Disease. Curr Probl Diagn Radiol. January/February 2012.
18. Kurt Barnhart, Norah M, van Mello, Tom Bourne, Emma Kirk, et al. Pregnancy of unknown location: A consensus statement of nomenclature, definitions and outcome. Fertil Steril. 2011;95(3):857-66.
19. Laparoscopic management of tubal ectopic pregnancy. RCOG. Consent advice No 8, June 2010.
20. Medical management of ectopic pregnancy, ACOG, 2008.
21. Medical treatment of ectopic pregnancy. Fertility and Sterility. Vol 90, Supplement 3, Nov 2008.
22. Mol F, Mol BW, Ankum WM, F Van der Veen and Hajenius PJ. Current evidence on surgery, systemic methotrexate and expectant management in the treatment of tubal ectopic pregnancy: a systematic review and meta-analysis. Human Reproduction Update, Vol.14, No.4 2008; pp. 309-19.
23. Rabbie K Hanna, John T Soper: The Role of Surgery and Radiation Therapy in the Management of Gestational Trophoblastic Disease. The Oncologist 2010;15:593-600.
24. Rinat Hackmon, Sachi Sakaguchi, Gideon Koren. Effect of methotrexate treatment of ectopic pregnancy on subsequent pregnancy. Vol 57: January 2011.
25. Ruijin Shao, Sean X Zhang, Birgitta Weijdega Rd, Shien Zou et al. Nitric oxide synthases and tubal ectopic pregnancies induced by Chlamydia infection: Basic and clinical insights. Molecular Human Reproduction. 2010;16(12):907-15.
26. Ruijin Shao. Understanding the mechanisms of human tubal ectopic pregnancies: new evidence from knockout mouse models. Human Reproduction. 2010;25(3):584-7.
27. Shaw JLV, Dey SK, Critchley HOD, and Horne AW. Current knowledge of the etiology of human tubal ectopic pregnancy. Human Reproduction Update. 2010;16(4):432-44.
28. The management of gestational trophoblastic disease. RCOG Green-top Guideline No. 38, 2010.
29. Undifferentiated vaginal bleeding/abdominal pain suggestive of ectopic pregnancy clinical pathways: department of emergency medicine, 2011, sep 7.

CHAPTER 5

Antepartum Hemorrhage in Late Gestation

Tania G Singh

Case: A patient with antepartum hemorrhage has arrived in the labor ward without any antenatal records which, in a state of hurry, were left at home. What would you like to ask and what will be your line of action?

Management of the Patient Presenting with Antepartum Hemorrhage

Complete History

- Enquire about all the risk factors (leading either to placental abruption or placenta previa)
- Most important is association with pain
- Is the pain continuous or intermittent?
- For how long did she bleed and the amount of bleeding?
- Is she perceiving fetal movements?
- Did she have any leaking per vaginam before the occurrence of bleeding?
- Were there any elevations of blood pressure in previous visits?
- Any previous episodes of bleeding in index pregnancy?
- If yes, was she ever admitted for the same and at what period of gestation?
- Did she have any such bleeding episodes in the previous pregnancies (in case she is a multigravida)?

On enquiring: Patient is a nulliparous woman, presenting with vaginal bleeding. She is not very sure of her dates, as her periods were irregular before pregnancy. She was given an EDD based on her scan, done at 5th month, according to which she is at present 35 weeks 5 days period of gestation. She noticed a small gush of blood and discovered a dark red stain in her underclothes. She denies acute abdominal pain but there is continuous lower abdominal discomfort. Fetal movements are present. BP throughout was normal. All trimesters were uneventful.

On examination
- Pulse rate: 94/min; BP: 158/87 mmHg
- Per abdomen: uterus ≈ 34 weeks size, contractions present, longitudinal lie, vertex presentation, head 2/5th palpable, FHS 130/min
- Per speculum: Internal os seems dilated; moderate vaginal bleeding present; no local cause of bleeding detected
- After these findings, a very gentle per vaginal (digital examination) was done, internal os was admitting 2 fingers, membranes bulging and vertex could be felt through the membranes with no evidence of placental tissue.

1. **What is your likely diagnosis?**
   Abruptio placenta

2. **Patient in this case had an uneventful pregnancy, still she has abruption. How do you explain this?**
   - Abruption is usually a sudden and unexpected obstetric emergency, not predictable by means of known reproductive risk factors
   - Approximately 70% of cases of placental abruption occur in low-risk pregnancies
   - There is no means by which it can be prevented
   - Even women taking antithrombotic therapy (low dose aspirin and low molecular weight heparins) for thrombophilia (a known risk factor for abruption) are also not protected
   - Precautionary measures that can be taken to reduce the risk:
     – Intake of folic acid and multivitamins during pregnancy
     – Though some reduction in incidence is shown by a recent observational study but further studies are required to authenticate the data
     – Smoking and cocaine misuse to be avoided during pregnancy
     – Domestic violence is to be stopped.

3. **What are the positive points in the history supporting your diagnosis?**
   Positive points
   - Continuous lower abdominal pain
   - Dark colored bleeding
   - Sudden and unexpected pain and bleeding, started almost at the same time
   - 3rd trimester of pregnancy
   - Increase in blood pressure (BP can be normal)
   - Vertex occupying the lower pole
   - Engaged head.

ANTEPARTUM HEMORRHAGE

Definition
- Any bleeding from or into the genital tract after mid-pregnancy
- Always first rule out placental bleeding (placenta previa or abruption, being the most important causes)
- Then think of various other causes of APH in late gestation:
  – Bloody Show
  – Vasa previa
  – Cervical lesion/injury
  – Vaginal lesion/injury
  – Uterine rupture
  – Hemorrhoids
  – Neoplasia
  – Circumvallate placenta
  – Marginal sinus bleeding
  – Marked decidual reaction
  – Coagulation disorder
  – Unexplained APH.

Death Toll due to APH
- Causes up to 50% of the estimated 500,000 maternal deaths that occur globally each year.

4. **Supposedly, this patient had a severe bleed with no records available and on per speculum examination internal os is closed. How will you investigate her?**

Blood tests:

If massive hemorrhage
- CBC
- Blood group and type
- Blood for cross match
- Kleihauer test, if Rh negative (to quantify fetomaternal hemorrhage)
- Renal function tests
- Liver function tests
- Platelet count, if low → complete coagulation profile.

If mild bleeding
- CBC
- Blood group and type
- Kleihauer test, if Rh negative (to quantify fetomaternal hemorrhage)
- Blood for crossmatch
- Platelet count.

USG
- To rule out placenta previa
- The sensitivity of ultrasound for the detection of retroplacental clot (abruption) is poor. However, when ultrasound suggests an abruption, the likelihood that there is an abruption is high
- To confirm IUD, if FHR is not detected by auscultation or even by CTG.

Fetal
- CTG → to rule out fetal distress.

5. **What complications can be faced due to bleeding in the 3rd trimester?**

Maternal complications
- Repeated episodes of bleeding can lead to:
    - Anemia
    - Infection
    - Prolonged hospital stay
- Acute hemorrhage:
    - Shock
    - Disseminated intravascular coagulopathy
    - Need for massive transfusions (and the associated complications)
    - Renal tubular necrosis/failure
- Rate of cesarean section and operative morbidity is increased
- Hysterectomy
- They are more prone to postpartum hemorrhage
- Couvelaire uterus (in cases of placental abruption)
- Maternal mortality.

Fetal and neonatal complications
- Intrauterine fetal death (if bleeding is severe)
- Fetal hypoxia
- Intrauterine growth restriction/Small for gestational age
- Preterm delivery/Prematurity
- Admission to NICU

- Increase in rates of hyperbilirubinemia
- Respiratory distress syndrome
- Hyaline membrane disease and the subsequent need for surfactant therapy (in cases of premature infants)
- Neonatal infections.

6. **What are the complications associated with unexplained APH?**

   There is increased risk of:
   - Preterm delivery
   - Stillbirth
   - Fetal anomalies
   - Induction of labor at term
   - Low-birth weight
   - Admission to NICU
   - Hyperbilirubinemia.

7. **Would you like to give steroids to your patient?**
   - Various studies from Cochrane data have shown that antenatal corticosteroids reduces neonatal death even when infants are born < 24 h after the first dose has been given
   - Another study has confirmed that incomplete courses of antenatal corticosteroids are beneficial
   - The exact time interval for steroids to become beneficial is unknown
   - There is a potential benefit commencing within hours of the first dose.

     In this case, though the gestational age is between 34–36 weeks and that delivery will occur within a few hours, still in author's opinion it is prudent to give a single dose of betamethasone, which is of no harm to the patient but may benefit the neonate.

8. **What mode of delivery would be appropriate for this patient?**
   - Since mother's vitals are stable, fetus is not compromised and patient is in established labor → vaginal delivery with simultaneous maternal resuscitation and continuous FHR monitoring would be the method of choice
   - Patient should not be left unattended
   - Measures to expedite delivery process should be undertaken
   - Cesarean section → in case the condition of mother or the fetus deteriorates or there is massive hemorrhage.

9. **How will you manage the 3rd stage of labor?**
   - Active management of third stage of labor should be anticipated, as this woman carries a risk factor for PPH
   - Oxytocics should be kept ready
   - Instead of oxytocin alone, use of ergometrine-oxytocin for AMTSL in cases of antepartum hemorrhage have shown small reduction in the risk of PPH
   - But as this patient's BP was on a higher side on admission, in spite of moderate bleeding, ergometrine should be avoided in her.

ABRUPTIO PLACENTA

Definition

- Partial or complete separation of a normally implanted placenta from its attachment on the uterine wall, after the 20th week of pregnancy but before delivery
- Peak rate of abruption occurs between 24–27 weeks.

Incidence

- 0.49–1.8%
- The incidence may be much higher than this, as cases which are not detected clinically but are diagnosed only after delivery of the placenta, are missed
- Maternal mortality in 1% of cases
- Perinatal mortality rates vary between 4.4–67%.

Risk Factors

- Prior abruption:
  - Risk is 4.4–5%, if one previous pregnancy was complicated by abruption
  - After two consecutive abruptions, risk increases to 19–25%
- Maternal hypertensive disorders:
  - Risk of abruption increases by 5-fold in cases of both preeclampsia and chronic hypertension
  - Cause: maternal vascular disease
  - Strongly associated with grade 3 abruptio, in which 40–50% cases have hypertensive disease
- IUGR (fetal growth restriction)
- Rapid uterine decompression:
  - Polyhydramnios
  - Twin gestation
    - 3-fold increase in the risk of abruption, mainly after the delivery of the 1st twin
- Non-vertex presentations
- Increasing parity and/or maternal age (though advanced maternal age being controversial)
  - Primiparous: frequency of placental abruption is <1%
  - Grand multipara: 2.5%
  - Postulated theories:
    - Damaged endometrium
    - Impaired decidualization
    - Aberrant vasculature
- Trauma (Blunt or penetrating)
  - Risk:
    - Minor trauma: 1.5%
    - Severe injury: risk of abruption increases to 50%
  - Two most important causes of trauma:
    - Road traffic accident
      - Uterine stretch, direct penetration, placental shearing from acceleration-deceleration forces → primary cause of abruption
    - Trauma as a result of domestic violence
- Bleeding in the 1st trimester
  - Threatened miscarriage → risk is 1.4%
  - Intrauterine hematoma on 1st trimester USG → increases the risk of abruption
- Preterm premature rupture of membranes
  - 2–5% of pregnancies with PPROM are complicated by abruption
- Low bodymass index (BMI)
- Inherited or acquired thrombophilia
  - Significant association is noted with:
    - Heterozygous factor V Leiden
    - Prothrombin gene mutation

- Uterine and placental factors:
  - Placental implantation over a uterine malformation (e.g. septum or fibroid)
  - Placental abnormalities (e.g. circumvallate placenta)
- Pregnancy following assisted reproductive technique
- Intrauterine infection
- Smoking:
  - Smoking causes decidual ischemia and necrosis
  - Smokers have 40% increased risk of fetal death from abruption with each pack of cigarette
- Cocaine abuse during pregnancy:
  - There is a 10% risk of abruption in the 3rd trimester
  - Cocaine causes vasospasm → decidual ischemia → reflex vasodilatation → vascular disruption within the placental bed.

Pathophysiology

Theory I

Hemorrhage at the decidual–placental interface → separates the decidua, leaving a thin layer attached to the placenta

↓

Hematoma enlarges → further separation and compression of the overlying intervillous space occurs

↓

Local destruction of placental tissue (seen as an organized clot lying on a depressed maternal surface of the placenta, if seen with naked eye)

Theory II

Abruptio placenta is often the final expression of a chronic placental disorder

↓

Activated neutrophils and macrophages → secrete cytokines and tumour necrosis factor

↓

These upregulate the production and activity of matrix metalloproteinases in the trophoblast

↓

Matrix metalloproteinases are presumed to have important functions in normal placental detachment

↓

Their ↑ production may result in destruction of extracellular matrices and cellular connections that secure the placenta

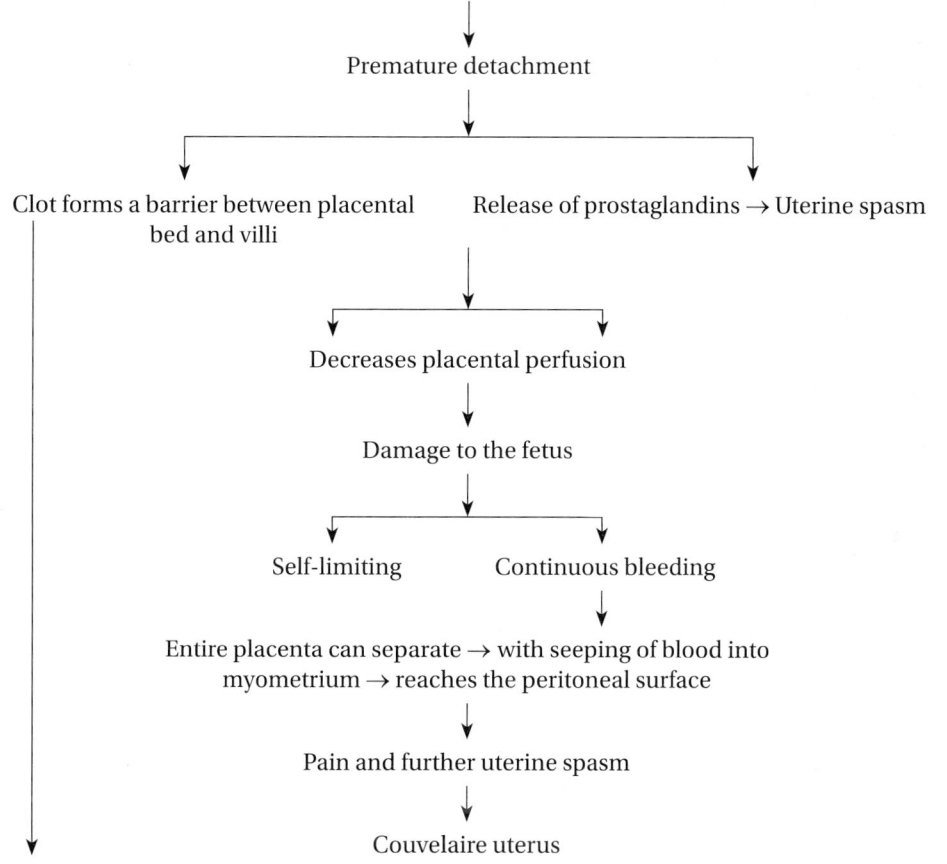

Classification

Ernest Page's Classification

There are four grades:

Grade 0
- No symptoms
- Retrospective diagnosis by finding an organized blood clot or a depressed area on the delivered placenta.

Grade I
- Mild abruption
- Variable bleeding per vaginam
- Slightly tender/irritable uterus

- Normal maternal BP and heart rate
- No coagulopathy
- No fetal distress
- Constitutes ≈ 40–48%.

Grade II
- Partial abruption
- Mild to moderate vaginal bleeding
- Moderate to severe uterine tenderness with possible tetanic contractions
- Maternal tachycardia with orthostatic changes in BP and heart rate
- Fetal distress
- Hypofibrinogenemia may be present
- Account for ≈ 45% of all placental abruptions.

Grade III
- Large to complete abruption
- Moderate to heavy vaginal bleeding
- Very painful tetanic uterus
- Maternal:
  - Shock
  - Coagulopathy
  - Anuria
- Fetal death → is a rule
- Constitutes 15%
- *Important observations:*
  - About 40% of patients will demonstrate signs of DIC
  - Within 8 hours of initial symptoms in such women, hypofibrinogenemia will be present
  - It will not recover without blood products
  - Time course for recovery from hypofibrinogenemia is 10 mg/dL per hour after delivery of fetus and placenta.

Sher's Classification

There are three stages:

Stage I
- Mild form with:
  - Unexplained vaginal bleeding
  - Retrospective diagnosis of a small hematoma postpartum.

Stage II
- Intermediate form with:
  - A hypertonic uterus
  - A live fetus.

Stage III
- Severe form with:
  - Intrauterine death of the fetus
    - IIIa → without coagulopathy
    - IIIb → with coagulopathy.

Clinical Features

- Although vaginal bleeding is the hallmark of placental abruption, in 10-20% cases, it may be occult or concealed
- Pain → prominent feature
  Pain may be due to:
  - Extravasation of blood into the myometrium
  - Overdistension of the uterus due to retroplacental bleeding, OR
  - Frequent contractions associated with the release of prostaglandins
- Uterine contractions may start causing additional, intermittent pain
- Contractions characteristically have a:
  - High frequency but
  - Low amplitude (5 per 10 minutes → "sawtooth" pattern)
  - An elevated baseline tone
- Uterus → extremely hard and tender, IT DOES NOT RELAX
- Fetal parts are difficult to palpate especially when blood is accumulating inside
- If the membranes are ruptured, blood stained liquor may be seen
- FHR inaudible, if death has occurred
- Fetal head may have entered the pelvic brim
- Preeclampsia may be associated in 1/3rd of cases
- Faintness and collapse, in severe cases.

Role of Sonography

- Early hemorrhage → Typically hyper or isoechoic
- Resolving hematomas → Hypoechoic within 1 week and sonolucent within 2 weeks of abruption
- Acute hemorrhage → May be misinterpreted as a thickened placenta or fibroid.

There are three predominant locations for placental abruption:

Retroplacental abruption
- Blood collection behind the placenta (between placenta and myometrium).

Subchorionic abruption
- Between placenta and membranes.

Preplacental abruption
- Between placenta and amniotic fluid
- Anterior to the placenta within amnion and chorion.

Clinical Relevance:
1. Retroplacental hematomas are associated with worse prognosis for fetal survival than subchorionic hemorrhage
2. Size → also predictive of fetal survival
   - Large retroplacental hemorrhage (> 60 mL) → ≥ 50% fetal mortality
   - Subchorionic hemorrhage (> 60 mL) → 10% mortality risk.

Management

Active Management

- Resuscitation:
  - IV access (large widebore cannulas)
  - Crystalloids followed by transfusion of blood and blood products
- O_2 by mask
- Investigations:
  - Hemoglobin
  - Hematocrit
  - Platelet count
  - LFT
  - RFT with electrolytes
  - Bloodgroup and typing
  - Coagulation profile
  - Fibrinogen
- Continuous FHR monitoring
- Expedite delivery, once mother stabilizes
- Prevention of complications.

Expectant Management

- If abruption is mild and self-limiting or diagnosis of abruption is not conclusive, *gestational age at the time of presentation is an important prognostic factor*
- < 20 weeks → 82% can be expected to have a term delivery, despite evidence of abruption
- >20 weeks → only 27% will deliver at term.

Management Proper

- Stabilization of mother is most important
- Maternal hemodynamic and clotting parameters must be followed closely

Scenario I
- Grade I abruption
- Preterm
- Mother and fetus → stable

  } Hospitalization, Tocolysis, Steroids

Studies have shown prolongation of pregnancy by > 1 week in > 50% of cases.

Scenario II
- Fetus is already dead (term or preterm) → aim for vaginal delivery
- Induction or augmentation of labor is not contraindicated but with close surveillance.

Scenario III
- Fetus is alive
- Not in labor
- Gestation not so early as to make fetal survival extremely unlikely

  } Deliver by cesarean section.

Scenario IV
- Fetus is alive
- Patient in established labor

  | Augmentation (ARM + oxytocin)
  Expedite delivery with strict monitoring and continuous CTG

Continuous FHR monitoring is recommended because 60% of fetuses may exhibit nonreassuring heart rate.

Disseminated Intravascular Coagulopathy (DIC)

Pregnancy is a hypercoagulable state.

	Normal changes in pregnancy
Non-pregnant	*Pregnancy*
Fibrinogen 200–400 mg%	300–600 mg/dL (↑ 50%)
Factor VII	↑ 10 times by term
Factor VIII	↑ 2 times by term
Factor IX and X	Increases
Factor XI	↓ by 60%
Factor XIII	↓ by 50%
Platelets (life span 9–12 days)	Width and volume ↑; ↓ platelet concentration due to hemodilution →↑number of younger and larger platelets
Clotting time	NO CHANGE
Fibrinolytic system	Depressed till 60 min after delivery of placenta (due to effect of placentally derived plasminogen activator inhibitor [Type 2])
Serum D dimer	Increases
Thromboxane A_2	↑↑ in mid pregnancy → it induces platelet aggregation

Naturally Occurring Anticoagulants

1. Antithrombin III:
   - Mainly inhibits thrombin and factor Xa
   - Synthesized in liver
   - Activity decreased in the following states:
     - DIC
     - Hypercoagulable states
     - Chronic liver disease
     - In OCP users
     - Cirrhosis of liver
   - During pregnancy, there is little change in level, but decreases during parturition with subsequent increase in puerperium.
2. Protein C and S:
   - Protein C
     - Inactivates factor V and VIII in conjunction with its cofactors, thrombomodulin and Protein S
     - Vitamin K dependent
     - Synthesized in liver
   - Thrombomodulin → stimulates protein C and protein S → binds to lipids and platelet surface → localization of reaction
   - Protein S → ↓ in pregnancy and puerperium.

Process of Fibrinolysis

Plasminogen activators
- Present in plasma after exercise, stress, surgery, trauma
- Are also present in tissue (uterus/ovaries)

Plasminogen Inhibitors
Antiplasminogen
- EACA
- Tranexamic acid
- Aprotinin

Antiplasmin
- Platelet
- Plasma
- Serum

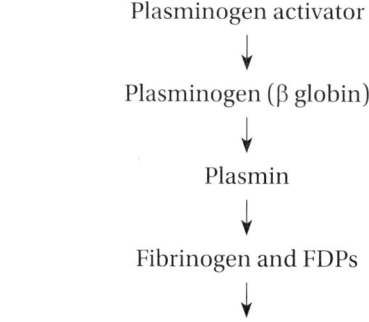

Plasminogen activator
↓
Plasminogen (β globin)
↓
Plasmin
↓
Fibrinogen and FDPs
↓
Normally, plasma antiplasmin levels exceed the levels of plasminogen.

What is DIC?

- It is a thrombohemorrhagic disorder occurring as a consequence of aberrant activation of coagulation cascade seen in association with well-defined clinical situations.

Conditions Associated with DIC

- Abruptio
- Amniotic fluid embolism
- Retained IUD fetus
- Puerperal sepsis and septic abortion
- Excessive blood loss
- Severe preeclampsia/eclampsia
- Induced abortion especially using hypertonic saline
- Acute fatty liver of pregnancy
- Molar pregnancy.

DIC is characterized by
- Intravascular coagulation
- Fibrinolysis
- Consumption of coagulation factors and inhibitors
- End organ damage.

In DIC, antithrombin III decreases.
Although fibrinolytic activity is present but level of this activity is too less to counteract ongoing coagulation.

Stimulation of Coagulation Activity and Possible Consequences

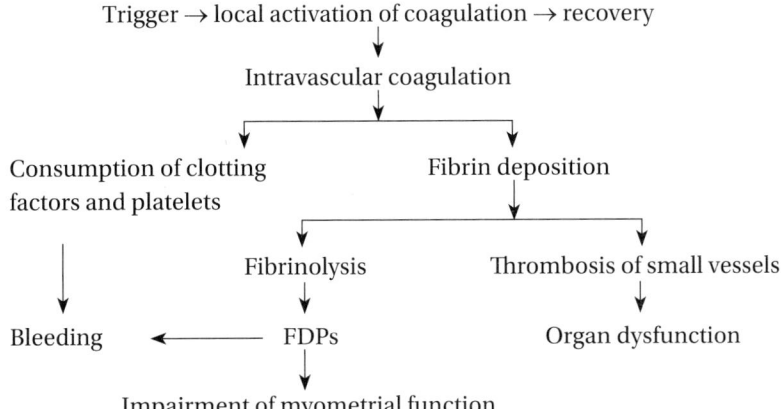

Clinical Features of DIC

- Petechiae
- Purpura
- Ecchymosis
- Hemorrhagic bullae
- Subcutaneous hematoma
- Bleeding from wound or venepuncture sites
- Variable degrees of shock and acidosis.

Diagnosis

Bedside tests
- Whole blood clotting time:
  - Normal 1–10 minutes
  - Take 5 mL of blood in glass tube and observe for clot formation
  - If prolonged, deficiency of clotting factors
  - If clot is not formed → fibrinogen is < 50 mg/dL
- Clot retraction time:
  - Normal 30–60 minutes
  - Weak friable clot → hypofibrinogenemia
  - Early dissolution → enhanced fibrinolysis.

Laboratory tests
- Peripheral smear:
  - Thrombocytopenia
  - Leukocytosis
  - Evidence of hemolysis

- DIC profile:
  - Prothrombin time (PT)
    - Normal 10–13 seconds
    - It tests the integrity of extrinsic and common pathway
    - When fibrinogen is < 100 mg/dL → PT is increased
  - INR (International normalized ratio):
    - Patient's PT: Laboratory's control PT
    - Normal → 0.9-1.2
    - Increased in deficiency of factors I, II, V, VII or X
    - Most sensitive to fall in factor VII
  - Partial thromboplastin time (aPTT):
    - Normal 25–35 seconds
    - Tests the integrity of intrinsic and common pathway
  - Thrombin time:
    - Normal is < 18 seconds
    - Extended when functional fibrinogen is < 100 mg/dL
    - Increases when FDPs are increased
  - Fibrinogen:
    - Bleeding occurs when levels fall below 100–150 mg/dL
  - D-dimer:
    - Measures cross-linked fibrin derivatives (i.e. those that have been in blood clot → 70% of fragment X is retained in the clot)
    - Fragments Y, D, E are retained to a lesser extent
    - Is a more specific FDP assay
    - Has been found to be the most useful test in diagnosing DIC
    - Normal < 0.5 mg/lit
  - FDP titer:
    - Normal is < 10 micrograms/dL
    - Increases in DIC
  - Platelets:
    - Normal is ≈1.5–4.0 lakhs
    - In DIC, platelets decrease.

Letzke's classification of severity of DIC			
Stage	Severity	Findings	Associations
I	Compensated	↑ FDPs ↑ soluble fibrin complexes ↑ vWF: Factor VIIc	Preeclampsia Retained dead fetus
II	Uncompensated but no hematocrit failure	Same as above + ↓ fibrinogen ↓ platelets ↓ factor V and VIII	Small abruption Severe preeclampsia
III	Very severe with ↑ derangements in blood values	↑↑ depletion of coagulation factors (particularly fibrinogen) and FDPs are ↑↑	Abruptio Amniotic fluid embolism Eclampsia

Management
- Correction of underlying problem
- Fluid resuscitation to restore the circulatory system, maintain BP and electrolyte balance
- Amount of blood loss should be estimated.

Crystalloids or Colloids?

Crystalloids
- Are more readily available and are less expensive
- Are to be infused in volume boluses calculated at 3 times the estimated blood loss because they remain in intravascular circulation for short time.

Colloids
- Have higher intravascular oncotic pressure with smaller amount as compared to crystalloids
- But as a disadvantage, there is delayed post-resuscitation diuresis and higher incidence of post-resuscitation hypertension.

Why dextrans can't be used?
- They affect platelet function
- Cause pseudoagglutination
- Interfere with interpretation of subsequent blood grouping and cross-matching
- They cause anaphylactic reactions.

Hemaccel
- Derivative of bovine gelatin
- Shelf-life of 8 years
- Can be stored at room temperature
- Isotonic and does not interfere with platelet function or blood grouping/cross-matching
- Renal function is improved when given in hypovolemic shock
- Generally non-immunogenic
- Reactions, if they occur, are due to histamine release.

Blood Component Therapy

Packed RBCs
- Volume – 300 mL
- Contain mostly red cells mixed with preservatives and anticoagulants:
  - Citrate
  - Phosphate
  - Dextrose
  - Adenosine
- Hematocrit of 70% (very viscous)
- For rapid transfusion, can be diluted with 100 mL normal saline
- RL should not be mixed with RBCs because its calcium content may precipitate when it interacts with citrate preservatives
- 1 unit of RBCs increases PCV by 3% points
- Packed RBCs have no platelets and only ≈ 10–15 mL of residual plasma
- Improves oxygen carrying capacity

- Increases hemoglobin by 1 gm/dL and PCV by 3% points
- For 4 units of PRBCs → give 1 unit FFP.

Fresh frozen plasma (FFP)
- Is a component of whole blood that remains once platelets and cellular elements are removed
- Prepared from single unit of whole blood (Random donor FFP with a volume of ≈ 250 mL) OR from plasma collected by apheresis technique (Jumbo FFP with volume ≈ 800 mL)
- Frozen at -18 to -30°C
- Contents: All coagulation factors + other proteins present in original blood
- FFPs should not be used as a source of albumin or other nutrients or as a volume expander
- Should be ABO compatible, not necessary Rh specific
- Hemostasis can be achieved when the activity of coagulation factors is at least 25% of normal because 1 unit random donor FFP will increase clotting protein levels by 8%, 2 units FFP is a good starting number to transfuse
- Plasma volume in adults is ≈ 40 mL/kg, this requires a dose of FFP of ≈ 15 mL/kg, therefore 2 units to be given at a time
- When to transfuse?
  When PT and/or aPTT is >1.5 times normal
- Can be preserved for 1 year at given temperature
- 1 unit FFP →↑ fibrinogen by 10 mg/dL.

Cryoprecipitate
- Prepared by thawing 1 unit of FFP at 4°C and collecting the formed precipitate in a concentrated volume of 10–15 mL/bag
- Each bag or unit contains:
  - 200–300 mg/dL fibrinogen
  - 100 units of factor VIII
  - vWF, factor XIII, and
  - 55 mg fibronectin in equal volume of 15–20 mL/bag
- Indication:
  - Fibrinogen < 75–100 mg/dL
  - 1U/10 kg of body weight with fibrinogen < 75 mg/dL
- Each unit increases fibrinogen by 10 mg/dL.

Platelets
- Obtained from whole blood from multiple donors or by apheresis collection (60–90 single unit equivalents)
  - 1 Random Donor Platelet (RDP) →↑ platelets by 5000–10000
  - 1 Single Donor Platelet (SDP) →↑ platelets by 50,000
- ABO typing is not essential but Rh typing is necessary
- In case Rh negative platelets are required and are not available, transfuse Rh positive platelets with a cover of Anti-D immunoglobulin
- Indication: < 50,000/mm^3 platelets
- Goal: Minimum 1 lakh/mm^3
- In non bleeding patients:
  - Cut off of 20,000/mm^3 is usually taken
  - Recent studies suggest a cut off as 10,000/mm^3 as the difference between the two, is clinically not significant.

10. **How will you manage DIC in case of antepartum hemorrhage?**
    - Coagulation studies and platelets should be urgently requested
    - By the time the reports are ready, up to 4 units of FFPs and 10 units of cryoprecipitate can be transfused
    - If the patient is on anticoagulant therapy with low molecular weight heparin (LMWH) and she bleeds, she is advised not to take any further doses unless she consults her obstetrician
    - She should be managed with intravenous, unfractionated heparin until the risk factors for hemorrhage have resolved.

PLACENTA PREVIA

Jauniaux and Campbell Classification

Type I (Low lying)
- Lower margin within 5 cm of the cervical os.

Type II (Marginal placenta previa)
- Reaches up to the margin of os but does not cover it.

Type III (Incomplete or partial placenta previa)
- Placenta partially covers the os.

Type IV (Central or Total)
- Placenta covers the os completely.

On the basis of placental localization on the anterior or posterior wall

Type A
- When placenta lies on the anterior wall.

Type B
- When placenta lies on the posterior wall
- Also known as *Dangerous placenta previa* because placenta on the posterior wall will get compressed by the presenting part → fetal asphyxia → even fetal death.

Major
- Placenta implanted across the cervix.

Minor/Partial
- Placenta not implanted across the cervix.

Risk Factors

- Previous placenta previa (recurrence rate is 4–8%)
- Previous cesarean sections:
  - One previous cesarean section (OR 2.2)
  - Two previous cesarean sections (OR 4.1)
  - Three previous cesarean sections (OR 22.4)
- Previous termination of pregnancy (OR 1.9)
- Multiparity (If > 5 → OR 2.3)
- Advanced maternal age (>40 years) (OR 9.1)
- Multiple pregnancy

- Smoking and cocaine use in pregnancy
- Congenital anomalies (OR 1.7)
- Deficient endometrium due to presence or history of:
  - Uterine scar
  - Endometritis
  - Manual removal of placenta
  - Curettage
  - Submucous fibroid
- Assisted conception
- Women with a large placenta from twins or erythroblastosis are at higher risk
- Placental pathology (velamentous insertion, succenturiate lobes, bipartite, i.e. bilobed placenta).

Etiopathogenesis

Various theories have been proposed but nothing is conclusive:
1. Dropping down theory
2. Persistence of chorionic activity
3. Defective decidua
4. Big surface area of placenta.

Placenta
- Large and thin
- Tongue shaped extension from main placental mass
- Degeneration with infarcts and calcification.

Cord
- May be attached to margins (Battledore) or to membranes (Velamentous)
- May be associated with vasa previa.

Lower uterine segment
- Increased vascularity
- Cervix is soft and more friable.

Why bleeding is Recurrent, Causeless and Painless?

Recurrent
- As lower uterine segment continues to grow in 3rd trimester, bleeding can occur again and again during its growth
- Now, this bleeding is controlled by:
  - Thrombosis of open sinuses
  - Mechanical pressure by presenting part
  - Placental infarction.

Causeless
- As this is a natural phenomenon (i.e. growth of lower uterine segment in 3rd trimester) and placenta is inelastic, with slower growth in later months whereas lower segment progressively dilates, the inelastic placenta is sheared off the wall of lower segment → opening up of uteroplacental vessels → bleeding episode.

Painless
- Because it is a physiological phenomenon
  Bleeding is almost always because of maternal bleed but trauma may become the cause of fetal bleed.

What is warning hemorrhage?
- Occurs somewhere in mid pregnancy
- Mild fresh bleed
- Little amount
- Lasting for 4–5 days, stopping in a weeks' time
- Not causing damage to mother or fetus
- Indicative of recurring bouts to come.

Clinical Suspicion
- The two classical presentations of placenta previa are:
  - As antepartum hemorrhage
    OR
  - As fetal malpresentation in late pregnancy
- Of late, a third important presentation is added to this → diagnosis of asymptomatic placenta previa by routine ultrasound examination
- Bleeding after 20 weeks of gestation and usually before term
- There is often repeated episodes of bleeding
- Maternal vitals corresponds to the amount of bleed
- Uterus relaxed, soft, nontender
- FHS → almost always present
- High presenting part
- Head cannot be pushed down in pelvis, its persistent displacement is highly indicative of placenta previa
- An abnormal lie
- Painless or provoked bleeding by sexual intercourse, irrespective of previous imaging results
- Painful only when labor accompanies
- Bleeding is bright red (indicative of fresh bleed) → because it occurs from separated uteroplacental sinuses close to cervical opening and escapes out immediately
- Stallworthy's sign: Drop the fetal head in the pelvic brim → FHS decreases → release the head → FHS normalizes.

Definitive Diagnosis

Ultrasonography: TAS or TVS?

TAS
Associated with high false positives. What leads to it?
1. Presence of myometrial contraction:
   - Contraction may mimic a placenta in appearance or may displace the placental edge low down
2. Over distended bladder:
   - Approximates anterior and posterior uterine walls, giving false impression of previa

3. Poor visualization of posterior placenta
4. Fetal head can interfere with visualization of lower segment
5. Obesity also interferes with accuracy
6. Phenomenon of placental migration:
   - Development of lower uterine segment in later part of pregnancy (10-fold growth of lower uterine segment compared to placenta)
   - Unusual placental expansion with marginal atrophy on one side and expansion on other

Note: Studies have shown that rate of placental migration:

- Is 0.1 mm/week → when it covers the os
- Is 4.1 mm/week → when placental edge is > 3 cm away from os
- Major degree placenta previa → is more likely to persist as previa at term, rather than the one away from it
- Cases in which placenta is more likely to migrate:
   - When it is posterior
   - When it is thicker
   - Lower edge is < 2 cm from os
   - When there is a history of previous cesarean section.

Advantages of TVS over TAS

- Considered gold standard
- More instructive than conventional transabdominal examination in cases of suspected placenta previa
- Imaging is better
- Even safe in presence of bleeding
- Woman does not need a full bladder → avoids both maternal discomfort and distortion of the anatomy of lower uterine segment and cervix
- Though some argue that probe insertion could provoke bleeding but an answer to this is, the insertion of probe to no more than 3 centimeters into the vagina will not come in contact with the cervix or lower uterine segment
- Has a:
   - Sensitivity of 87.5%
   - Specificity of 98.8%
   - Positive predictive value of 93.3%
   - Negative predictive value of 97.6%.

Few Observed Technical Difficulties

- In some cases, it can be difficult to establish whether there is a minor degree of placenta previa or a normally sited placenta
- Presence of an accessory lobe in the lower segment while the main bulk of the placenta can be clearly seen to be in the upper uterine segment.

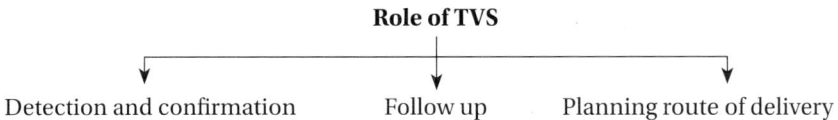

Detection and confirmation of placenta previa

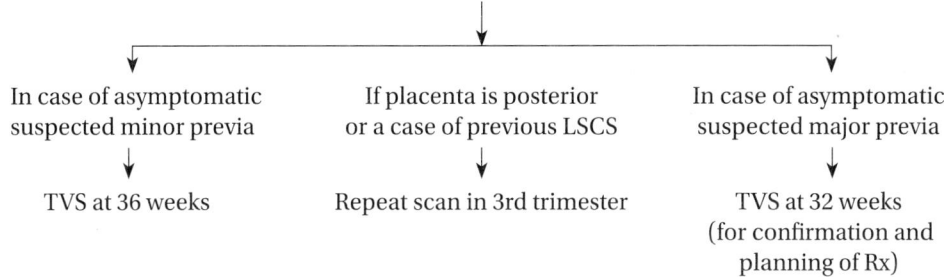

USG terminology:
i. When placental edge does not reach internal os → designated as "mm" away from internal os
ii. When placental edge overlaps internal os → distance is given as "mm of overlap"
iii. When placental edge exactly reaches internal os → measurement given as "0 mm".

Follow up

A. When placental edge overlaps or exactly reaches the internal os (between 18–24 weeks) → repeat TVS in the 3rd trimester
B. If it is between 20 mm away from internal os and 20 mm overlap after 26 weeks → repeat USG at regular intervals
C. If ≥ 20 mm at any time in 3rd trimester → there are ↑chances of cesarean section.

Planning route of delivery (After 35 weeks)
Depends upon the distance of placental edge from internal os:

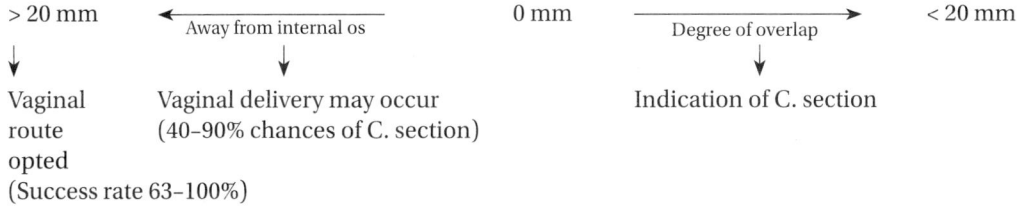

- It is recommended to defer elective cesarean section to 38 weeks to decrease neonatal morbidity
- If placental edge is between 20–35 mm away from os → Anticipate PPH.

Case of morbidly adherent placenta
- Previous LSCS with either placenta previa OR anterior placenta underlying the old cesarean scar are at ↑ risk of accreta.

Which women are most likely to bleed?
- Women with ↑ serum α fetoproteins at 15–20 weeks and placentas which encroach on the os
- Placenta which is thicker inferiorly
- Where placenta shows a turbulent flow at its lower margin on Doppler
- USG imaging shows echo free spaces at placental margins.

PLACENTAL INVASION (Accreta, Increta, Percreta)

Incidence

- Placenta accreta → 1 in 2500 deliveries
- Invasive placentation affects ≈ 2% of all singleton deliveries.

Definition

- Placenta accreta is typified by chorionic villi on the myometrial surface
- Placenta increta by villus infiltration into the myometrium
- Percreta by infiltration through the entire myometrium to breach the serosa and beyond.

Etiology

- Though exact reason is unknown, it has been postulated to be related to damage of the decidua basalis (destroying its barrier function), which allows for placental invasion into the myometrium
- This leads to invasion of the myometrium to varying depths, from the most superficial (placenta accreta) to deeper myometrial invasion (placenta increta)
- There can be breaches in the uterine serosa and possibly invasion into adjacent organs.

Risk Factors

- Placenta previa with or without previous uterine surgery
- Rising cesarean section rates
- Previous myomectomy
- Previous uterine curettage
- Evacuations associated with trauma or infection
- Asherman's syndrome
- Submucous fibroids
- Maternal age > 35 years
- Previous trophoblastic disease.

Complications of Placenta Percreta

- High maternal mortality (≈ 10%)
- Massive hemorrhage
- Disseminated intravascular coagulation
- Hysterectomy
- Bladder and ureteric trauma
- Acute respiratory distress syndrome
- Acute tubular necrosis
- They may present as acute abdomen and shock from:
  - Ruptured uterus
  - Antepartum hemorrhage

- Hematuria, if bladder is involved
- As a complication in the 3rd stage of labor.

Imaging Modalities in Placenta Accreta, Increta or Percreta

Grayscale Ultrasound

- Diagnostic criteria: when ≥ 1 of the following situations is present:
  - Placental lacunae
  - Obliteration of clear space
  - Interruption of bladder border
  - Myometrium of < 1 mm.

Placental lacunae
- These are multiple linear, irregular, vascular spaces within the placenta
- These placental lakes need not necessarily be in the area of invasion
- The likelihood of placenta accreta increases with the number of lacunae
- Gives placenta a moth-like appearance
- Do not have the highly echogenic borders that standard venous sinuses have
- Sensitivity → 80–93% between 15–40 weeks.

Obliteration of clear space
- Defined as the obliteration of any part of the echolucent area located between the uterus and the placenta
- Usually seen from 12th week onwards, corresponding to dilated vessels of decidua basalis
- Since the decidua basalis is absent in placenta accreta, it has been suggested that the absence of this line predicts placenta accreta but can only be used in conjunction with other USG findings, as alone it has poor sensitivity (57%).

Interruption of bladder border
- When interruption of the posterior bladder wall-uterine interface occurs, the usually continuous echolucent appearing line can instead appear as a series of dashes (intermittent interruptions or impression that bladder wall is bulging into uterine wall)
- This feature is a specific sign for placenta accreta
- It has a poor sensitivity of 21%.

Thin myometrium
- In patients with previous LSCS and low lying placenta.

2D Color Doppler

- Sensitivity → 82–100%
- Specificity → 92–97%
- Advantages over Power Doppler:
  - It can display the velocity and nature of the blood flow
  - High velocity and turbulent flow are always associated with placenta accreta
  - The placental vessels are usually large and this can only be picked up by using color Doppler rather than power Doppler ultrasonography
  - Color enhances the appearance of the vascular spaces
- Greyscale imaging is found to be equally good.

3D Power Doppler

- What can be seen?
  - Additional information provided by power Doppler:
    - Exact site
    - Extent of involvement
    - Depth of invasion by aberrant vessels over the uterine serosa-bladder junctional region
  - Hypervascularity
- Diagnostic performance:
  - Sensitivity 100%
  - Specificity 85%
  - PPV 88%.

MRI

- MRI is performed when the results of ultrasound are inconclusive
- The most common site for placenta accreta is anterior at the lower uterine segment → allowing a high frequency ultrasound transducer to evaluate this area with optimal resolution due to its superficial location
- When the abnormality is located in the posterior wall or in cases of fundal accreta or when the patient is obese, the resolution will be poor
- This is where MRI proves to be a better modality
- What can be seen?
  - Uterine bulging
  - Heterogeneous signal intensity within the placenta
  - Dark intraplacental bands on T2-weighted imaging
- Disadvantage: Very high cost of the machine and as a result testing is costlier, making it nearly impossible to use in all the cases.

Association with other markers

- Unexplained elevation of alpha-fetoprotein and creatine kinase have been linked with morbid adherence of the placenta
- In the absence of fetal anomalies, unexplained elevated maternal serum AFP may suggest the presence of placenta percreta
- AFP is more useful than creatine kinase and is more likely to be investigated in 2nd trimester.

Antenatal Management

Risks

Massive and/or Repeated hemorrhage
- Hospitalize the patient
- Written and informed consent
- General condition and vitals of the patient and assessment of degree of shock
- Estimation of amount of bleeding (number of pads used/soiled clothes)
- Wide bore cannula
- Immediately start IV fluids
- Draw blood for investigations

- Catheterize the patient
- Foot end elevation
- Per abdominal examination (uterine activity, tenderness, FHS)
- Give corticosteroids, if gestation is < 34 completed weeks
- Blood and blood products arranged and transfused according to laboratory reports
- If Rh negative, Kleihauer Betke test to know the amount of fetomaternal bleed and anti-D immunoglobulin accordingly

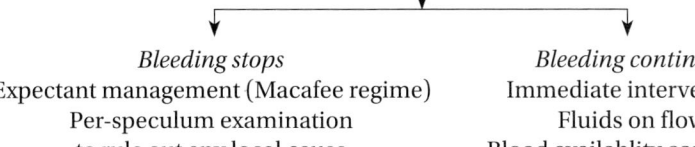

Bleeding stops
Expectant management (Macafee regime)
Per-speculum examination
to rule out any local cause

Bleeding continues
Immediate intervention
Fluids on flow
Blood availablity confirmed
Shift the patient to OT

- USG assessment of:
  - Fetal well-being
  - Placental localization and distance from internal os
  - Fetal abnormality (contraindication to expectant Rx).

In operation theater (Double set up examination)

Anesthetist with arrangements for general anesthesia ready

Lithotomy position – according to surgeon's preference

Per speculum examination: to rule out any local lesions

Per vaginal examination:

Index and middle fingers are introduced uptil fornices

Push fetal head into brim from above

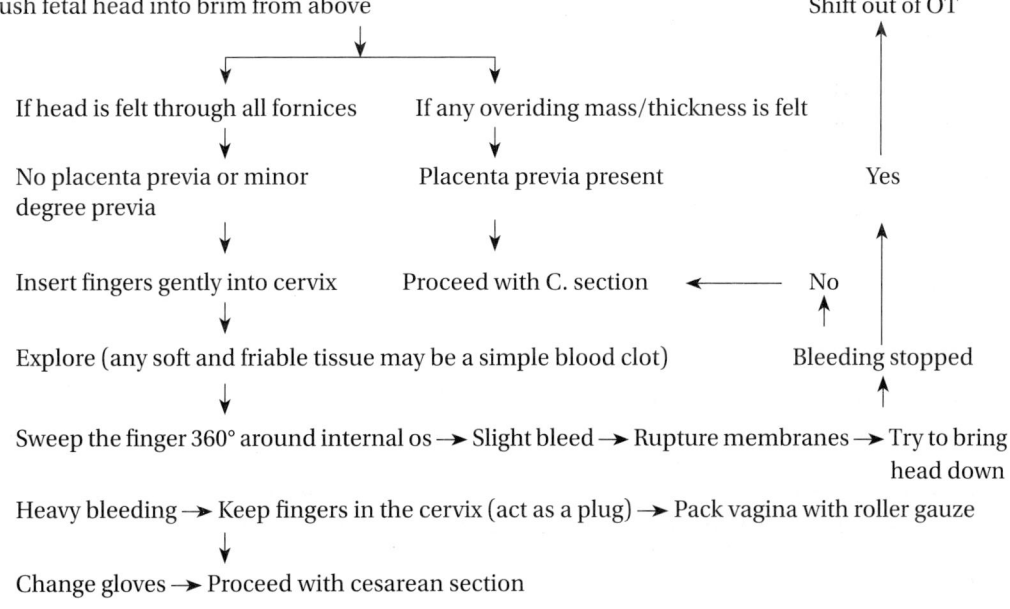

Preterm delivery
- Hospitalization:
  - Not recommended for placenta previa
  - Safety precautions should be taken at home (someone should be available to get the patient to hospital in case of emergency – bleeding, contractions, even minor suprapubic pain)
  - Not to stay too far from the hospital
- Cervical cerclage: No recommendations
- Tocolysis
  - For prophylaxis: No use
  - When presents with bleeding: Though studies have shown a positive response when 10 mg of ritodrine every 6 hours by intramuscular injections for 7 days was used. There was a prolongation of pregnancy by 2–3 weeks with an increase in birth weight but side effects have to be kept in mind. Each case needs to be individualized.

Thromboembolism
- For patients admitted to hospital for a longer time, following precautions should be taken:
  - Ambulation
  - Adequate hydration
  - Thromboembolic stockings
  - Anticoagulants → not recommended.

Uterine Perforation

Delivery

Mode of Delivery

Depends upon:
1. Clinical factors
2. USG findings → location of fetal head relative to leading edge of placenta
3. Whether fetal head has entered the pelvis
4. Thickness of the encroaching tongue of the placenta → if >1 cm, the chances are more in favor of cesarean section.

Time of Delivery

- Uncomplicated placenta previa → 38 weeks
- Uncomplicated placenta accreta → 36–37 weeks with corticosteroid cover.

Prerequisites before Delivery

1. Blood and blood products (Packed cells, FFP, Cryoprecipitate)
2. Detailed written and informed consent:
   - Risks of cesarean section in general
   - PPH (risk of massive hemorrhage is ≈12 times more likely with placenta previa)
   - Risks of blood transfusion
   - Need for hysterectomy
   - Leaving the placenta in situ
3. Senior obstetrician, neonatalogist and anesthetist should be readily available
4. Immediate access to operation theater in case of vaginal delivery.

Delivery by cesarean section
- Choice of skin and uterine incisions solely depends upon the location of placenta, hence the need for USG before surgery.

A low transverse skin incision
- Allows access to the lower half of the uterus
- Can be given in cases where the upper margin of the anterior aspect of placenta does not rise into the upper segment of the uterus.

Midline skin incision
- When placenta is anterior and is extending towards the level of the umbilicus
- Uterine incision → high upper segment longitudinal uterine incision or high transverse incision or a fundal incision
- The baby may also be delivered by passing a hand round the margins of the placenta, or by incising the placenta (careful ultrasound mapping of the placental site prior to operation is a must)
- Breech extraction can also be performed by grasping one of the baby's feet and pulling, which would be better than to struggle for quiet a high head
- If the placenta is cut, immediate clamping of the cord is recommended
- Troublesome separation of placenta:
  - Do not continue attempting separation of placenta, if it is not separating with the usual methods (which will eventually land up in hysterectomy)
  - Two options, that can be attempted:
    - Leaving the placenta in place and closing
    - Leaving the placenta in place, closing the uterus and performing hysterectomy
  - Consequences of leaving the placenta in situ can be any of the following:
    - Can have a normal subsequent pregnancy
    - Elective evacuation of retained products of conception
    - Increased chances of infection → can even lead to sepsis
    - Heavy bleeding requiring hysterectomy
- If the placenta separates partially (partial accreta):
  - Remove the separated part
  - Leave the non-separated part in situ
  - But massive hemorrhage may ensue → all measures to combat it should be ready, saving the patient from DIC
- Management of retained placenta:
  - Risks of increased bleeding and infection should be explained
  - Appropriate antibiotics started from the immediate postpartum period
  - Neither methotrexate nor arterial embolization helps in avoiding the above complications, therefore not recommended routinely
  - Follow up of the patient:
    - Patient should be followed up by serial USG and measurement of β hCG on weekly basis, to see for placental resolution
  - Prognosis for future pregnancies → insufficient data (may or may not recur).

Treatment of Massive Placental Invasion

1. Uterine preserving management
Literature was reviewed thoroughly and none of the following options was found to be superior to the other.

Expectant management
- Does not seem to be much effective without adjuvant therapy
- Balloon occlusion devices can be placed in both internal iliac arteries prior to surgery by an interventional radiologist
- The balloon occlusion devices can be inflated after the baby is delivered to minimize blood loss
- The balloon can also be retained for 24 hours post-operatively to prevent postpartum hemorrhage.

Embolization of uterine arteries
- Can be offered to a patient with stable vitals and not too excessive bleeding
- Shorter hospital stay and quicker recovery
- Disadvantages:
  - Iliac artery thrombosis
  - Uterine necrosis or sepsis resulting in multiple organ failure
  - Non-target embolization can cause ischemic damage to other organs.

Methotrexate therapy
- This approach was first described by Arulkumaran and colleagues in 1986 where systemic methotrexate 50 mg as an intravenous infusion was administered on alternate days and the placental mass was expelled few days after delivery
- Methotrexate disrupts the folic acid pathway in rapidly dividing cells such as trophoblasts
- However, the proliferation of trophoblasts in the later stages of pregnancy has been shown to have no role in placental growth
- Consequently, the use of methotrexate may not reduce placental volume
- This therapy might even be harmful: methotrexate has a immunosuppressive role and therefore, could increase the risk of infection or even sepsis, which is already increased in patients with abnormal adherent placentation
- Other specific adverse effects are methotrexate-related pancytopenia and nephrotoxicity.

Uterus preserving surgery
- Hemostatic sutures, arterial ligation and balloon tamponade, resection of invasive placentation are described, having different results which needs to be individualized.

2. Uterus removal (hysterectomy)
- The resultant loss of fertility is devastating if the patient is a young primigravida
- However, prompt hysterectomy has led to a reduction of maternal mortality to < 2%.

To summarize the management of placental invasion (placenta accreta/percreta)
High index of suspicion (all risk factors mentioned above)

USG color Doppler and/or MRI

Preoperative arrangements:
a. Written and informed consent (mentioning each and every risk in detail)
b. Arrangement of blood and blood products (Packed cells, FFPs, Platelets, Cryoprecipitate)
c. Operative team, consisting of:
  - Senior obstetrician
  - Neonatologist
  - Senior anesthetist
  - Urologist
  - Interventional radiologist

- Vascular surgeon (preferably)

Intraoperative: Locate the depth of invasion

Accreta/Increta	Percreta
Cesarean hysterectomy	Cesarean section with conservative management of placenta.

Vasa Previa

- Vasa previa is an uncommon condition in which fetal blood vessels traverse the lower uterine segment in advance of the presenting part
- Neither the umbilical cord nor the placenta supports the vessels
- A velamentous insertion of the cord is a prerequisite for vasa previa.

Incidence

- Reported incidence ranges from 1 in 1275 to 1 in 8333
- As high as 1 in 202 following IVF.

Risk Factors

- Velamentous cord insertion → in almost all cases
- Bilobed placenta (bipartite placenta)
- Succenturiate lobe
- Placenta previa
- Marginal insertion of the cord
- Pregnancies resulting from IVF
- Multiple pregnancy
- Palpable vessel or a suspected amniotic band is felt on vaginal exam
- Fetal anomalies associated with increased risk include:
  - Renal tract anomalies
  - Spina bifida
  - Single umbilical artery
  - Exomphalos
  - Prematurity
  - Antepartum hemorrhage
  - Fetal growth restriction.

Differential Diagnosis on USG

- Chorioamniotic membrane separation
- Normal cord loop (it is important to ascertain that the vessel is not displaced with maternal movement)
- Marginal placental vascular sinus
- Amniotic band.

Diagnosis

In the absence of bleeding
- Antepartum:
  - There is no method to diagnose it clinically
  - USG:
    - Gianopoulos and colleagues were the first to describe the diagnosis of vasa previa using ultrasound in a woman with a history of a low-lying placenta and a succenturiate lobe
    - Findings: Echogenic, parallel or circular lines over the internal os of the cervix with absent Wharton's jelly
    - Combined TAS and TVS gives a better diagnosis.
  - Color Doppler:
    - Nelson and colleagues were the first to report the use of color flow Doppler to diagnose vasa previa in a woman at 26 weeks' gestation
    - Can diagnose it accurately but even with the use of transvaginal ultrasound color Doppler, **vasa previa may be missed**
    - Aberrant vessels over os (pregnancy-associated varicosities of the uterine vessels may be mistaken for aberrant placental vessels)
    - Blood flow can be demonstrated through these umbilical vessels.
- Intrapartum:
  - Palpation of fetal vessels at the time of vaginal examination.
- Postpartum:
  - Presence of fetal vessels running through the membrane by simple clinical examination of placenta.

In the presence of bleeding
- Vasa previa presents with painless vaginal bleeding at the time of spontaneous rupture of membranes or amniotomy (AROM)
- Immediate changes on CTG: variable decelerations, bradycardia, sinusoidal pattern of fetal heart rate
- This bleeding is most of the times labelled as bleeding due to placental abruption, placenta previa or "Heavy show"
- Bleeding of even 100 mL is sufficient to cause fetal shock and death, which can occur rapidly
- Laboratory tests:
  - Kleihauer–Betke test and hemoglobin electrophoresis:
    - Fetal blood cells and fetal hemoglobin in vagina can be detected (concentrations as low as 0.01%)
    - These tests take a long time for detection, so can't be used actually in practice
  - Alkali denaturation tests
    - Basic principle: Fetal Hb is resistant to alkali denaturation unlike adult Hb
    - Requires the presence of at least 60% fetal hemoglobin to be positive, and requires centrifugation
    - Fast and reliable but insensitive tests
    Apt test
    Loendersloot test uses 0.1 N KOH
    Ogita test
    Lindqvist and Gren
     - Have recently described a much simpler bedside test using 0.14 M sodium hydroxide solution, which denatures adult hemoglobin, turning it into a brownish-green color, while fetal hemoglobin is resistant to denaturation and retains its red color
     - This method may have some applicability in the clinical situation but requires further validation.

Risks

- Fetal bradycardia when the velamentous vessels are compressed by the presenting part (in the absence of bleeding)
- Antepartum hemorrhage
- Low-birth weight (in case of preterm birth)
- Prematurity
- Perinatal mortality → 23-100% (because of asphyxia, hemorrhagic shock, fetal anemia)
- Admission to NICU after birth.

Management

Antenatally
- If diagnosed in 2nd trimester → reconfirm again in the 3rd trimester as ≈ 15% of cases are resolved as pregnancy advances
- If confirmed in the 3rd trimester → elective cesarean section between 35-37 weeks (prior to rupture of membranes)
- Administration of corticosteroids at 28-32 weeks would be a wise step, as premature delivery is most likely in these cases
- Though recommendations are for admission to hospital at 30-32 weeks but local hospital authorities should make a protocol so that adverse outcomes can be avoided
- In utero, laser therapy to ablate the vessels of vasa previa may prove to be of help in future.

During labor
- Fetus compromised (non-reassuring changes on CTG):
  - Emergency cesarean section
- Fetus not compromised and advanced labor:
  - Prompt delivery
  - Aggressive neonatal resuscitation.

Cervical Polyp

- During pregnancy → increased vascularity
- Confused with threatened abortion in early months and can become a cause of APH in later months
- Intermittent bleeding → most common
- Avulsion of polyp followed by persistent bleeding
- Treatment: removal → send for histopathological diagnosis
- Hemostatics and gentle local pressure with gauge, if bleeds.

Vulvovaginal Trauma

- History will confirm the cause
- Adequate pelvic exam → if required → under anesthesia
- Penetration of cul-de-sac → exploratory laparotomy
- Foreign bodies → removed
- Wounds → debrided, closed
- Hematoma → evacuated → hemostasis achieved → drains placed
- Tetanus prophylaxis given.

Hematuria

- Urine analysis.

SUGGESTED READING

1. Andre F Lijoi, Joanna Brady. Vasa Previa Diagnosis and Management. JABFP. November–December 2003; Vol. 16 No. 6.
2. Antepartum Hemorrhage. RCOG Green-top Guideline No. 63. November 2011.
3. Charlotte N Steins Bisschop, Timme P Schaap, et al: Invasive placentation and uterus preserving treatment modalities: a systematic review. Arch Gynecol Obstet. 2011;284:491-502.
4. Christina S Han, Frederick Schatz, Charles J. Lockwood, et al: Abruption-associated prematurity. Clin Perinatol. September 2011;38(3):407-21.
5. Dalia Adukauskienė, Audronė Veikutienė, Agnė Adukauskaitė, et al: The usage of blood components in obstetrics. Medicina (Kaunas) 2010;46(8):561-7.
6. David R Hall. Abruptio placentae and disseminated intravascular coagulopathy. Seminars in perinatology 2009.
7. Edwin WH Thia, Lay-Kok Tan, Kanagalingam Devendra, et al: Lessons Learnt from Two Women with Morbidly Adherent Placentas and a Review of Literature. Ann Acad Med Singapore 2007;36:298-303.
8. Giancarlo Maria Liumbruno, Chiara Liumbruno, Daniela Rafanelli. Autologous blood in obstetrics: where are we going now? Blood Transfus 2012;10:125-47.
9. Gülmezoglu AM, Azhar M: Interventions for trichomoniasis in pregnancy (Review). The Cochrane Library 2011, Issue 5.
10. Ivo Brosens, Robert Pijnenborg, Lisbeth Vercruysse, et al. The "great obstetrical syndromes" are associated with disorders of deep placentation. Am J Obstet Gynecol. 2011;204(3):193-201.
11. Karanth L, Barua A, Kanagasabai S, et al. Desmopressin acetate (DDAVP) for preventing and treating acute bleeds during pregnancy in women with congenital bleeding disorders (Review). The Cochrane Library 2013, Issue 4.
12. Management of Antepartum Hemorrhage: SLCOG National guidelines.
13. Neilson JP. Interventions for suspected placenta previa (Review). The Cochrane Library 2010, Issue 1.
14. Neilson JP. Interventions for treating placental abruption (Review). The Cochrane Library 2012, Issue 2.
15. Placenta previa, placenta previa accreta and vasa previa: diagnosis and management. RCOG Green-top Guideline No. 27. January 2011.
16. Robert Gagnon, et al: Guidelines for the Management of Vasa Previa. J Obstet Gynaecol Can 2009;31(8):748-53.
17. Roberto Romero, Juan Pedro Kusanovic, Tinnakorn Chaiworapongsa, et al: Placental bed disorders in preterm labor, preterm PROM, spontaneous abortion and abruptio placentae. Best Pract Res Clin Obstet Gynaecol. June 2011;25(3):313-27.
18. Thia EWH, Lee SL, Tan HK, et al: Ultrasonographical features of morbidly-adherent placentas. Singapore Med J. 2007;48(9):799.
19. Wagner KS, Ronsmans C, Thomas SL, et al: Women who experience obstetric hemorrhage are at higher risk of anemia, in both rich and poor countries. Tropical Medicine and International Health. January 2012; 17(1):9-22.
20. Walfish M, Neuman A and Wlody D: Maternal hemorrhage, Br J Anaesth 2009;103(Suppl. 1):47-56.
21. Xavier Miracle, Gian Carlo Di Renzo, Ann Stark, et al: Guideline for the use of antenatal corticosteroids for fetal Maturation. J Perinat Med. 2008;36:191-6.

CHAPTER 6

Uterine Size More than Expected

Tania G Singh

Case: A 34 years old G_2A_1, unbooked patient with 4 months period of gestation, comes for antenatal check up for the first time. Complains of swelling of the feet and continued vomitings since the 2nd month of her gestation. She has not received any dose of tetanus toxoid and is not taking any medications.

On examination:
BP: 130/88 mmHg   Weight: 70 kg   P/A: uterus 18–20 weeks POG
PR: 92/min   Height: 154 cm

How will you approach at the diagnosis?

Step 1. Calculate the dates properly (wrong dates—most common cause)

Step 2. Exclude distended bladder (ask patient to pass urine before examination)

Step 3. Obstetric examination:
- No fetus palpable/no FHS heard/no ballotment → vesicular mole → perform ultrasound
- 3 fetal poles → Conjoined twins

  OR

  Singleton pregnancy with uterine leiomyoma
- 4 fetal poles → twins
- > 4 fetal poles → triplets or higher order
- 2 fetal poles → singleton pregnancy → assess liquor → excessive → hydramnios

Step 4. Normal → Trendelenburg position (results in upward shift of structures free to do so–bowel, omentum, mobile ovarian tumour)

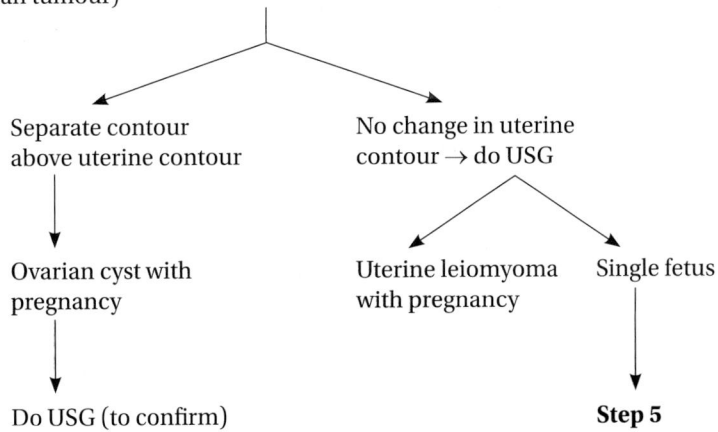

Step 5. Repeat USG after 3 weeks for fetal biometry

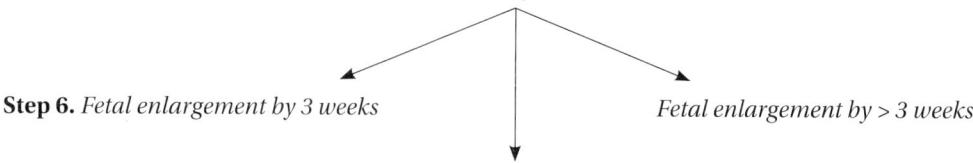

Step 6. *Fetal enlargement by 3 weeks*   *Fetal enlargement by > 3 weeks*

Hydrops fetalis or non-immune hydrops

Why three weeks for fetal biometry? Recommended interval between USG evaluation of fetal growth is 3 weeks because shorter intervals increase the likelihood of a false positive diagnosis of abnormal growth.

Trendelenburg position: a moderate to large sized cystic ovarian tumour may get included in uterine mass during clinical examination beyond 24 weeks. Trendelenburg position causes it to move cranially while uterus cannot do so. As a result, a transverse groove is seen in fundal contour, between tumour and fundus of uterus.

MULTIPLE GESTATION

How to Diagnose?

A. History:
- ART—ovulation induction drugs (esp. gonadotropins)
- Family history of twins (maternal >> paternal, especially for dizygous twins)
- If mother herself is a member of pair of dizygous twins, she has 2% chances of conceiving with twins as compared to dizygous husband whose wife has only 1% chance of giving birth to twins
- Increased age and parity
- Increased maternal body weight (not clear → may be because of increased circulating levels of pituitary gonadotropins)
- Race (highest—Nigeria and lowest in Japan).

B. Symptoms:
- Hyperemesis or increased nausea in early months
- Pressure symptoms:
  - Edema of legs [vulva/abdominal wall (may be)]
  - Shortness of breath
  - Palpitations
  - Varicose veins
  - Hemorrhoids
  - Digestive discomfort
- Undue uterine enlargement because of polyhydramnios
- Excessive fetal movements.

C. GPE:
- Anemia
- Unusual weight gain, not explained by preeclampsia/obesity
- Gestational: hypertension/preeclampsia.

D. Per-abdomen:
- Shape—Elongated shape of normal pregnant uterus → changed to barrel shape
- Abdomen—unduly enlarged

- Palpation:
  - Height of uterus > period of gestation (SFH)
  - ↑↑ Abdominal girth (at term)
  - Fetal bulk—disproportionately > in relation to fetal size
  - Palpation of at least 3 poles or 2 fetal heads (too many fetal parts)
- Auscultation:
  - Two separate FHS (heard simultaneously by 2 different observers) separated by a silent area with a discrepancy of at least 10 beats per minute → this may not be that easily heard because of presence of hydramnios (very commonly associated).

E. USG

Role of Ultrasound in Twin Pregnancy

- Twins make up > 98% of all multiple pregnancies
- Ultrasound is the only safe and reliable method for the diagnosis and assessment of twins
- Has a definitive role, right from the 1st trimester until delivery of the 2nd fetus
- Most common clinical uses of ultrasound:
  - Determination of chorionicity and amnionicity
  - Confirmation of gestational age
  - Diagnosis of anomalies and complications
  - Measurement of cervical length
  - Assessment of growth and amniotic fluid
  - Placental localization
  - Fetal position for intrapartum management.

DETERMINATION OF CHORIONICITY AND AMNIONICITY

Chorionicity (C)

- Relates to placentation
- More accurate before 14 weeks (accuracy is 96 to100% versus approximately 80% in the 2nd trimester)
- Clinical management depending on chorionicity:
  - Management of structural anomalies
  - Screening for and identification of aneuploidy
  - Determination of the etiology of fetal growth and/or fluid discordance
  - Early diagnosis of twin-to-twin transfusion syndrome
  - Management of the surviving twin following intrauterine demise of the other twin.

Amnionicity (A)

Before 8–10 weeks, separate and distinct amnions may be visible on USG as they have not enlarged sufficiently to contact each other and create inter twin membrane (they are extremely thin and delicate).

Assessment of C and A

Before 10 weeks gestation

- *Number of gestational sacs*
  - Each gestational sac forms its own placenta and chorion

- Therefore:
  - 2 gestational sacs → dichorionic
  - 1 gestational sac with 2 identified heartbeats → monochorionic.
- *Number of amniotic sacs within the chorionic cavity*
  - 2 amniotic cavities → diamniotic
  - 1 amniotic cavity → monoamniotic
    - Occurs in approximately 1% of all monozygotic twin pregnancies
    - They are at increased risk of fetal death due to cord entanglement
    - Therefore, early diagnosis is important
    - USG can predict virtually all cases of monoamniotic twins
    - Sonographic indicators in 1st trimester include:
      - Presence of a single yolk sac
      - Demonstration of cord entanglement from the placental or umbilical origin (most definitive sonographic finding which can be identified using color doppler).
- *Embryos per sac*
  - 1 embryo per sac in diamniotic dichorionic
  - 2 embryos per sac in monochorionic diamniotic
  - 2 embryos per sac in monochorionic monoamniotic.
- *Number of yolk sacs*
  - This may help diagnose the amnionicity:
    - 2 yolk sacs → diamniotic
    - A single yolk sac → in most cases indicate monoamniotic twins but a single yolk sac seen with dual embryos → a follow-up first trimester scan to definitively assign amnionicity.

After 10 weeks gestation
The above sonographic signs are no longer present.
The new sonographic findings determining chorionicity and amnionicity are:
- Fetal genitalia *(should not be done routinely)*
  - Phenotypic discordance → identifies dichorionicity in all except a few rare cases
  - Phenotypic concordance → does not rule out dichorionicity
  - Phenotypic concordance → always present in monochorionic twins.
- Placental number
  - Single placenta → mostly monochorionic (except where 2 placentas are fused to form one)
  - Two distinct placentas → dichorionic
  - Ability of USG to identify 2 discrete placental masses depends on proximity of implantation of 2 blastocysts
  - For example—when 2 blastocysts implant next to each other, the placentas often become fused along their borders, therefore 1 placenta is visualized.
- Chorionicity

  Twin peak or Lambda sign → Dichorionic diamniotic
  - A projecting zone of tissue of similar echotexture to the placenta, triangular in cross-section and wider at the chorionic surface of the placenta, extending into, and tapering to a point within, the intertwin membrane
  - Twin peak or Lambda sign at any gestation → 100% dichorionic placenta
  - Sensitivity 97%
  - Specificity 100%
  - Absence of the twin peak sign → monochorionic (especially before 20 weeks gestation)

  T-sign (Monochorionic diamniotic)
  - There is a 90° relationship between membrane and placenta with no apparent extension of dividing membrane

- Sensitivity 100%
- Specificity 98%.
- Membrane characteristics
  Dichorionic pregnancy
  - 2 layers of amnion
  - 2 layers of chorion
  - Membrane thicker and more reflective than the monochorionic diamniotic membrane
  - Membrane thickness of > 2 mm
  - Positive predictive value → 95%.
  Monochorionic pregnancy
  - Positive predictive value → 90%
  - Membrane thickness ≤ 2 mm.

Note:
- In the 2nd trimester, the number of membranes may be counted and if there are > 2, then dichorionicity is strongly suggested
- In ≈ 7% of dichorionic pregnancies, the twin peak sign disappears at 16–20 weeks. Therefore, its absence cannot exclude dichorionicity
- If intertwin membrane is not visualized, the possibilities include:
  - Monoamniotic
  - Normal twin gestation (diamniotic, in which membrane is present but cannot be identified owing to its thinness and orientation of the transducer)
  - Stuck twin secondary to severe oligohydramnios (less common)
- Monoamnionicity
  The diagnosis of monoamnionicity is made on the basis of the following criteria:
  - Single shared placenta
  - Fetal phenotype concordance
  - Absence of inter-twin membrane
  - Adequate amniotic fluid surrounding both fetuses
  - Free movement of both twins within the uterine cavity
  - 2 fetal poles within 1 chorionic sac
  - Entanglement of limbs or observation of a limb circumscribing the other is suggestive of monoamnionicity
  - Presence of conjoined twins
  - Single umbilical cord that contains >3 vessels
  - Visualization of 2 cord insertions into chorionic plate of placenta in very close proximity to one another.

Zygosity

- Genetic identity of each twin in the pregnancy
- Zygosity cannot always be inferred from the determination of chorionicity
- There are two types of twins, dizygotic (DZ) and monozygotic (MZ) twins

DZ Twins (Binovular)

- The mechanism(s) leading to DZ twins operate on the selection of developing follicles within the ovary where instead of one ovum being released mid-cycle, two follicles mature, releasing both oocytes, which are then fertilized by two sperms

- Have the same genetic relationship as ordinary brothers and sisters and on average share 50% of their genes
- They can be same sex (boy-boy or girl-girl) or opposite sex (boy-girl) twin pairs
- Number of placenta – 2 (except in cases where they are fused to form 1)
- Number of intervening membranes – 4
- There is no vessel communication
- Blood type will be different
- Usually discordant for chromosomal anomalies.

MZ Twins (Uniovular)

- Arise when an embryo splits soon after fertilization
- Carry essentially identical genetic instructions (share 100% of their genes)
- Are always of the same sex (boy-boy or girl-girl)
- Unknown mechanism(s) affect the early development of the embryo immediately after fertilization leading to separation of the cells into two or more embryos
- Number of placentae
  - In 75% cases - 1 placenta
  - In 25% - 2
- Number of intervening membranes depends upon the time of fertilization
- Reasons for the relatively high incidence of MZ twins in humans remain unclear
- There are no clear associations between MZ twinning and maternal, environmental or genetic factors and the mechanisms have not been identified, although families with a history of MZ twinning have been reported.

Useful Facts

Of all the twin pregnancies:

Dizygotic
- Constitute 70%
- They are always dichorionic diamniotic (DCDA)
- Sometimes 2 placentae may be fused to form 1

Monozygotic
- Constitute 30%
- These can be:
  - DCDA (33%)
  - MCDA (66%)
  - MCMA (<1%)

Now based on this, there are few other findings:
- Monochorionic can only be monozygotic with very rare exceptions that are due to post-zygotic changes
- Dichorionic can be dizygotic or monozygotic
- All dizygotic pregnancies are dichorionic
- Dichorionic twins with discordant sex are always dizygotic
- In the case of same-sex dichorionic twins, zygosity cannot be determined with confidence unless genetic testing is performed (using microsatellites or single nucleotide polymorphism techniques)
- In dizygotic, number of layers is always 4, but in monozygotic, number of layers depend on chorionicity and amnionicity

- Monozygotic: depends on time of division of fertilized ovum
  - Day 3
    - Chorion completes its differentiation
    - Rule: once any tissue has differentiated, it is no longer capable of splitting
  - Day 8
    - Amnion differentiation completed
  - Day 12
    - Differentiation of embryonic disc gets completed
  - After Day 13
    - Division usually incomplete → conjoined twins
  - Therefore, if cleavage occurs:
    - At < 3 days → dichorionic diamniotic (DCDA)
    - After 3 days but < 8 days → monochorionic diamniotic (MCDA)
    - After 8 days → monochorionic monoamniotic (MCMA).

COMPLICATIONS RELATED TO CHORIONICITY

Dichorionic Diamniotic

There are two main complications:
a. Discordant growth
b. Intrauterine fetal death (IUFD)

Discordant Growth

Criteria and causes
- Singleton growth curves currently provide the best predictors of adverse outcome in twins and may be used for evaluating growth abnormalities
- Determination of fetal growth discordance is important because studies have shown an association with increased mortality and morbidity when there are significant differences in birth weight
- Different definitions/criteria for discordance have been provided:
  - $$\frac{\text{EFW larger twin} - \text{EFW smaller twin}}{\text{EFW largest twin}} \times 100$$
    - Intertwin birth weight discordance of > 20% with reference to weight of larger twin
    - EFW is based on BPD and AC
    OR
    - AC and FL
    - Sensitivity (25–55%)
  - Difference in AC >20 mm
    - Sensitivity of 80%
    - Specificity 85%
    - Positive predictive value 62%
    OR
  - Difference in BPD > 8 mm
  - Mean intertwin birth weight difference ≈ 10%.
- Causes:
  - Twin to twin transfusion syndrome (most common → placental vascular anastomosis)
  - IUGR

- Structural anomalies occurring in 1 fetus only:
  - Weight discordance of ≥ 25% is significant (clinically important indicator of IUGR) but IUGR is more predictive of perinatal outcome than degree of discordance
  - Aim to undertake scans at intervals of < 28 days
  - IQ in smaller infant is less than in the larger one
- Due to different genetic growth potential
- One placenta with suboptimal implantation
- Indication for delivery depends upon:
  - Well being of fetuses
  - Gestational age
  - Serial growth velocity.

Intrauterine Death of One fetus

General overview
- Only 50% of twin pregnancies identified in the 1st trimester will result in 2 live born infants
- When the demise occurs early in pregnancy, the prognosis for the surviving fetus is excellent
- Demise of one fetus occurs in 2 to 5% of twin pregnancies during the 2nd and 3rd trimesters
- The occurrence of single fetal death is 3-fold to 4-fold higher in monochorionic twins than in dichorionic twins
- It is also more common in high-order multiples, complicating 14–17% of triplet pregnancies
- Adverse outcomes: the greatest risk to the surviving fetus, regardless of chorionicity, is
  - Preterm delivery (50-80% of surviving twins) and the associated complications of prematurity
  - Multi-organ damage (in surviving twin) in monoamniotic twins
  - Ischemic injury, which is thought to occur at the time of the demise, has been documented in the spleen, kidney, gastrointestinal tract, skin, and brain of the surviving twin
  - Neurologic injury (such as multicystic encephalomalacia) in upto 20% of surviving fetuses in monochorionic twins
  - These abnormalities may not be diagnosed by ultrasound until much later in pregnancy
- Immediate delivery may not prevent the development of such complications
- Offer women with uncomplicated:
  - Monochorionic twin pregnancies elective birth from 36 weeks, after a course of antenatal corticosteroids has been offered
  - Triplet pregnancies elective birth from 35 weeks, after a course of antenatal corticosteroids has been offered.

IUFD in Dichorionic Twins

Determining factors
- Cause of IUD
  and
- Gestational age

Consequences
- As placentas are separate, there is no worry of damage to surviving twin due to hypotensive or embolic phenomena, as in case of monochorionic pregnancy
- Risk is related to preterm labor
- Maternal DIC - rare
- Offer uncomplicated dichorionic twin pregnancies elective birth from 37 weeks onwards
- Risk → negligible in DC twins

- Perform:
  - NST
  - BPP
  - Give corticosteroids (between 24–34 weeks, if delivery anticipated within 7 days).

Monochorionic Diamniotic

1. TTTS
2. IUFD
3. TRAP

Twin to Twin Transfusion Syndrome (TTTS)

- Affects approximately 15% of these pregnancies
- Perinatal mortality is up to 80% if the syndrome is left untreated, particularly if problems develop before 28 weeks' gestation
- Accounts for 15 to 17% of the overall perinatal mortality in twins
- Results from abnormal shunting of blood between the circulations of the unborn twins through anastomoses of the vessels of the shared placenta
- Anastomosis can be:

Superficial
  - Bidirectional
  - Artery to artery anastomosis
  - Vein to vein anastomosis

Deep
  - Unidirectional
  - Artery to vein anastomosis
  - Arterial blood of 1 twin drains into venous system of the other

- Balanced blood flow across these connections occurs in most monochorionic twins
- Unbalanced transfusion from the donor to the recipient can occur in those placentas that have deep artery-to-vein connections, causing twin-twin transfusion syndrome
- *Does not occur in monoamniotic pregnancy.*

Antenatal criteria

- Same sex
- MCDA (with placental vascular anastomosis)
- Can be predicted as early as 10–14 weeks by discordantly increased nuchal translucency
- Folding of intertwin membrane at 15–17 weeks
- Absence of artery to artery anastomosis detected on serial Doppler USG from 14 weeks onwards
- Velamentous cord insertion at 18 weeks
- Discordance in fetal size with the larger twin seen often in the polyhydramnios sac (but is not essential for the diagnosis)
- 2 vessel cord, or unequal placental partition
- Doppler studies are also part of the diagnostic evaluation:
  - Absent or low end diastolic flow in the umbilical artery of the donor
  - Decreased ventricular function depicted by tricuspid regurgitation
  - Reversal of A wave in ductus venosus and/or
  - Cardiac chamber enlargement in the recipient are seen in more advanced stages of TTTS.

USG diagnosis

Features of recipient twin
- Excessive fluid (hydramnios)
- Normal structure
- Usually appropriately grown for gestational age
- Has a large distended bladder, visceromegaly
- May, if severely compromised, show tricuspid regurgitation or hydrops fetalis or heart failure (develops circulatory overload)
- Polycythemic
- Becomes plethoric
- Neurological sequelae
- Deepest vertical pocket <2 mm.

Features of donor twin
- Little or no fluid (oligohydramnios) or anhydramnios (the donor twin gets stuck against the wall of the uterus)
- This may lead to renal failure
- Separating membrane completely covering this fetus
- Normal structure
- Frequently severely growth restricted as it transfuses blood to the recipient twin → pulmonary hypoplasia
- Shows abnormal umbilical artery Doppler waveforms
- The bladder becomes non-visible
- Anemic
- Becomes pale
- Neurological sequelae
- Deepest vertical pocket
    a. > 8 cm prior to 20 weeks
    b. > 10 cm at 20-26 weeks
- Earlier criteria which was taken (now unreliable):
    a. Discordance ≥ 20% in weight
    b. Discordance of ≥ 5 gm/dL in hemoglobin level at birth.

The condition is now graded by the **Quintero staging system** (Quintero 1996) as follows:
Stage 1: Abnormal amniotic fluid levels alone with bladder filling in the donor
Stage 2: Collapsed bladder in the donor
Stage 3: Abnormal Doppler flow in the umbilical artery or ductus venosus of either twin
Stage 4: Hydrops in either twin
Stage 5: Intrauterine death of either twin.

All stages can further be subdivided depending upon presence or absence of artery to artery anastomosis:
a. If AAAs are absent, cases of fetal loss increased from 40 to 60% from stage I to stage IV
b. Survival better in presence of AAAs on USG.

Associated risks
- Although twin-twin transfusion is usually a gradual process, it can happen suddenly with the death of one twin, usually the recipient
- This can lead to the death of the co-twin or neurological handicap (cerebral palsy) occurring in 15% of the survivors

- Other co-morbidities among survivors include:
  - Cardiac
  - Renal
- Other risks:
  - Spontaneous miscarriage
  - PPROM
  - Preterm labor
  - Growth retardation.

Management: Even if 1st trimester scan is normal, routine USG at ≈ 2 weeks interval between 16 and 26 weeks is advised

Options include:
- Expectant management
- Repeated serial amnioreduction
- Endoscopic laser ablation of vascular anastomoses
- Amniotic septostomy
- Selective feticide.

Serial amnioreduction
- The repeated removal of excessive amniotic fluid by amniocenteses
- The most established method of treatment
- At >26 weeks:
  - Amniocentesis indicated if AFI > 40 cm or largest vertical pocket ≈ >12 cm
  - When laser therapy is technically difficult
  - When laser therapy is not available
- Different proposals of its effects are described:
  - There have been improvements in the color flow Doppler waveforms of the uterine artery
  - Reduction in the rate of fluid accumulation, which otherwise, would have compressed the placenta and increased the rate of transfusion to the recipient twin
  - Increase in fetoplacental blood volume with increasing gestation may reduce the effects of anastomoses, therefore, showing an improvement in the condition
- Advantages:
  - Prolongs pregnancy
  - Improves fetal survival (37–60%)
  - Some improvement in the risk of neurological damage (17–33%)
  - Does not require special equipment
  - Can be performed by most obstetricians specialized in fetal medicine
- Complications:
  - In around 10% of cases
  - IUFD within 48 hours of the procedure
  - Spontaneous abortion
  - Abruptio placentae has been reported.

Laser ablation
- It is the coagulation of the superficial blood vessels that cross the separating membrane of the placenta by means of laser
- Done at < 26 weeks
- Procedure:
  - Performed under regional analgesia or local anesthesia with maternal sedation
  - Under ultrasound guidance, a cannula and needle are inserted through the maternal abdominal wall, uterine wall and into the amniotic sac of the recipient twin

- Needle is removed and a fetoscope with a thin fibre to carry the laser energy is then inserted through the cannula
- The fetoscope is used to look at the blood vessels on the surface of the placenta
- Placental vessels are then coagulated using the Nd :YAG laser
- After completion of surgery, excess amniotic fluid in the recipient twin's sac is removed to achieve a normal volume
- Target AFI is <15 cm in order to prolong interval between the procedures
- Systematic coagulation of all these vessels should include the branches of these anastomoses and currently this remains the only method that can prevent transfusion between the placentas
- Survival rate is 55–73%
- Neurological handicap 4.2%
- Selective laser ablation is done on only those AVAs that are involved in TTTS
- Disadvantages:
  - Requires fetoscopic skills and therefore can only be performed in very few centers at present
  - It is a far more invasive procedure than amnioreduction
  - Maternal morbidity is much higher
  - Bleeding from the placental vessels is consistently reported
  - Further interventions like amnioreduction are required in around 20% of cases.

Septostomy
- It is the creation of a puncture in the inter-twin membrane by a 20–22G needle, improving the amniotic fluid dynamics → excess fluid passes from recipient sac to donor sac → normal volume in both
- Advantage:
  - Requires a single procedure
  - Survival rates as high as 83% can be achieved but no reliable figures for neurological outcome are available in literature
  - It equalizes the pressure in the two sacs thus relieving the pressure on the placenta
  - Relatively safe procedure
  - Does not require special equipment
- The major risk associated with amniotic septostomy is cord entanglement, as the procedure is effectively creating a monoamniotic pregnancy, within a single sac
- Procedure:
  - Under local anesthesia and ultrasound guidance, an amniocentesis needle is inserted through the maternal abdominal wall and uterine wall
  - The needle is then used to make a small hole in the membrane between the twins, allowing the fluid around the recipient twin to move into the donor twin's sac
  - Amnioreduction may also be performed before and/or after the septostomy.

Selective feticide
- At first it is very important to understand the difference between selective reduction and multi-fetal pregnancy reduction (MFPR)
  - In multi-fetal pregnancy reduction, the fetus(es) to be reduced are chosen on the basis of technical considerations, such as which is most accessible to intervention
  - In selective reduction, fetuses are chosen on the basis of health status or sex
  - Indications (Twins or Higher order gestation):
    - Usually >12 weeks
    - ↑NT in high order gestation for MFPR
    - Acardiac twin, anomalous fetus
    - TTTS

- In many cases, fetus that is chromosomally abnormal or affected by a genetic disorder would be preferentially selected for reduction
- Its entirely the decision of the pregnant woman to consent or not to consent for the procedure
- Dichorionic pregnancy
  Intracardiac KCl
  - Common method
  - Done as an outpatient procedure
  - USG guided at gestational age ≥ 24 weeks
  - Premedication (antibiotics, pethidine, antiemetics)
  - Clean maternal abdomen/ultrasound probe and cord
  - Procedure:
    - Obtain a 4-chamber view—record FHR
    - Free-hand technique/continuous ultrasound guidance
    - Local anesthetic → 5 mL of 2% lignocaine at entry site
    - 20 G 15 cm spinal needle—targeting left ventricle or most accessible chamber of fetal heart is selected
    - 15% KCl administered under direct vision—until asystole
    - Re-scan 30 mins later—confirm asystole
  Intracranial KCl injection
  - Newer technique—First case series reported in (2009) in Turkey
  - Difficulty in reaching the thorax due to fetal position
  - Fetal intracranial injection of KCl (2–3 mL)
  - Comment: Technically easier procedure than the intrathoracic approach
  - Technique should be reserved for selected cases by experienced operators
- Monochorionic pregnancy
  - Main Goal: Interrupt blood flow to candidate fetus while avoiding exsanguination of the co-twin
  - Different procedures:
    - *Bipolar cord coagulation*
    - *Cord ligation/compression*
    - *Radiofrequency ablation*
    - *Laser photocoagulation (Nd:YAG)*
    - *Cord embolization (thrombogenic coils/sclerosants)*
- Survival rate is ≈ 50%
- No figure has been provided for neurological outcomes
- Selective feticide has relative risks associated with the technique used.

Intrauterine Fetal Death

- 25% risk of death
- 25% risk of neurological handicap and multiorgan injury
- Multiple foci of encephalomalacia and ischemic changes in:
  - Spleen
  - Kidney
  - GIT
  - Skin
  - Brain
- (May be) because of embolization of thromboplastin material released from dead fetus, which goes to surviving twin through placental anastomosis

OR
- (May be) that acute bleeding from surviving to dead fetus occurs due to decreased pressure in dead twin → transient severe hypotension and ischemic damage in vital organs of surviving fetus
- Supported by occurrence of sudden anemia in surviving twin with normal coagulation profile after death of 1 fetus.

Treatment
Depends on:
- Gestational age, chorionicity and condition of surviving fetus
- If it is 1st trimester loss → no harm to surviving fetus
- If it is 2nd or 3rd trimester loss → outcome depends on chorionicity
  Previable
  - Termination
  Viable
  - Immediate delivery doesn't appear to change the outcome as injury could have occurred at the time of demise
  - Difficult to predict cerebral injury but multiple encephalomalacia can be diagnosed by USG or MRI (scheduled 2–3 weeks after the demise)
  - There may be transient increase in FDPs with hypofibrinogenemia, risk of clinically significant maternal coagulopathy → almost nil
  - Baseline maternal coagulation profile recommended
  - Follow up advised.

Twin Reversed Arterial Perfusion Syndrome (TRAP)

- Also known as acardiac twinning
- Occurs in 1 in 35,000 deliveries
- 1 in 100 monozyotic twins
- 1 in 30 monozygotic triplets
- Have a 90% risk of preterm birth and a 30% risk of congestive heart failure in the normal twin (also called pump twin)
- Understanding the syndrome:
  - Large artery to artery placental shunt can be seen in early 1st trimester
  - Imbalance in inter-fetal circulation and reversal of blood flow in umbilical vessels
  - Perfusion pressure of donor twin overpowers that in recipient twin
  - "Used" arterial blood reaching recipient twin preferentially goes to iliac vessels and thus perfuses only the lower part of body → disruption and deterioration of growth and development of upper body
  - High cardiac output in pump twin → decompensation
- It can be:
  - Acardius acephalus: failure or disrupted growth of head
  - Acardius myelacephalus: partially developed head with identifiable limbs
  - Acardius amorphous: failure of any recognizable structure.

Differential diagnosis includes
- Intrauterine fetal demise
- An abnormal monochorionic twin
- Placental tumours

Diagnosis
1. As early as 10 weeks
2. Arterial blood flows towards rather than away from affected fetus (reversal of blood flow within the abnormal fetus) on color Doppler → definitive diagnosis
3. Serial USG:
   - Grossly malformed fetus with amorphous cephalic pole
   - Poor definition of trunk and extremities (due to severe hypoxia)
   - Absence of cardiac pulsations
4. Fetal hemodynamic function should be assessed by fetal echocardiography; hydrops in the pump twin being a poor prognostic feature.

Treatment
- Goal:
  - Interruption of vascular communication
- Procedure:
  - Ultrasound guided
  - Needle used: 14 gauge radio ablation needle
  - Cauterization of umbilical vessels and termination of blood flow to the recipient twin at the site of cord insertion into umbilicus
  - Period of gestation at which performed: 18–24 weeks.

Monochorionic Monoamniotic

Conjoined Twins

- Incidence varies between 1 in 50,000 and 1 in 100,000 births
- Intrauterine fetal death in 60%
- Those born alive → die of anomalies
- Diagnosis can be made by ultrasound examination, even at less than 10 weeks period of gestation but again confirmation is required at 11–14 weeks
- Clues:
  - Bifid appearance of fetal pole
  - Lack of a separating membrane between the twins
  - Presence of > 3 vessels in the umbilical cord
  - Heads at the same level and body plane, extremities in unusual proximity
  - No change in fetal positions relative to each other
  - Inability to separate the fetal bodies and skin contours
  - Extended positions of spines
  - Monoamniotic
- Of all conjoined twins, only those who are omphalopagus have a reasonable chance of survival
- 2 varieties: equal or unequal (parasitic variety)
- Most frequent types:
  - Thoracopagus (anterior) - most common
  - Pygopagus (posterior)
  - Craniopagus (cranial)
  - Ischiopagus (caudal).

Management
- If termination between 18–24 weeks → hysterotomy may be required
- Close antenatal surveillance from 24 weeks onwards
- Elective cesarean section at 32–34 weeks

- Vaginal delivery includes risks of:
  - Dystocia
  - Trauma to uterus and cervix
  - Cord entanglement and sudden IUD.

Difference between TTTS and discordant growth

TTTS	Discordant
Hydramnios (DVP > 8 cm) in recipient sac	Normal amniotic fluid (DVP < 8 cm)
Stuck twin in donor	Stuck twin in growth restricted fetus

DETERMINATION OF GESTATIONAL AGE

- 1st trimester → ideal time to confirm or establish accurate gestational age dating
- But in twins, 2nd trimester dating is also considered acceptable and accurate (studies have proved)
- In the 1st trimester → crown–rump length (CRL)
- In the 2nd trimester, a combination of head circumference, abdominal circumference, and femur length provides the most accurate dating (rather than a single parameter)
- When twin pregnancy is the result of in vitro fertilization → accurate determination of gestational age should be made from the date of embryo transfer
- In general, about 95% of gestational age estimates in the 1st and 2nd trimester will be within 5 to 7 days of the "true" gestational age, regardless of the parameter or parameters used
- There is insufficient evidence to make recommendation of which fetus (when discordant for size) to use to date a twin pregnancy. However, to avoid missing a situation of early intrauterine growth restriction in one twin, most experts agree that the clinician may consider dating pregnancy using the larger fetus.

SCREENING FOR ANOMALIES

First Trimester

- Nuchal translucency for aneuploidy screening
- Risk of aneuploidy:
  - Chorionicity and zygosity can both affect the estimated risk of Down's syndrome in twins
  - Zygosity, rather than chorionicity, determines the degree of risk and whether or not the fetuses may be concordant or discordant for chromosomal anomalies
  - In monozygotic pregnancies, both twins are either affected or unaffected, with very rare exceptions, while in dizygotic pregnancies, the risk of aneuploidy for each twin is more or less independent of the risk for the other
  - The risk of aneuploidy in monochorionic twins appears similar to the risk in singleton pregnancies
- Nuchal translucency (NT) screening in twins:
  - NT distribution and therefore the Down's syndrome detection rates do not differ significantly between twins and singletons
  - NT measurement combined with maternal age has been the method of choice for prenatal aneuploidy screening in twins
  - Risk assessment can be calculated for each twin or for both together

In monochorionic twins:
- Each fetus has the same risk of being affected with Down syndrome and the overall risk is the same as in a singleton pregnancy

In dichorionic twin pregnancy:
- Each fetus is considered separately, and the risk for each fetus is calculated by using median NT values for singletons
- The prevalence of increased NT is higher in women with monochorionic pregnancies than in those with dichorionic pregnancies (8.4% vs. 5.4%), suggesting that increased NT in monochorionic twins may be an early manifestation of the twin-twin transfusion syndrome
- Map the fetal positions
- Use the combined screening test (nuchal translucency, β hCG, pregnancy-associated plasma protein-A) for Down's syndrome when CRL measures from 45 - 84 mm (at ≈11^{+0} to 13^{+6} weeks).

Second Trimester

A detailed scan should be performed for:
- Soft markers of Down's syndrome (if abnormal, a fetus specific risk is calculated according to soft marker detected)
- Congenital anamolies (1.2-2 times more common in twins): best performed between 18-22 weeks
- Most common structural abnormalities are:
  - Cardiac anomalies
  - Neural tube and brain defects
  - Facial clefts
  - Gastrointestinal and anterior abdominal wall defects
- Apart from structural defects, there are three types of congenital anomalies unique to twin pregnancies:
  - Midline structural defects, believed to be a consequence of the twinning process, exemplified by conjoined twins
  - Malformations resulting from vascular events as a consequence of placental anastomoses, leading to hypotension and/or ischemia. This can happen to a surviving twin after the demise of the other twin. Anomalies seen as consequence of such events include–
    - Microcephaly
    - Periventricular leukomalacia
    - Hydrocephalus
    - Intestinal atresia
    - Renal dysplasia
    - Limb amputation
  - Defects or deformities from intrauterine crowding:
    - Foot deformities
    - Hip dislocation
    - Skull asymmetry.

Fetal Surveillance

- Routine surveillance of twin pregnancies every 5 weeks appears to be beneficial
- More frequent surveillance will result in significantly higher false positive rates for IUGR

- The frequency of ultrasound evaluation in twin pregnancies is determined according to chorionicity and growth pattern:
  - Monochorionic twins are scanned more frequently to allow for earlier diagnosis of TTTS and/or growth restriction or discordance, which have greater implications for the non-affected twin than they do in dichorionic pregnancies
- Serial ultrasound assessments every 2 to 3 weeks, starting at 16 weeks of gestation for monochorionic pregnancies and every 3 to 4 weeks, starting from the anatomy scan (18 to 22 weeks) for dichorionic pregnancies
- Increased fetal surveillance should be considered when there is either growth restriction diagnosed in one twin or significant growth discordance.

CERVICAL LENGTH MEASUREMENT

- In asymptomatic women with a multiple pregnancy, measurement of 2nd trimester cervical length can be used to identify a group of women who are at increased risk for preterm birth
- Sensitivity, however, is low, indicating that a large percentage of women with a multiple pregnancy will deliver prematurely in spite of a long cervix in the 2nd trimester
- In view of the fact that cerclage is known to increase complications, a high specificity is also important, as a limited specificity would increase the exposure of women with a low risk of preterm delivery to unnecessary and potentially harmful interventions.

ASSESSMENT OF AMNIOTIC FLUID

- Best method of amniotic fluid assessment cannot be ascertained
- Various methods employed are:
  - Subjective assessment
  - Deepest vertical pocket
  - Modified amniotic fluid index
  - 2-dimensional pockets
  - Ascertain the presence of fluid, caudal and rostral, and determine to which fetus it belongs and subjectively estimate if normal
- When amniotic fluid volume appears reduced or increased, the vertical measurement of the largest pocket in each sac is taken. The condition is defined as oligohydramnios when the deepest vertical pocket is < 2 cm and as polyhydramnios when the deepest vertical pocket is > 8 cm
- These definitions correspond approximately to the 2.5th percentile and 95th percentile across all gestational ages
- This is also a common criterion used in defining TTTS, and for these reasons, this may be the clinically useful method for assessing amniotic fluid in twins.

Hellin's Rule

- Given in 1895
- Predicts the rates of multiple births
- If the rate for twins is 1 : 85, the rate for triplets is $1 : 85 \times 85$ and for quadruplets, $1 : 85 \times 85 \times 85$ and so on for higher orders.

Q. What is the average duration of pregnancy in multifetal gestation?
Average duration of pregnancy in:
- Singleton: 39 weeks
- Twins: 60% result in spontaneous labor before 37 weeks (uncomplicated twin pregnancy extending beyond 38 weeks increases the risk of fetal mortality)
    - Women with uncomplicated monochorionic twins—offered elective birth from 35 weeks (after administration of steroids)
    - Women with uncomplicated dichorionic twins—offered elective birth from 37 weeks
- Triplets: About 75% result in spontaneous labor before 35 weeks (fetal mortality rate is higher in triplets extending beyond 36 weeks)
- Quadruplets: 30 weeks.

Incidence of Multifetal Gestation

Multifetal Gestation

- Incidence varies worldwide: 6.7/1000 births in Japan to 40/1000 births in Nigeria
- Role of ART (IVF) in increasing the risk:
    - After transfer of 2 embryos: 17.9%
    - After transfer of 4 embryos: 24.1%
    - After transfer of 2 oocytes: 18.7%
    - After transfer of 3 oocytes: 25.8%.

Twin Gestation

Comprise approximately 1% of all pregnancies
- Monozygotic (33%)
    - Spontaneous
        - 3.5 – 4 per 1000 births (rate relatively constant)
    - After ART
        - 2 to 12 fold increase
- Dizygotic (66%)
    - Varies greatly with infertility treatments, maternal age and ethinicity
- Non-vertex presentation of the 1st twin or 2nd twin or both
    - Contributes about 60% of all twin pregnancies.

Factors Contributing to Twinning

- Iatrogenic twins:
    - Though ART is strongly suggested as the cause of iatrogenic twinning but maternal age plays a major role (as maternal age is usually higher in women taking ART treatment)
    - Studies have shown that greatest number of twin births occur due to *natural conception*
- Maternal age (first shown by Mathews Duncan) → increase in the frequency of dizygotic twins
- Parity:
    - Though maternal age and parity are highly correlated but their effects are independent of each other
    - They predominantly affect dizygotic twinning, which increases 4-fold from age 15 to 35 years, and not monozygotic twins

- Genetic factors: Inheritance of twins is seen on maternal side with very little or almost no effect from paternal side (a recent small study showing semen quality of father may play a role in twinning)
- Body composition:
  - Tall women (≥ 164 cm), have 1.5–2.0 times higher relative risk conceiving with twins than those with a shorter height (under 155 cm)
  - BMI < 20 is associated with a lower risk of twinning
  - BMI ≥ 30, associated with a higher risk
- Smoking: has a little effect on twinning
- Seasonal variation:
  - Influences dizygotic twinning
  - Various studies have reported higher rates of DZ twinning for conceptions during summer and autumn in several countries but this is not supported by all studies
  - Seasonal variation in day length may influence hormonal concentrations driving ovarian activity and influence fertility and multiple ovulation
- Preconceptional use of folic acid and oral contraceptives (results are conflicting for both):

Folic acid
  - Prolonged use of preconception folic acid, given for the prevention of neural tube defects, may increase the chance of successful implantation and survival of two embryos

Oral contraceptives
  - A theoretical reason for an increased risk of DZ twinning after taking oral contraceptives is that the hypothalamic-pituitary ovarian axis (HPO-axis) has to recover from the effects of exogenous steroids, causing a temporary increase of FSH levels
  - A clinical situation that mimics such a condition is when women with hypothalamic amenorrhea are treated with GnRH to induce ovulation where, in the first treatment only, this leads to higher FSH levels in association with multiple follicle growth and an increased risk of multiple pregnancies.

Q. What is superfetation and superfecundation?

Superfetation
- Separate ovulation
- By separate act of coitus
- During different menstrual periods
- Unproven in humans
- Fetuses with markedly different gestational ages.

Superfecundation
- Fertilization during same menstrual cycle
- By different act of coitus
- Not necessarily by sperms from same male.

Maternal Complications

- Anemia (iron deficiency and folic acid deficiency)
- Pressure symptoms:
  - Edema of legs
  - Shortness of breath
  - Increased varicose veins
- Hyperemesis

- Gestational hypertension and preeclampsia:
    - Advise women with twin pregnancies that they should take 75 mg of aspirin daily starting from 12 weeks upto 34 weeks, if they have one or more of the following risk factors for hypertension:
        - First pregnancy
        - Age 40 years or older
        - Pregnancy interval of > 10 years
        - BMI of 35 kg/m² or more at first visit
        - Family history of preeclampsia
- HELLP syndrome/placental abruption
- Placenta previa
- Polyhydramnios (in monochorionic twins, tends to occur in large twin sac), where increased cardiac output → increased renal excretion → preterm labor
    - Acute polyhydramnios → mainly in monoamniotic.

Fetal Complications

A. Vanishing twin syndrome:
- Arrest of development
- Subsequent resorption of fetus in 1st trimester
- USG—when 2 sacs are identified very early in pregnancy, the chances of resorption of 1 sac are as high as 40%, but once 2 embryos are seen, it is decreased to 7%

B. Malformations: structural defects
C. Chromosomal anomalies } Mentioned above
D. Complications based on chorionicity

E. Preterm labor
- More frequent ANCs (very increased risk)
- Serial evaluation of cervix
- < 34 weeks → (steroids and tocolytics together to be used with caution as these woman are at increased risk of pulmonary edema)

F. PPROM
- Rupture occurs in presenting sac
- Per speculum → swab taken for C/S
- Per vaginam → avoided
- Look for:
    - Infection
    - Abruption
    - Fetal death
- Antibiotics
- Steroids
- Conservative treatment till 34 weeks → approach individualized
- Median latency period – 1 day
- 90% will deliver in 7 days

G. IUGR
- Rate of growth in twins is same as singleton (till 32 weeks) followed by decrease in growth velocity
- Rate of growth in triplets → same as singleton till 28 weeks
- In last few weeks → competition for nutrients among fetuses.

Place of Invasive Procedures

Before any invasive procedure, determine chorionicity:
- In case of monochorionic → single sample of chorionic villi OR amniotic fluid is sufficient
- In case of dichorionic → sample from both sacs
  - Amniocentesis: Both amniotic sacs should be sampled in monochorionic twin pregnancies, unless monochorionicity is confirmed before 14 weeks and the fetuses appear concordant for growth and anatomy
  - After sample obtained from 1 sac, 1–2 mL of inert dye like indigo carmine is instilled to mark the sac, needle → removed → new needle used to sample next sac → clear, dye free fluid indicates entry into new sac → (same procedure for all present sacs)
  - Methylene blue is:
    - Not used
    - Associated with fetal small bowel obstruction and fatal fetal methemoglobinemia.

MANAGEMENT OF TWIN GESTATION

Prepregnancy (for any woman trying conception)

- Counseling of women undergoing ART
- Ideal BMI – 19.6–26.0 kg/m^2
- Laboratory testing:
  - CBC
  - Urinalysis
  - ABO Rh
  - VDRL
  - HIV
  - HbsAg
  - Rubella antibody titer
  - FBS/OGTT ⎫
  - TFT   ⎬ when indicated
  - TORCH   ⎭
- Folate-rich foods-fortified grains, spinach, lentils, chick peas, asparagus, broccoli, peas, brussels sprouts, corn, and oranges
- A multivitamin with folic acid (0.4–1.0 mg) × 2–3 months before conception
- Vitamin D intake of minimum 5 μg/day for nonpregnant women with limited exposure to sunlight (i.e. those whose hands and face are exposed to the open air for < 15 min/day) and 10 μg/day for pregnant women
- Avoid exposure to cat feces, raw/undercooked meats and unpasteurized milk
- Smoking and alcohol cessation
- Consumption of vitamin A to < 3000 μg/day.

Antenatal

First Trimester

- Documentation of chorionicity and amnionicity
- Nuchal translucency
- Treatment of exaggerated symptoms
- Folic acid—1 mg/day (1000 mcg/day)

- Diet: 300 kcal more than in singletons
- Increased proteins/vitamins/minerals/fiber rich diet
- Routine investigations (mentioned above)
- Multifetal pregnancy reduction—if required.

Second Trimester

- Iron and calcium supplementation (iron 100 mg/day) in early 2nd trimester
- Triple screen test at 16 weeks
- Tetanus toxoid injection (2 doses) 4–6 weeks apart
- Anomaly scan at 18–22 weeks
- If fetal cardiac abnormality is detected, fetal echocardiography at 24 weeks
- Rule out conjoined twins
- OGTT at 24 weeks
- Increased antenatal visits from mid pregnancy (every 2 weeks) for early detection of
  - Anemia (check hemoglobin minimum 4 times, once in each trimester and then before labor)
  - Preeclampsia (BP, weight measurement and urine analysis at each visit after midpregnancy)
  - Preterm labor
- Bed rest in left lateral position for minimum of 2 hours in morning or afternoon and minimum 10 hours at night, starting at 22 weeks gestation until 34 weeks
- In case of Rh negative pregnancy, consider anti-D at 28 weeks followed by serial ICT measurements
- Careful monitoring throughout antenatal period
- In cases of one fetal death, check well-being of second twin and look for coagulopathy (in case of monochorionic twins)
- If hydramnios develops—therapeutic amniocentesis.

Third Trimester

1. Serial USG (every 3–4 weeks but not > 5 weeks) for growth discordance, to assess liquor, to exclude placenta previa
2. Administration of 2 doses of betamethasone 12 mg IM, 24 hours apart in cases of threatened preterm or if delivery is planned before 34 weeks
3. Surveillance for hypertensive disorders
4. Fetal surveillance
5. Discuss with the couple the mode of delivery and methods of analgesia present.

Intrapartum

Optimal Time of Delivery

- Twins—37–38 weeks; no later than 39 weeks (risk of fetal death is lowest at this gestation)
- Triplets—36 weeks (no later than 37 weeks)
- Fetal lung maturity occurs at an earlier gestation in multiple pregnancy and therefore term gestation considered earlier than singleton
- Postmaturity—uncommon with multiple gestation.

Divide the 9 possible combinations of various presentations into three categories:
1. Vertex-vertex → 42%
2. Vertex -nonvertex → 45%
3. Nonvertex - nonvertex → 13%.

Before anticipating delivery, careful consideration of the following is deemed important:
- Gestational age
- Weight of each twin
- Chorionicity
- Lie and presentation of both twins
- Portable ultrasound machine
- CTG machine with dual probes
- IV access
- Blood crossmatch and availability
- Pediatrician and anesthetist—kept informed and that 2 obstetricians and 2 neonatologists are required at the time of delivery
- Labor analgesia (epidural)
- Delivery bed with lithotomy stirrups
- 5 cord clamps
- All oxytocics should be kept ready for active management of 3rd stage of labor and to combat PPH, if it occurs
- Working condition of vacuum should be checked well before and forceps made available
- Provision to carry out emergency cesarean section
- Last but not least, written and informed consent.

Indications for Cesarean Section

Accepted indications
1. Noncephalic presentation of twin 1
2. IUGR in dichorionic twins
3. Twin 2 significantly larger (>500 gm) than twin 1 including antepartum death of twin 1
4. Placenta previa
5. Fetal abnormality precluding safe vaginal delivery
6. Chronic TTTS in monochorionic twin
7. Monoamniotic twins.

Contentious indications
1. Maternal request
2. Unfavorable cervix at 39 weeks in nullipara
3. Death of twin 2
4. Uncomplicated monochorionic twins
5. Previous cesarean section.

Management Proper

Vertex–Vertex
1st twin
- Allow delivery by vaginal route
- Continuous CTG monitoring in active labor (> 4 cm dilatation)
- Discuss the options and benefits of intrapartum epidural analgesia
- An epidural is recommended due to increased risk of operative delivery in twins and the possibility of intrauterine manipulation in 2nd twin
- Patient should be kept on soft diet in latent phase and on liquid diet once active labor begins
- 1st twin delivered as in singleton pregnancy

- After delivery of first twin, clamp its umbilical cord with 2 clamps and do not deliver the placenta
- Withhold IM oxytocin after the delivery of 1st twin
- Main problems in 1st stage:
  - Over distension of uterus
  - Uterine inertia
  - Prolonged active phase
  - Increased frequency of contractions with lesser intensity
- In case of fetal distress, expedite delivery using vacuum or forceps
- Cesarean section is indicated in cases of:
  - Cord prolapse
  - Premature separation of placenta
  - Malpresentation.

2nd twin
- Repeat abdominal and per vaginal examination and reconfirm the presentation of 2nd twin by USG (as it may change)
- External version if necessary
- After the delivery of the 1st twin, uterine contractions may cease for sometime, therefore start oxytocin drip after 10 minutes and wait for contractions
- Continuous FHR monitoring
- Amniotomy of the 2nd sac once the head is engaged
- Time interval between deliveries of both fetuses is important
- Longer the interval between delivery, greater is the risk of hypoxia
- Umbilical cord blood gas deteriorates with increasing time interval – maximum time limit of 30 min with documentation of reassuring FHR pattern (average 10–15 minutes)
- But adverse outcome is not expected as long as FHR is continuously being monitored
- Use three clamps, leaving a double clamp on placental side for identification
- Give IM oxytocin.

Vertex-Non-vertex
- There are ongoing controversies to which mode of delivery should be opted, as rates of morbidity and mortality are the same for both vaginal delivery as well as cesarean section
- If vaginal delivery is anticipated, recheck the weight especially of the 2nd twin and managed as described below.

EFW >1500 gm

2nd twin is breech
- Vaginal delivery of twin 1
  ↓
- Twin 2 → attempt ECV → failed → breech extraction → failed → cesarean section

2nd twin is transverse
- ECV
- Internal podalic version (the only accepted indication of internal podalic version is breech extraction in case of 2nd twin when cervix is fully dilated)
- Prerequisites:
  - Skilled operator, well versed with the procedure
  - EFW > 1500 gms
  - Adequate liquor
  - Available anesthesia for effective uterine relaxation
  - Simultaneous preparation for emergency cesarean section.

EFW <1500 gm

- Perinatal outcomes same for both—cesarean section and vaginal delivery
- So, any mode can be selected.

Non-vertex—Non-vertex

- Cesarean section would be a better option
- Risk factors:
    - Twin 1 breech/twin 2 vertex
    - IUGR or fetal demise of one fetus
- Monoamniotic → elective cesarean section → why?
    - Cord of twin 2 may be inadvertently clamped during delivery of twin 1 in case of vaginal delivery.

Third Stage: Most Dangerous

Increased risk of PPH because of:
1. Large placenta, which may take longer time for complete separation
2. Larger placental site → capable of more profuse bleeding
3. Uterine inertia due to over-distension
4. As blood loss is more after twin deliveries, this blood may accumulate within the uterine cavity, hampering its further contraction
5. Placenta may occupy lower segment.

Employ the following:
1. AMTSL
2. Oxytocics
3. Scrupulous monitoring of vitals for a period of minimum 4 hours after delivery
4. Oxytocin drip should be continued.

Special Situations

Twins with Previous Scar

- Trial of labor is not an absolute contraindication if 1st twin has a vertex presentation
- Better to perform cesarean section in case of 1st nonvertex twin
- Success rate 30–75%
- Risk of uterine rupture is the same as VBAC in a singleton pregnancy.

Twin Entrapment

- Here, after coming head of twin1 (presenting as breech) is prevented from entering the pelvis by presenting part (head) of twin 2 → immediately induce anesthesia
- Push 2nd head out of the way so that 1st head can enter the brim (difficult manoeuver) → mostly twin 1 dies of asphyxia
- Decapitate twin 1
- Deliver body
- Retrieve head after delivery of twin 2
- Therefore better to go for elective cesarean section in case of MCMA twins.

Triplets or Higher Order
- Elective cesarean section
- Vaginal delivery can be planned if following criteria are fulfilled:
    - Non-contracted pelvis
    - Cephalic presentation of 1st triplet
    - Unscarred uterus
    - Gestation > 32 weeks
    - No fetal compromise.

POLYHYDRAMNIOS

Definition
- Excessive accumulation of amniotic fluid, more than that expected for that gestational age
- It is generally defined as:
    - Amniotic fluid index (AFI) > 20–25 cm
    - Largest fluid pocket depth (maximal vertical pocket (MVP)) > 8 cm
    - Overall amniotic fluid volume > 1500–2000 cc^3
    - Two diameter pocket (TDP) > 50 cm^2.

History
- Multigravida > primigravida
- If occurring in mid pregnancy → suspicion of monozygotic twins
- Acute or gradual onset
- To note in which trimester it has occurred.

Epidemiology
- It can occur in approximately 1–1.5% of pregnancies.

Classification
- Acute → within days, occurring usually in 2nd trimester
- Chronic → gradual, asymptomatic and occurs in 3rd trimester.

Causes
Maternal (25–30%)
- Diabetes: commonly gestational diabetes
- Hypertension/preeclampsia
- Maternal congestive heart failure

Fetal (10–20%)—listed below

Idiopathic (60–65%).

Chief Complaints
- Unmanageable girth
- Shortness of breath

- Digestive discomfort
- Edema of lower extremities
- Increasing troublesome varicose veins
- Hyperemesis (in late pregnancy).

Signs

- Dyspnea even in lying position
- Evidence of preeclampsia (hypertension, proteinuria/edema).

GPE

Inspection

- Abdomen markedly enlarged, globular, fullness at flanks (like in ascites)
- Skin—tense, shiny, large striae present.

Palpation

- Height of uterus > period of gestation
- Girth of abdomen (round umbilicus) > normal
- Fetus freely ballotted
- Fluid thrill present
- Fetal parts may not be easily palpable
- External ballottment → more easily elicited
- Malpresentation common
- Lie—unstable (may)
- If vertex presentation—head likely to be high.

Auscultation

- FHS not well heard.

Investigations

USG

- For diagnosis
- Any associated fetal malformations should be looked for:

CNS
1. Aneuploidy
2. Hydrocephaly
3. Hydranencephaly
4. Encephalocele
5. Microcephaly
6. Gastroschisis
7. Omphalocele
8. Cleft palate.

GIT
1. Astomia
2. Esophageal atresia
3. Diaphragmatic hernia
4. Duodenal stenosis
5. Annular pancreas.

Respiratory Tract
1. Cystic adenomatoid malformation of lung
2. Chylothorax.

Genitourinary
1. Fetal renal hamartoma
2. Unilateral PUJ obstruction.

CVS
1. Valvular incompetence
2. Valvular stenosis
3. Ebstein's anomaly
4. Arrhythmias
5. TTTS.

Musculoskeletal
1. Skeletal dysplasia
2. Myotonic dystrophy
3. Pena-Shokeir syndrome
4. Fetal akinesia/hypokinesia syndrome.

USG Criteria

- Ultrasound → modality of choice for assessing amniotic fluid volumes
- The AFV can be assessed by ultrasound by using 3 main indirect parameters:
  1. Single deepest (maximum vertical) pocket method
  2. Amniotic fluid index
  3. Two diameter pocket method.

Largest Vertical Pocket (Deepest Pocket)
- Considered the best method of assessing amniotic fluid volume
- Performed by assessing a maximal depth of amniotic fluid which is free of umbilical cord
- The usually accepted values are:
  - < 2 cm → indicative of oligohydramnios
  - 2–8 cm → normal but should be taken in the context of subjective volume
  - > 8 cm → indicative of polyhydramnios
    - 8–11 cm → mild
    - 12–15 cm → moderate
    - >16 cm → severe.

Amniotic Fluid Index
- Sum of deepest pocket in 4 cord and extremity free quadrants in gravid uterus (using external maternal landmarks of umbilicus and linea nigra)
  - Polyhydramnios if AFI > 24 cm
  - Phelan:

- Average AFI (at term) 12.9 ± 4.6 cm³ according to which AFI > 18 cm → excessive or hydramnios
- Carlson:
  - AFI > 2SDs of the mean (for late 2nd and 3rd trimester) → as 24 cm
- Best definition:
  - AFI > 95th percentile (for Indian women at term ≈ 18.2 cm).

Two-diameter Pocket Method (TDP)
- It is an alternative method of assessing amniotic fluid volumes on ultrasound
- It is, however, not thought to be good predictor of adverse neonatal outcome
- Assessment:
  - TDP < 15 cm²: indicative of oligohydramnios
  - TDP 15–50 cm²: usually taken as normal
  - TDP > 50 cm²: indicative of polyhydramnios.

Important Points

1. There is more fluid than fetus in 2nd trimester
2. At term → uterus totally occupied by fetus
3. Marked hydramnios: fetus seen lying on dependent surface with wide surrounding area of fluid over and about it → *"At the bottom of the sea"*
4. > 5 cm and < 18–20 cm → considered normal (by most).

How to Measure AFI?

1. Supine position
2. Divide uterus into four quadrants
   Maternal sagittal midline vertically

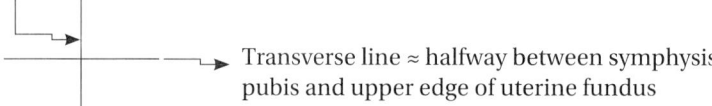

Transverse line ≈ halfway between symphysis pubis and upper edge of uterine fundus

3. Transducer → parallel to maternal sagittal plane and perpendicular to maternal coronal plane throughout
   - Sagittal plane (vertical plane parallel to midsagittal plane; divides body into right and left portion)
   - Coronal plane (known as frontal plane; vertical plane at 90° to sagittal plane; divides the body into anterior and posterior portions)
4. Deepest vertical pocket (free of umbilical cord and fetal parts) → chosen and image frozen
5. USG calipers → kept and measured in strictly vertical direction
6. Process repeated in all quadrants and summed up values give AFI in cm
7. If AFI < 8 cm, perform 4 quadrant evaluation thrice and give the average.

Rationale Behind Polyhydramnios and Oligohydramnios

- With GIT abnormalities—fluid swallowing is decreased → polyhydramnios
- With renal abnormalities—swallowed fluid not excreted → oligohydramnios.

Management Options

Usually minimal or no intervention required for idiopathic mild uncomplicated cases
Options include:
- Improved maternal diabetes control
- Cesarean section if there is profound macrosomia
- Therapeutic amniocentesis/amnioreduction
- Indomethacin.

Acute Polyhydramnios

- USG: Multiple fetuses or fetal abnormalities
- Management:
  - Spontaneous abortion occurs (most common)
  - Relieve distress—decompression done
  - Pregnancy terminated by low rupture of membranes → allow slow escape of fluid (head should be well-stabilized)
  - If very precious pregnancy *(though every pregnancy is precious)* → repeated abdominal amniocentesis after ruling out fetal congenital abnormalities.

HYDROPS FETALIS

Definition

The term hydrops fetalis comes from Latin meaning 'edema of the fetus'
Presence of extracellular fluid in at least 2 fetal body compartments:
- Scalp and body wall edema
- Pericardial effusion
- Pleural effusion
- Ascites
- Polyhydramnios (due to increased urine output → included by some)
- Placentomegaly
- Generalized fetal body edema – fetal anasarca
- Umbilical venous dilatation.

Classification

- Immune hydrops
- Non-immune hydrops

IMMUNE HYDROPS

- Do not occur until fetal hemoglobin falls to below 6 SDs from the mean for that particular gestational age
- Occurrence according to disease progression:
  - Small pericardial effusion (1st to come) > ascites and pleural effusion > scalp edema (last to appear)
- Early 2nd trimester
  Fetus severely anemic without overt hydrops
  This is because of ↓↓ in normal fetal lymph flow that occurs with advancing gestational age

- In 3rd trimester, fetus is rarely anemic without hydrops
- Exact mechanism why hydrops occurs secondary to fetal anemia is not known
- Few mechanisms which have been postulated:
  - Hypoproteinemia: hepatic dysfunction → ↓ production of serum protein OR extravasation of proteins from IVC secondary to endothelial damage
  - Myocardial failure
  - Lymphatic obstruction
- If placental hydrops is significant, an additional life threatening complication called BALLANTYNE Syndrome (also known as MIRROR SYNDROME; TRIPLE EDEMA; PSEUDO-TOXEMIA) is described.

Cause

- Feto-maternal blood group incompatibility (including rhesus incompatibility): Erythroblastosis fetalis.

Why Named Mirror Syndrome?

- Because mother mirrors the hydropic state of fetus
- Includes:
  - Maternal edema
  - Rapid weight gain
  - Mild proteinuria
  - Hypertension
  - Hematocrit and albumin decreases.

Difference with Preeclampsia

- Maternal intravascular volume appears to be expanded as opposed to typical hemoconcentration seen with preeclampsia
- Double lining of fluid filled intra-abdominal structures such as urinary bladder, gall bladder, stomach, bowel loops → earliest site of ascites. In male fetus, hydrocele may suggest hydrops.

NONIMMUNE FETAL HYDROPS (NIFH)

- Accumulation of extracellular fluid in tissues and serous cavities in conditions other than Rh incompatibility
- Generalized skin edema → 1st feature (revealed in early pregnancy)
- Where? At level of fetal head and more specifically at back of neck (rationale for measurement of nuchal translucency) → >5 mm
- Other features:
  - Ascites
  - Pericardial and pleural effusion
  - Placental enlargement
  - Polyhydramnios
- Ascites in presence of urinary and GIT abnormalities shouldn't be considered an early sign of hydrops
- Increased peak systolic velocity of MCA → fetal anemia even in nonimmune hydrops.

Note:
In absence of:
- Cardiac abnormalities (structural or rhythm)
- Suspected anemia
- Viral infection
- Suspected chromosomal abnormalities

≤ 2 mm pericardial fluid → Normal finding

Causes and Associations of NIFH

I. Focal abnormalities:
- Cranial
  - Intracranial hemorrhage
  - Vein of Gallen aneurysm.
- Cardiac
  - AV septal defect with or without Down's syndrome
  - Tricuspid dysplasia with Ebstein's anamoly
  - RVOT obstruction (because of pulmonary stenosis/pulmonary atresia)
  - Premature closure of foramen ovale.
- Thorax
  - Rhabdomyoma/hemangioma/hamartoma
  - Cardiomyopathy (dilated/restrictive)
  - Myocarditis
  - Arrhythmias/SVT
  - Complete heart block
  - Sinus bradycardia.
- GIT
  - Diaphragmatic hernia
  - Meconium peritonitis
  - Intestinal hemorrhage because of bowel perforation.
- Renal
  - Congenital nephrosis (Finnish type)
  - Urethral obstruction with rupture of bladder
  - PCKD
  - Renal vein thrombosis.
- Tumour and vascular disorders
  - Teratoma
  - Mediastinal fibrosarcoma
  - IVC thrombosis
  - Renal vein thrombosis.

Generalized abnormalities
- Hematological
  - Extrinsic hemolysis (fetomaternal hemorrhage)
  - Intrinsic hemolysis
    - α thalassemia
    - G6PD deficiency
    - Pyruvate kinase deficiency.

- Infection
  - Parvovirus B19 (Fifth disease; Slapped-cheek disease)
  - CMV
  - Syphilis
  - Toxoplasmosis
  - HSV
  - Adenovirus
  - Hepatitis A
  - Rubella.
- Skeletal dysplasias
  - Achondrogenesis type I and IA
  - Short Rib-Polydactyly syndrome
  - Osteogenesis Imperfecta type II
  - Achondroplasia
    - Metabolic disorder.
- Lysosomal storage disease.
- Glycogen storage disease.
- Syndromes:
  - Autosomal dominant
    - Opitz Frias syndrome
    - Noonan's syndrome
    - Congenital myotonic dystrophy.
  - Autosomal recessive
    - Arthrogryposis
    - Multiplex congenita.
- Chromosomal aberration:
  - Trisomy 13,18, 21
  - Tri and tetraploidy
  - Turner's syndrome.
- Placental and umbilical abnormalities:
  - Chorioangioma
  - TTTS
  - True knots of cord.

II. Idiopathic (20%).

III. Maternal diseases.
- Uncontrolled Diabetes Mellitus
- Severe anemia
- Thyrotoxicosis.

MYOMA

- Hypoechoic solid mass
  - Distinguish it from myometrial contraction
  - If mass disappears during course of an examination or on repeat ultrasound → it is a contraction rather than myoma
- Not always found in same location (owing to rotation of uterus)
- Most myomas do not change in size, only they become more prominent and sharply outlined, due to decreased echogenicity during pregnancy.

OTHER PELVIC MASSES

- Corpus luteum cyst
  - Usually declines after 1st trimester but may occasionally be present.
- Cystadenoma
  - Most common mass to enlarge during pregnancy
  - Usually multiloculated, cystic mass.

VESICULAR MOLE

- Typical appearance may not be present in 1st trimester
- Undue enlargement of uterus and occurrence of theca lutein cysts, with extremely high β-hCG levels in complete molar pregnancy
- USG (for early detection):
  - Early: Irregular anechoic mass
  - Late 2nd trimester: "Snowstorm appearance"
  - Areas of increased echogenicities associated with mole do not cause shadowing suggesting absence of calcification
  - Invasive mole: Echogenic areas seen within the uterine wall on ultrasound → when it invades the myometrium → complete mole.

Differential Diagnosis

1. Degenerating fibroid: presence of calcification unlike mole
2. Ovarian tumour: confusion occurs when mass is large and it is not possible to determine site of origin → do CT
3. β hCG levels are not increased with ovarian tumour or fibroid. Also cystic spaces in the above two and incomplete abortion are not as regular and uniform as vesicles of molar tissue
4. Multiseptated ovaries: Theca lutein cysts are bilateral and frequently > 5 cm in diameter.

MACROSOMIA

Generalized Fetal Enlargement

Definition

- Refers to fetal growth where EFW has surpassed a specific weight (4000 gms) regardless of gestational age, whereas large for gestational age is where the EFW is > 90th percentile for gestational age
- Rare before 37 weeks of gestation and is more common in post-dated pregnancy (≥ 42 weeks).

Causes

- Size of parents (especially mother → obesity)
- Poorly controlled diabetes melleitus/GDM
- Postmaturity (> 42 weeks)
- Multiparity
- Male fetus
- Erythroblastosis fetalis and other causes of hydrops
- Prior macrosomic infant.

USG

- Early clue to macrosomia may be provided by decreased FL/AC ratio (N → 22% ± 2). This ratio is quiet accurate provided abnormally small femur is ruled out
- Increased subcutaneous fat (may) → as a sonolucency separating scalp from skull by ≥ 4 mm (Diabetic Halo)
- Baby weight assessment remains the only accurate way to diagnose macrosomic infant
- USG still remains unreliable for prenatal detection of macrosomia.

Fetal Hazards

- Surprise dystocia due to CPD
- Shoulder dystocia
- Brachial plexus injury
- Asphyxia
- Birth trauma
- Meconium aspiration
- Clavicle fracture
- Humerus fracture
- HI encephalopathy
- Death.

Maternal Hazards

- Injury to maternal soft tissues (vagina, perineum)
- PPH
- Puerperal sepsis
- Increased rate of cesarean section.

Treatment

1. Prophylactic (preterm) induction of labor to decrease risk of shoulder dystocia
2. Elective cesarean section in diabetic mother with big baby.

WRONG DATES

- Menstrual age = Gestational age
- Fetal age = Conceptional age → begins at conception (e.g. in IVF/artificial insemination)
- Menstrual age → Conceptional age + 14 days.

Methods for Determining Menstrual Age

- IVF ± 1 day
- Ovulation induction ± 3 days
- Artificial insemination ± 3 days } To conceptional age
- Single intercourse ± 3 days
- BBT record ± 4 days

Good Dates

1. Patient is certain of LMP
2. Regular menses
3. No exposure to hormonal contraceptives (for ≥ 3 regular immediate preconceptional cycles)
4. No unusual bleeding
5. Patient didn't conceive in lactational amenorrhea.

Bad Dates

1. Uncertain of LMP
2. Unusual bleeding (oligomenorrhea, abnormal bleeding)
3. Use of hormonal contraceptives (ovulation may be delayed for 4–6 weeks)
4. Became pregnant in 1st ovulation cycle after a recent delivery
5. Ovulation very early (< day 11) or very late (>21 days).

Prediction of Gestational Age

Patient's Statement

- Date of fruitful coitus
    - Add 266 days to it (± 7 days)
- Naegele's formula: ± 7 days
    - If interval of cycles is longer, extra days are to be added
    - If interval is shorter, lesser days are to be subtracted to get EDD
- Date of quickening
    - Add 22 weeks in primigravida and 24 weeks in multi (to it).

Previous Records

Required weeks to be added to make it 40 weeks
- Clinical
    - Size of uterus <12 weeks ≈ period of amenorrhea
    - Palpation of fetal parts by 20th week
    - Auscultation of FHR by 18-20 weeks (by stethoscope) and by Doppler by 10th week
- Investigation record of 1st half of pregnancy
    - UPT +ve at first missed period by earliest
    - USG: visualization of gestational sac at 5th week
    - CRL → 10 mm (at 7 weeks)
        34 mm (at 10 weeks)
  (CRL in cm + 3.5 = week of pregnancy).

Objective Signs

- Height of uterus above symphysis pubis (or SFH)
- Lightening: labor commences approximately at or within 3 weeks
- Size of fetus, change in uterine shape, volume of liquor amnii, hardening of skull and girth of abdomen.

USG

Gestational age (1st and 2nd trimester) should be compared with menstrual age
- When difference in gestational age and menstrual age is < 7 days → EDD by LMP is taken
- When >7 days → EDD by USG age is taken.

SUGGESTED READING

1. Chantal Hoekstra, Zhen Zhen Zhao, Cornelius B Lambalk, et al. Dizygotic twinning. Human Reproduction Update. 2008;14(1):37-47.
2. Charlotte N Steins Bisschop, Tatjana E Vogelvang, Anne M May. Mode of delivery in non-cephalic presenting twins: a systematic review. Arch Gynecol Obstet. 2012;286:237-47.
3. Crowther CA, Han S. Hospitalisation and bed rest for multiple pregnancy (Review). The Cochrane Library, 2010, Issue 7.
4. Dodd JM, Crowther CA. Elective delivery of women with a twin pregnancy from 37 weeks' gestation (Review), The Cochrane Library 2010, Issue 1.
5. Dodd JM, Crowther CA. Reduction of the number of fetuses for women with a multiple pregnancy (Review), The Cochrane Library 2012, Issue 10.
6. Dodd JM, Crowther CA. Specialised antenatal clinics for women with a multiple pregnancy for improving maternal and infant outcomes (Review). The Cochrane Library 2012, Issue 8.
7. François Audibert, Alain Gagnon. Prenatal Screening for and Diagnosis of Aneuploidy in Twin Pregnancies. JOGC, July 2011.
8. Hofmeyr GJ, Barrett JF, Crowther CA. Planned cesarean section for women with a twin pregnancy (Review). The Cochrane Library 2011, Issue 12.
9. Intrapartum management of a planned vaginal twin birth. Clinical Guidelines OGCCU, King Edward Memorial Hospital, Perth Western Australia, July 2012.
10. Intrauterine laser ablation of placental vessels for the treatment of twin-to-twin transfusion syndrome: National Institute for Health and Clinical Excellence, December 2006.
11. Joachim W Dudenhausen, Rolf F Maier. Perinatal Problems in Multiple Births, Dtsch Arztebl Int. 2010;107(38):663-8.
12. Lim AC, Hegeman MA, Huisin MA, Veld T, et al. Cervical length measurement for the prediction of preterm birth in multiple pregnancies: a systematic review and bivariate meta-analysis, Ultrasound Obstet Gynecol. 2011;38:10-7.
13. Lucie Morin, Kenneth Lim. Ultrasound in Twin Pregnancies. JOGC June 2011.
14. Management of monochorionic twin pregnancy: RCOG Dec 2008.
15. Mark I, Evans a Lau TK: Making Decisions When No Good Choices Exist: Delivery of the Survivor after Intrauterine Death of the Co-Twin in Monochorionic Twin Pregnancies. Fetal Diagn Ther. 2010;28:191-5.
16. Multiple pregnancy: The management of twin and triplet pregnancies in the antenatal period: NICE clinical guideline 129, September 2011.
17. Roberts D, Neilson JP, Kilby M. Interventions for the treatment of twin-twin transfusion syndrome (Review). The Cochrane Library 2008, Issue 3.
18. Septostomy with or without amnioreduction for the treatment of twin-to-twin transfusion syndrome. National Institute for Health and Clinical Excellence, December 2006

CHAPTER 7

Uterine Size Less than Expected

Tania G Singh

Case: A primigravida with 6 years married life, conceived after infertility treatment, visits the outpatient department for antenatal checkup. She had a history of irregular periods since the time of marriage, so was not very sure of her dates. This was her 2nd visit. On examination: vitals were stable, weight gain was normal. Per abdomen: uterus 26 weeks size, relaxed, FHS present

She was carrying a normal ultrasound report (done at 20 weeks according to which patient should have been 30 weeks period of gestation now). What can you think?

Possibilities:
1. As this patient had irregular periods and has conceived after infertility treatment, her dates must be wrong but as uterine height is also not corresponding according to the scan report, she can have a fetus with intrauterine growth restriction (if fetal abnormalities have been ruled out)
2. She can also have reduced liquor but less liquor at this gestational age may either be associated with some congenital abnormality or with IUGR
3. Since her level II scan is normal and also FHS can be heard on clinical examination, the diagnosis points towards IUGR.

Such cases where uterine height seems less than the period of gestation can be managed according to the following algorithm:

Most common cause → WRONG DATES but first exclude other possibilities:
Step I → Check gestational age
Step II → Confirm whether fetus is alive or dead by USG
Step III → FHS absent

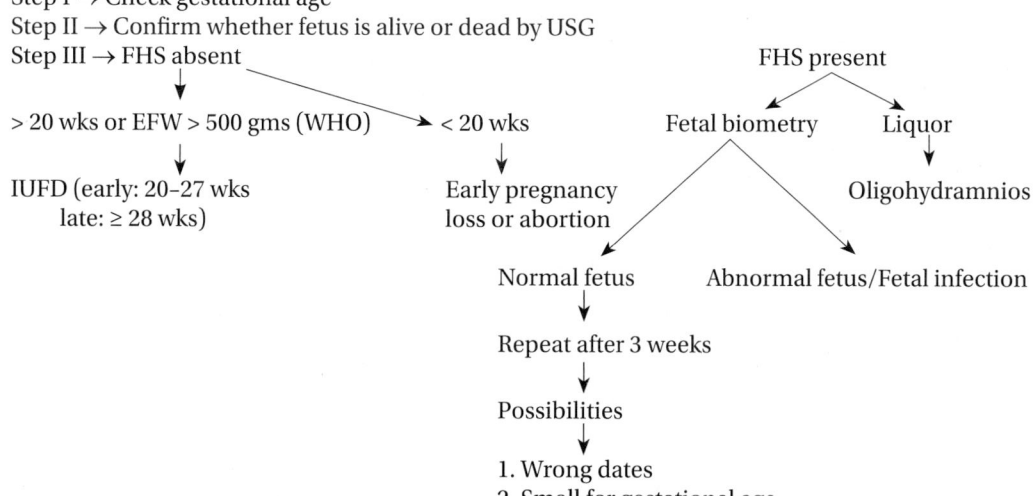

BRIEF DESCRIPTION OF ALL POSSIBILITIES

Wrong Dates

- Menstrual age = Gestational age
- Fetal age = Conceptional age → begins at conception (e.g. in IVF/Artificial insemination).

Good Dates

Criteria

- Patient is certain of LMP
- Previous regular menses
- No exposure to hormonal contraceptives for ≥ 3 regular cycles
- No unusual bleeding
- Patient didn't conceive in lactational amenorrhea.

Bad Dates

Criteria

- Uncertain of LMP
- Unusual bleeding/Oligomenorrhea/Abnormal bleeding
- Use of hormonal contraceptives (ovulation may be delayed by 4–6 weeks)
- Became pregnant in 1st ovulatory cycle after a recent delivery
- Ovulation very early (< D11) or very late (>D21).

After excluding wrong dates, the 2nd thing which comes to our mind is that the fetus must be small. But one should be able to differentiate between the 3 entities, i.e. Small for gestational age/ Symmetrical IUGR and Asymmetrical IUGR.

Constitutionally Small Fetus (Small for Gestational Age)

Criteria

- These fetuses are constitutionally small
- Growth rate is usually below but parallel to normal
- Always symmetrical
- No anatomical abnormality is found
- Amniotic fluid is normal
- Normal BPP and umbilical artery Doppler
- No other additional evaluation is required
- Anticipate term delivery
- They have normal Ponderal index
- Normal subcutaneous fat
- Uneventful neonatal period.

Symmetrical IUGR

Criteria

- Growth rate is markedly below normal but growth pattern is 'symmetrical'
- It indicates that, in them, the cell size is normal but they have fewer cells
- On USG:
  - All fetal biometric parameters are below the 10th centile for the given gestational age
  - Both length as well as weight parameters are reduced
  - They have near normal
    - HC/AC ratio
    - FL/AC ratio
- Usually occurs in first half of pregnancy
- Anatomy is usually abnormal owing to:
  - Fetal infection (TORCH; Malaria; HIV)
  - Structural defects (Anencephaly, GI atresia, CNS abnormalities, etc.)
  - Chromosomal abnormality (Trisomy 13, 18, 21)
  - Autoimmune diseases (Antiphospholipid syndrome; SLE; Thrombophilia)
  - Genetic disorders
  - Drugs (Antiepileptics, warfarin, steroids, antineoplastic)
  - Radiation
  - Smoking/alcohol consumption
  - Nutritional deficiency/Low maternal weight
  - Uncontrolled Type I DM
- Amniotic fluid is either normal or they have hydramnios (Liquor is decreased in the presence of renal agenesis or urethral obstruction)
- BPP is variable but usually have normal umbilical artery Doppler
- Karyotype may be required
- Time of delivery depends upon etiology
- They have normal Ponderal index.

Asymmetrical IUGR

Criteria

- Growth rate is variable, with asymmetric growth pattern
- It indicates that, in them, there is decrease in cell size, but have less effect on total cell numeric
- This usually occurs in 2nd half of pregnancy
- Pathological growth restriction is due to:
  - Uteroplacental insufficiency
  - Chronic hypertension /Hypertensive disorders of pregnancy
  - Renal disease/Cyanotic heart disease/Respiratory disease (cyanotic, asthma, bronchiectasis)
  - Vasculopathy (Long-standing Diabetes mellitus)
  - Placental disorders (multiple infarcts; aberrant cord insertion; single umbilical artery; small placenta)
  - Nutritional deficiency/Low maternal weight
  - Idiopathic
- Brain growth is spared, which is pathologically characterized by an increased brain to liver ratio

- USG:
  - The parameter classically affected is the abdominal circumference (AC) which is reduced out of proportion to other fetal biometric parameters and is below the 10th centile
  - BPD, HC and FL may be normal
  - ↑ FL : AC
  - ↑ HC : AC
    - Negative predictive value of 98%
    - Sensitivity of 82%
    - Specificity of 94%
  - Unexplained oligohydramnios
  - EFW is also < 10th centile
    - Negative predictive value of 99%
    - Sensitivity of 89%
    - Specificity of 88%
- A paradoxical rare situation is, with maternal cocaine use, where the head circumference is reduced out of proportion to others
- Anatomically these are normal
- BPP score decreases and umbilical artery Doppler is evident of vascular resistance
- Fetal lung maturity testing may be indicated
- Time of delivery entirely depends on Doppler changes and/or liquor volume
- Low Ponderal index
- Decreased subcutaneous fat
- Increased rates of neonatal complications and need of admission to NICU.

OLIGOHYDRAMNIOS

Definition

Quantitatively

- Defined as amniotic fluid volume < 300–500 mL after midtrimester (≈ 24 weeks) because before that normal AFV is < 500 mL
- AFI < 5 cm
- Single vertical pocket < 2 cm
- Two diameter pocket method < 1 × 1 cm or < 15 cm².

Subjectively

- Obvious lack of fluid
- Poor fluid fetal interface
- Marked crowding of fetal parts.

Incidence

- 0.5 to 5%
- In postdated pregnancy → 11%.

Causes

Fetal

I. Renal Tract Abnormalities

Renal and urinary tract pathologies → directly affect fetal urine production, therefore, should be considered first.

Bilateral Renal Agenesis

- Amniotic fluid volume will be normal until 20 weeks (due to other sources)
- After 20 weeks, as fetal urine is the prime source of amniotic fluid → amniotic fluid volume begins to decrease (although fetal lungs produce fluid, adequate volume of amniotic fluid is required for normal fetal lung development)
- Number of dysmorphic characteristics develop over remaining weeks, mentioned as follows:
    - Potter's Facies
    - Marked pulmonary hypoplasia   } Oligohydramnios
    - Limb deformities   } Sequence
    - Generalized growth retardation

Potter's Facies

- Proximal epicanthal folds
- Flattened nose
- Low set ears
- Previously referred to as Potter's Syndrome, is now divided into:

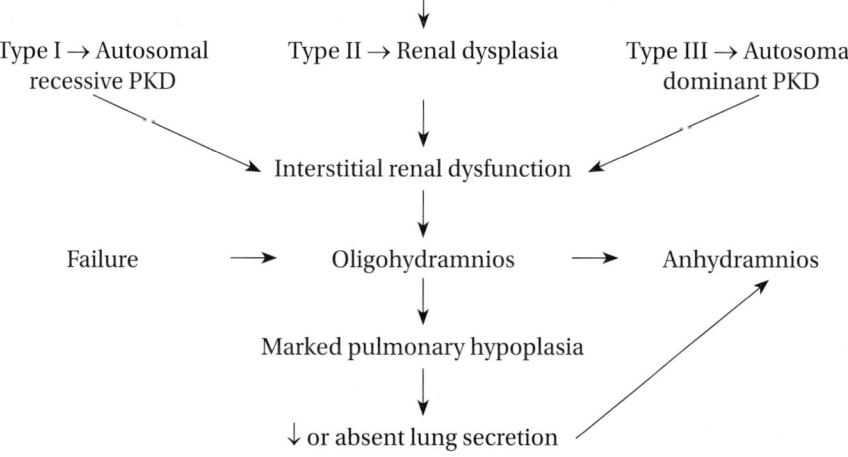

Diagnosis

- Inability to visualize fetal kidneys and bladder → confirms the diagnosis
- But what may confuse you?
    - Expansion of adrenal glands into renal fossa, as adrenals may be mistaken for kidneys

- Doppler: Visualization of fetal renal arteries with color Doppler helps to determine whether organs identified are infact the kidneys.

Note: Severe oligohydramnios, for whatever etiology up to 26 weeks (the end of canalicular phase of fetal lung development) → is associated with severe pulmonary hypoplasia.

Urinary Tract Obstruction

Urethral obstruction and PUJ obstruction → bladder overdistention (Megacystitis) with back pressure upon the kidneys

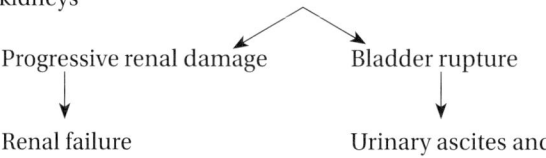

Progressive renal damage → Renal failure

Bladder rupture → Urinary ascites and Prune Belly Syndrome or Triad Syndrome
- Deficient abdominal muscles
- Undescended testis
- Urinary tract abnormalities
} Oligohydramnios and pulmonary hypoplasia

II. Genetic Abnormalities
- Smith Lemli Opitz syndrome
- Meckel-Gruber syndrome.

III. GI Conditions

IV. Aneuploidies, chromosome abnormalities, genetic and structural defects and metabolic disorders

V. IUGR and placental insufficiency

VI. Presentation (breech)

VII. Isolated (≈ 50%).

Maternal

- Postdated pregnancy
- PROM (25% of cases) → but not all cases of PROM will have less liquor
- Hypertension
- Indomethacin (especially when used for prolonged periods) →↓ in fetal urine production
- Autoimmune disorders
- Maternal hydration.

Clinically

- Uterus appears small for dates (with moderate to severe oligohydramnios)
- If IUGR is also present:
  - Fetal parts easily palpated
  - Uterus feels as if clamped over fetal parts
  - Little ballottment.

USG

Oligohydramnios diagnosis → may be difficult → amnioinfusion with normal saline
↓
Detailed examination
↙ ↘
Fetal anatomy (mainly renal tract)   Fetal growth, parameters (for IUGR)

Doppler: Umbilical artery (must be performed) → If ↑ S/D ratio → fetus at risk
If normal →↓ iatrogenic morbidity.

Management

- Depends on severity of oligohydramnios
- Gestational age
- Associated pregnancy complication

Remote from term → prolong pregnancy if possible with close fetal monitoring

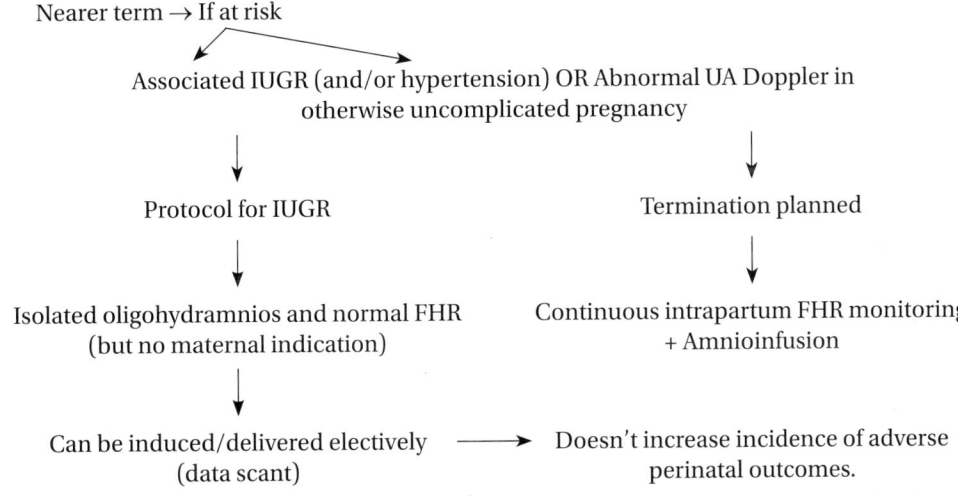

Role of Maternal Hydration

- Oral or IV → increases AFI up to 30% (but temporary)
- Oral → 2–4 liters of water/day
- IV → 2 liters of hypotonic (diluted) Ringer's lactate, but not isotonic (undiluted)
- Amino acid infusion (e.g. alamine SN) IV thrice/week. May be repeated after 3–4 weeks, if necessary
- Amnioinfusion: 250–500 mL RL
  - Transabdominally → antepartum
  - Transcervical → intrapartum
  - Uses → increases accuracy of USG diagnosis.

Antepartum Amnioinfusion

In cases of PPROM
- PPROM delivery interval ⎤
- Pulmonary hypoplasia   ⎬ Significantly better with serial amnioinfusions
- Neonatal survival   ⎦
- No increase in infections → during pregnancy or in puerperium
- Risk of abnormal neurologic outcome is much decreased (though proved by very few studies).

Intrapartum Amnioinfusion

- For meconium stained liquor
- There is reduction in:
  - Heavy meconium staining of liquor
  - Variable decelerations
  - Cesarean section rates
  - NICU admissions
  - Neonatal ventilation and hypoxic ischemic encephalopathy
- Prophylactic amnioinfusion in labor
  - Significantly improved neonatal outcome
  - Decreased cesarean section rates
- Because it is an invasive technique and indiscriminate and improper use can have higher complications.

Role of Vesico-amniotic Shunt

- For bladder outflow obstruction → will allow obstruction to be relieved
- Risks:
  - PPROM
  - Increase intrauterine loss rate
  - Increased risk of severe renal dysfunction
  - Increased risk of renal transplantation in surviving neonates
- Others:
  - Open fetal surgery
  - Fetal cystoscopy
  - Electrocautery of posterior urethral valves.

Complications

- Fetal distress
- Fetal death
- Pulmonary hypoplasia
- Prematurity
- Pressure effects
- Talipes
- Dislocated hips
- Ankylosis of joints
- Intrauterine constriction of limb or amputation.

INTRAUTERINE FETAL DEMISE

Definition
"Unplanned and/or unexpected death of fetus after the period of viability but prior to the complete expulsion or extraction from its mother".

Incidence
- In 2009, the estimated global number of stillbirths was 2.64 million.

Risk Factors
- Maternal:
    - Maternal age > 35 years
    - Obesity
    - Black race
    - Low socioeconomic status
    - Low education status
    - Smoking/tobacco
    - Nulliparity
- Fetal:
    - Congenital malformation
    - Male sex
- Pregnancy complications:
    - IUGR
    - Preeclampsia
    - Abruptio
    - Rh negative/Nonimmune hydrops
    - Multiple pregnancy
    - Post-term pregnancy
    - Infection
    - Antepartum asphyxia
    - Previous history of stillbirth
    - Nuchal cord or knotted cord
- Medical disorders:
    - Diabetes mellitus
    - Hypertensive disorders
    - Chronic nephritis
    - SLE
    - Thrombophilias
    - Cholestasis of pregnancy
    - Hyperpyrexia
    - Severe anemia
    - Drugs (Quinine beyond therapeutic levels)
- Infection:
    - Parvovirus B_{19}
    - CMV
    - *Listeria monocytogenes*

- E. coli
- Group B streptococcus
- Ureaplasma urealyticum.

Prepregnancy overweight females have a significantly higher risk of fetal death (term stillbirth), probably due to greater placental dysfunction.

Morbid Pathology

Maceration (aseptic degenerative process) of epidermis (first structure to undergo degeneration) → Blistering and peeling off the skin (between 12–24 hours after death)

↓

Softening of ligamentous structures   and   Liquefaction of brain matter.

Diagnosis (2 steps)

I. To confirm IUD
II. To find cause of IUD.

To Confirm IUD

- Symptoms: fetal movements absent (which were present earlier)
- Signs: retrogression of positive breast changes
- Per abdomen:
  - Fundal height
    - Less than gestational age
    - Regress compared to previous documentation
  - Uterine tone → diminished
  - Uterus → flaccid
  - Fetal movements → absent
  - FHS → absent (on Auscultation/Doppler)
  - Egg shell crackling feel of fetal head → late feature.
- Ultrasound:
  - Fetal movements + fetal cardiac activities absent. To be observed for a period of 10 minutes
  - Look for oligohydramnios and collapsed cranial bones.
- Straight X ray abdomen (rarely done)
  a. Appearance of gas shadow → Robert's sign (in chambers of heart and great vessels) as early as 12 hours
  b. Spalding sign → Liquefaction of brain matter + softening of ligamentous structure (supporting the vault) [can be seen on USG] → Irregular overlapping of cranial bones (7–10 days after death)
  c. Hyperflexion of spine (common) → due to loss of muscle tone (Ball sign)
  d. Hyperextension of neck (less common)
  e. Crowding of ribs shadow → loss of normal parallelism
  f. Accumulation of fluid in subaponeurotic space → elevation of thin, dark fat line around the head (Halo sign)

↓

IUD confirmed.

To Find Cause of IUD

Antepartum

1. Complete history (exclude all risk factors)
2. Investigations (Lab.):
   - FBS/RBS
   - HbA_1C
   - TORCH
   - VDRL
   - APLA
   - Thyroid profile
   - Mini renals (urea/creatinine)
   - Kleihauer Betke tests
3. Cytogenetic studies

Amniocentesis (if not done during pregnancy) → 10–25 mL of amniotic fluid taken.

Cord blood or cardiac blood for:
1. Cytogenetic studies
2. Bacterial culture
3. TORCH.

Postpartum

Newborn

1. Photographs of unclothed infant:
   - Views of whole body in frontal, dorsal and lateral views
   - Close up of face and any grossly abnormal part
2. X ray:
   - Single AP view of whole body (including hands and feet) with limbs extended
   - If dwarfism is present, additional AP and lateral views of infant limbs, head and spine
3. Autopsy:

Grade of maceration	Features	Time since fetal death
0	"Parboiled" reddened skin	< 8 hours
I	Skin slippage and peeling	>8 hours
II	Extensive skin peeling; red serous effusions in chest and abdomen	2-7 days
III	Liver yellow-brown; turbid effusion	≥ 8 days

4. MRI:
   - If autopsy consent denied.

Placenta

- Gross and microscopic examination
- Culture for bacteria and viruses (with sterile sticks, cultures taken from under the amnion).

Management

- Spontaneous expulsion occurs in 80–90% (within 2 weeks)
- Refractory cases or cases where early termination is indicated:
  - Psychological
  - Infection (if membrane ruptured)
  - ↓ Fibrinogen level
  - Retained > 2 weeks

  - Hospitalization
  - Proper counseling
  - Investigations (Hb, blood group, PT /aPTT)
  - Options for induction (prostaglandins/oxytocin)
  - Place of cesarean section:
    - Major degree placenta previa
    - ≥ 2 previous LSCS
    - Transverse lie.

IUGR

The term intrauterine growth **restriction** has largely replaced the term intrauterine growth **retardation**.

Prevalence

- 10% of all pregnancies
- 3–5% in healthy mothers
- ≥ 25% in high-risk groups.

Diagnosis

Clinical Examination

Weight Gain

- Pre-pregnancy weight < 40 kg and BMI < 19 kg/m² are more prone for IUGR
- Ideal weight gain depends upon pre-pregnancy BMI
- Weight and BMI correlation:
  Underweight: BMI <18.5
  Normal weight: 18.5 to 24.9
  Overweight: 25.0 to 29.9
  Obese: > 30.0
- Ideal weight gain should be:

Weeks	Weight gain (Pounds)	Weight gain (kg)
0-10 weeks	No weight gain	No weight gain
10-14 weeks	3-4 pounds	1.5 kg
14-20 weeks	4-6 pounds	2.5 kg
20-30 weeks	10-12 pounds	4.5 kg
30-36 weeks	6 pounds	2.7 kg
36-38 weeks	2 pounds	1.0 kg
38-40 weeks	Almost no weight gain	Almost no weight gain
Total	**25-30 pounds**	**12-14 kg**

Out of the total weight gain,
- Reproductive weight gain (6 kg):
  - Fetus 3.3 kg
  - Placenta 0.6 kg
  - Liquor 0.8 kg
  - Uterus 0.9 kg
  - Breasts 0.4 kg.
- Net maternal weight gain (6 kg)
  - Increase in blood volume 1.3 kg
  - Increase in extracellular fluid 1.2 kg
  - Accumulation of fat and protein 3.5 kg.

Maternal Blood Pressure

- Check for any rise in BP (suggestive of hypertensive disorders)
- For ideal method of BP recording, *refer to chapter 1*

Fundal Height by (McDonald's Rule)

- It is a measure of the size of the uterus used to assess fetal growth and development during pregnancy. It is measured from the top of the mother's uterus to the top of the mother's pubic bone in centimeters.

Gestational age	Fundal height
40 weeks	1-2 finger width below subcostal arch
36 weeks	At costal arch
32 weeks	Between umbilicus and xiphoid process
28 weeks	3-finger widths above umbilicus
24 weeks	At umbilicus
20 weeks	3-finger widths below umbilicus
16 weeks	3-finger widths above symphysis

- In IUGR: fundal height < period of gestation (lag of ≥4 weeks) → but this is less sensitive.

Symphysis Fundal Height

Measurement by Tape
- To determine:
  - Period of gestation
  - Growth of the fetus
  - Multiple pregnancies
  - Complications of pregnancy, e.g. amniotic fluid disorders, hydatidiform mole and fetal growth disturbances
- Between 20 to 34 weeks gestation, the height of the uterus correlates closely with measurements in centimeters (except in obesity).
  Refer to chapter 1 for correct method of measurement.

In IUGR, there is:
- Lag of ≥3 cms (≈ ≥ 3 weeks)
  - Lag of 4 weeks → moderate IUGR
  - Lag of > 6 weeks → severe IUGR.

Investigations

< 28 weeks (Usually Symmetrical)
- Congenital abnormality → USG
- Chromosomal abnormality → Karyotyping.

>28 weeks (Usually Asymmetrical)
- Rule out hypertensive disorders of pregnancy.

Common Investigations (To Both Symmetrical and Asymmetrical IUGR)
- TORCH
- Urine culture/sensitivity
- Rule out malaria
- Investigate for present maternal status:
  - Chronic hypertension
  - Chronic renal disease
  - Chronic DM
- Send antiphospholipid antibodies (APLA) → if clinical profile of patient suggests
- History based → smoking, alcohol or other substance abuse.

Ultrasonography
1. Dating: Ist trimester

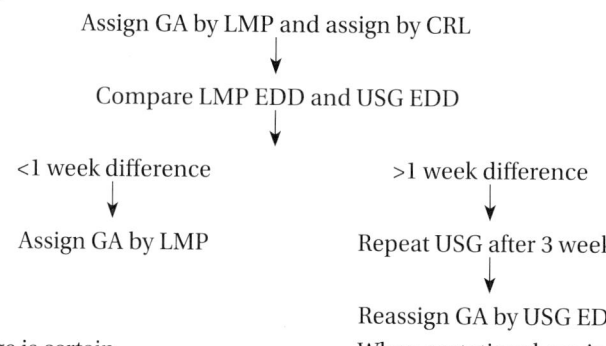

2. When gestational age is certain
   - EFW and AC → most accurate
   - HC/AC >1 after 32 weeks → IUGR

   When gestational age is uncertain
   TCD/AC → most accurate
   FL/AC>23.5 → IUGR
   Fetal PI < 7

3. Gestational age independent parameters:
   - FL/AC (in asymmetrical IUGR)
     - 22+/- 2 → normal
     - >23.5 → IUGR
   - HC/AC
     - >1 (<32 weeks)
     - = 1 (32–34 weeks) } normal
     - < 1 (after 34 weeks)

NOTE: *HC/AC >2 SD and FL/AC >23.5 indicates asymmetrical IUGR and differentiates IUGR from SGA.*

4. Transcerebellar diameter (TCD):
   - To determine gestational age
   - Up to 25 weeks → *TCD (in cms) = gestational age (in weeks)*
5. If brachycephaly (very round) OR dolichocephaly (very elongated) is present:
   - Measure cephalic index (CI) → age independent
   - CI → BPD: occipitofrontal diameter.

Interval Growth (on USG)

- Most sensitive indicator of IUGR
- To be seen after 3 weeks → if no growth → ominous.

Treatment Proper

2 basic steps

I. Antepartum fetal surveillance (APFS)
II. Determination of optimum time of delivery.

APFS

- Start at ≈ 32 weeks or 1–2 weeks before stillbirth in previous pregnancy.

Methods

- **Fetal Movement Count**
  - From 28 weeks onwards
  - Loss of fetal movement is followed by disappearance of FHR within next 24 hours
  - A number of methods have been described in literature but superiority of one over the other is not proved
  - Most commonly used is Cardif 'count 10' formula:
    - Start counting from any particular time
    - Count ends when 10 movements are perceived
    - Report if,
      - < 10 movements during 12 hours on 2 successive days
        OR
      - No movement is perceived even after 12 hours in a single day.
- **NST:**
  Reactive NST:
  - Baseline FHR 110–160 bpm
  - At least 2 accelerations of ≥ 15 beats lasting at least 15 sec
  - If nonreactive in 20 min → extended to 40 min → if still nonreactive → BPP
  - At 28 weeks → only 65% of healthy fetuses have reactive NST
  - At 32 weeks → 85%
  - At 34 weeks → 95%.

  Consistent with fetal hypoxia:
  - Fixed baseline heart rate
  - Poor baseline variability

- Loss of acceleration
- Spontaneous fetal heart decelerations.
- **BPP (Manning score)**
  - Time consuming
  - Does have a role in cases in which UA Doppler is abnormal
  - Time required = 30 min (at least)
  - Interpretation:
    - Score: 0 → if absent; 2 → if present; maximum → 10/10
    - Score: ≥ 8/10 → no fetal asphyxia
    - Score: 6/10 → repeat test within 24 hours
    - Score: 0/10 to 4/10 → ↑ hypoxia
    - In 30 min:
      - Tone: 1 episode of active extension with return to flexion of limbs or trunk → 7th week (First to come and last to go)
      - 3 discrete body/limb movements in 30 min → 8–9 weeks
      - 1 episode of breathing at least 30 sec → 18–19 weeks
      - Amniotic fluid (1 pocket ≈ 2cm in 2 perpendicular planes)
      - NST: reactive (last to come and first to go, so if NST is there, everything is there).
- **Modified BPP**

Note: Keeping amniotic fluid as an independent important risk factor for fetal mortality and that NST is last to come and first to go, therefore MBPP is recommended.

DOPPLER

CHANGES IN NORMAL PREGNANCY

Normal Fetal Circulation

Maternal blood rich in oxygen and substrates → fetal umbilical vein → left lobe of liver (also receiving depleted portal blood from splanchnic circulation via portal vein) → ductus venosus → inferior vena cava → right atrium.

Venous Tributaries Entering Right Atrium

1. Ductus venosus and left hepatic vein (carrying oxygenated blood with higher nutritional content)
2. Inferior and superior vena cava
3. Right and middle hepatic veins
4. Coronary sinus.

Venous Tributaries Entering Left Atrium

1. Pulmonary veins (deoxygenated blood from lungs)
   - Due to the different directions and velocities of tributaries, the position of the crista dividens and valve of the foramen ovale:
     - Right atrium (saturated blood from the ductus venosus) → reaches the left atrium → left ventricle → through aorta → brachiocephalic circulation → myocardium and brain

- Right atrium (relatively depleted blood) → right ventricle → lungs
- Ductus arteriosus – conduit where the 2 bloodstreams from right and left ventricles meet (inserts into aorta distal to left subclavian artery) → at aortic isthmus shunting takes place → descending aorta carries oxygenated blood to the rest of the body
- Umbilical artery → depleted blood → placenta for exchange.

Fetal Hemodynamics in Growth Restriction

- There is increased vascular resistance and uteroplacental insufficiency → reflected on ultrasound Doppler by uteroplacental blood flow assessment.

Uteroplacental Blood Flow Assessment

- An important part of fetal wellbeing assessment and evaluates Doppler flow in the uterine arteries and rarely the ovarian arteries.

Physiology

In a nongravid state and at the very start of pregnancy, the flow in uterine artery is:
- Of high pulsatility
- Has a high systolic flow
- A low diastolic flow
- A physiological early diastolic notch may be present
- Resistance to blood flow gradually decreases as pregnancy advances due to greater trophoblastic invasion of the myometrium
- If resistance is low, it has an excellent negative predictive value with a < 1% chance of developing either preeclampsia or IUGR
- A high resistance often equates to a 70% chance of preeclampsia and 30% of IUGR.

Doppler Assessment

The rationale for performing a Doppler study in the diagnosis of IUGR is that, many cases of growth restriction are thought to be associated with small vessel disease in the fetoplacental or uteroplacental circulation. Numerous Doppler criteria have been proposed for diagnosing IUGR. These involve at least 3 of the following waveform indices:
- Systolic/diastolic (S/D) ratio
- Pulsatility index (PI)
- Resistive index (RI)
- Spectral waveform of the umbilical, uterine, and fetal internal carotid arteries and the fetal descending thoracic aorta
- Spectral waveform of the ductus venosus and inferior vena cava.

Resistive Index (Pourcelot Index)

Calculated as:
- **RI** = (PSV − EDV)/PSV = (peak systolic velocity − end diastolic velocity)/peak systolic velocity
- Normal (low resistance) RI → < 0.55–0.8.

Systolic/Diastolic Ratio (S:D ratio)

Calculated as:
- **S:D** = peak systolic velocity (PSV)/end diastolic velocity (EDV)
- 2–3 is normal after 32 weeks
- >3 after 30 weeks → abnormal
- <30 weeks → higher values can be accepted, but need to be correlated to normal reference charts.

Pulsatility Index (PI) (Gosling Index)

Calculated as:
- **PI** = (peak systolic velocity - end diastolic velocity) / time averaged velocity = (PSV - EDV) / TAV.

Abnormal Patterns Include

- Highest uterine artery PI – lowest uterine artery PI >1.1 (persistence of high resistance)
- Persistence of protodiastolic notch, unilateral or bilateral, after 23 weeks is suggestive of IUGR or preeclampsia
- RI > 0.55 with bilateral notches
- RI > 0.65 with a unilateral notch
- RI > 0.70 with or without notches
- RI > 90th percentile for a given gestational age regardless of notches
- An S/D ratio of > 3 after 30 weeks of gestation is abnormal
- The reversal of flow in ductus venosus is suggestive of a fetus with severely compromised IUGR and reflects fetal metabolic acidemia
- Umbilical venous blood flow, both absolute flow (in mm/min) and corrected blood flow (in mL/min/kg) are reduced in IUGR
- Presence of pulsations in umbilical vein waveform between 8 and 12 weeks is normal, and its persistence is abnormal
- The presence of umbilical vein pulsations is associated with an increased risk of an adverse perinatal outcome.

Doppler in IUGR

Gives information regarding vascular resistance by studying blood flow in the following vessels:
I. Uterine artery in mother
II. Umbilical artery and MCA in fetus.

Method

- Vessel to be studied → 1st visualized by B-mode real time USG
- Place the Doppler gate over selected vessel
- Switch USG to pulse wave Doppler mode
- Doppler waveform obtained
- Measure peak systolic and diastolic velocities
- Indices (related to vascular resistance) independent of angle of insonation:
  - S/D ratio (systolic/diastolic ratio)
  - PI (pulsatility index)
  - RI (resistance index).

Uterine Artery Doppler

- In normal development of human placenta, trophoblast cells invade intradecidual portion of spiral arteries (early in pregnancy) → destroy first the endothelial and then muscular and spiral tissue → replace it with fibrinoid material → completed by end of 1st trimester
- Between 14–16 weeks, same process involves intramyometrial part of maternal artery → converts muscular arterial system into low resistance uteroplacental unit → capable of immense dilatation → accommodates increased blood flow to uterus and placenta → reflected by Doppler as high end diastolic blood flow → S/D ratio or RI values significantly decrease with advancing gestation until 24 to 26 weeks.

Umbilical Artery (UA)

Normally

- Most commonly performed in normal pregnancy
- Should be obtained in a free loop of cord midway between site of placental insertion and fetal insertion
- ↑ blood flow ↔ ↓ S/D ratio
- ↑ resistance ↔ ↓ blood flow → ↑ S/D ratio
- During normal pregnancy, flow in UA ↑ and resistance ↓ → Lowest around 36 weeks (just opposite to MCA waveforms)
- Blood flows from UA to placenta both in systole and diastole
- Umbilical arterial waveform usually has a "saw tooth" type pattern with flow always in the forward direction
- The 95% confidence interval limits (CI) slowly decrease for both the resistive index (RI) and pulsatility index (PI) through the course of gestation due to progressive maturation of the placenta and the increase in the number of tertiary stem villi.

DIAGRAM

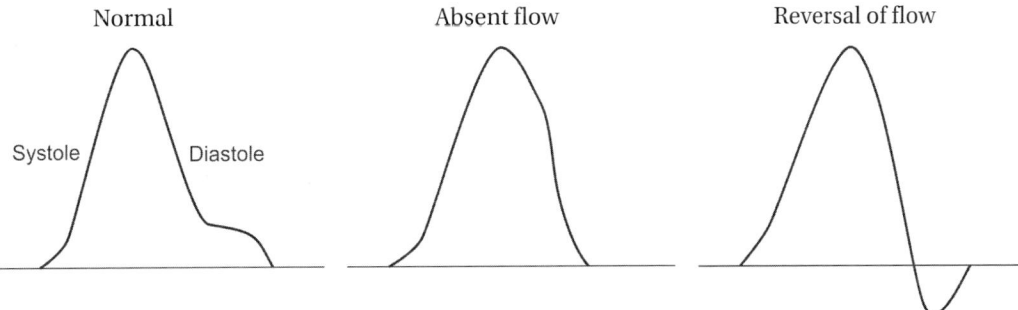

In Placental Insufficiency

Resistance to blood flow increases in placental vessels, reflected by:
- ↑ S/D ratio ⎫
- ↑ R/I   ⎬ in umbilical artery
- ↑ PI   ⎭

Sequence of Changes Occur in the following Manner

- ↑ S/D ratio (does not signify fetal hypoxia or acidosis) → absent end diastolic flow → reversal of diastolic flow (i.e. 70% of placental arteries are obliterated).

Absent end diastolic flow (AEDF → RI=1)

- Classified as Class II in severity in abnormal umbilical arterial Doppler
- Its presence can be normal in early pregnancy (up to 16 weeks)
- In mid to late pregnancy → usually occurs from placental insufficiency when the diastolic flow first reduces, then becomes absent and finally goes into reverse
- On Doppler ultrasound → umbilical arterial velocity is seen reducing to zero at the end of diastole
- The capillaries in placental terminal villi are decreased in number and they have fewer branches
- 80% of fetuses with absent diastolic flow are hypoxic and 46% are acidemic
- Absent end-diastolic flow has an associated 40% perinatal mortality
- Usually associated with:
  - Intra uterine growth restriction (IUGR)
  - Increased risk of neonatal thrombocytopenia
- At or near term → deliver
- Remote from term → daily NST and BPP (till maturity or if severe fetal compromise).

Reversal of end diastolic flow (REDF)

- During first 16 weeks, it can be a normal finding due to the low resistance arcuate arteries and intervillous spaces not yet being formed
- Flow reversal can also be detected in the fetal aorta
- Ominous, if detected after 16 weeks (represents 'tip of the iceberg')
- Classified as Class III in severity in abnormal umbilical arterial Doppler
- Ideally a low wall filter setting (< 100 Mhz) and an acute insonation angle of < 30% is recommended
- The severity can be quantified by the ratio of the maximum antegrade velocity versus the maximum retrograde velocity
- Immediate delivery, if salvageable
- Associated with significant perinatal mortality → up to 70%.

When flow in the umbilical artery becomes abnormal, this can be further worked up by evaluating flow in other vessels which usually include:
- Fetal MCA Doppler assessment
- Umbilical venous flow assessment
- Ductus venosus flow assessment.

Middle Cerebral Artery (MCA)

Normally

Vessel of choice to assess the fetal cerebral circulation.
- Easy to identify
- Has a high reproducibility
- Provides information on the brain sparing effect
- Can be studied easily with an angle of zero degrees between the ultrasound beam and the direction of blood flow and, therefore, information on the true velocity of the blood flow may be obtained

   Normally MCA has high resistance flow therefore, blood flows in MCA in systole and very low in diastole.

DIAGRAM

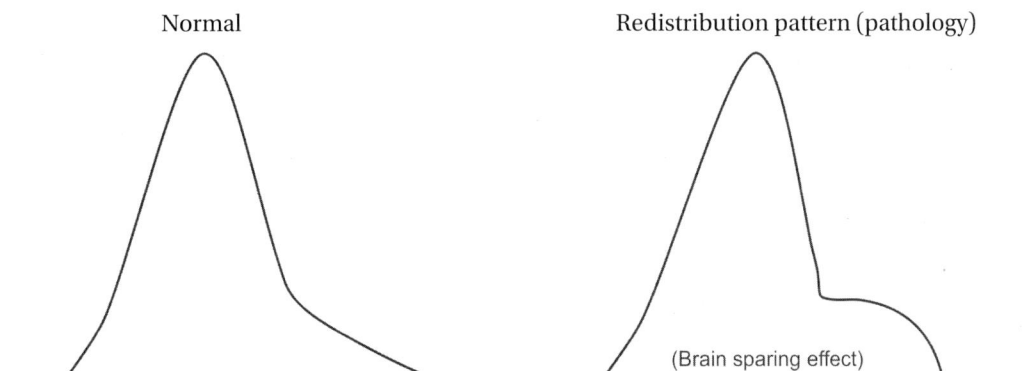

Normal — Redistribution pattern (pathology) (Brain sparing effect)

In Placental Insufficiency

- UA/MCA ratio reverses → redistribution of flow (by vasoconstriction of somatic, renal and hepatic vessels and increase blood supply to vital organs like brain, heart and adrenals → this increased blood flow (preferential) is seen in MCA) → Brain sparing effect or centralization of flow → this does not indicate fetal hypoxia or acidosis. Only indicates that fetus is under ↑ resistance to flow and compensating it by brain sparing effect
- Cerebral vasodilatation is limited. The nadir of the MCA PI is reached 14 days or more before fetal compromise
- With the onset of hypercapnia, vascular dilatation is suppressed by cerebral edema, resulting in a "normalization" of the MCA PI. The reversal of adaptation in a growth restricted fetus is considered a poor prognostic sign
- MCA peak systolic velocity becomes elevated as a late finding in severe IUGR prior to a non-reassuring heart rate tracing, i.e. continuous late decelerations or a biophysical profile score < 4
- The increase in the MCA peak systolic velocity is due to an ↑ left cardiac output, associated with increased placental vascular resistance
- Delivery should be considered when there is a 20–30% increase in the MCA PI per day for 2 days (trend towards normalization)
- Since changes in the middle cerebral artery pulsatility index may occur daily, some of the changes noted above may be missed in an individual case. Because of the wide variability in MCA indices, a single operator will have better and more consistent results.

Reflected as:
- ↑ end flow in diastole →↓ S/D ratio
- ↓ PI
- ↓ RI
- MCA PI: UA PI < 1.0–1.1 → Diagnostic of brain sparing effect.

Fetal Venous Circulation

Most commonly studied vessels:
I. Umbilical vein
II. IVC
III. Ductus venosus (DV)

- Fetal hypoxia → compensatory hemodynamic changes → if hypoxia remains uncorrected, fetal decompensation occurs at some point →↑↑ CVP → abnormal Doppler waveforms in fetal venous system, which reflects status of RV function
- Blood flow in venous circulation of healthy fetus is essentially non-pulsatile with occasional interruptions due to fetal movements and fetal breathing. If pulsatile flow appears →↑ morbidity and mortality
- The farther, the veins demonstrating this are, from the heart, the worse is the prognosis.

Umbilical Vein

- Flow in the physiological situation → monophasic nonpulsatile with a mean velocity of ~ 10–15 cm/s
- The presence of pulsatility implies a pathological state unless in the following situations:
  - Up to ~ 13 weeks gestation
  - In chromosomally abnormal fetuses
  - In presence of:
    - Fetal movements
    - Fetal breathing
    - Fetal hiccups

Perinatal mortality is highest when pulsations are seen in umbilical vein.

IVC

- Has wide variations and therefore limited role.

DV Flow

Abnormal waveforms can occur in a number of situations:
- Aneuploidic anomalies
  - Down syndrome: ~ 80% are thought to have abnormal waveforms
- Intrauterine growth restriction (IUGR)
- Congenital cardiac anomalies
- Fetal pulmonary arterial anomalies:
  - Congenital pulmonary stenosis
  - Pulmonary atresia
- Fetal arteriovenous malformations leading to shunting:
  - Vein of Galen malformation
- Fetal tumours that lead to arterio-venous shunting:
  - Sacrococcygeal teratoma
  - Epignathus
- Twin to twin transfusion syndrome: recipient twin
- Maternal diabetes: may exhibit increased PI values.

Doppler Assessment (Normal)

- The only venous vessel with forward flow during all phases of the cardiac cycle
- Of all the pre-cardial veins, this allows the most accurate interpretation of fetal cardiac function as well as myocardial hemodynamics

- The average shunting of blood through the DV decreases from 30% at 18–20 weeks to 18% at 31–34 weeks
- Flow in ductus venosus has a characteristic triphasic waveform, always in the forward direction (i.e. towards the fetal heart) and has 2 distinct peaks corresponding to systole and diastole
- Nadir corresponding to atrial contraction phase of cardiac cycle
- The triphasic waveform comprises of:
  - S wave: corresponds to fetal ventricular systolic contraction and is a highest peak, reflects the pressure gradient between the peripheral venous system and the right atrium
  - D wave: corresponds to fetal early ventricular diastole and is a second highest peak, represents the opening of the atrial ventricular valves and passive early filling of the ventricles
  - A wave (or rather trough): corresponds to fetal atrial contraction and is the lowest point in the waveform

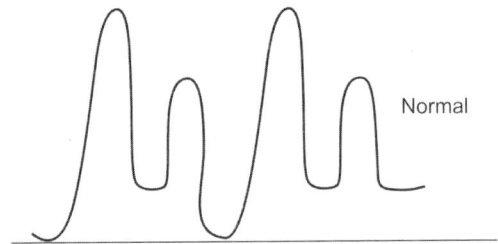

- The pulsatility index is utilized to quantitate ductus venosus flow
- PI of ductus venosus normally declines with advancing gestation
- Hypoxemia →↑ in umbilical venous flow through the DV and a ↓ in hepatic blood flow (Normal ductal flow suggests continued fetal compensation)
- Further deterioration → reversed flow during the atrial contraction of the ductus venosus and a markedly increased pulsatility index. This indicates a failure of compensatory mechanisms and the onset of right heart failure. Fetuses with reverse flow in the A-wave of the ductus venosus are not necessarily acidemic, and may survive for days to weeks in utero. Hence, the main goal of antepartum surveillance, when the gestation age is < 30 weeks, is to differentiate fetuses with ductal venosus reversed flow who require intervention, from those whose delivery can be delayed from days to weeks. Intermittent reversed flow in the ductus venosus may occur from 2 to 57 days
- Once reverse flow is constant, it may persist from 1 to 23 days before delivery is mandated by non-reassuring fetal testing
- Abnormal waveforms include:
  - Reduced flow in A wave
  - Absent flow in A wave
  - Reversal of flow in A wave
  - Abnormal indices:
    - Abnormal pulsatility index (PI)
    - Abnormal S wave to A wave ratio (S : A)
    - Abnormal peak velocity index.

DIAGRAM

↓ in forward flow during atrial systole

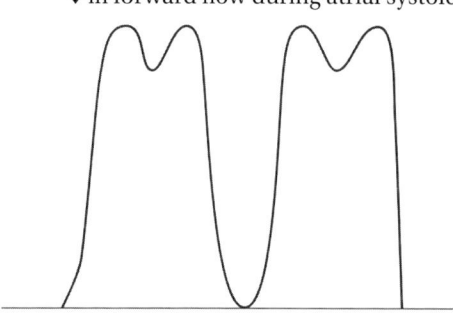

Reversal of flow during atrial systole

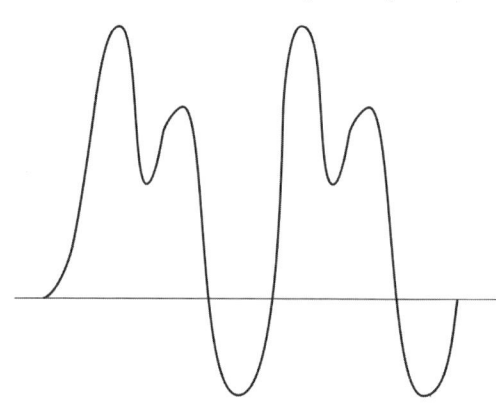

Abnormal Waveform (Proximity to Fetal Death)

I. Interrupted forward flow
II. Reverse flow during atrial contraction
III. Presence of end diastolic pulsations in UV (mortality → 63–100%).

Sequence of Doppler Changes in IUGR

1. Elevated umbilical artery S/D ratio
2. Middle cerebral artery PI < 5th percentile (brain-sparing)
3. Umbilical artery → absent diastolic flow
4. Umbilical artery → reversed diastolic flow
5. Ductus venosus → elevated pulsatility index
6. Ductus venosus → reversed a-wave
7. Ductus venosus → decreased IVR, reversed a-wave
8. Umbilical vein double pulsations
9. Umbilical vein triple pulsation with reversed a-wave flow

- The farther a compromised vein is from the heart, the higher is the perinatal mortality risk. For example, perinatal mortality is 8 times greater with an abnormal ductus venosus waveform pattern and 18 times greater with pulsations in the umbilical vein
- In 70% of cases, Doppler deterioration occurs 24 hours before a decline in the biophysical profile score
- When both a multi-vessel Doppler study and the biophysical profile score are abnormal, an expeditious delivery is mandatory.

DETERMINATION OF OPTIMUM TIME OF DELIVERY

>28 weeks

I. Investigations + APFS
II. Steroids.

Follow Up

- UA/MCA Doppler weekly
- AFI weekly
- NST weekly (if gestation age >32 weeks)
- USG every 2 weeks for growth.

If RI/PI ↑

- UA and MCA Doppler biweekly
- NST biweekly
- AFI biweekly.

Indications for Termination

- Gestational age at 37 weeks
- Absent diastolic flow in UA
- Reversal of flow in UA
- AFI <3 cm
- Absent 'a' wave on DV Doppler
- Nonreactive NST (>32 weeks).

*DV Doppler to be done, if UA shows absent or reversal of flow (for benefits of steroids).

Modes of Termination

- ↑ resistance to flow ⎫
- Absent diastolic flow ⎬ Termination of induction
- Severe oligohydramnios ⎭
- Reversal of flow ⎫
- Abnormal DV Doppler (i.e. absent 'a' wave and/or ⎬ Termination by
  pulsations in umbilical vein) ⎭ Cesarean section.

Important Points

I. Suspect IUGR even if USG predicts a normal weight or EFW in not <10th percentile but clinical suspicion is high
II. Even if BPP score is 6/10 or 8/10 with abnormal amniotic fluid → there are still↑ chances of perinatal mortality (as AFI is an independent risk factor for fetal mortality).

Following has No Role

I. Bed rest
II. β mimetics
III. Ca^{2+} channel blockers → no role for improving weight of fetus
IV. TENS (Transcutaneous electrical nerve stimulation therapy)
V. Estrogens (thought to increase blood flow)
VI. O_2 therapy
VII. Nutrient supply (carnitine → amino acid which releases energy from fat, solcoseryl–protein free calf blood extract, glucose and galactose → fruit, meat and milk sugars)
VIII. Plasma volume expansion.

SUGGESTED READING

1. Andrea Lausman, Fergus P McCarthy, et al: Screening, Diagnosis, and Management of Intrauterine Growth Restriction, J Obstet Gynaecol Can. 2012;34(1):17-28.
2. Eliza Berkley, Suneet P Chauhan, Alfred Abuhamad: Doppler assessment of the fetus with intrauterine growth restriction. American Journal of Obstetrics and Gynecology, April 2012.
3. Gomez R ponce de leon, wing D, Fiala C: Misoprostol for intrauterine fetal death. International Journal of Gynaecology and Obstetrics. 2007;99:S190-3.
4. Late Intrauterine Fetal Death and Stillbirth: RCOG Green-top Guideline No. 55, October 2010.
5. Nourah Al Qahtani: Doppler Ultrasound in the Assessment of Suspected Intra-uterine Growth Restriction, Webmed central Obstretics and Gynaecology, 2010;1(10).

CHAPTER 8

Diabetes in Pregnancy

Tania G Singh

Physiological changes in pregnancy

Pregnancy is a diabetogenic state.

Early Pregnancy

- Basal glucose—unchanged
- Insulin secretion—unchanged
- Glucose tolerance—normal
- FBS falls gradually, reaches the nadir at the end of the first trimester
- Basal hepatic glucose production—unchanged (till 12-14 weeks)

As Gestation Advances

- Basal glucose ↑
- Postprandial insulin ↑
- Lipogenesis ⎫ under influence of ↑
- Fat storage ⎭ estrogen, progesterone and insulin

Third Trimester

- Basal glucose 10-15 mg/dL lower than prepregnancy levels
- Basal and postprandial insulin ↑2 folds
- ↑insulin resistance (max. at 34-36 weeks) → due to hormones
  - Human chorionic somatomammotropin
  - Estrogen
  - Progesterone
  - Prolactin
  - Cortisol
- Insulin action is 50-70% lower than nonpregnant levels
- FBS↓
- ↑↑PPBS with prolonged glucose peak
- Hepatic gluconeogenesis ↑ by 16-30% ←→ Insulin is not able to suppress this production
- Glucose production increases with maternal body weight, such that glucose production/kg body weight does not change throughout pregnancy
- Under the influence of human chorionic somatomammotropin
  ↓
  Lipolysis and fat mobilization

Changes in GDM

Same
Same

Marked
↑↑↑ plasma glucose
↑↑ fetal weight
  ↓
↑ fetal and neonatal complications

GESTATIONAL PREDIABETES

- Absence of diabetes before pregnancy and the presence of blood glucose levels above normal but not high enough to meet the diagnostic criteria for GDM when tested in early pregnancy
- Together they should be considered as risk factors for diabetes. This would help to prevent GDM if timely modifications are made
- Modifications:
  1. Diet therapy with better nutrition and focused calorie intake
  2. Adequate physical activity
  3. Proper check on weight gain.

PREGESTATIONAL DIABETES (OVERT DIABETES)

- Diabetes present before pregnancy (irrespective of the type).

GESTATIONAL DIABETES (GDM)

- Carbohydrate intolerance of variable severity with onset or first recognition during the present pregnancy
- GDM is accompanied by alterations in fasting, postprandial and integrated 24-hour plasma concentrations of amino acids, glucose and lipids. These changes include:
  - 3-fold↑ in plasma triacylglycerol concentrations during 3rd trimester
  - ↑ of plasma fatty acids
  - Delayed postprandial clearance of fatty acids
  - ↑ of branched-chain amino acids

Prevalence

- Worldwide—1 in 10 pregnancies
- Of those—90% are GDM
- Among high-risk group—30% may have diabetes
- Indian scenario—prevalence of GDM is 14–15%
- In Asians 5–8%.

Screening Based on Risk Factors

Ideally all antenatal women (irrespective of risk factors) should be screened for GDM (ADA 2011 → changed recommendations).

Risk factors are classified as follows:

Low Risk

- Young (age < 25 years)
- Non-Hispanic white
- Normal BMI (≤ 25 kg/m^2)
- No history of previous glucose intolerance
- No history of adverse pregnancy outcomes associated with GDM
- No first-degree relative with known diabetes.

Moderate Risk

- Do not satisfy all criteria of women at low risk, but they lack two or more risk factors for GDM

High Risk

Usually defined as having two or more risk factors:
- Age > 35 years
- BMI > 30 kg/m^2
- GDM in previous pregnancy
- Unexplained IUD in previous pregnancy
- Previous macrosomic baby (weight ≥ 4.5 kg)
- First-degree relative with DM
- Previous bad obstetric history
- Large baby in present pregnancy
- Member of ethnic group with high prevalence (South Asians, Black Caribbean, Middle Eastern countries)
- Polycystic ovary syndrome
- Polyhydramnios in present pregnancy
- Hypertension (more recently noted).

Screening and Diagnosis Based on Laboratory Values

1. 75 gm anhydrous glucose (5 level teaspoons, not heaped). Juice of half lemon can be added to avoid nausea and vomiting, when taken on empty stomach
2. Fasting is defined as no calorie intake for at least 8 hours
3. Unrestricted diet (carbohydrate ≥ 150 gm/day) and routine physical activity before testing
4. Patient should preferably remain seated
5. Refrain from smoking throughout the test.

IADPSG (International Association of Diabetes and Pregnancy Study Group)

- Glucose—75 gm (after an overnight fasting of 8 hours) in 250–300 mL of water
- Criteria—when any one or more of the following is met or exceeded:
  - FBS → 92 mg/dL (5.1 mmol/L)
  - 1 hour → 180 mg/dL (10 mmol/L)
  - 2 hour → 153 mg/dL (8.5 mmol/L).

Carpenter and Coustan

2-step procedure
1. GCT (glucose challenge test) → with 50 g glucose (irrespective of the last meal) → after 1 hour → if > 140 mg/dL → OGTT
2. OGTT → 4 samples are taken (any 2 values above cut-off) with 100 g glucose
   - Fasting → 95 mg/dL
   - 1 hour → 180 mg/dL
   - 2 hour → 155 mg/dL
   - 3 hour → 140 mg/dL.

WHO/NICE

- Glucose—75 g
- Fasting ≥ 126 mg/dL (≥ 7 mmol/L)
- 2 hour → ≥ 140 mg/dL (≥ 7.8 mmol/L)

DIPSI (Diabetes in Pregnancy Study Group India)

- Approved by Ministry of Health, Government of India
- Glucose—75 g (irrespective of fasting or nonfasting state)
- 2 hours → ≥ 140 mg/dL (≥ 7.8 mmol/L)
- Advantages:
  - Requires only 1 blood sample
  - Less costly as compared to IADPSG
  - No fasting required
  - Both screening and diagnostic
  - Best for low-resource settings.

Prediabetes

Impaired Fasting Glucose
- FBS 100–125 mg/dL (5.6–6.9 mmol/L)

    OR

Impaired glucose tolerance
- After 75 g glucose load
- 2-h plasma glucose → 140–199 mg/dL ((7.8–11.0 mmol/L)

    OR

- HbA_1C → 5.7–6.4%

Prediabetes, in itself, is not a disease, but considered as risk factor for diabetes.

Overt Diabetes

If any of the following is found in pregnancy:
- FBS ≥ 126 mg/dL
- RBS > 200 mg/dL
- HbA_1C ≥ 6.5% (adopted as criteria by ADA in 2010).

GDM

- FBS > 92 mg/dL but < 126 mg/dL.

Screening: Many criteria!! What is to be followed in routine practice??
- Ideally all women, irrespective of risk category, should be screened for diabetes in the 1st trimester by FBS (very important period for organogenesis)
  - If ≥ 126 mg/dL → overt diabetes
  - If > 92 but < 126 mg/dL → GDM
  - If < 92 mg/dL → no diabetes
- Advantages:
  - No need for taking glucose
  - Early detection of overt diabetes
  - GDM and overt diabetes can be easily differentiated
- For those at high risk, screen using OGTT at first prenatal visit
- Those presenting for the first time in 2nd trimester, screen with OGTT at 24–28 weeks
- Role of HbA_1C-only in predicting risk of fetal malformations when performed periconceptionally
- Overt diabetes is diagnosed if any time in pregnancy the following are found:

- FBS ≥ 126 mg/dL OR
- HbA$_1$C ≥ 6.5 OR
- RBS ≥ 200 mg/dL (with further confirmation with either of the above two).

Classification of Diabetes

This includes 4 clinical classes:

Type 1 Diabetes

- β-cell destruction → absolute insulin deficiency.

Type 2 Diabetes

- A progressive insulin secretory defect on the background of insulin resistance.

Other Types (Due to Other Causes)

- Genetic defects in β-cell function
- Genetic defects in insulin action
- Diseases of the exocrine pancreas (such as cystic fibrosis)
- Drug or chemical-induced (such as in the treatment of HIV/AIDS or after organ transplantation).

GESTATIONAL DIABETES MELLITUS (GDM)

1. **Why is GDM screening done at 24–28 weeks?**
   - During pregnancy, an increase in insulin resistance occurs
   - Euglycemia is maintained through a compensatory increase in insulin secretion
   - The key factor which results in the development of gestational diabetes appears to be a failure to compensate with increased insulin secretion
   - As the increase in insulin resistance is greatest in the 3rd trimester, GDM usually develops going into this period
   - Therefore, screening for GDM usually occurs around 24–28 weeks.

Pedersen Hypothesis

- ↑ glucose in mother →↑ glucose in fetus →↑ insulin →↑ growth of fetus →↑ fat deposition → macrosomia → organomegaly (mainly liver and heart) →↑ erythropoietin production and ↓ surfactant production.

Recent Advances

- ↑ insulin → may lead to biochemical diabetic nephropathy defined as hypoglycemia and biochemical dysregulation in the newborn, occurred when 3rd trimester amniotic fluid insulin levels were > 17 µU/mL. It is not widely accepted due to involvement of invasive procedure
- ↑ growth → significantly accelerated growth of fetal AC (with normal growth of HC and FL):
  - Clinical measure of **somatic fetopathy**
  - More frequent assessment of AC growth would permit earlier therapeutic intervention and provide more time to normalize fetal growth by adjusting glycemic targets

- Considered a simple and practical measure
- Categorized as:
    - Low risk (< 75th percentile for gestational age)
    - High risk (≥ 75th percentile for gestational age).

Risks to Mother

1. Preeclampsia/gestational hypertension
2. Increased weight gain in pregnancy
3. Increased risk of cesarean section
4. Labor inductions are increased
5. Obstructed labor
6. Traumatic vaginal delivery
7. PPH (traumatic)
8. Interventional delivery
9. Complications associated with coagulopathy (in cases of prolonged retention of dead fetus)
10. Risk of developing postpartum prediabetes, Metabolic syndrome and Type 2 diabetes in future.

Risks to Fetus

1. Fetal macrosomia/large for gestational age
2. Fetal malformations (Type 1 DM)
3. Stillbirth
4. Preterm labor
5. Prematurity
6. Intrapartum asphyxia
7. Birth trauma:
    - Shoulder dystocia
    - Bone fracture (clavicle)
    - Nerve palsy (brachial plexus injury).

Risks in Newborn

1. Respiratory distress syndrome
2. Admission to NICU
3. Hypoglycemia (because of high insulin levels in fetus)
4. Hypocalcemia
5. Hypomagnesemia
6. Hyperviscosity
7. Polycythemia
8. Hyperbilirubinemia
9. Hyperinsulinemia
10. Cardiomyopathy.

Risk to Children Born to Diabetic Mothers

1. Obesity
2. Impaired glucose tolerance
3. Type 2 diabetes in adulthood
4. Metabolic syndrome.

Treatment in Pregnancy

- Treat even a milder form of GDM.

Diet and Nutrition Therapy

1. *Nutritional therapy—for 2 weeks*
   - Diet plan with visit to dietician every 4 weekly
   - Blood glucose is reassessed for 2-3 days with checking of FBS, premeal and postmeal monitoring (1-2 hours)
   - If it fails, i.e. FBS ≥ 90 mg/dL and/or postmeal ≥ 120 mg/dL → start insulin or oral hypoglycemic agents
   - If blood sugars are in range, wait for another 2 weeks and reassess
   - Recommended calorie intake:
     - Underweight: 35-40 kcal/kg
     - Normal weight: 30-35 kcal/kg
     - Overweight: 25-30 kcal/kg.

2. *Medical Nutrition Therapy (MNT)*

Definition: "Carbohydrate-controlled meal plan that promotes adequate nutrition with appropriate weight gain, normoglycemia and the absence of ketosis."
Primarily targets postprandial glucose levels.

Recommended Weight Gain in Pregnancy
- Normal BMI (19.8-26.0 kg/m^2) → 11.4-15.9 kg
- Overweight (BMI 26.1-29.0 kg/m^2) → 6.8-11.4 kg
- Obese women (BMI >29 kg/m^2) → upto 7 kg

Recommended Calorie Intake According to Trimester
- 1st trimester → no increase in calories
- 2nd trimester → an additional 340 kcal/day
- 3rd trimester → an additional 452 kcal/day

Modest calorie restriction, 1600-1800 calories/day or a 33% reduction in intake, does not lead to ketosis but controls weight gain and glucose levels in obese women and has been more successful.

Recommended Calorie Intake According to Body Weight
- Underweight → 35-40 kcal/kg
- Normal BMI → 30-35 kcal/kg
- Overweight → 25-30 kcal/kg
  60 : 20 : 20 → carbohydrate : protein : fat

Carbohydrate
- One of the most important components especially playing a role in diabetic patients
- Requirements:
  - In nonpregnant state—130 g/day
  - Pregnancy—175 g/day (this addition is for fetal brain development and functioning)
- In GDM, the carbohydrate intake has to be manipulated by:
  - Controlling the total amount of carbohydrate
  - Its distribution over several meals and snacks
  - Type of carbohydrate

- Role of glycemic index:
  - Even if total carbohydrates are controlled, low glycemic index (<55) foods produce a lower postmeal glucose elevation, whereas foods with a high glycemic index (>70) show higher postprandial values.

Diet in Diabetes

- High-fiber foods:
  - Whole grains
  - Oats
  - Chana aata
  - Millets
- Must contain milk without cream (minimum 2 servings) → right combination of carbohydrates and proteins
- Fruits high in fiber:
  - Apple
  - Orange
  - Pear
  - Guava
- Fruits avoided or eaten in moderation:
  - Mangoes
  - Bananas
  - Grapes
- High-fiber green vegetables:
  - Peas
  - Beans
  - Broccoli
  - Spinach
  - Green-leafy vegetables
- Pulses
- Good fats:
  - Omega 3
  - MUFA.

Exercise

Recommendations:
- Physical activity ≈ 30 minutes/day is recommended
- Brisk walk or arm exercises while sitting on a chair for at least 10 minutes after each meal.

Insulin therapy

Chemistry

- Consists of 51 amino acids
- Arranged in two chains ('A' and 'B') linked by disulfide bonds/bridges
- 'A' chain has 21 while 'B' chain has 30 amino acids
- Molecular weight—6000 Da → cannot cross placental barrier but can be transported across the placenta as part of antibody-insulin complex (anti-insulin antibodies)

- Stored crystals consists of 2 atoms of zinc and 6 molecules of insulin
- Contain 8 mg of insulin/human pancreas (= 200 units).

Secretion: By β-cells in pancreatic islet (respond to a variety of stimuli—glucose, mannose, leucine, arginine and vagal activity).

Degradation: Liver and kidney (hydrolysis of disulphide bond)
- Endogenous: Liver (60%) and kidney (35-40%)
- Exogenous: Liver (35-40%) and kidney (60%).

$t^{1/2}$ in plasma: 3-5 minutes.

Physiological and Pharmacological Actions

1. Sugar metabolism:
   - Stimulates hepatic glucose uptake and use by cells
   - Inhibits gluconeogenesis and glycogenolysis
   - Blood sugar↓
2. Fat metabolism:
   - Improves fatty acid transportation and fat anabolism
   - Inhibits fat catabolism
   - Inhibits fatty acid and acetone body generation
3. Protein metabolism:
   - Improves amino acid transportation and protein anabolism
   - Inhibits protein catabolism and amino acid utilization in the liver
4. Potassium:
   - Stimulates K^+ entering cells → blood K^+↓
5. Long-term action:
   - Improves or inhibits the synthesis of some enzymes.

Mechanism of Action

Insulin receptor in cell membrane mediates the effect.
Insulin receptor consists of:
- 2α subunits, which constitutes the recognition site
- 2β subunits, which contains a tyrosine kinase.

Sources of Exogenous Insulin

- Three types exist: Bovine, Porcine and Human insulin
- Pork insulin is more homologous to human insulin
- Only difference between them is that the 30th amino acid in the β-chain in pork insulin is alanine, whereas it is threonine in human insulin
- Human insulin:
  - Made by replacement of 30-alanine in β-chain of porcine insulin by threonine
  - Less expensive, less immunogenic
  - Production by recombinant DNA technology in *E. coli* and in yeast or by enzymatic modification of porcine insulin
  - More water-soluble and hydrophobic than porcine or bovine insulin
  - More rapid subcutaneous absorption
  - Has an earlier and more defined peak
  - Has slightly shorter duration of action

Administration

- Subcutaneous route
- Intravenous (only regular insulin).

Disadvantages/Adverse Reactions

- Insulin allergy (IgE antibodies): itching, redness, swelling, anaphylaxis shock
- Pain at the injection site
- Need for multiple injections
- Insulin resistance (IgG antibodies)
- Need for refrigeration
- Potential for hypoglycemia: nausea, hunger, tachycardia, sweating
- Skilful handling of syringes (problem in low resource countries)
- High cost
- Poor patient compliance
- Lipodystrophy at injection site: atrophy.

Concentration in Pregnancy

Not always same in different trimesters
- ↑ in very early pregnancy
- ↓ in second half of 1st trimester
- ↑ in 2nd and 3rd trimester
- After 32 weeks, stays constant or even declines, which may manifest as hypoglycemia.

Available Types

1. Short-acting insulin (regular or soluble):
   - Onset of action: 30 minutes-1 hour after injection
   - Therefore, it should be injected 30 minutes before planned meal
   - Peak action → in 2–4 hours
   - Duration of action → 6–8 hours
   - Vial has a yellow color strip for identification
   - Brand names: Actrapid, Huminsulin, Insugen R
2. Intermediate acting:
   Lente insulin (insulin zinc suspension)
   - Mixture of 30% semilente with 70% ultra lente insulin → provide a combination of relatively rapid absorption with sustained long action
   - Onset of action: 1–2 hours
   - Peak action: 8–10 hours
   - Duration of action: 20–24 hours

   Isophane insulin (neutral protamine hagedorn, NPH)
   - Absorption and onset of action is delayed by combining appropriate amounts of insulin and protamine
   - 6 molecules of insulin per molecule of protamine
   - Onset of action: 1–2 hours after injection
   - Peak action: 8–10 hours
   - Duration of action: 20–24 hours
   - Vial has a green color strip for identification

3. Ultra short-acting (modified insulin with minor changes):
   - Onset of action: within few minutes after injection (very fast)
   - Permit more physiologic prandial insulin replacement
   - Injected just before meal or sometimes immediately after the meal
   - Peak in 30 minutes
   - Duration of action: 2 hours
   - The only type that should be administered intravenously
   - Brand names: Lispro and Aspart
4. Ultra long acting:
   - Not approved to use in pregnancy
   - Concern: They bind with IGF-1 receptor and possible teratogenicity
   - Brand names: Glargine and Detemir
a. *Extended insulin zinc suspension (Crystalline)*
   - Slower onset: 4-6 hours
   - Prolonged peak of action: 14–18 hours
   - Duration: 24–36 hours
b. *Protamine zinc insulin (Ultralente)*
   - Onset (4-6 hours) and a prolonged peak (14–20 hours)
   - Duration: 24–36 hours
   - Recommended dose to be taken in 2 or more divided doses
c. *Glargine*
   - Soluble, peakless, ultra long-acting insulin analog
   - Designed to provide reproducible, convenient, background insulin replacement
   - Has a slow onset of action (1–1.5 hours)
   - Achieves a maximum effect after 4–5 hours and maintained for 11–24 hours or longer
   - Given once a day.

Regimens for Administration of Insulin

Requirements according to trimesters:
- 1st trimester → 0.7–0.8 U/kg/d
- 2nd trimester → 0.8–1 U/kg/d
- 3rd trimester → 0.9–1.2 U/kg/d.

Targets to achieve:
- FBS ≤ 95 mg/dL (5.3 mmol/L)
- 1-hour postprandial ≤ 140 mg/dL (7.8 mmol/L)
- 2-hour postprandial ≤ 120 mg/dL (6.7 mmol/L).

Regimen I (Split Mix Regimen)
Total dose → 2/3rd in morning and 1/3rd in evening (with ≈ 12 hours' gap). Check before lunch—if out of target range, give 4–8 units of regular insulin.

Out of the total dose to be given in the morning (before breakfast):
   - 2/3rd—isophane (long-acting)
   - 1/3rd—actrapid (regular)

Out of 1/3rd in the evening (before dinner):
   - 1/2—isophane
   - 1/2—actrapid.

Try to start with 0.2–0.4 U/kg body weight, i.e. 12–24 units:
- 24 units → 16 units in the morning and 8 units in the evening
- 16 units → 10 units long-acting
  6 units regular-acting
- 8 units → 5 units long-acting
  3 units regular-acting

Regimen II (Multiple Subcutaneous Injections)
- Before meals → short-acting
- Bedtime → long-acting or intermediate-acting
- Try to start with 0.2–0.4 units/kg body weight
- Start Inj. Actrapid 4 units before meals
- Bedtime → 6–10 units Inj. Insulatard
- Check FBS, pre and post each meal sugars
  - Observe for 2–3 days
- Dose can be increased by 2 units at a time.

Key Points

Insulin Adjustment
1. If fasting is high → increase insulin at bedtime. Start intermediate-acting instead of long-acting insulin
2. If postmeal value is high, increase premeal value before that particular meal
3. Late night hypoglycemia → reduce bedtime insulin.

Glucose Monitoring
1. Check at home by glucometer
2. Check FBS, pre- and postmeal sugars
3. Check late-night sugars between 2 am and 4 am (2–3 times/week)
4. Charting of each day's value
5. In between, confirm the accuracy of glucometer by checking sugar levels with laboratory values.

Future Researches
- Trials on making oral, buccal and inhaled insulin are in progress with satisfactory results.

Intrapartum Management

- Usually insulin is not required during labor as the uterine muscle contractions reduce the need for insulin by increasing its sensitivity
- Planned induction—start in morning
- Not to skip the night dose
- Goal during labor—to maintain sugars between 70 and 110 mg/dL because if maternal hyperglycemia occurs at this time, it will lead to neonatal hypoglycemia
- Insulin chart.

Immediate Postpartum

- If the patient has delivered by cesarean section, give insulin according to the sliding scale for the first 24 hours, checking sugars every 4–6 hourly

- If delivered vaginally:
  - Type I—reduce dose of insulin by 1/3rd to 1/2 → Start oral meals
  - Type II—may not require any medications
  - GDM—check FBS
  - If FBS<126 mg/dL → they can continue with diet therapy and exercise with regular check on sugar levels.

Recurrence of Gestational Diabetes

- In ≈90% of the cases, GDM resolves after pregnancy but there is still a high risk of glucose intolerance or development of GDM in subsequent pregnancies
- There is a wide range of 30–84% in whom GDM occurs in subsequent pregnancies owing to different studies involving different populations.

Oral Hypoglycemic Agents (OHAs)

Main groups:

Sulphonylureas

- Introduced in 1956 (tolbutamide)
- Insulin secretagogues

Mechanism of action
- These stimulate pancreatic insulin secretion → reduces hepatic glucose output → increases peripheral glucose disposal
- They are potassium channel blockers → allow influx of calcium into pancreatic β-cells →↑ in the release of insulin
- Slow down the rate at which the liver releases glucose into the blood stream
- Increase the number of insulin receptors on cell membranes → increase insulin efficiency
- The pathogenesis of both GDM and Type 2 diabetes are insulin resistance and inadequate insulin secretion; therefore, beneficial in both
- For them to act, patient must have residual β-cell function; therefore not useful in Type 1 diabetes.

First generation
Rarely used:
- Acetohexamide
- Chlorpropamide
- Tolazamide
- Tolbutamide

Second generation
- Glibenclamide
- Glyburide
- Glipizide
- Glicazide
- Glimepiride

Advantages of second-generation over first-generation sulfonyl ureas:
- More potent on a per milligram basis
- Fewer side effects
- Their pharmacokinetics allow for more effective once-a-day dosing, which enhances compliance

Side effects
Mild and uncommon with second generation:
- Severe or recurrent, mild episodes of hypoglycemia
- Mild gastrointestinal upset (nausea, vomiting, diarrhea or constipation, flatulence, headache)
- Skin reactions: rashes, purpura, pruritus
- Weight gain (least with glimepiride due to its insulin-sparing effect)
- Hyponatremia and fluid retention when taken in large doses
  Chlorpropamide
    - Longer lasting hypoglycemia
    - Seen more often because of its long half-life and duration of action
  Glipizide
    - Lower risk of hypoglycemia because it is metabolized to inactive by products that do not have hypoglycemic activity
- Hematologic reactions: transient leukopenia, thrombocytopenia, hemolytic anemia
- Cholestasis (with and without jaundice)—with chlorpropamide
- Secreted in breastmilk.

Glyburide

- Category B drug
- Metabolized in liver
- Potent but slow-acting
- Metabolite excreted in urine and bile
- Peak action → 2–4 hours after intake } therefore should be administered
- Peak in glucose in GDM → occurs at 90 minutes, after food } at least 1 hour before meal
- Plasma t½ → 4–6 hours
- Duration of action: 18–24 hours
- Daily dosing: 5–15 mg
- Crosses placenta in negligible amounts (99.8% is protein bound)
- Fetal malformations and hypoglycemia are not found in various studies—therefore, it is suitable for use in pregnancy
- There have been contradicting results from various studies regarding its safety in the 1st trimester and neonatal morbidity
- Almost not found in breastmilk.

Biguanides (insulin sensitizers)

- Introduced in 1957
- Also known as antihyperglycemic agents (do not stimulate endogenous insulin secretion → hypoglycemia does not occur)

Mechanism of action
- Suppress hepatic glucose production → ↑ glucose utilization in peripheral tissues to a lesser degree → insulin resistance in muscle cells
- Food intake is ↓ → ↓ intestinal glucose absorption

Metabolism
- Not metabolized, excreted unchanged by kidneys

Metformin
- Second generation biguanide

- Category B drug
- It does not stimulate endogenous insulin secretion; therefore, hypoglycemia does not occur with it
- Hypoglycemia may occur when metformin is taken with:
  - Insulin
  - A sulfonylurea
  - Excessive amount of alcohol
- Beneficial effects:
  - Lowers triglyceride and LDL cholesterol
  - Increases HDL cholesterol
  - Weight loss or no weight gain
  - Useful in PCOS patients
- Side effects:
  - GI upset (diarrhea, bloating)—start with low dose, increase gradually and take with meals
  - Metallic taste
  - Effect on vitamin B_{12} levels
  - Decrease in appetite
  - Lactic acidosis (rare)—excreted by kidneys; therefore, serum creatinine is to be monitored periodically
  - Serum creatinine >1.4 mg% → stop medication
- Contraindicated in:
  - Significant hepatic disease
  - Cardiac insufficiency
  - Alcohol abuse
  - Hypoxic conditions
  - History of lactic acidosis
- Temporarily discontinued 1 to 2 days before any dye studies
- t½ : 1.5–3 hours
- Duration of action: 6–8 hours
- Cleared by kidneys
- Not bound to plasma proteins
- Daily dose: 0.5–2.0 g
- Not metabolized at all
- GFR increases in pregnancy; therefore, dose adjustment is required as its excretion is mainly through renal tubules
- Crosses placenta
- Studies have proved its role in PCOS patients, who got pregnant while on metformin. Rates of early pregnancy loss, gestational diabetes, neonatal morbidity and mortality were significantly lower in metformin group
- Metformin-exposed fetuses, when followed at 2 years of age, showed more subcutaneous fat and less visceral fat (a pattern showing increased insulin sensitivity)—MiG TOFU trial
- Concentration in breast milk is low, making it safe while breastfeeding

Phenformin
- Almost removed from the market after reports of fatal lactic acidosis.

Alpha Glucosidase Inhibitors

Acarbose
- Higher failure rate in the few trials → further research is needed before implementation.

Miglitol
Voglibose
- Breakdown of disaccharides and polysaccharides into monosaccharides is made slow
- Glucose absorption → delayed →↓ postmeal blood glucose values.

Thiazolidinediones (insulin sensitizers)

- Newer class (commercially known as glitazones)
- Developed in 1997
- They enhance insulin sensitivity by reducing peripheral insulin resistance
- Do not stimulate the pancreas to produce more insulin
- Metabolized in liver; therefore, can be used safely in patients with renal dysfunction

Troglitazone
- First glitazone, linked with hepatocellular injury and death secondary to liver failure; hence removed from the market.

Rosiglitazone
- Not approved for use in pregnancy
- Category C drug
- Very high risk of placental transfer when exposed in 1st trimester, leading to fetal abnormalities.

Pioglitazone
- No data available of use in pregnancy.

Meglitinides (insulin secretagogues)

Repaglinide

Nateglinide
- A very recent addition
- Ultra-short t½ (1 hour)
- Structurally different but similar in action to sulphonylureas
- Acts directly on pancreatic β-cells by blocking potassium channels and causing an influx of calcium →↑ secretion of insulin
- Pulsatile release of insulin is also corrected
- Much lower incidence of hypoglycemia
- It allows for flexible timing and missed meals
- Combination of repaglinide and metformin is very effective.

Note: *Only glyburide and metformin can be considered in pregnancy.*

Management Proper

Prepregnancy Counseling (in cases of pre-existing diabetes)

1. Pregnancy needs to be started with a good glycemic control
2. Explain the patient the:
   - Risks (maternal and fetal)
   - Fetal malformations with Type 1 diabetes
3. In cases of PCOS well-controlled on metformin, the drug need not be stopped at conception
4. Weight reduction in cases of obese patients
5. Folic acid 4 mg/day at least 3 months prior to conception

6. Oral hypoglycemics to be switched over to insulin (studies on complete safety of glyburide still awaited)
7. To lay stress on diet and exercise
8. Systemic examinations to be done (in case of Type 1 diabetes)
   - Fundus
   - Renal function tests
   - Hypertension
   - Any infections to be treated well beforehand (UTI, dental caries)
9. Immunity to rubella should be checked
10. Patients with IGT, IFG or an HbA_1C of 5.7–6.4% should undergo the following interventions before pregnancy:
    - Weight loss ≈ 7% of body weight
    - Increasing physical activity to at least 150 minutes/week of moderate activity, such as walking
    - Metformin therapy for prevention of type 2 diabetes may be considered in those with:
      - BMI > 35 kg/m^2
      - Women with prior GDM.

Antenatal management

First trimester

(Prediabetics)
1. All routine investigations (CBC, ABO Rh, HIV, HbsAg, Anti HCV, Urine routine)
2. HbA_1C and OGTT
3. Kidney function tests with electrolytes
4. 24-hour urine albumin and creatinine
5. Fundus examination
6. Metformin to be continued
7. ACE inhibitors to be discontinued and switch on to safer drugs
8. Folic acid 4 mg/day
9. Regular BP monitoring (in case of hypertensive patients)
10. Oral hypoglycemics to be switched over to insulin
11. Diet/exercise
12. USG for nuchal translucency and congenital anamolies
13. Dental check-up (optional, if required)
14. BP, weight and urine examination to be done at each visit
15. ANCs:
    - 1st and 2nd trimesters → every 15 days
    - 3rd trimester → weekly

FBS (in all antepartum women, irrespective of risk category):
- To exclude any hidden cases of pregestational diabetes
- To rule out cases of gestational prediabetes so that proper management, to avoid their progression to GDM, can be done timely.

Second trimester
1. Triple screen at 16–18 weeks
2. Level II scan at 18–22 weeks
3. Fetal echocardiography at 20–24 weeks (especially in cases of overt diabetes)
4. USG for growth and liquor at ≈ 26–28 weeks
5. Injection → tetanus toxoid

6. Iron and calcium supplements
7. Fundus examination in Type 1 diabetes
8. Signs and symptoms of hypoglycemia to be explained
9. Hypocare.

Third trimester
1. Serial USG to exclude:
   - Large for date fetus
   - Excessive liquor
   - IUGR (in cases of diabetic vasculopathy)
2. Fetal macrosomia or polyhydramnios is not an indication to start insulin in patients of GDM, being managed on diet alone
3. In patients with uncontrolled diabetes, risk of sudden IUD should be kept in mind and well explained to the patient beforehand
4. Fetal monitoring (in all cases):
   - DFKC
   - NST twice weekly from 32 weeks onwards
   - BPP weekly
   - Doppler in cases of IUGR

Delivery
- Wait for spontaneous onset of labor:
  - Till 40 weeks in cases of GDM well-controlled on diet
  - Till 38–39 weeks in cases of GDM on insulin
  - Till 38 weeks in case of well-controlled pre-existing diabetes
  - Uncontrolled pre-existing diabetes can be terminated earlier, when indicated
    - If glucocorticoid is given for lung maturity, caution is adviced with close glycemic control during three days after the first dose
    - The steroid effect begins approximately 12 hours after the first dose and lasts for five days
- Cesarean section→ in case where EFW is ≥ 4 kg or for other obstetric indications
- Risks at the time of vaginal delivery:
  - Shoulder dystocia
  - Brachial plexus injury
  - Clavicle fracture
  - Need for Roberts maneuver
  - Birth asphyxia
  - Need for interventional delivery.

Labor

Spontaneous labor
- Patient to be kept NPO
- GDM patients well controlled on diet do not require insulin or sugar monitoring during labor
- Secure 2 IV lines.

1st IV line
- Insulin infusion with 1 unit/mL (50 units of Insulin + 50 mL of Normal saline)
- Infusion rate 1 mL/hour
- 2 hourly sugar monitoring and titrate infusion as per the table below

Blood glucose levels (mg/dL)	Insulin (unit/hour)	Infusion rate (mL/hour)
≤ 100	No insulin	–
101–140	1	1
141–180	1.5	1.5
181–220	2	2
>250 → 5%Dextrose changed to Normal saline	–	–

2nd IV line
- Start 5% dextrose @ 100–125 mL/hr (to meet the calorie demands)

Induced labor
- With prostaglandins (after assessing Bishop's score)
- To be started early morning
- Give night dose of insulin and omit the morning dose
- Monitoring as mentioned above
- Strict FHS monitoring
- Partograph (to avoid obstructed labor) which is even more worse in a diabetic patient.

Postpartum

Screening required—why?
- GDM confers a 7-fold risk for future Type 2 diabetes
- Up to 1/3rd of women with Type 2 diabetes have been diagnosed with GDM
- GDM patients should be screened for diabetes at 6 to 12 weeks postpartum, using nonpregnant OGTT criteria or by using FBS.

Screening at 6 to 12 weeks postpartum
- Which is more suitable—OGTT or FBS?
  OGTT:
  - Sensitivity → 100%
  - Results can identify overt diabetes mellitus, impaired fasting glucose (IFG), impaired glucose tolerance (IGT) or normal glycemia
  - More time-consuming
  - Need for glucose administration
  FBS:
  - Sensitivity → 67%
  - Can identify IFG but not IGT
  - Requires less time
  - No need for glucose administration.

Further follow-up:
- GDM patients with normal postpartum screening
  - Rescreened with OGTT every 3 years
- GDM found to have IFG or IGT or both (prediabetes)
  - Lifestyle interventions or metformin to prevent diabetes
  - OGTT at 1 year postpartum
  - FBS yearly
  - OGTT at 3 years

- HbA₁C is not recommended postpartum
- Breastfeeding should be encouraged.

Contraception

Barrier Methods (Condoms, Diaphragm, Cervical Cap, Spermicides)
- Accepted well
- No systemic side effects
- No influence on glucose tolerance
- Failure rate is high ≈20% per year
- Strong motivation required among both the partners
- Good in cases where there is risk of STIs and HIV

Intrauterine devices
Ideal contraceptive for women with prior GDM—why?
- Very effective
- Reversible
- No metabolic disturbances
- No increased risk of pelvic inflammatory disease (with copper or LNG IUDs)
- Failure rates <1%
- No restriction in any type of diabetes
- Low frequency of bleeding disturbances and very low failure rate makes LNG IUDs the contraceptive of choice in patients with prior GDM or overt diabetes
- No influence on blood glucose, HbA₁C or insulin levels

Combined oral contraceptives (ethinyl estradiol + progestin)
Ethinyl estradiol (EE)
- Has no effect on glucose tolerance and insulin sensitivity
- Has a positive effect on bleeding control →↑ patient compliance
- But risk of thrombosis and ↑ in BP is very high even with lowest doses (due to adverse effect of EE on hemostasis and renin angiotensin system)
- Effect on lipid metabolism:
   - ↑ triglycerides and HDL
   - ↓ LDL

Progestin
- Main components:
   - Second-generation (e.g., levonorgestrel or norgestimate) OR
   - Third-generation (e.g., desogestrel or gestodene)
- ↓ glucose tolerance and insulin sensitivity
- No influence on BP or clotting factors
- Effect on lipids:
   - ↓ triglycerides and HDL
   - ↑ LDL cholesterol

Note:
- COCs containing lowest dose of EE (20–35 µg) and progestin can be used but with caution, keeping in mind the other side effects related to oral use of these hormones
- Overall the metabolic effects will depend on type and dose of each component

Nonoral combined hormonal methods (monthly injection, transdermal patch or intravaginal ring)
Very few studies are available with conflicting results; therefore, safety is still debated upon.

Progesterone-only oral contraceptives
- Advantages:
  - No influence on diabetes control
  - No ↑ in globulin production; therefore, do not ↑ BP or coagulation factors
- Disadvantages:
  - Irregular bleeding
  - No off (all days of the month)
  - Strict timings
  - In cases of missed pill, doubling the dose will not compensate
  - Higher failure rates as compared to COCs
- Well suited for:
  - Type 1 DM patients ⎱ where estrogen is
  - Patients with prior GDM with cardiovascular risk factors ⎰ contraindicated
- Not suited for:
  - Lactating women with prior GDM (Breastfeeding inhibits endogenous estrogen and. in such cases, unopposed progestin together with insulin resistance and β-cell dysfunction will lead to an ↑↑ risk of diabetes)—according to various studies.

Intramuscular or subcutaneous progestin methods (Norplant, Implanon, DMPA)
- Limited studies
- DMPA (Depot medroxyprogesterone acetate)— better avoided as ↑↑ risks associated.

Sterilization

- Best method in diabetics with completed families or not desiring more children.

SUGGESTED READING

1. Akadiri Yessoufou, Kabirou Moutairou: Maternal Diabetes in Pregnancy: Early and long-term outcomes on the offspring and the concept of 'Metabolic Memory'. Experimental diabetes research. September 2011.
2. Alison Tovar, Lisa Chasan-Taber, Emma Eggleston, et al: Postpartum screening for diabetes among women with a history of gestational diabetes mellitus. Prev Chronic Dis. 2011;8(6):A124.
3. Balaji V: Use of oral hyperglycemic agents in pregnancy diabetes. Medicine Update. 2011.
4. Catherine Kim, Diana K. berger, Shadi Chamany: Recurrence of gestational diabetes mellitus. Diabetes care. May 2007; Volume 30, Number 5.
5. Counterpoint:Oral hypoglycemic agents should be used to treat diabetic pregnant women. Diabetes care. November 2007; Volume 30, Number 11.
6. Diagnosis and treatment of gestational diabetes. Royal College of Obstetricians and Gynaecologists. Scientific Impact Paper No. 23. January 2011.
7. Donald R Coustan: Pharmacological management of gestational diabetes. Diabetes Care. July 2007, Volume 30, Supplement 2.
8. Gestational Diabetes Mellitus. American diabetes association. Diabetes care. Jan 2003; Volume 26, Supplement 1.
9. Joel G Ray, Howard Berger, Lorraine L. Lipscombe, et al: Gestational prediabetes: a new term for early prevention? Indian J Med Res. 2010;132:251-5.
10. Joel G Ray, Howard Berger, Lorraine L Lipscombe, Mathew Sermer: Gestational prediabetes: A new term for early prevention? Indian J Med Res. 2010;132:251-5.
11. Kavitha Nagandla, De Somsubhra, Kanagasabai Sachchithanantham: Oral Hypoglycemic Agents in Pregnancy: An Update. The Journal of Obstetrics and Gynecology of India. 2013;63(2):82-7.
12. Lisa Hartling, Donna M Dryden, Alyssa Guthrie et al: Screening and diagnosing gestational diabetes mellitus. AHR Qpublication. October 2012;No. 12(13):E021-EF.

13. Michael Plevyak: The Role of Oral Agents in the Treatment of Gestational Diabetes, The Female Patient. April 2011;Volume 36.
14. Nancy F Butte: Carbohydrate and lipid metabolism in pregnancy: normal compared with gestational diabetes mellitus. Am J Clin Nutr. 2000;71 (suppl):1256S-61S.
15. New consensus criteria for GDM. Diabetes Care. March 2010; Volume 33, Number 3.
16. N Wah Cheung: The management of gestational diabetes. Vascular Health and Risk Management. 2009;5:153-64.
17. Peter Damm, Elisabeth R Mathiesen, Kresten R Petersen, et al: Contraception after gestational diabetes. Diabetes Care. July 2007; Volume 30, Supplement 2.
18. Point: Yes, It Is Necessary to Rely Entirely on Glycemic Values for the Insulin Treatment of All Gestational Diabetic Women: Diabetes care. March 2003; Volume 26, Number 3.
19. Seth Hawkins J.: Glucose Monitoring During Pregnancy, Curr Diab Rep. 2010;10:229-34.
20. Siri L Kjos, Ute M Schaefer-Graf: Modified therapy for gestational diabetes using high-risk and low-risk fetal abdominal circumference growth to select strict versus relaxed maternal glycemic targets. Diabetes care. July 2007; Volume 30, Supplement 2.
21. Standards of medical care in diabetes 2013. Diabetes care. Jan 2013;Volume 36, Supplement 1
22. Thomas R Moore: Glyburide for the treatment of gestational diabetes. Diabetes Care. July 2007; Volume 30, Supplement 2.
23. Waugh N, Royle P, Clar C, Henderson R, et al: Screening for hyperglycaemia in pregnancy: A rapid update for the national screening committee. Health Technology Assessment. 2010;14:45.

CHAPTER 9

Hypertensive Disorders in Pregnancy (HDP)

Tania G Singh

Case: An elderly primigravida, conceived after infertility treatment, is admitted in the labor room with 19^{+3} weeks period of gestation with BP measurements of 150/104 mmHg. She has a family history of hypertension and diabetes. This is her 2nd visit of antenatal checkup. Taken 1 dose of tetanus toxoid and is taking iron and calcium as prescribed. How will you work up this case?

Step I → Patient presents with hypertension

Step II → Assess gestational age

Step III → ≤ 20 weeks

Step IV → Check urinary proteins

It can either be:
a. Chronic hypertension OR
b. Early manifestation of preeclampsia in any one of the following:
   - Multiple pregnancy
   - Anti phospholipid antibody syndrome
   - Molar pregnancy
   - Preeclampsia supcrimposed on chronic hypertension
   - Hydrops
   - Acute polyhydramnios

Step V →

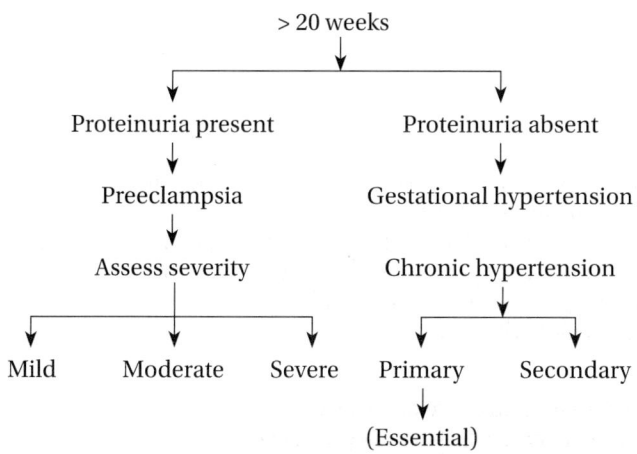

IMPORTANT POINTS IN THE HISTORY

Present and Past History of BP Elevation

- Earlier in the course of present pregnancy
- Previous history of BP elevation, if yes:
  - Since how long
  - On which medications
  - What is the highest reading
  - What is the working BP of the patient
  - Any complications ever encountered
  - Any investigations done ever
  - Taking treatment regularly or only symptomatically
  - Any side effects of the on-going drug.
- BP in previous pregnancies:
  - Was the pregnancy singleton or was it a multiple gestation
  - In which period of gestation was it revealed
  - Which antihypertensives were started
  - What was the highest reading encountered
  - Any complications of the mother or the fetus
  - Was the delivery before time or in time
  - When were the antihypertensives stopped
  - Did it continue after delivery
  - Were antihypertensives restarted after delivery.

Family History

- Hypertension or diabetes.

Physical Examination

Blood Pressure Recording in Pregnancy–Ideal Method

First one should be familiar with the *5 phases of Korotkoff sounds*
Phase I: 1st appearance of sounds marking systolic pressure
Phase II and III: Increasing loud sounds
Phase IV: Muffling of sounds
Phase V: Disappearance of sounds.

Position
- Rest – 5 minutes
- Sitting with feet supported on flat surface (avoid supine position)
- Remove all tight clothing from the arm
- Arm well supported at the level of the heart (different arm positions can alter the BP significantly)
- Measure BP on both the arms at first visit (this excludes rare vascular disorders)
- BP of the arm giving higher reading is to be taken
- In labor → left recumbent position.

Cuff
- Length - 1.5 times the circumference of the arm
- Wide enough to cover at least 2/3rd of the upper arm

- Arm circumference >33 cm → use larger cuff
- *Smaller cuff size will overestimate BP*
- *Larger cuff will underestimate BP*
- Lower edge of the cuff should be 2-3 cm above the point of brachial artery pulsation (easy access to antecubital fossa)
- Application should be firm.

Measurement apparatus
- Mercury sphygmomanometer is still considered as best for measuring BP in preeclamptic patients
- Automated devices may underestimate BP by 10-15 mmHg.

Measurement
- Do not kink or twist the tube on the cuff
- Inflated and deflated smoothly
- Korotkoff V is taken for diastolic BP
- Korotkoff IV only when sounds are audible as level approaches "0"mm Hg (due to hyperdynamic circulation of pregnancy).

AN OVERVIEW

Hypertension in Pregnancy (PIH is an Obsolete Term and should not be Used)

- SBP ≥ 140 mmHg
- DBP ≥ 90 mmHg (using Korotkoff V)
- Based on an average of minimum 2 readings using the same arm.

Classification

- Preeclampsia – eclampsia
- Gestational hypertension
- Transient hypertension
  - Late onset hypertension, without proteinuria or pathologic edema
- Chronic hypertension
  - Essential (primary)
  - Secondary
  - White coat
- Preeclampsia superimposed on chronic hypertension
- Unclassifiable antepartum.

Incidence and Prevalence

- Preeclampsia affects 5 to 10% of all pregnancies worldwide, but can be higher (up to 18% in developing countries)
- In India, it is 8–10%
- Responsible for about 50,000–60,000 maternal deaths worldwide every year (10–15% of maternal deaths).

Predictive Testing

Role of Uterine Artery Doppler in Prediction of Preeclampsia

- Despite the analysis of more than 100 methods, there is still no reliable and certain test for predicting HDP
- The most useful method is uterine artery Doppler ultrasonography
    - If abnormal uterine flow (specifically the bilateral notch or high resistance index) is present between weeks 22 and 24, there is a 60% risk of developing preeclampsia and/or IUGR later in pregnancy
    - The predictive value of Doppler ultrasound is particularly high for the development of severe preeclampsia before 34 weeks and for preeclampsia with IUGR
    - However, routine screening of all pregnant women is not recommended; uterine artery Doppler is beneficial as a test in pregnant women who are at high risk for preeclampsia
    - According to recent meta analysis an increased pulsatility index with notching (after the 16th week) is the best predictor of preeclampsia in women with established risk factors (positive likelihood ratio: 21.0)
    - This test should, therefore, be used in clinical practice
- Research is on-going to determine the relevance of combinations of maternal risk factors, early biochemical markers (such as placental protein 13) as well as Doppler results from the 1st and 2nd trimester.

Role of Mean Arterial Pressure

- When blood pressure is measured in the 1st or 2nd trimester of pregnancy, the mean arterial pressure is a better predictor for preeclampsia than systolic blood pressure, diastolic blood pressure, or an increase of blood pressure
- Mean arterial pressure (MAP) = (DBP + 1/3) × (SBP–DBP).

Can Proteinuria be Used as A Predictor of Complications?

- The only known cure for preeclampsia is delivery of the placenta
- Proteinuria has been proposed and studied as both an indicator of severity of disease and as a predictor of outcome in preeclampsia and many clinicians even today make major management decisions based on the degree of proteinuria
- But recent advances suggests that proteinuria is a poor predictor of either maternal or fetal complications in women with preeclampsia
- Maternal and fetal clinical condition and gestational age, complemented by hematologic and biochemical parameters, should for the time being remain the primary determinants for timing delivery in women with preeclampsia.

Testing for Proteinuria

- Exclude UTI
- Clean catch urine sample
- Measure using automated reagent strip first
- Quantitation by laboratory methods if urine dipstick test is ≥ "1+"
    - Spot urine protein: creatinine can be used to detect significant proteinuria (>30 mg/mmol)
    - 24-hour urine collection is not necessary in routine clinical management but is gold standard in severe preeclampsia

- But automated reagent strip method is not suggested in severe preeclampsia or high-risk cases as it can be affected by:
  - Variable excretion
  - Maternal dehydration
  - Bacteriuria
- When compared with a 24-hour urine collection, the sensitivity of dipstick testing for proteinuria is only 61%, with a specificity of 97%.

Readings of Dipstick

Trace → 0.1 g/L
1+ → 0.3 g/L
2+ → 1 g/L
3+ → 3 g/L
4+ → 10 g/L.

How Much BP is to be Lowered?

In Mild and Moderate Cases

Without comorbid conditions:
- SBP 130–155 mmHg
- DBP 80–105 mmHg.

With comorbid conditions:
- SBP 130-139 mmHg
- DBP 80-89 mmHg.

In Severe Cases

- SBP <160 mmHg
- DBP <110 mmHg.

Fundus Changes in Hypertensive Disorders

Grade I

- Mild arteriolar constriction
- Broadening of light reflex.

Grade II

- Attenuation of vessels
- Deflection at A-V crossings (Salu's sign).

Grade III

- Salu's sign
- Banking of veins (Bonnet)
- Tappering of veins (Gunns)

- Copper wire vessels
- Cotton wool spots
- Hard exudates.

Grade IV

- Silver wire papilloedema.

BEFORE MOVING ONTO THE ACTUAL MANAGEMENT, LETS DISCUSS THE ROLE OF FEW DRUGS

How is Calcium Important in Hypertensive Disorders?

- Low dietary calcium intake or no calcium supplementation can cause increase in blood pressure by stimulating the release of parathyroid hormone and/or renin → increased intracellular calcium concentration in vascular smooth muscle cells and causes vasoconstriction
- Role of calcium supplementation in reducing hypertensive disorders in pregnancy can possibly be explained by ↓ in parathyroid calcium release and intracellular calcium concentration, thereby ↓ smooth muscle contractility and promoting vasodilatation
- Calcium supplementation could also prevent preterm labor and delivery by reducing uterine smooth muscle contractility directly and indirectly by increasing magnesium levels
- Second explanation could be – malnutrition. It had been proposed that hormones involved in blood pressure control are altered during malnutrition and can lead to significant morbidity in malnourished pregnant women
- Recent studies have shown that calcium supplementation during pregnancy reduces all gestation related hypertensive disorders
- Reduces neonatal mortality by decreasing the risk of birth asphyxia due to severe preeclampsia/eclampsia
- Studies have quoted reduction in childhood hypertension whose mothers were supplemented with calcium during pregnancy
- Measures taken to improve calcium intake (especially in developing countries)
  - Calcium intake from dairy products
  - Calcium supplementations
  - Food fortification with calcium.

How is Acetyl Salicylic Acid Helpful in Preeclampsia?

Acetylsalicylic acid has been implicated in the physiological transformation of spiral uterine arteries: it inhibits thromboxane-mediated vasoconstriction more than prostacyclin-mediated vasodilatation, and may thereby offer protection against vasoconstriction and pathological blood coagulation in the placenta. Its use prevents failure of physiological spiral artery transformation as well as the development of preeclampsia.

- A significant affect is observed if administered especially before 16 weeks
- According to recent Cochrane review:
  - It reduces the rate of preeclampsia by 17%, neonatal mortality by 14%
  - Pregnancies with pre-existing risk factors (particularly severe preeclampsia in previous pregnancies) benefit most from aspirin

- Aspirin is not recommended after 23 weeks if a pathological Doppler flow is present
- Aspirin is not recommended in cases of manifest preeclampsia or gestational hypertension.

Use of Diuretics During Pregnancy

Mechanism of Action

Short-term effects:
- The initial hypotensive response is mediated by a simple reduction in plasma volume and cardiac output.

Long-term effects:
- Long term effect of low blood pressure is associated with partial reversal of the initial hemodynamic changes; the plasma volume and cardiac output partially rise toward the baseline level, while the systemic vascular resistance falls.

Adverse effects on neonates:
- A meta-analysis of almost 7000 neonates exposed to diuretics during pregnancy did not find an increased risk of adverse effects, such as birth defects, fetal growth restriction, thrombocytopenia, or diabetes, among neonates exposed to diuretics in utero.

ACE Inhibitors during Pregnancy

- Widely used as 1st line therapy for chronic hypertension in non-pregnant females
- Captopril, enalapril and lisinopril cross the human placenta in pharmacologically significant amounts.

Use in 1st trimester

- Studies have shown that when used in 1st trimester, there is no increased risk (as some women already on ACE inhibitors get pregnant unplanned) in the rate of congenital malformations
- Recent studies strongly suggest that the original report by Cooper et al might reflect uncontrolled confounding.

Use in 2nd and 3rd Trimester

Associated with:
- Oligohydramnios
- Hypocalvaria
- Anuria
- Renal failure
- Neonatal hypotension
- Patent ductus arteriosus
- Aortic arch obstructive malformations
- Some of these infants exhibit severely impaired renal function and hypoplastic lungs owing to oligohydramnios, and they might progress to death or end-stage renal failure
- Cause of these defects appears to be related to inhibitory effects on the renin-angiotensin-aldosterone system
- Morbidity is estimated to be quite high; it is between 10% and 20% of infants exposed.

DRUGS FOR HYPERTENSIVE DISORDERS

Drug	Dose	Action	Route	Onset of action	Contra-indication	Side effects
Nifedipine	5-10 mg capsule	Calcium channel antagonist	Oral	10-20 minutes Repeat dose after 30 - 60 min	Aortic stenosis	Severe headache associated with flushing and tachycardia. Peripheral edema, orthostasis, constipation May inhibit labor and have synergistic action with magnesium sulfate in BP lowering
	10-20 mg tablet		Oral	30-45 min Repeat after 45 min		
Labetalol	20 mg IV initially, then 20 to 80 mg every 20 to 30 minutes, maximum of 300 mg	β adrenergic blocker with mild α vasodilator effect	IV bolus over 2 min	5 min Repeat after 15-30 min Peak effect: within 10-20 min	Asthma, congestive heart failure	Bradycardia, bronchospasm, headache, nausea, tremulousness, scalp tingling (which usually resolves within 24-48 hours)
	Infusion: 1 to 2 mg/min 100-400 mg bid daily (for mild hypertension)		Oral			
Methyldopa	250-750 mg tid	Central (false neurotransmitter) Primary action is on CNS Has some peripheral effect	Oral	Slow onset of action (max. drug effect 4-6 hours after ingestion) Persists for 10-12 hours	Hepatic disorders Congestive cardiac failure, Depression	Postural hypotension, dry mouth, sedation, depression, headache, blurred vision, swelling of feet (safety after 1st trimester well-documented; including 7 years follow up of offspring)
Hydralazine	5 mg, IV or IM, then 5 to 10 mg every 20 to 40 minutes; once BP controlled, repeat every 3 hours; max 30 mg If BP not controlled after 3 doses: start infusion if PR is <120/min Infusion: 0.5 to 10.0 mg/h; (50 mg drug + 50 mL NS) start at 10 mL/hr, after 15 min, rate ↑ by 5 mL/hr	Direct Vasodilator (Releases noradrenaline, which is a potent vasoconstrictor of uteroplacental circulation, therefore monitor FHS meticulously)	IV bolus	20 min Repeat after 20 min		Flushing, anxiety, restlessness, headache, nausea, hypotension, oliguria, may cause abruption, stillbirth May cause marked tachycardia – sympathetic effect of hydralazine May cause neonatal thrombocytopenia and low Apgar scores at 1 min

Contd...

Contd...

Diazoxide	30-50 mg (max 300 mg) every 5-15 min	Direct vasodilator	IV rapid bolus	3-5 min Repeat after 5 min	Hypotension, hyperglycemia, may arrest labor, use is waning
Prazosin	0.5-5 mg tid	Alpha blocker			1st dose effect- orthostatic hypotension
Hydrochl-orthiazide	12.5-25 mg daily	Diuretic	Oral		
Atenolol	25-50 mg bid	β Receptor blocker			May decrease uteroplacental blood flow; may impair fetal response to hypoxic stress; risk of growth restriction when started in 1st or 2nd trimester (atenolol); may be associated with neonatal hypoglycemia at higher doses
Nitro-prusside (relatively contra-indicated)	Constant infusion 0.25 to 5.0 μg/kg/min (only in refractory cases) Max. dose 8 μg/kg/min	Short-acting direct vasodilator of both arterial and venous smooth muscles	IV	1-2 min Has short duration of action (1-3 min)	Hypotension, cyanide toxicity if used > 4 hours; agent of last resort

Maternal Antihypertensive Medications Usually Compatible with Breastfeeding

- Captopril
- Diltiazem
- Enalapril
- Hydralazine
- Hydrochlorothiazide
- Labetalol
- Methyldopa
- Minoxidil
- Nadolol
- Nifedipine
- Oxprenolol
- Propranolol
- Spironolactone
- Timolol
- Verapamil.

Anesthesia and Fluid Management

- Anesthetist kept informed
- In all severely hypertensive patients, platelet count should be done prior to induction or when they come in labor
- Regional analgesia or anesthesia is appropriate in the following conditions:
  - Platelet count > 75,000 (unless there is a coagulopathy)
  - Falling platelet concentration
  - Coadministration with antiplatelet agent (aspirin) or anticoagulant (heparin)
- If no other contraindications, epidural can be inserted for pain relief
- Bolus fluids should not be administered before anesthesia
- In the absence of contraindications, all types of anesthesia (epidural, spinal, combined spinal/epidural and general anesthesia) can be given
- In cases of oliguria, bolus fluids or administration of diuretics is not recommended.

Do not use the following to prevent hypertension

- Bed rest
- Nitric oxide (NO) donors
- Progesterone
- Diuretics especially thiazides
- LMW heparins
- Magnesium
- Folic acid
- Antioxidants (vitamin C and E)
- Fish oils/algal oils
- Garlic
- Salt restriction
- Vitamin D supplementation
- Calcium supplementation reduces the risk of developing preeclampsia in high-risk women and those with low dietary calcium intakes. Prevention through routine supplementation is ineffective.

Reducing the Risk of Hypertensive Disorders in Pregnancy

Following women at high risk of preeclampsia should take 75 mg of aspirin (low dose acetylsalicylic acid) and calcium supplementation (1.5–2.0 gm elemental calcium) daily from 12 and 14 weeks respectively until the birth of the baby:
- Hypertensive disease during a previous pregnancy
- Chronic kidney disease
- Autoimmune disease such as SLE or APAS
- Type 1 or type 2 diabetes
- Chronic hypertension
- Multiple pregnancy.

GESTATIONAL HYPERTENSION

- New onset of hypertension arising after 20 weeks gestation
- No additional features of preeclampsia
- Resolves within 3 months postpartum.

Following risk factors require additional assessment and follow-up:
- Nulliparity
- Age ≥ 40 years
- Pregnancy interval of > 10 yrs
- Family history of preeclampsia
- Multiple pregnancy
- BMI of ≥35 kg/m^2
- Gestational age at presentation
- Previous history of preeclampsia or gestational hypertension
- Pre-existing vascular disease
- Pre-existing kidney disease.

Maternal Monitoring

Mild Hypertension (140/90 to 149/99 mmHg)

- Do not admit
- No treatment required
- Measure BP once a week
- Measure proteinuria at each visit (using automated reagent-strip reading device) or urinary protein:creatinine ratio (taking midstream urine sample)
- Only routine investigations.

Moderate Hypertension (150/100 to 159/109 mmHg)

- Do not admit
- Treat with oral labetalol (1st line drug) to keep DBP between 80–100 mmHg and SBP< 150 mmHg
- Measure BP twice a week
- Measure proteinuria at each visit
- Blood tests:
  KFT with electrolytes
  CBC
  LFT → only transaminases and bilirubin.

*Do not carry out further blood tests if no proteinuria at subsequent visits.

Severe Hypertension (≥160/110 mmHg)

- Recheck BP after 15 min of rest before making diagnosis
- Admit (until BP is ≤159/109 mmHg)
- Manage with oral labetalol (1st line drug) to keep DBP between 80–100 mmHg and SBP< 150 mmHg
- Measure BP at least 4 times/week
- Measure proteinuria daily
- Investigate at presentation and then monitor weekly: KFT with electrolytes
  CBC
  LFT-only transaminases and bilirubin.

*2nd line management: Methyldopa, nifedipine
*Follow up: BP and proteinuria twice weekly
  Blood tests weekly.

Fetal Monitoring

Mild and Moderate Hypertension

- If <34 weeks- USG for growth, AFI
                    Umbilical artery Doppler
- If >34 weeks- above not required
- NST only if DFKC not adequate.

Severe Hypertension

- NST at diagnosis and weekly
- USG for growth, AFI and umbilical artery Doppler at diagnosis and every 2 weekly.

Time of Delivery

- For mild and moderate hypertension → at 37 completed weeks
- In refractory cases → at 34 weeks after a course of steroids.

Postnatal

BP measurement
- Daily × 2 days
- At least once between day 3 and day 5
- As clinically indicated if antihypertensive drugs are changed after birth.

Antihypertensives
- Continue use of antenatal antihypertensive Rx (↑or ↓ according to BP)
- Stop methyldopa within 2 days of birth.

Physician reference
- After 2 weeks of delivery and at 6–8 weeks, if required.

PREECLAMPSIA (PE)

Onset at >20 weeks' gestational age of:
- 24-hour proteinuria ≥ 300 mg/day or, if not available, a protein concentration ≥30 mg (≥1+ on dipstick) in a minimum of two random urine samples collected at least 4–6 hours but no more than 7 days apart
- A systolic blood pressure >140 mmHg or diastolic blood pressure ≥ 90 mmHg as measured twice, using an appropriate cuff, 4–6 hours and less than 7 days apart and
- Disappearance of all these abnormalities before the end of the 6th week postpartum, in a woman who was normotensive prior to pregnancy.

NOTE:
- Raised BP is commonly but not always the first manifestation
- Proteinuria is also common but should not be considered mandatory to make the clinical diagnosis.

Diagnosis can also be made when:

Hypertension arises after 20 weeks gestation (confirmed on 2 or more occasions).

Accompanied by one or more of the following:
- Significant proteinuria:
  - Random urine protein/creatinine ratio ≥ 30 mg/mmol, OR
  - A validated 24 hour urine collection shows > 300 mg protein OR
  - ≥ 3+ in dipstick test
- Renal involvement
  - Serum or plasma creatinine ≥ 90 micromol/L OR
  - Oliguria (< 500 mL/24 hours)
- Hematological involvement
  - Thrombocytopenia (platelets < 1 lakh/mm^3)
  - Hemolysis
  - DIC
- Liver involvement
  - Raised transaminases
  - Severe epigastric or right upper quadrant pain
- Neurological involvement
  - Severe headache
  - Persistent visual disturbances (photopsia, scotoma, cortical blindness, retinal vasospasm)
  - Hyper-reflexia with sustained clonus
  - Convulsions (eclampsia)
  - Stroke
- Pulmonary edema
- Intrauterine fetal growth restriction (IUGR)
- Placental abruption.

Also classified as:
- Mild hypertension 140–149/90–99
- Moderate hypertension 100–109/150–159
- Severe hypertension ≥ 160/110.

Severe hypertension in pregnancy → BP ≥ 160/110. Why chosen this value?
- This represents a level of blood pressure above which cerebral autoregulation is overcome in normotensive individuals, which may lead to cerebral hemorrhage and hypertensive encephalopathy
- For severe hypertension, a repeat measurement should be taken after 15 minutes for confirmation.

Risk Factors for Preeclampsia
- Preeclampsia in a previous pregnancy
- Family history of preeclampsia
- Poor outcome in a prior pregnancy (placental abruption, IUGR, fetal death in utero)
- Interdelivery interval >10 years
- Nulliparity
- Pre-existing medical conditions:
  - Chronic hypertension
  - Diabetes (pre-existing or gestational)
  - Renal disease

- Thrombophilias:
  - Antiphospholipid antibody syndrome
  - Protein C and S deficiency
  - Antithrombin III deficiency, and
  - Factor V Leiden
- Maternal age ≥ 40 years
- BMI >35 kg/m^2
- Multiple pregnancy
- Raised BP at booking
- Gestational trophoblastic disease
- No midtrimester fall in BP
- Finger and facial edema
- Fetal triploidy
- High altitude has also been shown to increase the incidence of preeclampsia which is credited to greater placental hypoxia, smaller uterine artery diameter and lower uterine artery blood flow.

Note:

- The relevance of inherited thrombophilia in the development of preeclampsia is unclear
- Routine antenatal thrombophilia screening is not recommended
- According to recent guidelines, anti phospholipid antibodies should be determined in patients with a
  - Previous history of severe or recurrent preeclampsia/HELLP syndrome < 34 weeks' gestation OR
  - Intrauterine growth restriction (IUGR)
- A recent consensus paper recommends investigating inherited and acquired thrombophilias in these cases
- The most frequent pregnancy-associated risk factors for developing preeclampsia are: "Bilateral notch" (diagnosed by uterine artery Doppler), multiple pregnancies and gestational diabetes mellitus.

Though Gestational Age is Considered an Important Criteria for Planning Line of Action but the Actual Management and Time of Delivery Depends Solely on Severity of Disease

Does Edema has Any Significance in Preeclampsia?

- Though edema is no longer included in the definition of preeclampsia but rapid development of generalized edema should alert the clinician.

Management

Mild PE (140/90 to 149/99 mmHg)

- Admit to hospital
- No treatment required
- Measure BP at least 4 times/day
- Measure proteinuria everyday (mid-stream urine sample)
- Investigations: twice/week
  - KFT with electrolytes
  - CBC
  - LFT: transaminases and bilirubin

- Delivery at 37 completed weeks
- At 34–37 weeks: In labor
  - Nonreassuring NST } deliver
  - Other obstetric indication

Moderate PE (150/100 to 159/109 mmHg)

- Admit to hospital
- Rx with oral labetalol (1st line drug) to keep DBP between 80–100 mmHg and SBP< 150 mmHg
- Measure BP at least 4 times/day
- Measure proteinuria daily
- Investigations: 3 times/week
  - KFT with electrolytes
  - CBC
  - LFT- only transaminases and bilirubin
- Delivery at 37 completed weeks
- At 34-37 weeks: In labor
  - Non-reassuring NST } deliver
  - Other obstetric indication

Outpatient Management (once BP stabilizes)

- Regular diet (no salt restriction)
- Counsel woman and family about danger signals of PE and eclampsia
- Do not give anticonvulsants, sedatives and diuretics
- Maternal evaluation: Biweekly follow up
  - BP recording every visit
  - S/S of severe PE
  - Investigations biweekly
- Fetal evaluation: USG every 15 days
  - DFKC
  - NST weekly.

Severe PE

- Admit to hospital (≥160/110 mmHg)
- No need for *strict* bed rest
- Rx with oral labetalol (1st line drug) to keep DBP between 80–100 mmHg and SBP< 150 mmHg
- Measure BP > 4 times/day
- Measure proteinuria
- Investigations: 3 times/week
  - KFT with electrolytes
  - CBC
  - LFT- only transaminases and bilirubin
- Deliver at 34 completed weeks after course of corticosteroids or earlier if indicated.

Postnatal Management

Measure BP
- 4 times/day till patient in hospital, then every 1-2 days till 2 weeks and antihypertensives according to BP.

Physician reference
- After 2 weeks of delivery and at 6–8 weeks, if required.

Investigations
- Platelet count, transaminases and serum creatinine at 48–72 hours after birth
- If normal → do not repeat
- If reducing but still abnormal → measure at 6–8 weeks or as clinically indicated
- If not improving → measure as clinically indicated
- Measure proteinuria everyday when in hospital, thereafter at each visit and at 6–8 weeks
- If abnormal → further review at 3 months and specialist opinion.

IMPENDING ECLAMPSIA

Symptoms/Signs of Impending Eclampsia

- Severe hypertension with proteinuria
- Persistent neurological symptoms → headache (occipital or frontal), restlessness, agitation, phosphene signals, tinnitus, and brisk, diffuse, polykinetic tendon reflexes
- Visual disturbance → blurred vision, photophobia
- Fundoscopy → marked retinal edema, severe hemorrhages, exudates and papilloedema
- Epigastric and/or RUQ pain
- Nausea/vomiting
- Oliguria
- Renal impairment: serum creatinine >106 µmol/L
- Laboratory evidence of DIC/HELLP syndrome
- Sudden swelling of face, hands or feet
- Signs of clonus (≥ 3 beats)
- Platelets <1 lakh
- Liver enzymes >70 IU/lit
- Pulmonary edema
- "Preeclamptic angina" – severe epigastric pain and/or vomiting with abnormal liver enzymes.

But eclampsia may not develop even in the presence of the following signs:
- Severe headaches (especially occipital)
- Brisk reflexes > 3+
  - 3+ is hyperactive without clonus
  - 4+ is hyperactive with unsustained clonus
  - 5+ is hyperactive with sustained clonus
- Visual disturbances.

Management

- Main aim: to prevent seizures
- No role of ambulatory management
- Expectant management at tertiary care center
- If symptoms developed at home:
  - Keep in bed
  - Sedated
  - Transferred

On admission:
- Quiet darkened room
- Sedated, if required
- IV access
- Antihypertensives:
  - At '0' hrs:
    - Inj. Labetalol 20 mg IV (over 2 min)
  - At '20' min.:
    - If BP > 150/100 mmHg, double the dose every 20 min (20 mg, 40 mg, 80 mg, 80 mg) till a maximum dose of 220 mg/hour
- Prophylactic $MgSO_4$ (after catheterization)
  - Pritchard regime (for 24 hrs) or stat dose according to progress
  - Look for signs of magnesium toxicity (respiratory rate, urine output and patellar reflexes)
- Investigations
- Maintain O_2 saturation
- Fluid management:
  - Excessive fluid administration can result in pulmonary edema, ascites and cardiopulmonary overload, whereas too little fluid exacerbates an already constricted intravascular volume and leads to further end-organ ischemia
- Urine output should be > 30 mL per hour and intravenous fluids limited to 100 mL/hour ($\approx$ 1 mL/kg/hr, using present weight) unless there are other ongoing losses (input/output charting)
- If oxytocin is indicated, it should be concentrated and this fluid should be considered as intake.

Maternal
- CBC with platelets
- Urine protein (mid-stream urine sample)
- 24 hr urinary protein
- KFT with electrolytes
- LFT (AST, ALT, LDH and bilirubin)
- If platelet count is < 1 lakh → coagulation profile and peripheral smear
- Fundoscopy.

Fetal
- NST if gestational age is > 32 weeks
- USG (gestational age, AFI, abruption, IUGR)
- Doppler, if IUGR.

Depending Upon Gestational Age

< 28 weeks (EFW<1 kg) or > 34 weeks
- Antihypertensives
- Prophylactic $MgSO_4$
- Termination (induction with prostaglandins).

28–34 weeks
- Antihypertensives
- Prophylactic $MgSO_4$
- Investigations

- Steroids
- After 48–72 hrs, manage as mentioned below, depending upon BP readings:

BP controlled → expectant management

Maternal
- 4 hrly BP
- Daily I/O charting
- Daily LFT, KFT, platelet count
- Daily urine albumin
- Bed rest

Fetal
DFKC
Daily NST
Biweekly Doppler and AFI
USG for fetal growth every 2 wks

Stable → terminate at 34 weeks.

BP uncontrolled → termination.

Factors Mandating Immediate Delivery

Maternal
- Uncontrolled hypertension
- Progressive deterioration of hepatic and/or renal function
- HELLP syndrome
- Eclampsia/Persistent neurologic signs
- Labor
- Gestational age ≥ 37 weeks
- Acute pulmonary edema.

Fetal
Nonreassuring NST
Severe IUGR with abnormal Doppler
Placental abruption
AFI< 5 cm

Labor Management in Hypertensive Disorders

- Written and informed consent (explaining all complications and associated risks) is very important in all hypertensive cases (as complications may occur at low BP readings)
- Vaginal delivery unless cesarean section is required for other reasons
- Steroids should be covered
- Cervix unfavorable → cervical ripening with prostaglandins and augmentation using oxytocin and amniotomy
- Antihypertensive treatment should be continued throughout labor and birth to maintain systolic BP at <160 mmHg and diastolic BP < 110 mmHg
- Much lower values of BP are not recommended due to risk of placental abruption and hypoperfusion
- IV access
- Attention to administration of fluids
- Epidural can be given
- Vitals charting (every 2 hourly in latent phase and ½ hourly in active phase)
- For all cases of severe preeclampsia, blood should be kept arranged
- Strict vigilance on signs of impending eclampsia
- Anesthetist and pediatrician to be informed beforehand
- Assistance with 2nd stage is not routinely required but may be necessary, if:
  - BP is poorly controlled
  - Progress is inadequate
    There are premonitory signs of eclampsia

- Active management of 3rd stage is recommended due to the increased risk of postpartum hemorrhage
- Ergometrine or syntometrine should not be given as it may produce an acute rise in BP.

CHRONIC HYPERTENSION

- Hypertension which is detected at <20 weeks period of gestation or was present preconceptionally.
- Can be:

Essential (Primary)

- Idiopathic
- Present in 90–95% of cases
- There is no accompanying proteinuria
- BP >140/90 mmHg preconceptionally or prior to 20 weeks without an underlying cause
OR
- BP < 140/90 entering pregnancy on antihypertensives
- Other features:
  - Mainly present in multiparous women of little older age group
  - Family history often present
  - Blood parameters usually remain unchanged
  - Ophthalmic changes: may present as silver wiring of arterioles/hypertensive retinopathy.

Secondary

- Hypertension due to:
  - Chronic kidney disease (e.g. glomerulonephritis, reflux nephropathy and adult polycystic kidney disease)
  - Renal artery stenosis
  - Pyelonephritis, tuberculosis or neoplasm
  - Systemic disease with renal involvement (e.g. diabetes mellitus, systemic lupus erythematosus)
  - Endocrine disorders (e.g. pheochromocytoma, Cushing's syndrome and primary hyperaldosteronism)
  - Coarctation of the aorta
- Other features:
  - Can present at any age
  - Parity is unrelated
  - There is no family history
  - Persists even after pregnancy
  - Blood urea and creatinine often found elevated
  - Urinary changes:
    - Low specific gravity
    - Presence of albumin and granular casts
  - Ophthalmic changes:
    - Albuminuric retinopathy
    - Cotton wool patches
    - Flame-shaped hemorrhages.

Note: Diagnosis of chronic hypertension can be missed, if:
- Patient approaches the doctor after mid-pregnancy, when physiologic decrease in blood pressure may incorrectly label the patient as normotensive, and
- When these physiologic effects will go, it will be labelled as gestational hypertension in 3rd trimester
- Such patients should be reassessed after 6 weeks of delivery to reclassify them.

Preeclampsia Superimposed on Chronic Hypertension

Diagnosed where a woman with pre-existing hypertension develops:
- Systemic features of preeclampsia or proteinuria
- After 20 weeks gestation
- Occurs in ≈ 20% of women with chronic hypertension
- Risks for both mother and fetus are greater than for preeclampsia or chronic hypertension alone
- Risk increases, if:
    - Hypertensive for ≥ 4 years
    - History of preeclampsia in previous pregnancy
    - Baseline diastolic BP > 100 mmHg.

WHITE COAT HYPERTENSION

- Defined as hypertension in a clinical setting but normal blood pressure in non-clinical settings when assessed by 24 hour ambulatory blood pressure monitoring or home blood pressure monitoring, using an appropriately validated device
- Women with this condition present early in pregnancy with apparent chronic hypertension, but their outcomes are better than those of women with true chronic hypertension
- They may generally be managed without medication by using repeated ambulatory or home blood pressure monitoring. A small proportion will go onto develop preeclampsia
- Defined as office diastolic BP of ≥ 90 mmHg but home BP of < 135/85 mmHg.

Management of Chronic Hypertension

Maternal

- Preconceptional counseling
- Stop ACE inhibitors/ARBs (angiotensin receptor blockers) or chlorthiazides (increased risk of congenital abnormalities) within 2 days of pregnancy detection
- Start other antihypertensives:
    - Labetalol – drug of choice   ⎫ Start in
    - Nifedipine   ⎬ 1st trimester
    - Methyldopa   ⎭
- Do not give:
    - Atenolol → associated with IUGR
    - Diuretics → not teratogenic, but may restrict the natural plasma volume expansion of pregnancy
- Maintain BP <150/100 mmHg
- Low sodium intake
- USG whole abdomen
- Spot urine protein: creatinine ratio where there is doubt about proteinuria on dipstick, i.e., 1+ or 2+ proteinuria

- Serum electrolytes
- 24 hour urine catecholamine, if there is severe hypertension
- Specialist opinion
- Ophthalmic examination
- Delivery at 37 completed weeks if BP<160/110 mmHg or earlier, if high
- Continue antenatal antihypertensives for 2 weeks after delivery
- If a woman has taken methyldopa to treat chronic hypertension during pregnancy, stop within 2 days of birth and restart the antihypertensive treatment taken before pregnancy
- Review long-term antihypertensive treatment 2 weeks after birth
- Medical review at 6-8 weeks after delivery.

Fetal

- USG and Doppler at 28-30 weeks and between 32-34 weeks. If results are normal, do not repeat further
- NST weekly from 30 weeks onwards or if ↓ DFKC.

Postpartum Management of Hypertensive Disorders

- If diastolic BP is > 100 mmHg after 48-72 hours → restart antihypertensives
- In many women, BP is unstable for 1-2 weeks after delivery (particularly high on 3rd to 6th day)
- Do not restart methyldopa if patient was taking it during pregnancy
- All other agents mentioned earlier are compatible with breastfeeding, including ACE inhibitors, enalapril and captopril
- Confirm that end organ dysfunction of preeclampsia has resolved
- NSAIDs should not be given postpartum in following cases:
  - If BP is not controlled
  - High creatinine ≥ 100 microm
  - Platelet count <50000/mm^3
  - Oliguria
- Screening after 6 weeks
  - Screen for preexisting hypertension, if present, tests to be done:
    - Urine analysis
    - Electrolytes and creatinine
    - FBS
    - Lipid profile
    - ECG
  - Overweight patients are advised to lose weight
  - Gap between subsequent pregnancies should not be < 2 years or > 10 years
- Contraception
  - Low dose progesterone only pills
  - Puerperal tubal ligation → avoided especially in cases of severe hypertension because of
    - Anesthetic complications
    - Thromboembolic disorder
    - Pulmonary embolism.

Breastfeeding while on Antihypertensive Rx

- Allow breastfeeding postpartum
- Avoid diuretic therapy

- Following drugs have no adverse effects on baby:
  - Labetalol, nifedipine, enalapril, captopril, atenolol, metoprolol
- Insufficient evidence on safety of following antihypertensives:
  - ARBs, amlodipine and ACE inhibitors (except enalapril and captopril).

Future Pregnancy

Risk of Recurrence

- Transient hypertension recurs in 80–90% of cases
- Preeclampsia recurs in 25% of women
- Eclampsia recurs in 2% cases.

Women at High Risk of Preeclampsia

USG and uterine artery Doppler starting between 28 and 30 weeks (or at least 2 weeks before previous gestational age of onset if earlier than 28 weeks) and repeating 4 weeks later, is to be done in women with previous:
- Severe PE
- PE that needed birth before 34 weeks
- PE with a baby whose birth weight was < 10th centile
- IUD
- Placental abruption.

SUGGESTED READING

1. Aamer Imdad, Afshan Jabeen, Zulfiqar A Bhutta: Role of calcium supplementation during pregnancy in reducing risk of developing gestational hypertensive disorders: a meta-analysis of studies from developing countries. BMC Public Health. 2011;11(Suppl 3):S18.
2. Adriana Magalhaes Ribeiro Salles, Tais Freire Galvao, Marcus Tolentino Silva, Lucilia Casulari Domingues Motta, and Mauricio Gomes Pereira. Antioxidants for Preventing Preeclampsia: A Systematic Review. Scientific World Journal. 2012;2012:243-476.
3. Almundher Al-Maawali, Asnat Walfisch, Gideon Koren: Taking angiotensin-converting enzyme inhibitors during pregnancy. Is it safe? Canadian Family Physician. Vol 58: Jan 2012.
4. BCRCP obstetric guidelines for hypertension in pregnancy:June 2006.
5. Chronic hypertiesion in pregnancy: ACOG Feb 2012.
6. Emmanuel Bujold, Anne-Maude Morency, Stéphanie Roberge, et al. Acetylsalicylic acid for the prevention of preeclampsia and intra-uterine growth restriction in women with abnormal uterine artery Doppler: A systematic review and meta-analysis. J Obstet Gynaecol Can. 2009;31(9):818-26.
7. Eric M George, Joey P Granger: Endothelin: Key Mediator of Hypertension in Preeclampsia. Am J Hypertens. 2011;24(9):964-9.
8. G Justus Hofmeyr, Michael Belfort. Proteinuria as a predictor of complications of preeclampsia. BMC Medicine. 2009;7:11.
9. Gordon CS. Smith: Researching new methods of screening for adverse pregnancy Outcome: lessons from preeclampsia, PLoS med, July 2012, Med 9(7).
10. Hypertension in pregnancy: The management of hypertensive disorders during pregnancy: NICE Aug 2010.
11. Hypertension in pregnancy – Medical Management: Clinical Guidelines: OGCCU, King Edward Memorial Hospital, Perth Western Australia, Aug 2011.
12. Hypertensive disorders of pregnancy: Queensland Maternity and Neonatal Clinical Guideline. August 2010.
13. Hypertensive disorders of pregnancy: Queensland Maternity and Neonatal Clinical Guideline Supplement 2013.

14. Jacques WM Lenders: Pheochromocytoma and pregnancy: a deceptive connection. European Journal of Endocrinology. 2012;166:143-50.
15. Jeltsje S Cnossen, Karlijn C Vollebregt, Nynke de Vrieze, et al. Accuracy of mean arterial pressure and blood pressure measurements in predicting preeclampsia: systematic review and meta-analysis. BMJ, Online first, 30 March 2008.
16. Jeltsje S Cnossen, Rachel K Morris, Gerben ter Riet, et al: Use of uterine artery Doppler ultrasonography to predict preeclampsia and intrauterine growth restriction: a systematic review and bivariable meta-analysis. CMAJ. 2008;178(6):701-11.
17. Jennifer Uzan, Marie Carbonnel 1, Olivier Piconne, Roland Asmar, Jean-Marc Ayoubi. Preeclampsia: pathophysiology, diagnosis, and management. Vasc Health Risk Manag. 2011;7:467-74.
18. J Moodley. Potentially increasing rates of hypertension in women of childbearing age and during pregnancy – be prepared! Cardiovasc J Afr. 2011;22:330-4.
19. John CP. Kingdom and Sascha Drewlo: Is heparin a placental anticoagulant in high-risk pregnancies? Blood, 3 November 2011, Volume 118, Number 18.
20. Laura A Magee, Chris Cham, Elizabeth J Waterman, et al: Hydralazine for treatment of severe hypertension in pregnancy: meta-analysis. BMJ. 2003;327:955.
21. Laura A Magee, Edgardo Abalos, Peter von Dadelszen, et al: How to manage hypertension in pregnancy effectively. Br J Clin Pharmacol. 2011;72(3):394-401.
22. Laura A Magee, Michael Helewa, Jean-Marie Moutquin, et al. Treatment of the Hypertensive Disorders of Pregnancy. JOGC, Volume 30, Number 3, March 2008, S 24-36.
23. Laura A Magee, Michael Helewa, Jean-Marie Moutquin, et al:, Prediction, Prevention, and Prognosis of Preeclampsia. JOGC, Volume 30, Number 3, March 2008, S 16-23.
24. Laura A Magee, Michael Helewa, Jean-Marie Moutquin, et al: Diagnosis, evaluation and management of hypertensive disorders of pregnancy: JOGC, Volume 30, Number 3, March 2008, S 9-15.
25. Lawrence Leeman, Patricia Fontaine: Hypertensive Disorders of Pregnancy. American Family Physician. Volume 78, Number 1, July 1, 2008.
26. Lowe SA, Brown MA, Dekker G, Gatt, et al: Guidelines for the management of hypertensive disorders of pregnancy. Society of Obstetric Medicine of Australia and New Zealand 2008.
27. Michelle Hladunewich, S Ananth Karumanchi, Richard Lafayette: Pathophysiology of the Clinical Manifestations of Preeclampsia. Clin J Am Soc Nephrol. 2007;2:543-9.
28. Mosa'b Al-Balas, RPh Pina Bozzo R, Adrienne Einarson: Use of diuretics during pregnancy, Canadian Family Physician. Vol 55: Jan 2009.
29. Nelson Sass, Caroline Harumi Itamoto, Marina Pereira Silva, et al: Does sodium nitroprusside kill babies? A systematic review. Sao Paulo Med J. 2007;125(2):108-11.
30. RK Morris, RD Riley, M Doug, JJ Deeks, MD Kilby. Diagnostic accuracy of spot urinary protein and albumin to creatinine ratios for detection of significant proteinuria or adverse pregnancy outcome in patients with suspected preeclampsia: systematic review and meta-analysis. BMJ. 2012;345:e4342.
31. Shakila Thangaratinam, Arri Coomarasamy, Steve Sharp, et al:Tests for predicting complications of preeclampsia: A protocol for systematic reviews. BMC Pregnancy and Childbirth. 2008;8:38.
32. Stéphanie Roberge A Pia Villa D Kypros Nicolaides, et al: Early administration of low-dose aspirin for the prevention of preterm and term preeclampsia: A systematic review and meta-analysis. Fetal Diagn Ther 2012;31:141-6.
33. Thais Alquezar Facca, Gianna Mastroianni Kirsztajn, Nelson Sass. Preeclampsia (marker of chronic kidney disease): from genesis to future risks. J Bras Nefrol. 2012;34(1):87-93.
34. Tiina Podymow and Phyllis August: Update on the Use of Antihypertensive Drugs in Pregnancy, Hypertension. 2008;51:960-9.
35. Werner Rath, Prof. Dr. med.* 1 and Thorsten Fischer, Prof. The Diagnosis and Treatment of Hypertensive Disorders of Pregnancy. Dtsch Arztebl Int. 2009;106(45):733-8.
36. WHO recommendations for prevention and treatment of preeclampsia and eclampsia: WHO 2011.
37. Yves Gigue` re, Marc Charland, Emmanuel Bujold: Combining Biochemical and Ultrasonographic Markers in Predicting Preeclampsia: A Systematic Review. Clinical Chemistry. 2010;56:(3):361-74.

CHAPTER 10

Previous Cesarean Section

Tania G Singh

A 25 years old $G_2P_1L_1$, delivered 3 years back by emergency cesarean section (Indication: failure to progress in labor due to occipito posterior position). Pelvis was assessed and was adequate. Pregnancy had been uncomplicated and she had gone into spontaneous labor at 40 weeks 5 days. She had contractions for 24 hours and during this time, she underwent AROM and was given oxytocin infusion for 8 hours. Cervix became 6 cm dilated but had no further progress, despite regular strong contractions. Baby was well after emergency C.S., but the woman was readmitted to hospital after 7 days because of infected wound hematoma for which she required IV antibiotics. She now feels anxious that she might have to go through the same experiences again. At present she is 16 weeks gestation and has had a normal nuchal scan. Booking blood tests are normal.

1. **Would you like to assess pelvis in this patient again - when and how?**

    Pelvic assessment
    - In vertex presentation: Assessment is done at any time beyond 37th week but better at the beginning of labor as softening of tissues makes assessment better
    - Empty bladder
    - Dorsal position
    - Aseptic precautions
    - Sterilized gloved fingers once taken out should not be reintroduced.

    Sacral promontory
    - Attempt should be made to tip the sacral promontory
    - Try to establish the length of the diagonal conjugate
    - Method:
        - Fingers are to follow anterior sacral curvature
        - In normal pelvis, it is difficult to feel sacral promontory (or felt with difficulty)
        - To reach it, elbow and wrist are to be depressed sufficiently and fingers are mobilized in upward direction
        - Point at which bone receds from fingers is sacral promontory
        - Fingers are then mobilized under symphysis pubis and a marking is placed over gloved index finger by index finger of left hand
        - Internal fingers are removed
        - Distance between marking and tip of middle finger gives measurement of diagonal conjugate
        - Practically: If middle finger fails to reach promontory or touches it with difficulty → conjugate is adequate for average size head to pass through
    - If it is easily tipped, it should alert one to the possibility of a contracted pelvis.

Curvature of the sacral curve
- It is next assessed to see if it is flat or well curved
- A well curved sacrum allows for internal rotation of the fetal head.

Pelvic side walls
- Assessed next to see if they are parallel or convergent
- Normally not easily palpable.

Ischial spines
- Should next be palpated to see if they are prominent and sticking in (that is decreasing the space in mid pelvis)
- Normally these are everted.

Sacro-sciatic notch
- Sufficiently wide to place 2 fingers over sacro-spinous ligament covering the notch
- Gives information of the capacity of posterior segment and side walls of lower pelvis.

Posterior surface of symphysis pubis
- Smooth rounded curve
- Angulation/beaking → abnormal.

Pubic arch
- Normally rounded
- Should accommodate palmar aspect of 2 fingers
- Configuration more important than pubic angle.

Sub pubic angle
- Before the fingers are removed from the vagina, the sub-pubic angle is assessed to see if it is acute or obtuse.

Now take out your fingers

Inter Tuberous Diameter
- Having removed the fingers, the inter tuberous diameter is assessed to see if it accommodates more than four knuckles.

Conclusion

The most suitable pelvis for vaginal delivery is that of a gynaecoid type that has adequate dimensions. Features of a gynaecoid pelvis include:
- A wide diagonal conjugate
- A well curved sacrum
- Parallel side walls
- Ischial spines that are not prominent
- A wide sub-pubic angle and lastly
- A wide inter tuberous diameter.

2. **In this case, do you think there is some factor which may have weakened the scar?**

   Factors for weakening of scar

   Two most important factors playing a major role:
   I. Infection and
   II. Placental site in the index pregnancy
   - Patient had infected wound hematoma after previous section

- Cesarean section was done late in labor: lower segment was
  - Stretched
  - Thinned out
  - Friable
- Previous cesarean section requiring induction or augmentation of labor.
  Other factors of prime importance in impaired healing:
  - Imperfect apposition of cut margins
  - Pressure of sepsis
  - Pressure of hematoma in wound
  - Implantation of placenta over site of old scar (anterior placenta previa).

3. **Does the risk of rupture depends on site and type of previous uterine incision? Which is a better scar and why?**

Risk of rupture
- 4-9% → classical and T-shaped scar
- 1-7% → low vertical incision
- 0.2- 1.5% → low transverse incision.

Advantages of the lower segment over the upper segment incision:
- Less blood loss: due to less vascularity and the placental bed is away from the incision
- Easier to repair
- Though both upper and lower uterine segments heal by primary intention, forming a fibrous tissue that has 80% of the tensile strength of the surrounding tissue but lower segment being thinner, better coaptation of the edges is achieved and maintained
- Better healing as the lower segment is more 'at rest' than the upper segment in the postpartum period (however the lower segment also undergoes dramatic cellular atrophy and diminution in size)
- Where there has been prior classical cesarean section, the placenta is likely to be found implanted over the scar (i.e. on the anterior uterine wall) in approximately 40% of pregnancies, which might account for a higher rate of rupture of classical scars (2% in upper segment versus 0.2% in lower segment)
- Less subsequent adhesions to the bowel and omentum
- Less liability to acute gastric dilatation and paralytic ileus
- Less liability to peritonitis due to better peritonization and healing.

Indications of upper segment cesarean section
- Dense adhesions, extensive varicosity or myoma in the lower uterine segment making its exposure or incising through it difficult
- Impacted shoulder presentation
- Anterior placenta previa
- Defective scar in the upper segment
- Rapid delivery is indicated
- Previous successful repair of high vesico-vaginal or cervico-vaginal fistula
- Cancer cervix
- Post-mortem hysterectomy.

Incidence and types of hematoma after cesarean section
Incidence of hematoma → 2.4-5.6%
  a. Retrovesical hematoma
   - Common after lower segment operation
   - (May) cause pyrexia
   - Not much troublesome

b. Hematoma in abdominal incision
      - May cause dehiscence or infection
   c. Rectus sheath hematoma
      - Rare
      - May present with hypovolemic shock or consumptive coagulopathy → surgery.

4. **What is the success rate of planned vaginal birth after cesarean (VBAC)?**
   - 60-82%.

5. **What is the success rate of VBAC if patient has had a vaginal delivery before?**
   - 87-90%.

6. **Who should be offered VBAC?**

   VBAC can be offered to the following:
   - Gestational age: 37-40 weeks
   - Adequate pelvis
   - Previous C.S. for non-reassuring indication:
     - Breech
     - Fetal distress
     - Maternal hemorrhage
   - Prior lower segment cesarean section (transverse)
   - Vertex presentation
   - Patient's consent
   - Facility to carry out immediate LSCS.
     The hospital should have the following facilities:
     - Access to an emergency C.S.
     - Continuous intrapartum monitoring
     - Advanced neonatal resuscitation
     - On site blood transfusion
     - Staff experienced in advanced analgesic techniques
   - Women with 2 previous low transverse scars, who wish to attempt VBAC can also be considered if they had a vaginal delivery in the past
   - Blood transfusion facilities are available.

   Contraindications to VBAC
   - Previous classical or inverted T-shaped or J- shaped uterine incision
   - Previous uterine surgery (myomectomy) or prior low vertical incision
   - Previous extensive transfundal uterine surgery
   - Previous history of uterine rupture
   - Contracted pelvis
   - Medical or obstetric complications that precludes vaginal birth:
     - Placenta previa
     - Elderly patient
     - Long standing 2° infertility
     - Previous perinatal deaths
   - Two prior uterine scars with no vaginal delivery
   - Inability to perform emergency LSCS
   - Previous significant sepsis post cesarean section.

Predictors for VBAC success or failure
Increased chance of success:
- Maternal age < 40 years
- Adequate pelvis
- Prior vaginal delivery
- Prior VBAC
- Spontaneous labor
- Nonrecurrent indication
- Favorable cervix (Bishop's score > 6).

Reduced chances of success:
- Gestational age > 40 weeks
- Increased number of cesarean sections
- Estimated fetal weight > 4 kg
- Previous C.S. requiring induction/ augmentation of labor
- Previous postpartum wound infection
- Maternal obesity (BMI >30)
- Diabetes milletus
- Multiple gestation
- Induction of labor
- Recurring indication (CPD/failed 2nd stage)
- Short maternal stature
- Interval < 19 months after last delivery
- No previous VBAC
- Previous preterm C.S.
- No epidural anesthesia
- Advanced maternal age
- Female child.

Benefits of vaginal delivery over repeat cesarean section
- Shorter hospital stay
- Early ambulation and resumption to work
- Economical
- Less chance of bleeding
- No contamination of peritoneal cavity
- No pulmonary/wound complications
- Less infection
- Damage to internal organs and major vessels avoided
- Scar related remote complications are avoided:
  – Keloid
  – Hypertrophy
  – Incisional hernia
  – Adhesions
  – Scar endometriosis
- Successful VBAC → subsequent obstetric career improves.

7. **Why is it necessary to know placental location in a case of previous LSCS?**
   - Placental localization over the site of previous scar is one of the major causes making the scar weak resulting in uterine rupture

- If placenta is low lying and anterior → placenta accreta should be sought on USG with color Doppler
- Trial of labor → not indicated in these patients.

8. **What is the role of induction of labor in trial of VBAC?**
   - Induction of labor → not a contraindication but chances of success are less
   - Oxytocin safer than prostaglandins
   - Risk of uterine rupture ↑↑ when prostaglandins were followed by oxytocin (sequential use)
   - Misoprostol should NOT be used [even dinoprostone (E2) is not recommended] in 3rd trimester inductions in such cases.

9. **Does the technique of repeat cesarean different from standard lower segment operation?**
   Does not differ much:
   - Peritoneum → open as high as possible with great care because:
     - Bladder may be displaced upwards
     - Intestines may be adherent to original wound
   - Uterovesical pouch → much shallower than in fresh case and more adherent to uterus
   - Reflecting down bladder from lower segment
     - Be extra careful because it may be adherent
     - Safer to dissect this down by sharp dissection in proper plane than by blunt dissection.

10. **What are the risks of failed VBAC?**
    Risks
    - Uterine rupture with increased perinatal mortality
    - Hysterectomy
    - Operative injury
    - Postoperative infection
    - Need for blood transfusion
    - Hypoxic ischemic encephalopathy in newborn.

11. **What are the various risks for infant in a case of elective repeat cesarean section and trial of VBAC?**

    Elective repeat cesarean section
    - Transient tachypnea
    - RDS
    - Hyperbilirubinemia
    - Increased neonatal lacerations
    - Iatrogenic prematurity (if dates not reliable).

    VBAC
    - Cord blood gas pH < 7
    - 5′ apgar score < 7
    - Sepsis
    - Hypoxic ischemic encephalopathy.

12. **If a patient does not have any previous records available and uterine scar is not known, what will be the decision?**
    This is a case of *unknown scar*
    - Always elicit the history
    - Under which circumstances, cesarean section was done
    - Majority of unknown scars will be lower segment transverse incisions (92%)

- Trial of induction of labor is NOT contraindicated in patients with an unknown scar, unless there is a high clinical suspicion of a previous classical incision.

13. **If this patient wants to go for a trial of labor, how will you manage the case antenatally and intrapartum?**

    ### Antenatal management in women attempting trial of labor (TOL)
    1. It is a high risk pregnancy, requiring special ANCs
    2. Obtain records or information regarding previous cesarean, its indication, previous uterine scar
    3. Correct dating of pregnancy is essential, from
        - History
        - Clinical examination
        - USG
    4. Early detection of other obstetric (esp. placenta previa, PIH etc.) and medical complications (anemia etc).
    5. All routine investigations to be done
    6. If VBAC is to be considered, rule out the following:
        - Malpresentations
        - Multiple pregnancy
        - Macrosomia
    7. Ultrasound:
        - Fetal maturity especially when LMP is not certain
        - Fetal weight
        - Placental localization
        - Scar integrity assessment
    8. In 3rd trimester: at every visit, enquire about:
        - Fetal movements
        - Suprapubic pain
        - Palpate for scar tenderness
        - Vaginal bleeding
    9. For TOL → pelvic assessment at 37 weeks and again in early labor
    10. Proper counseling for risks and benefits
    11. Patients staying far → admit at 38 weeks
    12. Spontaneous labor has high success rates
    13. Trial of labor, should not be attempted if hemoglobin is ≤ 9 gm% or blood is not arranged (correction of anemia is very important)
    14. Induction of labor (IOL) → not a contraindication but the risks should be explained:
        - Risk of uterine rupture is increased 2-3 fold
        - Likelihood of repeat cesarean section with IOL -1.5 fold
        - Misoprostol should NOT be used in 3rd trimester for cervical ripening or labor induction in cases of previous LSCS
    15. Written and informed consent (all risks and benefits)
        Risks
        - Uterine rupture
        - Shock
        - Need for blood transfusion
        - Operative delivery →↑ chances of surgical injury
        - In adverse circumstances, hysterectomy

- Increased fetal morbidity and in few cases mortality
- Increased rate of admission to NICU
- Long separation of mother and baby
- Delayed resumption of breastfeeding
- Risk of postoperative infection
- Longer hospital stay.

Benefits
- Overall success rates are high
- Shorter hospital stay
- Less postpartum pain
- Less postpartum infections
- Fewer chances of blood transfusions
- Early initiation of breastfeeding
- Reduced chances of respiratory problems requiring admission to NICU
- Less chances of placenta previa accreta in subsequent pregnancy.

16. Proper counseling and consent for sterilization (if appropriate at that time).

Assessment of Scar Integrity

- TVS is better than TAS with a difference of < 1 mm in the intraobserver and interobserver variability
- A scar 'defect' or 'niche' is defined by the presence of a wedge-shaped cystic or hypoechogenic area within the myometrium of the LUS, at the site of a previous C.S
- Various studies have concluded that myometrial scar tissue takes at least 3 months to form and that complete involution and recovery of the zonal anatomy is not achieved until 6 months later
- In general,
    - There are three layers that can be identified in the LUS in pregnancy using B-mode 2D TVS:
        - The chorioamniotic membrane with the decidualized endometrium;
        - The middle muscular layer; and
        - The uterovesical fold (peritoneal reflection seen as a hyperechoic line juxtaposed with the muscularis and musosa of the bladder)
- Essentially, the uterine scar should be easily identified with TVS by applying the following approach:
    - Set the USG to 1st trimester routine setting or any gynecology settings
    - Obtain panoramic view of the lower segment, including the cervical canal up to the external os, where possible
    - Identify the scar (should occupy at least 75% of the image)
    - The sector width is set to full range, where the axis of the cervical canal can be demonstrated in relation to the lower segment and the uterine fundus
- The C.S scar should be well delineated as a hypoechoic indentation at the anterior wall of the LUS, measurable in three dimensions and lying between the uterovesical fold and the internal cervical os
    - In cases of previous elective C.S the scar will appear halfway between the uterovesical fold and the internal cervical os
    - In cases following emergency C.S → the scar could well be below, or at the level of the os
- Because of the heterogeneity of the various available studies, no ideal cut-off value can yet be recommended which can describe a strong or a weak scar.

MANAGEMENT IN LABOR

Delivery → always where facility for emergency cesarean section is present.

1st stage

1. Blood group and cross match
2. Patient kept NPO or on a liquid diet
3. IV line secured
4. Anesthetist and neonatologist kept informed
5. Monitoring done meticulously:
   - FHS
     - If facilities available → CTG
     - If not, intermittent auscultation or use of doppler
   - Partograph– for progress of labor (PR, BP, FHS, contractions and scar tenderness)
   - Oxytocin – can be used for augmentation but judiciously. Once good uterine contractions start, cervical dilatation should be minimum 1 cm/hour
   - Amniotomy can be performed once cervix is 3-4 cm dilated
   - Slow IV fluids started (avoid dehydration)
   - Epidural analgesia is not contraindicated in VBAC
   - Watch for symptoms and signs of scar dehiscence and impending rupture.

   SIGNS:
   - Non reassuring FHR pattern → 1st sign of uterine rupture
     - FETAL BRADY CARDIA → most consistent finding
     - Others – prolonged and variable decelerations
   - Scar tenderness (suprapubic pain and tenderness)
   - Unexplained tachycardia
   - Hypotension
   - Sudden onset of shortness of breath
   - Suprapubicbulge
   - Rarely, chest pain or shoulder tip pain.

   SYMPTOMS:
   - Suprapubic pain persisting in between contractions and aggravated during contractions
   - Slight fresh vaginal bleeding
   - Loss of station of presenting part
   - Changes in uterine contour
   - Bladder tenesmus
   - Development of in coordinate uterine action in active labor and complete cessation of contractions
   - There can be development of frank hematuria.
6. Scar dehiscence can be totally SILENT (detected at the time of cesarean section only)
7. Impending rupture → earliest finding is fetal distress.

2nd Stage

1. Should not be prolonged
2. Bladder should be emptied
3. Patient should be allowed to bear down on her own (NO FUNDAL PRESSURE)

4. Episiotomy to cut short 2nd stage
5. Vacuum and outlet forceps application is not a contraindication in VBAC, but used with caution.

3rd Stage
1. Exploration of the uterine scar is not warranted unless there is post partum hemorrhage which fails to settle with appropriate medication

14. **The previous delivery was a case of prolonged labor. What are the stages of normal labor?**
    Labor stages and durations should be thoroughly understood prior to making dysfunctional labor as an indication for cesarean section.
    Stages of normal labor
    1st stage
    - Begins with onset of true labor pains and ends with full dilatation of cervix
    - "Cervical stage"
    - Duration: 12 hours in a primi and 6 hours in multigravida.

    2nd stage
    - Defined as the interval between achieving full cervical dilatation and the birth of the baby
    - The optimal duration remains undefined, but a mean of 70 minutes, with 79% of women experiencing a 2nd stage of less than two hours has been reported
    - Duration: 2 hours in primigravida and 30 minutes in a multigravida
    - Subdivided into:
      - A passive phase (Propulsive phase)
        - Where the woman has no urge to push
        - The presenting part descends to below the ischial spines and the fetal head usually rotates to an occipito-anterior position
        - Can be affected by the use of analgesia, especially epidural, that may remove the urge to push
        - Directed pushing should be discouraged until the presenting part descends below the spines.
      - An active phase (Expulsive phase)
        - When the woman is bearing down during contractions
        - Associated with fetal acidosis and denervation injury to maternal perineal muscles and there are recommendations for this to be shortened
        - Active phase should not exceed an hour in primigravida and should be shorter in multiparous women.
    - Failure to progress in the 2nd stage may be due to:
      - Malposition of the fetal head
      - Ineffective uterine contractions → oxytocin infusion can help
      - Feto-pelvic disproportion.

      NOTE: The recent NICE guidelines for intrapartum care recommend that birth would be expected to take place within three hours of the start of the active second stage for primagravida, and two hours for multiparous women.

    3rd stage
    - Begins after expulsion of fetus and ends with expulsion of placenta and membranes (afterbirths)
    - Duration: 15 min in both primi and multigravida.

    4th stage
    - "Stage of observation" for atleast 2 hours, after expulsion of after births.

15. What is prolonged labor? Was it prolonged in this woman?

Prolonged labor: when combined duration of 1st and 2nd stage is more than arbitrary time limit of 18 hours

WHO: When cervical dilatation is < 1 cm/hr and descent of presenting part < 1 cm/hr for a period of minimum 4 hours observation

Causes	1st stage	2nd stage
Fault in Power	Abnormal uterine contraction (inertia etc.)	Uterine inertia Inability to bear down Epidural anesthesia Constriction ring
Fault in Passage	Contracted pelvis Cervical dystocia Pelvic tumour Full bladder	CPD/android/contracted pelvis Spasm or old scarring → undue resistance of pelvic floor Soft tissue pelvic tumour
Fault in Passenger	Malpresentation Malposition Congenital anamolies of fetus	Occipito posterior position Malpresentation Big baby Congenital anamolies

Yes, labor was prolongedin this woman.

16. What is prolonged latent phase?

- Normal duration
  - Primigravida – 8 hours and 4 hours in a multigravida
- Prolonged
  - Primis >20 hrs and in multis > 14 hrs
- There is sometimes a difficulty to determine time of onset of latent phase because of increased uterine activity (false labor) that occurs 3-4 days before onset of spontaneous (true) labor
- Latent phase is complete: when cervical dilatation reaches 4 cm with variable cervical effacement
- Causes:
  - Unripe cervix
  - Malpresentation/malposition
  - CPD
  - PROM.

17. What if latent phase is prolonged. Would you like to go for cesarean section?

Prolonged latent phase
- Per se is NOT an indication for cesarean section
- Worrisome to patient but does not endanger mother or fetus

Management
- Expectant Rx → rests and analgesics
- Augmentation → oxytocin or prostaglandins
- Amniotomy → usually avoided.

18. What is "protracted active phase"?

- When the rate of dilatation in a primi is <1.2 cm/hr and <1.5 cm /hr in multigravida
- Adequate contractions MUST BE present

- Minimum of 2 per vaginal examinations done 1 hr apart.

19. **When is the 1st and 2nd stage of labor said to be prolonged?**
    - Prolonged 1st stage → >12 hrs (in both primi and multigravida)
    - Dilatation <1 cm/hr in primigravida and <1.5 cm/hr in multigravida
    - Descent (of presenting part) <1 cm/hr in a primi and < 2 cm/hr in a multi
    - Diagnosis and further monitoring is done by partograph.

20. **What do you mean by failure of descent, protracted descent and arrest of descent?**
    Failure of descent
    - No descent (during 2nd stage)
    - Diagnosis: 2 vaginal examinations 1 hr apart during stage 2

    Protracted descent
    - < 1 cm/hr in primi and < 2 cm/hr in multigravida
    - Normally 3.3 cm/hr in primigravida and 6.6 cm/hr in a multigravida

    Arrest of descent
    - Cessation of descent for ≥ 1 hr in stage 2
    - Diagnosis: 2 pelvic exam 1 hr apart.

21. **What is secondary arrest (of cervical dilatation)?**
    - Cessation of dilatation for ≥2 hrs in active phase of labor with evidence of adequate contractions i.e. it commences normally
    - Most common cause : malposition or CPD.

22. **What is prolonged 2nd stage?**
    - Prolonged: >2 hr (P) and >1 hr(M)
    - Diagnosis:
        - Protraction
        - Moulding/caput
    - Protraction of descent: failure of head descent within 1 hr of full dilatation.

23. **What is precipitate labor?**
    - Dilatation and descent: > 5 cm/hr (P) and >10 cm/hr (M)
    - Definition: combined duration of 1st and 2nd stage is < 2 hrs.

24. **How will you diagnose prolonged labor?**
    - Find a cause (proper history)
    - Pelvic assessment at 37 weeks and at onset of labor
    - Leopold's maneuvers before and at onset of labor
    - In labor: on P/V exam., if finger is accommodated in between cervix and head during uterine contraction, pelvic adequacy can be reasonably established
    - Partograph (at 4 cm dilatation)
    - USG (to know the cause).

25. **What are the dangers of prolonged labor?**
    Fetal
    - Hypoxia (↓es uteroplacental circulation especially after rupture of membranes
    - Intrauterine infections
    - Intracranial stress or hemorrhage
    - Increased operative delivery
    - Variable and late decelerations on CTG (prolonged 2nd stage).

Maternal
- Distress
- PPH
- Trauma of genital tract
  - Concealed : undue stretching of perineal muscles
  - Revealed : cervical tear, rupture uterus
- Increased operative delivery
- Puerperal sepsis
- Subinvolution.

Management of prolonged labor
1. Try and find out the cause
2. Use of partograph
3. Selective and judicious augmentation
4. AROM (in active phase) → f/b oxytocin
5. Change in posture (other than supine)
6. Avoid dehydration
7. Adequate analgesia
8. If referred from outside - prompt correction of ketoacidosis by rapid IV RL
9. 1st stage delay:
   - Pelvic assessment
   - Fetal presentation/position/station
   - AROM followed by oxytocin
   - Pain relief
10. 2nd stage delay:
    - Short period of expectant management, provided FHR is reassuring
    - Assisted vaginal delivery or cesarean section
11. Secondary arrest:
    - (Esp. in multi) → very careful while using oxytocin
    - Cesarean section (if indicated).

Physiology of uterine contractions
- Named after Braxton –Hicks (1st described its entity during pregnancy)
- Starts very early in pregnancy and can be detected on bimanual examination
- P/A : uterus firm at one moment and soft at another
- Can be excited by rubbing the uterus
- Irregular, infrequent, spasmodic, painless w/o any effect on dilatation of cervix
- Patient not conscious of it
- Near term: frequent, ↑in intensity, some discomfort present
- Labor → contractions become painful
- Intrauterine pressure below 8 mmHg
- Physiology: during contraction → complete closure of uterine veins with partial occlusion of arteries in relation to intervillous space → stagnation of blood in space →↓ placental perfusion → transient fetal hypoxia → fetal bradycardia coinciding with contraction
- In abdominal pregnancy: Braxton- Hicks contractions not felt.

CESAREAN SECTION

The first modern Cesarean section, introducing the transverse incision, was performed by German gynecologist Ferdinand Adolf Kehrer in 1881.

Average Rate of Cesarean Section Worldwide

- Approximately 15%
- In India: 8-20%.

Types of Cesarean Section

According to Timing

- Elective cesarean section: Preplanned, which means it is indicated to do it
- Selective/Emergency cesarean section: The operation is done after onset of labor or may be before it, as an instant decision.

According to the Site of Uterine Incision

- Upper segment cesarean section (classical C.S.): The incision is given in the upper uterine segment and it is always vertical
- Lower segment cesarean section (LSCS): It is the commoner type. The incision is made in the lower uterine segment and may be transverse (the usual) or vertical in the following conditions:
  - Presence of lateral varicosities
  - Constriction ring to cut through it
  - Deeply engaged head.

According to the Number of Operations

- Primary cesarean section
- Repeat cesarean section.

According to the State of Peritoneal Cavity

- Transperitoneal: The usual type, where peritoneum is opened before incising the uterus
- Extraperitoneal: The peritoneal cavity is not opened and the lower uterine segment is reached either laterally or inferiorly by reflecting the peritoneum of the vesico-uterine pouch
  - Usually not done
  - Indication: e.g. chorioamnionitis (to avoid infection).

26. **Why do you think the incidence of cesarean section is increasing?**

   There are a number of reasons:
   - Delayed childbearing
   - Rising obesity rates
   - Increase in multiple birth deliveries due to increase number of patients approaching infertility clinics
   - Sharp decline for VBAC by women with previous cesarean sections
   - "Clinical impatience" - Longer labor times due to increase in number of induced labors
   - Many obstetricians themselves refuse to attempt a vaginal delivery in cases of previous cesarean sections
   - A very important role is being played by CTG – though hard to believe, many obstetricians lack thorough knowledge of CTG – over diagnosed cases of fetal distress and injudicious use of CTG machine should be avoided. Clinical knowledge and experience – is still the best today

- Breech presentation has become almost a permanent indication for cesarean section
- With better neonatal facilities, more preterm babies are being better delivered by cesarean section
- To avoid legal process for alleged neglect in vaginal delivery, obstetricians prefer cesarean section for even the smallest indication.

Indications for Cesarean Section

Cragin's famous phrase of 1916 'Once a cesarean always a cesarean' was coined because Cragin believed that the only indication for Cesarean section was pelvic contraction. But, if seen today, the scenario is entirely different.

Common Indications

- Failure to progress in labor
- Suspected fetal distress
- Previous classical (longitudinal) cesarean section
- Very low birth weight
- Fetal macrosomia
- Fetal malpresentation (e.g. breech, transverse lie)
- Placenta previa/accreta
- Placental abruption
- Multiple pregnancy
- Suspected fetopelvic disproportion
- Failed induction
- Failed instrumental delivery
- Cord prolapse
- Severe preeclampsia, HELLP syndrome or eclampsia
- Maternal infections (e.g. HIV, active Herpes simplex)
- Uterine rupture (previous or in index pregnancy)
- Previous IUD of the fetus (ante- or intrapartum)
- Mother's choice
- Improper use of electronic fetal monitoring.

Less Common Indications

- Fetal coagulation defects
- Lack of obstetric skill.

Anesthesia in Cesarean Section

Types of anesthesia that can be used in cesarean section:

Spinal Anesthesia

Anesthesia of choice (block required is till T4 level).

Benefits
- May reduce the need for systemic opioid administration postoperatively
- Mother remains conscious

- Simple technique
- Rapid onset
- Low failure rate
- Very less drug use
- Excellent muscle relaxation.

Drawbacks
- Inferior vena cava compression due to gravid uterus
- Decreased venous return
- Complete sympathetic block.

$\left.\right\}$ Hypotension (SBP ≤ 90-100 mmHg) →↓ cardiac output

Risks to Mother
- Unconsciousness
- Pulmonary aspiration
- Apnea
- Cardiac arrest.

Risks to Fetus
- Impaired placental perfusion leading to hypoxia
- Fetal acidosis → weak rooting and sucking reflexes → hampering early initiation of breastfeeding
- Neurological injury.

Prevention of Hypotension
- Infusion of IV fluids to increase blood volume before anesthesia
- Proper maternal position with the uterus displaced off the vena cava
- Administration of ephedrine → causes vasoconstriction in peripheral circulation and ↑ in heart rate
- Leg wrappings → minimizes venous pooling of blood in the legs.

Epidural

- Given during labor, can be extended in case of emergency C. section
- Mother remains conscious.

General Anesthesia

- Most common type that can lead to maternal mortality
- Other risks:
  - Failed endotracheal intubation
  - Failed ventilation
  - Aspiration pneumonitis
  - Dental trauma
  - Postoperative nausea and vomiting
  - Delayed breastfeeding and sedation of baby.

Techniques of Cesarean Section

Preoperative Preparation (In Any Type)

- Clinical assessment
- Routine blood tests

- Anesthetic assessment
- Oral intake restriction when cesarean section is anticipated
- Interventions to reduce the volume or acidity of stomach contents (Antacid and Antiemetic)
- Intravenous fluids (avoid excessive dextrose)
- Antibiotic prophylaxis
- Antiretroviral prophylaxis for HIV-positive women not yet receiving antiretroviral therapy
- Insertion of a urinary catheter
- Shave and prepare parts.

In the operating theatre
- Fetal lie
- Presentation
- Position and
- FHS are checked
- Indication for cesarean section – reviewed
- Regional analgesia (spinal or epidural)
- Prevention of spinal hypotension (supine position with a lateral tilt).

Types of Incisions and Various Techniques for Cesarean Section

Over the years, many variations in the technique of cesarean section have been developed.

Pfannenstiel

- Described by Pfannenstiel in 1900
- Located two fingers- breadth above the symphysis pubis
- Skin opened transversely with sharp dissection, the incision curving upwards (the "smile" incision/Pfannenstiel incision)
- Rectus sheath → opened transversely with sharp dissection and freed from the underlying rectus abdominis muscles
- Peritoneum → opened longitudinally with sharp dissection
- Uterus → opened with a transverse incision on lower segment
- Uterine incision → closed with two layers of continuous sutures
- Both peritoneal layers are closed with continuous sutures
- Rectus sheath → closed with continuous or interrupted sutures
- Skin → interrupted or continuous intracutaneous suture
- Difficulty in delivery of the fetus is minimal with Pfannenstiel incisions measuring at least 15 cm in length, the length of a standard Allis clamp - the 'Allis clamp test'.

The Pelosi-type Cesarean Section

- Skin → transverse with sharp dissection (Pfannenstiel incision)
- Subcutaneous layer and rectus sheath → electrocautery used to divide them transversely
- Rectus muscles are separated bluntly → both index fingers then inserted to free the fascia vertically and transversely
- Peritoneum → opened by blunt finger dissection → all layers of the abdominal wall are then stretched manually
- Bladder not reflected inferiorly

- Uterus → a small transverse incision on lower segment is made → extended laterally, curving upwards, bluntly with finger or sharp dissection with scissors
- Spontaneous delivery of placenta
- Uterine closure → with continuous locking suture in single layer
- Neither peritoneal layer is sutured
- Rectus sheath → closed with a continuous synthetic absorbable suture
- Subcutaneous layer → if thick, interrupted 3-0 absorbable sutures are used
- Skin is closed with staples.

Maylard Procedure

- Length of the incision is usually longer than the Pfannenstiel incision to allow greater access to the abdomen
- The rectus abdominus muscles → divided either sharply or by electrocautery
- Disadvantage:
  - There is decent amount of tissue damage
  - Underlying artery may be entered.

The Cherney Procedure

- Lower fascia is reflected exposing the tendinous attachment of the rectus abdominus muscle bodies to the fascia of the pubis
- The muscle is severed as low as possible
- Proximal and distal ends suture ligated
- One or both muscle attachments may be divided as required.

Mouchel Incision

- Similar to the Maylard incision but is lower than the latter
- It is a transverse incision
- Runs at the upper limit of the pubic hair
- In this, the muscles are divided above the openings of the inguinal canals.

The Joel-Cohen technique

- Skin → straight, transverse, sharp, ≈ 3 cm below the level of anterior superior iliac spine (higher than the Pfannenstiel incision) → 'Joel Cohen' abdominal incision
- Subcutaneous tissues → opened only in the middle 3 cm, then blunt along with rectus sheath
- Rectus sheath → fascia is incised transversely in the midline, then extended laterally with blunt finger dissection
- Rectus muscle → by finger dissection, muscles are separated vertically and laterally
- Peritoneum is opened bluntly
- All layers of the abdominal wall are stretched manually to the extent of the skin incision
- Bladder → reflected inferiorly
- Myometrium is incised transversely in the midline, then opened and extended laterally with finger dissection
- Uterus closed by interrupted sutures
- Peritoneum is not closed
- Rectus sheath closed by continuous sutures.

The Misgav-Ladach Technique

- A modification of the Joel-Cohen technique
- Developed by Stark and colleagues
- The Joel-Cohen abdominal incision is used, except that the fascia is opened blindly with slightly opened scissor-tips
- Uterus is opened as for the Joel-Cohen method
- Placenta is removed manually → uterus is exteriorized → myometrial incision is closed with a single-layer locking continuous suture → peritoneal layers are not sutured
- The fascia is sutured with a continuous suture → skin is closed with two or three mattress sutures. Between these sutures, the skin edges are approximated with Allis forceps, which are left in place for about five minutes while the drapes are being removed
- Advantages include:
  - Shorter operating time
  - Less use of suture material
  - Less intraoperative blood loss
  - Less postoperative pain
  - Less wound infection
  - Fewer adhesions at repeat surgery
- Classical Joel-Cohen incision is associated with less postoperative blood collection (than the modified incision) in the:
  - Abdominal wall
  - Pouch of Douglas
  - Lower uterine segment.

Modified Misgav - Ladach Technique

Different from original technique in the following ways:
1. Skin incision can be given as Pfannenstiel due to cosmetic reasons
2. Visceral peritoneum is not opened
3. Uterine closure can be in a single layer as in original one or can be closed with two continuous suture layers
4. Skin closure can be by subcutaneous suture or various skin closure methods.

Traditional Vertical (Midline and Paramedian)

- Skin, subcutaneous layer and rectus sheath opened by sharp vertical incision
- Rectus muscle opened by blunt or sharp dissection
- Peritoneum opened by sharp longitudinal incision
- Bladder reflected inferiorly
- Uterine incision → transverse in lower uterine segment, opened bluntly or by sharp dissection
- Closure of uterus can be in a single or double layer by either continuous or interlocking sutures
- Both layers of peritoneum closed by continuous sutures
- Rectus sheath → interrupted sutures
- Subcutaneous layer → interrupted sutures
- Skin closed by interrupted or continuous sutures.

Midline Vertical or Subumbilical Midline Incision

Advantage
- Requires very less time in entering the abdomen
- There is less bleeding
- Vertical midline incision may be extended upwards if more space is required for access
- May be used if a cesarean delivery is planned under local anesthesia.

Disadvantage
- Increased risk of postoperative wound dehiscence
- Increased chances of developing incisional hernia
- Scar is cosmetically less pleasing.

Paramedian incision

- Skin incision is made to one side of the midline (usually right)
- The anterior rectus sheath is opened under the skin incision
- Rectus abdominus muscle is then retracted laterally and the posterior rectus sheath and peritoneum are opened.

Advantage
- The stress on the scar is supposed to be less
- Stronger than the midline scar
- Cosmetically – the same.

Upper Segment Cesarean Section

- Abdominal incision → vertical
- Uterine incision: 10 cm vertical incision is made in the midline of upper uterine segment without incising the peritoneal coat separately as it is adherent in the upper segment
- Extraction of the fetus: as a breech in cephalic presentation
- The last layer of the uterine incision closure includes the superficial part of the myometrium with the peritoneal covering
- The remainder of the procedure is as lower segment cesarean section.

The Extraperitoneal Cesarean Section

- Historically the extraperitoneal approach was used in septic cases in an attempt to limit the spread of sepsis prior to the advent of effective antibiotics
- It is seldom used today.

Porro's Operation

- Cesarean section followed by removal of the uterus, ovaries, and oviducts.

Porro-Müller Operation

- Cesarean section in which the uterus is lifted from the abdominal cavity before the fetus is extracted.

Porro-Veit Operation

- Cesarean section by Porro's method, in which the stump is ligated and returned to its place.

Wound Drainage for Cesarean Section. Required?

- Though peritoneum heals extremely rapidly and reabsorbs blood, still some prefer to put sub-rectus sheath drains, or drains between the sheath and the skin (subcutaneous).

Advantages

- Removes the extra collections (blood and serous fluid)
- Irritation of the peritoneal lining of the abdomen can be minimized
- Reduces postoperative pain
- Blood can provide a medium for bacteria to culture
- Blood and fluid loss can be measured externally.

Disadvantages

- Blood clots in the abdominal cavity cannot be removed by a drain
- Quiet uncomfortable for the patient – carrying a suction bottle each time during ambulation is troublesome
- Pain while removing the drain
- Site of insertion on the skin can act as a nidus for infection.

Methods of Removal of Placenta after Cesarean Section

There are 3 main methods:
- Placental drainage with spontaneous delivery
  - The end of the umbilical cord is left unclamped → placental blood is drained and the placenta delivers spontaneously through the uterine incision
  - This method is not widely used.
- Cord traction
  - Involves gentle traction on the umbilical cord with external uterine massage after giving oxytocin
- Manual removal
  - Placenta is separated with a gentle sawing action from its implantation site
  - A quicker way to deliver the placenta than awaiting spontaneous separation
  - But it may cause more bleeding
  - Introduction of a possibly contaminated hand into the uterus may increase the risk of infection.

Is there any Role of Mechanical Dilatation of Cervix at Elective Cesarean Section?

- A mechanical dilatation of the cervix at cesarean section is defined as an artificial dilatation of the cervix performed by finger, sponge forceps or other instruments at non labor cesarean section
- Very few studies have been done on this issue
- There are both pros and cons of mechanical dilatation.

- Pros
  - Dilatation helps in the drainage of blood and lochia in the postpartum period avoiding collection of blood in the intrauterine cavity and distended uterus
  - Reduces intrauterine infection (postoperative endometritis)
  - Reduces the risk of PPH.
- Cons
  - Dilatation using sponge or finger may result in contamination by vaginal micro-organisms, increasing chances of infection
  - Risk of cervical trauma is increased.

Extra-abdominal versus Intra-abdominal Repair of the Uterine Incision at Cesarean Section

There are two schools of thought.

Exteriorization of the Uterus

- It is a boon when incision is not clearly seen and approached, which may lead to tearing of uterine angle leading to increased bleeding
- It is found easier to suture when it is exteriorized
- Bleeders and oozers can be visualized clearly
- Less blood loss
- Associated with a smaller reduction in postoperative hematocrit value.

The Other Side

- There can be increased nausea and vomiting with uterine traction especially when spinal or epidural anesthesia is given
- Hemodynamic instability
- Fallopian tubes can be traumatized easily
- Increased chances of infection
- There can at times be possible rupture of the utero-ovarian veins upon replacing the uterus and pulmonary embolism.

Complications of Cesarean Section

Operative

- Primary maternal mortality is 4 times that of vaginal delivery which may be due to:
  - Shock
  - Anesthetic complications particularly Mendelson's syndrome
  - Hemorrhage usually due to extension of the uterine incision to the uterine vessels, atony of the uterus or DIC
- Injuries to the bladder or ureter
- Transient tachypnea of the newborn is more common after cesarean section. Why?
  - Certain hormonal and physiological changes associated with labor are necessary for lung maturation in neonates
  - In elective cesarean sections, where the patient has not gone into labor at all, there is a lack of the physiological catecholamine surge and fluid retention in the lungs ('Wet lungs'), which would otherwise be removed by the pressure of contractions

- It is currently recommended that whenever possible, elective cesarean section should be deferred to 39 weeks
- Recent evidence indicates that lung epithelial sodium channels promote alveolar fluid drainage, which become active only during the process of labor
- Glucocorticoids appear to increase the number and function of sodium channels, as well as the responsiveness to catecholamines and thyroid hormones, providing a rationale for their exogenous administration in cases of elective cesarean section
- Though not routinely recommended at term, the author doesn't find any harm in giving corticosteroids which would otherwise save unnecessary NICU admissions, increasing the overall costs and delaying breastfeeding
- Fetal injuries (from either direct trauma to the baby, or secondary to there being a delay in the timing of birth with subsequent reduction in oxygen delivery)
    - The most common form of injury to the baby at the time of cesarean section is → laceration to the skin (incidence is 0.74% to 3.12% of all cesarean births)
    - Difficult cesarean birth may result in:
        - Fractures
        - Peripheral nerve damage
        - Spinal cord injury
        - Subdural hematoma.

Post-operative

Early:
- Thrombosis and pulmonary embolism
- Acute dilatation of the stomach and paralytic ileus
- Wound infection, puerperal sepsis and burst abdomen
- Chest infection.

Late:
- Rupture of the uterine scar
- Incisional hernia
- An increased risk of placenta previa, placental abruption and placenta accreta (in subsequent pregnancies).

Postoperative Care and Complications

- Strict monitoring of:
    - Vital signs
    - Urine output
    - Signs of uterine relaxation and hemorrhage
- Restricting oral intake for a minimum of 6 hours, though Cochrane does not support this (There was no evidence to justify a policy of withholding oral fluids after uncomplicated cesarean section as bowels are not usually exposed or handled during the operation, and one would therefore not expect bowel function to be disturbed)
- Early ambulation
- Skin-to skin contact with the baby and breastfeeding are encouraged.

Few Very Important Points Regarding the Post Operative Period Need a Special Mention

Fluid Management

- Total body water content in females = 50% of body wt.
- Total body fluid is mainly divided into 2 compartments
  - ICF: 2/3rd of body wt.
  - ECF: 1/3rd of bodywt.
    - Interstitial fluid (3/4th of ECF)
    - Plasma or intravascular vol. (1/4th of ECF)
- Transcellular fluid- includes synovial, peritoneal, pericardial, cerebrospinal and intraocular spaces (1-2 liters).

Electrolytes	ECF	ICF
Sodium	142	10
Potassium	4.3	150
Chloride	104	2.0
Bicarbonate	24	6.0
Calcium	5.0	0.01
Magnesium	3.0	40
Phosphate and sulphate	8.0	150

IV Fluids

- Daily fluid requirement = U.O. +700 mL
- 700 mL = insensible loss

Ringer's Lactate

- 1 lit of fluid supplies:
  - Na^+ 130 mEq
  - K^+ 4 mEq
  - Cl^- 109 mEq
  - Ca^{2+} 3 mEq
  - HCO_3 28 mEq
- Most physiological fluid
- As sodium concentration is high, it expands intravascular volume very effectively
- Useful in correction of metabolic acidosis.

Isotonic saline (0.9% NaCl-Normal saline)

- 1 lit. of fluid contains:
  - Na^+ 154 mEq
  - Cl^- 154 mEq

- Provides major EC electrolytes
- Increases intravascular volume substantially.

Dextrose Saline (DNS)

- 1 lit of fluid contains:
  - Glucose 50 gm
  - Na$^+$ 154 mEq
  - Cl$^-$ 154 mEq
- Has advantage of both 5% dextrose (to provide energy) and isotonic saline (to provide salt)
- Increases only ECF volume.

5% Dextrose

- 1 liter of fluid contains – glucose 50 gms
- Corrects dehydration and supplies energy
- After consumption of glucose, remaining water is distributed in all compartments proportionately
- Therefore, best agent to correct intracellular dehydration
- Selected when there is a need of water but not electrolytes.

Fluid and Electrolyte Therapy

- Standard "cookbook" approach for every patient should be avoided
- Post operative fluid administration is based on:
  - Estimated blood loss
  - Urine output
  - Vitals
- 24 hour maintenance therapy includes:
  - 1 liter of NS or RL (to provide for renal solute excretion)
  - 600-900 mL 5% dextrose (to replace insensible losses).

Normal Physiology Post Operatively

- Stress of surgery →↑ ADH + ↑aldosterone
  ↓
  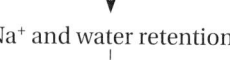
  ↓
  Weight gain (in 1st 24-48 hours)

- Kidney lacks the capacity for retention of potassium
- Kidneys will continue to excrete a min. of 30- 60 mEq/L of K$^+$ daily, irrespective of serum K$^+$ level and total body K$^+$ stores
- During 1st postoperative day, tissue damage and catabolism results in release of sufficient intracellular potassium but beyond that, supplementation is necessary.

Complications with Fluid and Electrolytes

- Most common fluid and electrolyte disorder- fluid overload
- Over enthusiastic excessive infusion of intraoperative fluid or blood transfusion or large volume of blood loss replaced exclusively with 3 times volume of crystalloid can cause volume excess
- Volume excess due to blood-pulmonary congestion

- Excessive saline- weight gain, periorbital puffiness
- Excess of hypotonic saline like 5% dextrose → hyponatremia → mental confusion, drowsiness
- **Oliguria**
  - Urine output < 0.5 mL/kg/h rather than U.O.< 30 mL/h
  - Reflects intravascular volume depletion
  - Dry tongue, ↓ skin turgor, sunken eyeballs, low volume pulse with tachycardia, postural hypotension and concentrated urine
  - Rapid infusion of 250 mL of NS or RL results in prompt ↑ in urine production
  - Diuretic therapy to be given in patient who has normal intravascular volume and ↓ output secondary to ↑ ADH or in a hypertensive patient who is diuretic dependent.

Hypokalemia

- Most common electrolyte abnormality
- Important causes:
  - Gastrointestinal loss (diarrhea, vomiting)
  - Prolonged administration of K^+ free fluids
  - Post operative infusion of diuretics
- Consequences:
  - Extreme weakness (muscular hypotonia)
  - Ileus
  - Arrhythmias (especially on digitalis therapy)
- Symptomatic hypokalemia occurs at serum levels < 2.5mEq/L.

Hyponatremia

- Mild hyponatremia –common observation
- Stress of surgery → ↑ADH + ↑aldosterone
  ↓
- ↓free water clearance with retention of water relative to sodium
- Patient drowsy, weak, confused or gets convulsions → always rule out hyponatremia
- Na^+<130 mEq /L → treated with water restriction and diuretics.

How to Calculate Rate of Fluid Infusion?

- 15 drops = 1 mL
- RULE OF TEN (24 HRS)
  - From fluid volume, how to calculate drop rate?
  - IV fluid in liter/24 hours x 10 = Drop rate/min
  - Drop rate/min ÷ 10 = IV fluid in liter/24 hours
- RULE OF FOUR (1 hour)
  - Volume in mL/hour ÷ 4 = drop rate/min
  - Drop rate/min × 4 = vol. in mL/hour.

Post operative Infections

Risk Factors

- Altered immunocompetence
- Obesity

- Absence of perioperative antibiotics
- Excessive intraoperative blood loss
- Prolonged operative time
- Low socioeconomic status
- Diabetes Milletus
- Poor nutrition
- Surgery in an infected operative site
- Poor surgical technique.

Fever

- All febrile morbidity is not infectious morbidity
- Definition:
  - Presence of temperature ≥ 100.4°F (38°C) on two occasions at least 4 hours apart during postoperative period, excluding first 24 hours

  OR
  - 2 consecutive temperature elevations > 101°F (38.3°C)
- In early postoperative period, it is often self-limited, resolves without therapy and is usually non-infectious in origin
- Overzealous evaluations of early postop. fever are time consuming, expensive and uncomfortable for the patient.

Non Operative Site Infections

UTI

- Incidence <4%
- Even a single dose of perioperative prophylactic antibiotic decreases the incidence of postop. UTI from 35% to 4%
- E. Coli – most common organism
- Others – klebsiella, proteus and enterobacter
- Catheterization of urinary tract → main cause of contamination
- Treatment- hydration and antibiotics.

Vascular

Phlebitis
- IV line to be inspected daily
- Catheter to be removed if, associated fever, pain, redness or induration or a palpable venous cord
- Incidence increases after 72 hours
- Therefore, should be changed every 3 days
- Usually resolves within 3-4 days
- Treatment -warm,moist compresses and removal of catheter from infected vein.

Respiratory

- Not a very common site for infection after cesarean section
- Basilar atelectasis → most common pulmonary complication

- Adversely affected by inhalational anesthetics
- Retention of pulmonary secretions → alveolar collapse → atelectasis → possibly pneumonia
- Early ambulation and aggressive management of atelectasis are most important preventive measures
- Pneumonia (rare) → may be hospital acquired caused by gram negative organisms.

Operative Site Infections

Wound complications

Factors that increase the likelihood:
- Systemic factors:
  - Obesity
  - Anemia
  - Infection
  - Malnutrition
    - Vitamin C –Maintains capillary wall integrity
    - Vitamin A- counteracts the effects of corticosteroids in wound healing
    - Vitamin B complex- permits effective cross-linking of collagen fibers required for progressive increase of tensile strength of healing incision
    - Iron supports O_2 transport and is a co-factor for collagen synthesis
    - Zinc, which can be quickly depleted by stress, small bowel fistula drainage and weight loss, is a co-factor for collagen formation and protein synthesis
  - Infection.
- Surgical factors:
  - Excessive use of cautery → results in thermal injury of normal tissue
  - Tissue trauma
  - Excessive suture tension → should be avoided
  - Suture to incision length ratio > 4
    - Ratio < 4 → 2.5 fold higher incidence of hernia.
- Post operative factors:
  - Abdominal distension
  - Vomiting
  - Coughing
  - Straining
  - Hematoma
  - Wound infection.

Physiology of Wound Healing

a. Inflammation
b. Epithelialization
c. Fibroplasia
d. Scar maturation.

Inflammation (3-5 days)

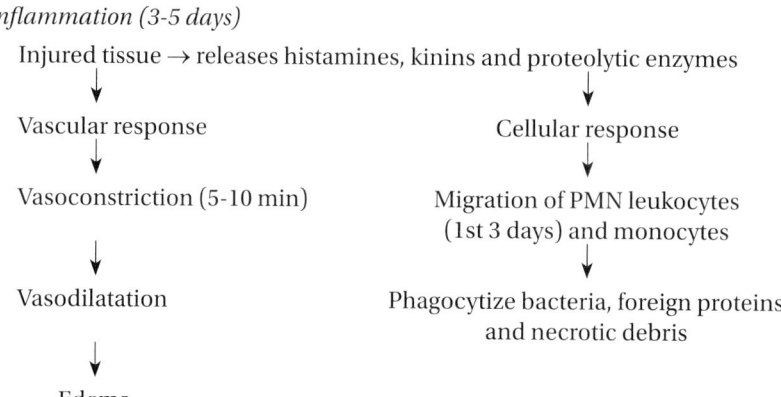

Proliferative Phase
- Wound defect fills with new connective tissue and gets covered with epithelium
- In wounds that have been closed primarily, minimal tissue synthesis is required
- In wounds that heal by secondary intention - granulation tissue appears
- Granulation tissue- composed primarily of capillaries, which explains its red color and propensity to bleed after minimal surface trauma.

Epithelialization

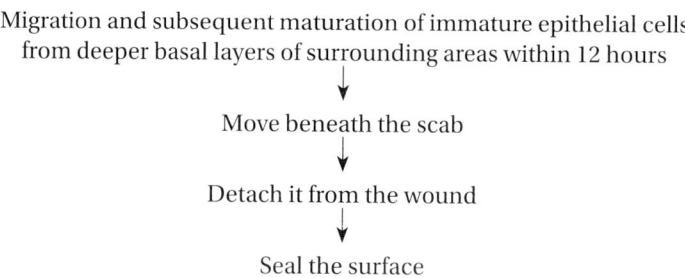

Total Duration → within 24 hours of injury.

Fibroplasia
- Process by which wound regains strength
- Results in production of collagen

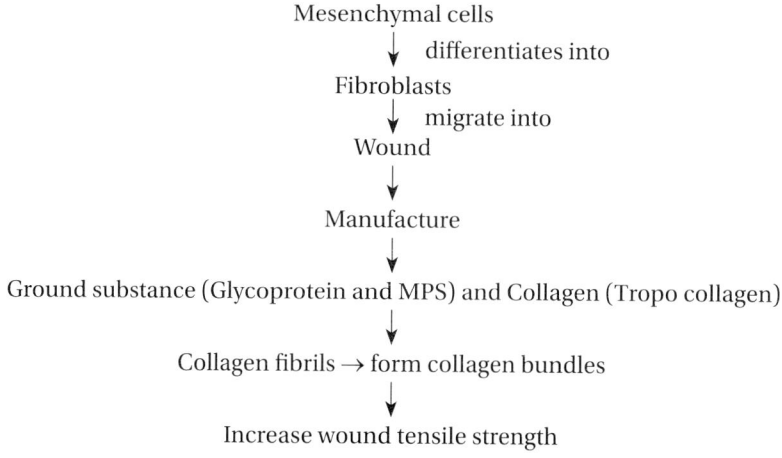

- Induration surrounding the incision reflecting accumulation of collagen is normally palpated on 6th through the 10th postoperative day
- Its absence indicates increased risk of superficial wound separation.

Scar Maturation
- Continues for up to 1 year or even longer
- Collagen maturation and remodelling occurs
- During this, break down of old disordered collagen slightly exceeds production of new organised collagen
- However, if collagen production exceeds breakdown, then keloid or hypertrophied scar results.

Post Operative Wound Complications

- Superficial wound separation:
  - Separation of skin and subcutaneous tissue
  - Fascia is intact
  - Consequence of:
    - Hematoma
    - Premature removal of skin clip
    - Excessive distracting forces on the wound edges
    - Infection
  - Studies reported that use of s/c sutures for wounds > 5 cm in depth decrease the occurrence of superficial separation.
- Dehiscence:
  - Separation of fascia with variable separation of superficial tissues
  - Sentinel WARNING sign → serosanguinous drainage from the wound after 1st postoperative day
  - Factors increasing the risk:
    - Wound infection
    - Obesity
    - Hypoproteinemia
    - Hypertension
    - Excessive tension on suture line
    - Sutures placed within 0.5 cm of cut fascial edge
    - Elderly
    - Pulmonary disease
    - Ascites
- Infection:
  - Most common complication
  - Diagnosis:
    - Erythema
    - Purulent drainage
    - Leucocytosis
    - Fever
  - Bacteriodes – most common anerobes that infect necrotic wounds
  - Pseudomonas and staph aureus – most common pathogens in absence of nonviable tissue
  - >10,000 organisms /gm of tissue are necessary for clinical diagnosis of wound infection.

Surgical Wound Healing

Depending on the manner of wound closure, 3 types of surgical wound healing are recognised:
- Primary intention:
  - Healing occurs by primary intention, if wound layers are reapproximated following injury
  - Healing occurs in a minute of time, with no separation of wound edges and with minimal scar formation.
- Secondary intention:
  - Surgical wounds when left unapproximated and allowed to close spontaneously
  - More complicated and prolonged than primary
  - Wound heals by combination of contraction and formation of granulation tissue
  - Slow and characterized by formation of excessive scar tissue.
- Third intention:
  - Also known as delayed primary closure
  - Refers to technique of wound closure after a period of delay
  - Often used after postop. wound breakdown or as an alternative to healing by secondary intention of wounds that should not be closed primarily (infected or contaminated).
  - Closure on or after 4th day is ideal
  - After 7-8 days → approximation is difficult
  - Between 3-6 days → lowest infection rates.

Bowel Obstruction

- Stomach remains atonic for 18-24 hours after surgery
- Small bowel exhibits return of normal peristaltic activity within hours of lower abdominal surgery
- Colon regains function, based on passage of flatus, ≈ 48 hours after abdominal surgery.

Paralytic Ileus

- Most patients experience some degree of ileus
- Exact mechanism- not known
- Associated with opening of peritoneal cavity and aggravated by manipulation of intestinal tract and prolonged surgical procedures
- Features: abdominal distension, absence of bowel sounds and flatus, abdominal tenderness, nausea, vomiting
- Abdominal radiography in flat (supine) position and in upright position – useful in diagnosis
- Most common finding- dilated loops of small and large bowel as well as air –fluid levels while the patient is in upright position
- Fluid and electrolyte replacement
- Treatment – nasogastric tube to evacuate stomach of its fluids and gaseous contents
- If no improvement within first 48-72 hours → other causes of ileus should be sought.

Adhesion Formation after Cesarean Section

- Adhesion - defined as abnormal fibrous connection between 2 anatomically different surfaces
- Adhesio genesis is a culmination of increased extracellular matrix (ECM) production associated with diminished matrix degradation, combined with decreased fibrinolytic activity

- Rate of adhesion formation after cesarean section:
  - 2nd cesarean section → 24-46%
  - 3rd cesarean section → 43-75%
  - 4th cesarean section → upto 83%
- Most common site after cesarean section → anterior cul-de-sac.

Pathology of Adhesion Formation

Normal process

Surgery → bleeding → leakage of lymphatic fluid from transected vessels with histamine release → tissue hypoxia

↓

Accumulation of RBCs and WBCs, platelets, clotting factors, growth factors and cytokines → coagulate → form a fibrin clot overlying the injured tissue

↓

Normal healing

For removing and stopping the further migration of above mentioned cells into fibrinous clot, the tissue plasminogen activator (tPA) system, which is present in the peritoneal mesothelium works → therefore no adhesions form.

How adhesions form?

In cases where there is increased tissue hypoxia → ↓ in tPA → ↓ fibrinolytic activity → ↑ production of nitrous oxide, superoxide and lipid peroxidation → fibrinous mass persists → fibroblast ingrowth occurs → deposition of ECM material including collagen → forming abnormal connections between tissue surfaces (which possibly become vascularized and innervated) to form adhesions.

Prevention of Adhesions after Cesarean Section

1. Good surgical technique:
   - Strict adherence to the basic surgical principles minimizing tissue trauma
   - Meticulous hemostasis
   - Minimization of ischemia and desiccation
   - Prevention of infection and foreign body retention
   - Peritoneal closure - much debate has occurred with inconclusive results. Review of the literature does not support the closure of peritoneum to prevent adhesions.
2. Antiadhesive barriers:
   The ideal adhesion barrier should meet the following criteria:
   - Achieves effective tissue separation
   - Has a long half-life within the peritoneal cavity so that it can remain active during the critical 7-day peritoneal healing period
   - Is absorbed or metabolized without initiating a marked proinflammatory tissue response
   - Remains active and effective in the presence of blood
   - Does not compromise wound healing
   - Does not promote bacterial growth.

Barriers
- Expanded Polytetrafluorethylene (Gore-Tex Surgical Membrane)
- Oxidized-regenerated cellulose (Interceed)
- Modified sodium hyaluronate/carboxymethyl cellulose (Seprafilm)

When selecting the most appropriate adhesion barrier, following things are taken into consideration:

1. Half-life of the barrier in the abdomen to ensure that it remains biologically active for at least 5 to 7 days
2. Its ability to be absorbed
3. The inert metabolic products that need to be excreted.

Literature does not support hydro floatation and use of NSAIDs for adhesion prevention after C.section.

SUGGESTED READING

1. AC Lim, MA Hegeman, MA Huisin T Veld. Cervical length measurement for the prediction of preterm birth in multiple pregnancies: a systematic review and bivariate meta-analysis, Ultrasound Obstet Gynecol 2011;38:10-7.
2. Agustina Mazzoni, Fernando Althabe1, Nancy H Liu, et al. Women's preference for cesarean section: a systematic review and meta-analysis of observational studies, BJOG. March 2011;118(4):391-9.
3. Anorlu RI, Maholwana B, Hofmeyr GJ. Methods of delivering the placenta at cesarean section (Review), The Cochrane Library 2008; Issue 3.
4. Awoniyi O Awonuga, Nicole M Fletcher, Ghassan M Saed, et al. Postoperative Adhesion Development Following Cesarean and Open Intra-Abdominal Gynecological Operations: A Review, Reproductive Sciences 2011;18(12):1166-85.
5. Caroline de costa. Vaginal birth after classical Cesarean section, Australian and New Zealand Journal of Obstetrics andGynaecology 2005;45:182-6.
6. Cesarean section for placenta praevia: Consent Advice 12, RCOG, Dec 2010.
7. Cesarean section: NICE clinical guideline 132, August 2012.
8. Classification of urgency of cesarean section – a continuum of risk: Royal College of Obstetricians and Gynaecologists, Good Practice No. 11, April 2010.
9. Dan Farine, Debra Shepherd. Classification of Cesarean Sections in Canada: The Modified Robson Criteria, J ObstetGynaecol Can 2012;34(10):976-9.
10. Daniel Robert Reilly. Cesarean Section on Maternal Request: How Clear Medical Evidence Fails to Produce Ethical Consensus, JOGC, Dec 2009.
11. Jacobs-Jokhan D, Hofmeyr GJ. Extra-abdominal versus intra-abdominal repair of the uterine incision at cesarean section (Review), The Cochrane Library 2011; Issue 2.
12. James Low. Cesarean Section—Past and Present, J Obstet Gynaecol Can 2009;31(12):1131-6.
13. Jon Barrett, Alan Bocking, et al. Management of Twin Pregnancies (Part 1), SOGC July 2000.
14. Julie van Schalkwyk, Nancy Van Eyk, et al. Antibiotic Prophylaxis in Obstetric Procedures, JOGC Sep 2010.
15. Mangesi L, Hofmeyr GJ. Early compared with delayed oral fluids and food after cesarean section (Review), The Cochrane Library 2009; Issue 1.
16. Maria Regina Torloni1, Ana Pilar Betran, Joao Paulo Souza, et al. Classifications for Cesarean Section: A Systematic Review, PLoS ONE Volume 6, Issue 1, January 2011.
17. National institutes of health consensus development conference statement: vaginal birth after caserean: new insights: NIHMar 2010.
18. O naji, Y abdallah, AJ bij de vaate, et al. Standardized approach for imaging and measuring Cesarean section scars using ultrasonography, Ultrasound Obstet Gynecol. 2012;39:252-9.
19. Rahim Ostovar, Arash Rashidian, Abolghasem Pourreza. Developing criteria for Cesarean Section using the RAND appropriateness method, BMC Pregnancy and Childbirth 2010;10:52.

20. Rebecca Kukla, Miriam Kuppermann, et al. Finding Autonomy in Birth, Bioethics. January 2009;23(1):1-8.
21. Vaginal birth after cesarean section (VBAC): Queensland Maternity and Neonatal Clinical Guideline, November 2009.
22. Vaginal Birth After Cesarean:New Insights, AHRQ Publication No. 10-E003March 2010.
23. Vaginal birth after previous caserean section: ACOG Aug 2010.
24. Víctor Hugo González-Quintero, Francisco E Cruz-Pachano. Preventing Adhesions in Obstetric and Gynecologic Surgical Procedures, Rev Obstet Gynecol. 2009;2(1):38-45.
25. Women with a previous Cesarean section: Clinical Guidelines: OGCCU, King Edward Memorial Hospital, Perth Western Australia, September 2010.

CHAPTER 11

Pain Abdomen during Pregnancy

Tania G Singh, Earl Jaspal

Step I → Establish whether the patient is pregnant or not
Pregnancy established
↓
Determine POG (because many conditions are more common at a particular period of gestation)
↓
Step II → Obtain a detailed history regarding pain:
- Time of onset (when and how did it occur last/gradual or sudden)
- Duration
- Intensity
- Character of the pain (dull aching, cramp like, sharp, stabbing)
- Localization (radiating/nonradiating)
- Association with meals (before or after meals or entirely unrelated to it)
- Did it awaken the patient from sleep
- Association with movement (any relief on lying down or on walking)
- Any associated symptoms (especially vaginal bleeding/show)
- Does anything make it worse.

Remember, few symptoms are experienced in normal pregnancy
- Nausea
- Vomiting
- Constipation
- Increased frequency of micturition
- Pelvic or abdominal discomfort.

Ask the patient to differentiate these normal pregnancy changes from the acute event for which she is present.

Before moving onto **STEP III** (physical examination), let us first be able to differentiate causes of pain in abdomen on the basis of symptoms
- Because the patient is pregnant, the first thing which always comes to our mind is pregnancy-related problems/complications
- And the search will further be simplified if we know which conditions occur in which trimester (though certain conditions are common to both 2nd and 3rd trimester).

OBSTETRIC CAUSES

Trimester	Presentation
Trimester I (Week 1-12)	
Implantation pain	• Low, period-like pain or cramps for a day or so early in pregnancy • This usually happens around the time the embryo is implanting itself in the endometrium.
Abortion	
Threatened abortion	• Pain abdomen/backache → mild pain/cramping • Vaginal bleeding → minimal / moderate
Inevitable abortion	• Pain abdomen- moderate/ severe • Vaginal bleeding – moderate → becomes severe at the time of expulsion
Incomplete abortion	• Vaginal bleeding – moderate/severe • Pain abdomen – moderate/severe • History of having passed products of conception but not complete.
Due to a growing hemorrhagic corpus luteum cyst	• Pain will be mild/moderate but once it ruptures, pain becomes acute.

Ectopic pregnancy	• Most common gestational age → 6–10 weeks
	• Classic triad of ectopic:
	  – Abdominal pain
	  – Vaginal bleeding Present in only
	  – Adnexal mass 45% of patients
	
	Note:
	  – 25–30% patients will not have vaginal bleeding
	  – 10% will have palpable adnexal mass
	  – ≈ 10% have negative pelvic examination
	  – Profuse vaginal bleeding is suggestive of incomplete abortion rather than ectopic
	  – Abdominal pain + vaginal bleeding → 39%
	  – Abdominal pain + vaginal bleeding + other risk factors → 54%

Unruptured	• Mild/moderate pain • Minimal vaginal bleeding.
Ruptured	• Acute pain • Mild/Moderate bleeding • Patient may appear pale, if large bleed present.
Trimester II (Week 13–28)	
Stretching of ligaments/Round ligament pain	• Due to stretching of ligaments as the uterus grows with time • Can be dull aching or may present as sharp pain on one side or on both sides • Pain is mostly felt while getting up from bed or may be on coughing or sudden change in positions • Any pain which disappears after resting → is of no consequence.
Abortion	• Mentioned above.
Molar pregnancy	• Pain usually occurs secondary to the enlarging uterus and ovarian theca lutein cysts late in 1st trimester or in 2nd trimester (though the classic appearance is not of pain).
Threatened preterm labor	• Pain can be dull aching/cramp-like or just a feeling of pelvic pressure or lower abdominal heaviness • May or may not be associated with vaginal leak.

Contd...

Contd...

Preterm labor	• Pain lower abdomen radiating to back and thighs • Increasing in frequency and duration • Associated with 'Show' • May be associated with leak per vaginum.
Acute polyhydramnios	• Extremely rare • Usually < 20 weeks period of gestation • Usually associated with uniovular twins or chorioangioma of placenta • Onset: acute and fluid accumulates within few days • Symptoms: abdominal pain, nausea, vomiting → acute abdomen.
Abdominal pregnancy	• Abdominal pregnancy, in which the fetus grows in the peritoneal cavity, occurs in about 1.0 of 10,000 pregnancies • It usually arises from intraperitoneal rupture of a tubal pregnancy • Rarely, the blastocyst implants on the liver or spleen • Common symptom → pain abdomen.
Trimester III (Week 29-40)	
Threatened/Established preterm labor	• Mentioned above.
Placental abruption	• May occur in 2nd trimester • Continuous pain • Associated dark colored bleeding (which sometimes may not be present in cases of concealed hemorrhage) in 78% of cases • Uterine contractions – 22% • Uterine tenderness and back pain - 66%.
False labor pains (Braxton Hicks)	• Mild discomfort/pain • Contractions: rhythmic, involuntary, spasmodic without cervical dilatation.
True labor pains	• Occurring at regular intervals • Intermittent, radiating to back and thighs • Increases in intensity and duration • "Show" present.
Uterine rupture	• Rare in pregnancy • Mainly occurs during labor • Severe abdominal pain • Vaginal bleeding • Patient may present in shock.
Severe preeclampsia/Impending eclampsia	• Epigastric or right upper quadrant pain • Nausea/vomiting • Blurring of vision • Headache.
HELLP syndrome	• Malaise (in 90% of cases) • Epigastric or right upper quadrant pain (90%) • Nausea and vomiting (50%) • Jaundice-rare.
Acute fatty liver of pregnancy	• Nausea, vomiting, anorexia, malaise • Mid-epigastric or right upper abdominal pain • Jaundice – characteristic (up to 5–15 mg/dL).

Medical/Surgical Causes

Acute cystitis	• Presence of the following without evidence of systemic infection: – Dysuria – Urgency – Frequency of urination • Suprapubic pain, pyuria, nocturia and hematuria can also be accompanied.
Acute pyelonephritis	• Occurs beyond 16 weeks • Usually bilateral, if unilateral, present more on right side • Lower urinary tract symptoms (e.g., frequency, urgency, dysuria) • Upper urinary tract symptoms (e.g., flank pain) • Constitutional symptoms (e.g., fever, chills, malaise) • Gastrointestinal symptoms (e.g., nausea, vomiting, anorexia, abdominal pain).
Acute cholecystitis	• History of previous episodes present • Most reliable symptom → acute (moderate/severe) epigastric or right upper quadrant pain which may radiate to the back • Pain lasts for a longer time • Vomiting occurs in ≈ 50% of cases • Fever only occasionally • Jaundice is rare • Cholecystitis can mimic appendicitis in the 3rd trimester.
Cholelithiasis/Biliary colic	• More common • Most gallstones are asymptomatic in pregnancy • Biliary colic → most common symptom • Location of pain: epigastrium or RUQ → radiating to back, shoulders and flanks • Nausea/vomiting accompanied • Pain can be spontaneous or elicited after a fatty meal • Fever- absent • Pain generally lasts < 3 hours (settles well with oral /injectable analgesics) • Jaundice is rare.
Acute pancreatitis	The presentation is similar to that in nonpregnant patients: • Occurs most commonly in 3rd trimester and postpartum • Acute abdominal (epigastric) pain - Observed in 75% of cases • Onset - Usually sudden • May radiate to back, shoulders and flanks • Nausea and vomiting - Usually present and may be severe, occurring after meals • Low-grade fever - May be present • Jaundice - Observed in a few patients • Most common cause- gallstones (in 70% of cases) • Mostly occurs in 3rd trimester due to increase in intra-abdominal pressure on biliary ducts.
Acute appendicitis	• Abdominal pain always present • Location of pain according to different trimesters – 1st trimester→ pain and tenderness located in the right lower quadrant – 2nd trimester→ appendix is located at the level of the umbilicus (periumbilical pain) – 3rd trimester → pain is diffuse or in the right upper quadrant • Other symptoms: – Nausea - Present in nearly all cases – Vomiting - Present in 2/3rd of pregnant patients – Anorexia - Present in only 1/3rd to 2/3rd of pregnant patients • Patients usually lie down, flex their hips, and draw their knees up, to reduce movements and to avoid worsening their pain • Fever and tachycardia - Variably present; they are not sensitive signs • Vomiting that precedes pain is suggestive of intestinal obstruction, and the diagnosis of appendicitis should be reconsidered.

Contd...

Contd...

Intestinal obstruction	• Rarely occurs during the 1st trimester
	• Occurs most commonly:
	  – In the 3rd trimester, due to mechanical effects of enlarged gravid uterus
	                      OR
	  – At term, due to descent of fetal head and sudden decrease in uterine size at delivery
	• Abdominal pain → in 90% of patients
	• Classical triad: abdominal pain, emesis and constipation
	• Description of pain:
	  – May be constant or periodic, mimicking labor
	  – Pain may radiate to the flank, imitating pyelonephritis
	  – Its severity may not reflect the severity of disease
	  – Small bowel obstruction is more painful than colonic obstruction
	• Vomiting → highly variable symptom. If the obstruction is more proximal (small intestine involvement), vomiting occurs earlier in the course
	• Severe obstruction can be present with no vomiting
	• Constipation is different from the usual constipation in pregnancy → Patients experience a complete cessation of stool and flatus
	• Bowel sounds are high-pitched and hypoactive in early intestinal obstruction and are absent in late obstruction.

Urolithiasis	• History of a prior episode - In 25% of patients • Pain, usually in the flank - Almost always the presenting complaint • Nausea and vomiting • Dysuria • Urgency • Fever • Gross hematuria • History of a prior episode - In 25% of patients • Usually occurs during 2nd and 3rd trimesters • May also present with lower abdominal pain radiating to the groin or labia.
Acute hydronephrosis	• Most common after 20th week of gestation; frequently asymptomatic • May mimic nephrolithiasis • Right or left flank pain may occur, which can be unremitting, extreme, and recurrent • Occasionally associated with nausea and vomiting.

GYNECOLOGICAL CAUSES

Rupture of ovarian cyst	• Occurs in 1 in 81 to 1 in 1000 cases of pregnancy • Rupture of ovarian cyst is rare • There may be a history of mild trauma (due to fall, intercourse, or a vaginal examination), but may occur spontaneously • The patient may have mild, chronic lower abdominal discomfort that suddenly intensifies.
Degenerating myoma	• Red degeneration occurs in 5–10% of pregnant women with myomas • Often occurs between 12 and 20 weeks' gestation • Acute onset • Significant, localized abdominal pain • Vomiting present • Low-grade fever may be present • Constipation.

Contd...

Contd...

Hemorrhagic ovarian cyst	• Localized abdominal pain • Nausea/vomiting • If rupture, patient may be in hypovolemic shock.

Adnexal torsion	• Occurs most frequently in the 1st trimester, occasionally in the 2nd, and rarely in the 3rd
	• Occurs more frequently on the right than on the left, with a ratio of 3:2
	• Variable presentations of pain:
	  – The lower abdominal pain is often sharp and sudden in onset and may last from several hours to days
	  – Intermittent pain may indicate detorsion or devitalization of sensory nerves
	• There may be a history of prior, intermittent episodes of similar pain
	• Nausea and vomiting – in 2/3rd cases
	• Fever - low-grade
	• Adnexal mass – present in 90% cases, tenderness present with adnexal torsion.

Step III → General physical examination

Why assessment of pain is more difficult in pregnancy?

ABDOMINAL EXAMINATION WILL HAVE THE FOLLOWING CHANGES DURING PREGNANCY

- Clinical presentation and natural history of many abdominal disorders are altered during pregnancy
- Findings may be less prominent than those in non-pregnant patients with the same disorder
- Uterine enlargement may hide classical signs
- Peritoneal signs are often absent in pregnancy, because of the lifting and stretching of the anterior abdominal wall
- The underlying inflammation has no direct contact with the parietal peritoneum, which precludes any muscular response or guarding that would otherwise be expected
- The uterus can also obstruct and inhibit the movement of the omentum to an area of inflammation, distorting the clinical picture
- To help distinguish extrauterine tenderness from uterine tenderness, performing the examination with the patient in the right or left decubitus position, thus displacing the gravid uterus to one side, may prove helpful
- When performing a physical examination of the gravid abdomen, it is essential to recall the changing positions of the intra-abdominal contents at different gestational ages. For example, the appendix is located at:
  – Mc Burney point in patients in early pregnancy and in nonpregnant patients
  – After the 1st trimester, the appendix is progressively displaced upward and laterally until, in late pregnancy, it is closer to the gallbladder
- Few possibilities must be borne in mind:
  – Intra-abdominal infection or inflammation can be associated with premature labor or fetal loss
  – Acute conditions such as appendicitis carry higher risks in pregnancy
  – Where assessment is difficult, surgeon must be consulted and risks of exploratory surgery must be balanced against the risks of delayed diagnosis.

OBSTETRIC CAUSES

Abortion	
Threatened abortion	• Vitals stable • Per-speculum: minimal bleeding/spotting through os present • Uterine size corresponds to period of gestation • Cervix uneffaced • Internal os closed.

Inevitable abortion	• Vitals stable
	• General condition proportionate to visible blood loss
	• P/S: bleeding through os present
	• P/V:
	  – Uterine size corresponds to period of gestation
	  – Uterus tender, firm
	  – Cervix → effaced
	  – Internal os open
	  – Products of conception → felt at os
	• Miscarriage unavoidable.

Incomplete abortion	• Vitals may be stable or patient is in hypovolemic shock
	• P/S: profuse bleeding through os present
	• P/V
	  – Uterine size < period of gestation
	  – Uterus tender, firm
	  – Cervix → effaced; internal os partly closed
	  – Products of conception felt at os
	• Most likely to occur in 2nd trimester.

Ectopic pregnancy	• Abdominal tenderness (97.3%) • Adnexal tenderness (98%) • Amenorrhea with vaginal spotting/bleeding (60–80%) • Tachycardia or orthostatic changes • Cervical motion tenderness → in 3/4th of patients but may be present prior to rupture • Uterine tenderness (from blood irritating the peritoneal surfaces) • A palpable mass • Rebound tenderness or peritoneal signs • Pallor • Abdominal distension • Enlarged uterus • Shock /collapse. Other, less commonly reported symptoms: • Breast tenderness • Gastrointestinal symptoms • Dizziness, fainting or syncope • Shoulder tip pain (secondary to diaphragmatic irritation) • Urinary symptoms • Passage of tissue • Rectal pressure or pain on defecation.

Contd...

Contd...

Molar pregnancy	• Though classical scenario is not of pain, but undue pressure and associated abdominal discomfort is seen in complete molar pregnancy
	• Other features which may be present:
	  – Vaginal bleeding in 80–90%
	  – Undue enlargement of uterus in ≈ 28%
	  – Anemia in ≈ 5%
	  – Preeclampsia (H. mole to be considered when preeclampsia develops in 1st and 2nd trimester) in 1%
	  – Hyperemesis (8%)
	  – Hyperthyroidism.

Threatened preterm labor	Per-abdomen: • Contractions present Per-speculum: • There may be copious, thin, greyish or curdy white discharge present (suggestive of infection) Per-vaginal examination: • Internal os closed.
False labor pains	• No associated cervical changes • "Show" – not present.
True labor (Term or preterm)	Per-vaginal examination: • "Show" present • Progressive cervical dilatation and effacement • Formation of bag of waters • Presenting part felt through os.
Severe preeclampsia/ Impending eclampsia	• Severe hypertension with proteinuria • Persistent neurological symptoms – Headache (occipital or frontal), restlessness, agitation, phosphene signals, tinnitus, and brisk, diffuse, polykinetic tendon reflexes • Visual disturbance- blurred vision, photophobia • Epigastric and/or RUQ tenderness • Nausea/vomiting • Oliguria • Sudden swelling of face, hands or feet • Signs of clonus (≥3 beats) • Pulmonary edema.

Uterine rupture	Signs:
	• Nonreassuring FHR pattern → 1st sign of uterine rupture
	• Fetal bradycardia → most consistent finding
	• Others → prolonged and variable decelerations
	  – Scar tenderness (suprapubic pain and tenderness)
	  – Unexplained tachycardia
	  – Hypotension
	  – Sudden onset of shortness of breath
	  – Suprapubic bulge
	  – Rarely, chest pain or shoulder tip pain

Contd...

Contd...

	Symptoms:
	• Suprapubic pain persisting in between contractions and aggravated during contractions
	• Slight fresh vaginal bleeding
	• Loss of station of presenting part
	• Changes in uterine contour
	• Bladder tenesmus
	• Development of incoordinate uterine action in active labor and complete cessation of contractions
	• There can be development of frank hematuria
	• Scar dehiscence can be totally silent (detected at the time of cesarean section only)
	• Impending rupture → earliest finding is fetal distress.
Placental abruption	• Fundal tenderness
	• High frequency of contractions or hypertonus - 34%
	• General condition: out of proportion to visible blood loss
	• High BP (found in 1/3rd cases)
	• Nonreassuring fetal heart rate - 60%
	• Intrauterine fetal demise - 15%
	• Head may be engaged
	• In advanced cases, shock, evidence of disseminated intravascular coagulation, or renal failure possible.
Acute polyhydramnios	• Ill patient
	• Absence of shock
	• Edema of legs or other associated features of preeclampsia present
	• Abdomen hugely enlarged > period of amenorrhea (wall tense, skin shiny)
	• Fluid thrill present
	• Fetal parts (not felt) and FHS - not audible
	• Internal examination: taking up of cervix or dilated cervix through which bulging membrane are felt.
Abdominal pregnancy	• Abdominal tenderness
	• Per-vaginal examination:
	– A closed uneffaced cervix
	– A palpable mass distinct from the uterus.

Medical/Surgical Causes

Acute cystitis	• Lower abdominal and/or supra-pubic tenderness.
Acute pyelonephritis	• Fever (temperature > 100.4°F [38.0°C])
	• Tachycardia
	• Hypotension
	• Costovertebral angle tenderness
	• Possible abdominal or suprapubic tenderness.

Contd...

Contd...

Cholelithiasis/Biliary colic	• Unremarkable, except for occasional upper quadrant tenderness • May not require hospitalization • Murphy sign may not be elicited Murphy sign: • Ask the patient to breathe in • Place your hand below right coastal margin in mid clavicular line (i.e. at ≈ location of gallbladder) • Patient is asked to take a deep breath • Positive: if there is sudden accentuation of pain during inspiration and inspiration is inhibited • During inspiration, inflamed gallbladder touches examiner's fingers → sudden cessation of inspiration.
Acute cholecystitis	• Rebound tenderness is rare • Cholecystitis can mimic appendicitis in the 3rd trimester • Hospitalization is definitely required • Murphy sign may not be elicited.
Acute pancreatitis	• Epigastric tenderness - Most reliable physical finding • Occasional rebound tenderness • Abdominal guarding • Abdominal distension • Bowel sounds - diminished (hypoactive).

Acute appendicitis	• Rebound tenderness - Present in 55–75% of cases
	• Abdominal muscle rigidity - Observed in 50–65% of patients
	• The Rovsing sign - observed as frequently in pregnant patients with appendicitis as in nonpregnant persons
	• Psoas irritation - Observed less frequently in pregnancy than it is in nonpregnant states
	• Rectal tenderness - Usually present, particularly in the 1st trimester
	Examination
	Palpation: 2 important things:
	  1. Hands warm
	  2. Fingers placed flat on abdominal wall. Forearm kept horizontal along the level of abdomen (if vertical, they will poke the abdominal wall).
	Hyperesthesia: if there is inflamed organ underneath → cutaneous hypersensitivity
	Method:
	• Gently pick up a fold of skin and lift it off the abdomen OR
	• Simply scratch the abdominal wall with finger
	  – Hyperesthesia in Sherren's triangle (formed by lines joining umbilicus, right ASIS & symphysis pubis) → Gangrenous appendicitis
	  – Hyperesthesia between 9th and 11th ribs posteriorly on right side (at s/o radiation of pain to back, typically below scapula) → Boar's sign → acute cholecystitis.
	Tenderness
	• Pointing test: ask patient to show site of pain
	• In acute cholecystitis:
	  – Just below the tip of 9th coastal cartilage on lateral margin of right rectus.
	• In acute appendicitis:
	  – Mc Burney's point → at junction of lateral 1/3rd and medial 2/3rd of right spino-umbilical line joining right anterior superior iliac spine (ASIS) and umbilicus

Contd...

Contd...

	• Appendicular tenderness: with pointing test, marks the most tender spot. Patient now turned to her left. Keep in this position for 1 min → viscera will shift to left exposing the appendix to direct palpation and abdominal wall also becomes relaxed in this position
	• If there is shifting of tenderness → there is uterine pathology.
	* Keep in mind – pyelitis and cystitis
	Rebound tenderness (Blumberg's sign or Release sign):
	• Suspected area palpated → with each expiration, hand on abdomen is gradually pressed down → now withdrawn suddenly and completely → abdominal musculature + parietal peritoneum (which is also inflamed because of underlying inflamed organ) springs back to its original place → very painful.
	Rovsing's sign: very important test
	• If left iliac fossa is pressed → pain in right iliac fossa → Acute appendicitis (because coils of ileum shift slightly to right and press on inflamed appendix).
	Muscular rigidity (muscle guard)
	• Voluntary: by patient, due to fear of being hurt
	• Involuntary: indicates underlying parietal peritonitis
	   – Gently move fingers all over the abdomen or use both hands, one above the other
	      - Hand (in contact with abdominal wall) → passive, only feels the abdominal musculature
	      - Hand (which is above) → give slight and steady pressure with it
	   – Muscle guard usually responds to area of tenderness
	• Appendicitis varies according to position of appendix
	   – If paracecal → rigidity over right iliac fossa
	   – Retrocecal → over loin
	   – Pelvic → no rigidity of abdominal wall
	• Obturator sign
	   – Present when the internal rotation of the thigh elicits pain (i.e., pelvic appendicitis)
	• Psoas sign
	   – Present when the extension of the right thigh elicits pain (i.e. retroperitoneal or retrocecal appendicitis).

Urolithiasis	• Patient extremely restless • Costovertebral angle tenderness - Almost always present • Abdominal tenderness (upper quadrant); tenderness in flanks - May be observed.
Intestinal obstruction	• Classic distended, tender abdomen with high-pitched bowel sounds is the exception in pregnancy • Abdominal tenderness may be absent • Pressure on the uterus often causes pain due to transmitted pressure to the bowel, misleading the clinician to consider a uterine process • Bowel sounds are often normal on presentation • A tender cystic mass can sometimes be palpated • Rebound tenderness, fever, and tachycardia occur late in the course.
Acute hydronephrosis	• Pyrexia • Loin tenderness on one or the other side.

GYNECOLOGICAL CAUSES

Rupture of ovarian cyst	• Occurs in 1 in 81 to 1 in 1000 cases of pregnancy
	• Rupture of ovarian cyst is rare
	• Lower abdomen may demonstrate peritoneal signs
	• Tenderness and guarding may be present
	• Peritonism may be present in lower abdomen and pelvis
	• Adnexal size → unremarkable due to collapsed cyst
	• Pelvic ultrasound:
	  – Complex mass appearance
	  – Fluid in the pouch of Douglas.

Adnexal torsion	Signs include: • Unilateral lower quadrant tenderness • A palpable tender adnexal mass in 90% of cases • Cervical motion tenderness OR • Rebound tenderness from peritonitis • Fever → low-grade.
Degenerating myoma	Features: • Tenderness and rigidity over tumour • Malaise or increased temperature • Dry or furred tongue • Rapid pulse • Constipation.

Step IV → Management
Before discussing the management, laparoscopic approach of surgery in a pregnant patient should be highlighted
- Initially, laparoscopic surgery in pregnancy was felt to be more dangerous and, in fact, was contraindicated due to the following reasons:
  - Injuring the pregnant uterus
  - Elevating the CO_2 level in the fetus
  - An increase in spontaneous abortion
  - The risk of preterm labor
  - Anesthetic complications
- These concerns have proven to be false as surgical skills have increased, more experience has been gained, and the envelope has continued to be pushed with ever more elegant instrumentation
- In fact, the laparoscope has made it possible to make a difficult diagnosis in pregnancy earlier, if one is comfortable with the use of this formidable tool.

Physiological Changes in Pregnancy

- The minute ventilation in pregnant women is 50% higher than that in nonpregnant women → this results in a marked decrease in carbon dioxide in the arterial concentration → resulting in mild respiratory alkalosis
- The fetus has a mild respiratory acidosis in the normal state that may facilitate the delivery of oxygen
- Many other physiological changes in pregnancy:
  - A normal mild anemia
  - Increased cardiac output

- Increased heart rate
- Increased oxygen consumption that allows the mother and fetus to be adequately oxygenated
- These changes are most remarkable, but must be considered when planning general anesthesia
- On the other side of the picture, there are certain hematological changes in pregnancy which increase the risk of venous thromboembolism:
  - Increase in fibrinogen
  - Increase in factor VII and factor XII
  - A decrease in antithrombin III
- When considering the acute abdomen in pregnancy, making the correct diagnosis is even more difficult:
  - Nausea and vomiting are common
  - Leukocytosis is the norm
  - Low-grade fever, mild hypotension, and anorexia are common
  - The gravid uterus pushes the abdominal contents cephalad → alters the various landmarks by displacing the organs and possibly inhibiting the migration of the omentum
  - The gravid uterus often causes a decrease in gastric motility and an increase in the risk of gastroesophageal reflux disease, including aspiration (Mendelson's syndrome), a life-threatening phenomenon.

Timing of Surgery

- If surgery is not that urgent, it would be prudent to wait until after the pregnancy is completed
- If surgery is deemed necessary during pregnancy, best time to perform it would be in the 2nd trimester, as the risk of preterm labor and delivery is lower in the 2nd trimester than in the 3rd, and the risk of spontaneous loss and risks due to medications such as anesthetic agents are lower in the 2nd trimester than in the 1st.

Laparoscopy during Pregnancy

- The Hasson technique, an open approach to entering the abdomen, has been suggested, to avoid potential injury to the gravid uterus with the Veress needle or trocar
- CO_2 insufflation of 10–15 mmHg is concerned safe
- Due to the CO_2 exchange in the peritoneal cavity and concerns over the effects of acidosis on the fetus, the use of capnography during laparoscopy in pregnant patients is recommended
- Advantages of laparoscopy over laparotomy include:
  - Shortened hospital stay
  - Less need for narcotics
  - Easier postoperative ambulation
  - Earlier postoperative tolerance of oral intake
- Care must be taken to minimize manipulation of the uterus
- Adjust the location of trocar based on uterine size
- Monitor fetal heart tones during the procedure
- The surgeon must work closely with the obstetrician to maintain fetal well-being during the surgical procedure
- An experienced laparoscopist is important to keep surgical times as short as possible
- Several studies have indicated, however, that laparoscopic surgery can be safely performed on pregnant patients during any trimester, without an appreciably increased risk to the mother or fetus

Note: Obstetric causes are discussed separately in individual chapters in detail (except preterm labor).

MEDICAL AND SURGICAL CAUSES

Acute Cystitis

- Relates to infection of the bladder, very often involving the urethra
- The major distinguishing feature of acute cystitis from asymptomatic bacteriuria is the presence of dysuria, urgency and frequency
- Most mothers may not be aware that they are having the infection because urgency and frequency are common symptoms in a normal pregnancy.

Why there is increased chances of UTI in females than in males?

Owing to the following factors:
- Short urethra
- Close proximity of external urethral meatus to areas (vulva or lower 1/3rd vagina) contaminated heavily with bacteria
- Catheterization
- Sexual intercourse
- Pregnancy:
  - Pregnancy increases the risk of UTI
  - At around 6th week of pregnancy, due to the physiological changes of pregnancy the ureters begin to dilate → this is also known as "hydronephrosis of pregnancy", which peaks at 22–26 weeks and continues to persist until delivery
  - Both progesterone and estrogen levels increase during pregnancy and these will lead to decreased ureteral and bladder tone
  - Increased plasma volume during pregnancy leads to decrease urine concentration and increased bladder volume
  - The combination of all these factors leads to urinary stasis and uretero-vesical reflux
  - Glycosuria in pregnancy is also another well-known factor which predisposes mothers to UTI.

Incidence
- 1%

Investigations
- Urine analysis:
  - Leukocyte esterase positive
  - Nitrite positive
  - Pyuria
  - Bacteriuria
  - Hematuria
- Urine culture and sensitivity:
  - Bacteriuria (a bacterial count of $> 10^2$ CFU/mL of urine in a symptomatic patient is diagnostic).

Management
- Oral antibiotics:
  - Nitrofurantoin 100 mg at bedtime x 10 days
  - Cephalexin 250 mg 2–4 times daily x 7–10 days
  - Fosfomycin 3 gm sachet stat
- Repeat urine culture 1–2 weeks after completing antibiotic therapy.

Acute Pyelonephritis

- Acute pyelonephritis is infection of the kidney and the pelvic ureter
- A serious systemic illness affecting 1–2% of all pregnancies and the most common non-obstetric cause of hospital admission during pregnancy
- Without treatment, it can cause preterm labor and maternal septicemia
- Recurrent pyelonephritis → a cause of IUGR and IUD
- Recurrence → ≈ 2–3% and it can recur during the same pregnancy.

Investigations

- Same as in acute cystitis
- Urine culture growing ≥ 10^5 colony-forming units/mL of urine.

Management

- Hospitalization
- Indications for admissions include:
  - Severe distress (septicemia)
  - Dehydration
  - Poor oral food tolerance
  - Maternal and fetal complications
  - Where intravenous antibiotic is necessary
- IV hydration
- Vitals charting (PR, BP, temperature, urine output)
- Antibiotics:
  - Ampicillin
  - Gentamycin
  - Cefazolin or ceftriaxone.

Cholelithiasis/Acute Cholecystitis

- Gallstones are present in > 95% of patients with acute cholecystitis
- Pregnancy promotes bile lithogenicity and sludge formation because estrogen increases cholesterol synthesis and progesterone impairs gallbladder motility
- But pregnancy does not increase its complications
- Acute cholecystitis:
  - It is a chemical inflammation usually caused by cystic duct obstruction and supersaturated bile
  - Not very common in pregnancy (1 to 8 cases/10000 pregnancies)
  - It is the 3rd most common nonobstetric surgical emergency during pregnancy.

Both the above conditions share almost the same management as gallstones are the most common cause of acute cholecystitis in pregnancy.

Investigations

- Blood tests → of limited value
  - Leukocytosis → observed in normal pregnancy
  - Serum alkaline phosphatase levels → normally elevated in pregnancy
  - Aspartate transferase and alanine transferase levels → may help to distinguish cholecystitis from hepatitis

- Serum amylase levels → elevated transiently in up to 1/3rd of patients
- A markedly elevated amylase level suggests pancreatitis
- Serum electrolyte evaluations → needed if vomiting has been persistent
- Ultrasonography → diagnostic and safe
  Features:
  - Markedly distended thick walled gallbladder
  - Sludge
  - Sonolucent layer of halo around gallbladder wall due to fluid acoustic shadowing from an immobile stone impacted at gallbladder neck
  - Positive **sonographic** Murphy sign.

Management

- Initial treatment:
  - IV fluids
  - Nasogastric suction – in case of ↑ vomiting
  - Analgesia - morphine may produce spasm of the sphincter of Oddi
  - Broad spectrum antibiotics - ampicillin, cephalosporins and clindamycin.

Surgery

- Indications:
  - If patient does not tolerate the above therapy
    OR
  - Has recurrent bouts
- Timing of surgery:
  - For acute cholecystitis it is controversial
  - Some promote performing surgery during pregnancy, while others prefer delaying it until the postpartum period.
- Approach:
  - Laparoscopic cholecystectomy
  - Can be safely performed at any time with intense fetal monitoring during the 1st and the 3rd trimester
  - Tocolysis may be required, when operating in the 3rd trimester.

Prognosis

- Complications can occur, including:
  - Empyema
  - Perforation
  - Pancreatitis
  - Failure to respond to medical management.
- If surgery is delayed, there is increased chances of:
  - Hospitalization
  - Spontaneous abortion
  - Preterm labor
  - Preterm delivery
  - Prematurity

- Low-birth weight
- Admission to NICU
- Maternal and fetal mortality is < 5% in case of acute cholecystitis.

Recurrence

- Symptomatic cholelithiasis during the 1st trimester has recurrence rate of 92%
- During the 2nd trimester, the recurrence rate is 64%
- During the 3rd trimester → 44%.

Acute Pancreatitis

- Whether pregnancy predisposes patients to pancreatitis is controversial
- Risk factors include the following:
  - Cholelithiasis - Most common risk factor in pregnant patients with pancreatitis, being observed in 90% of pregnancy-associated pancreatitis
  - Viral infections
  - Abdominal trauma
  - Hyperlipidemia
  - Hyperparathyroidism
  - Alcohol use
- Pancreatitis during the 1st trimester is associated with fetal wastage and during the 3rd trimester is associated with preterm labor.

Investigations

- Most useful markers:
  - Serum amylase (During normal pregnancy, however, amylase levels are slightly elevated), and
  - Lipase (lipase level is unchanged during pregnancy)
- Serum amylase can increase in conditions like intestinal perforation, infarction, intestinal obstruction but serum lipase and amylase-to-creatinine clearance ratio will be normal in them
- Ultrasound upper abdomen → helpful in confirming cholelithiasis and bile duct dilatation.

Management

- Usually mild in pregnancy
- Medical management remains the mainstay of treatment:
  - NPO
  - IV fluids for hypovolemia
  - Correction of electrolyte imbalances
  - Analgesia
  - Gastric acid suppression
  - Correction of glucose levels
  - Correction of calcium disturbances
  - Continuous nasogastric suctioning → with severe disease
- Total parenteral nutrition → in case if disease prolongs.

Surgery
- If gallbladder disease is causative, surgery can be performed when the patient's condition stabilizes.

Prognosis
- Acute symptoms last for ≈ a weak
- Maternal mortality rate ranges from 0-37%
- Perinatal mortality rate is ≈ ≤ 11% (risk increases with severity).

Intestinal Obstruction
- Acute intestinal obstruction is the 2nd most common nonobstetric abdominal emergency, with an incidence of 1 in 1500 pregnancies.

Causes
- Simple obstruction:
  - Most common type
  - Is most likely due to prior surgery and adhesions (cause 60-70% of small bowel obstruction during pregnancy)
- Volvulus:
  - Second most common
  - Predominantly due to adhesions
- Small intestinal and cecal or sigmoid volvulus may be present in the absence of prior adhesions owing to increased mobility of the bowel and its displacement into the upper abdomen by the growing uterus
- Intussusception → less common
- Incarcerated inguinal or femoral hernia and carcinoma → extremely rare.

Investigations
Radiography:
- Upright and supine films of the abdomen are the best initial study and are very essential for diagnosis
- Do not avoid diagnostic radiography out of concern for fetal effects
- Sequential films may be needed.

Laboratory tests:
- Leukocytosis - May be present (but is commonly observed in normal pregnancy)
- Electrolyte abnormalities
- Hemoconcentration
- Elevated serum amylase levels.

Management
- Decision should be very quick as the fetus and the intestine both are at risk
- Correction of fluid and electrolyte imbalances - Fluid management is critical during pregnancy because uterine blood flow depends on normal maternal blood volume
- Medical management is offered to patients with intermittent or partial obstruction

- Surgery is recommended for unremitting and complete intestinal obstruction:
  - Decompression of the bowel → nasogastric suction
  - Resection of nonviable tissue
  - A midline abdominal incision is optimal.

Prognosis

- Serious complication, with maternal mortality rates ranging from 5–15%
- Perinatal mortality rates range from 20–30%.

Appendicitis

General Overview

- Defined as an inflammation of the inner lining of the vermiform appendix that spreads to its other parts
- Most important factor contributing to appendicitis is the obstruction of the appendiceal lumen
- More common in the 2nd trimester
- Normally in pregnancy, appendix is displaced upwards and laterally, may reach right flank
- Severity of appendicitis may be increased in pregnancy
- Incidence of perforation is 25% in pregnancy, which increases to 66%, if surgery is delayed for > 24 hours.

Anatomy

- Wormlike extension of the cecum, therefore known as vermiform appendix
- Average length is 8–10 cm (ranging from 2–20 cm)
- Appears during the 5th month of gestation
- Supplied by appendicular artery, a terminal branch of the ileocolic artery
- Venous drainage is via the ileocolic veins and the right colic vein into the portal vein
- Generally has no fixed position
- Originates 1.7–2.5 cm below the terminal ileum
- Dorsomedial location is the most common.

Diagnosis

- Clinical examination – diagnostic
- Lab tests generally do not help.

Management

- Surgery (*Appendectomy*) → definitive treatment
- Laparoscopic appendectomy is the preferred method
- Intra-abdominal pressure 10–12 mmHg
- Tilt the operating table 30º to the patient's left to help bring the uterus away from the surgical site and to improve maternal venous return and cardiac output
- Even if the appendix appears normal, there are two reasons to remove it:
  - Early disease may be present despite its grossly normal appearance, and
  - Diagnostic confusion can be avoided if the condition recurs.

Prognosis

- Perforation and abscess formation are more likely to occur in pregnant patients with appendicitis
- The rate of generalized peritonitis relates directly to the interval of time from symptom onset to diagnosis
- Maternal and fetal morbidity and mortality rates increase once perforation occurs.

Urolithiasis

Investigations

- There may be coexisting UTI
- Microscopic hematuria → observed in 75% of cases, although the absence of hematuria does not exclude a stone
- Strain the patient's urine to help determine whether a stone is present
- USG (KUB) → to check for evidence of obstruction
- Remember the physiologic dilatation of the right side in the 2nd half of pregnancy.

Management

- Depends on the:
    - Size and location of the stone
    - Degree of obstruction
    - Severity of symptoms
    - Presence of infection
- Most stones pass with hydration
- Minimally invasive procedures can be considered, including:
    - Ureteral stent placement
    - Ureteroscopic retrieval
    - Percutaneous nephrostomy
- Extracorporeal shock-wave lithotripsy has not been approved for use in pregnancy.

Prognosis

- A good perinatal outcome is expected, unless a severe infection is present.

Acute Hydronephrosis

- Renal ultrasound: Dilated ureteral calyceal system may reveal severe hydronephrosis and hydroureters
- A positive leukocyte esterase test indicates pyuria, suggesting the presence of infection or a stone, as does a urine pH of 4.7 and 5.5 respectively
- Hematuria is present in 95% of patients of nephrolithiasis
- Urine culture and sensitivity: negative
- Presence of bacteriuria> 10^2 CFU/mL suggests a concomitant UTI.

GYNECOLOGICAL CAUSES

Adnexal Masses

- Incidence → 2%
- The pathology ranges from asymptomatic non-neoplastic ovarian cysts to the surgical emergencies like ovarian torsion, ruptured ovarian cyst, and tubo-ovarian abscess

- According to size:
  - About ½ of adnexal masses are < 5 cm in diameter
  - About ¼ are between 5 and 10 cm in diameter, and
  - About ¼ are > 10 cm in diameter
- 95% are unilateral
- Most common are non-neoplastic cysts, including the corpus luteum cyst and the follicle cyst, both of which usually involute by midterm
- Most adnexal masses are asymptomatic and are incidentally detected by sonography
- Even ovarian cancer is often asymptomatic
- Symptoms can include:
  - Vague abdominal pain
  - Abdominal distension
  - Urinary frequency
- Severe pain present in:
  - Torsion
  - Hemorrhage
  - Rupture
- 10–15% of adnexal masses undergo torsion
- The management of an ovarian mass during pregnancy is controversial
- Abdominal sonography is highly sensitive at mass detection but is insufficiently accurate at distinguishing malignant from benign lesions
- Asymptomatic ovarian masses with benign sonographic features are usually followed closely by serial sonography into the 2nd trimester, the optimal time for abdominal surgery in terms of maternal and fetal safety
- 1st trimester surgery is associated with fetal wastage, and 3rd trimester surgery is associated with premature labor
- Laparoscopy often suffices to extirpate the mass while preserving the pregnancy
- Patients with malignancy detected during late pregnancy are candidates for prompt cesarean section
- Prognosis depends on the histologic grade and pathologic stage of the cancer.

Ovarian Tumours

- Most common in pregnancy: Dermoids followed by cystadenoma
- Effect of tumour on pregnancy:
  - Impaction → retention of urine
  - Mechanical distress
  - Malpresentation
  - Non-engagement at term
  - Obstructive labor
- Effect of pregnancy on tumour:
  - Torsion of pedicle at
    - 8–10 weeks (tumour out of pelvis)
    - Early puerperium (lax abdominal wall)
  - Intracystic hemorrhage because of increased vascularity
  - Rupture (during labor)
  - Infection
  - Mechanical pressure (necrosis, infection)

- In early months:
  - Palpated separately from uterus
  - USG: cyst along the side of gravid uterus with its internal echoes
- Later months: (HINGORANI SIGN)
- Per-vaginal examination:
  - Head down Trendelenburg position
  - To elicit groove between 2 swellings (e.g. gravid uterus and ovarian tumour)
- Differential diagnosis:
  1. RV gravid uterus esp. when bladder is distended and painful → pass catheter and examine
  2. Hematocele in pouch of Douglas or peritubal (but margins are less discrete)
  3. Fibroids in pregnancy (when pedunculated)
  4. Double uterus
- Management:
  - Uncomplicated: operate between 14–18 weeks. Why?
    - Decreased risk of abortion
    - Assess to pedicle is easy
  - Beyond 35–36 weeks: cesarean section and removal of cyst at term OR in early puerperium
  - Complicated:
    - Removed irrespective of period of gestation
    - Puerperium: as early as possible
  - During labor:
    - Well above the presenting part → hope for vaginal delivery
    - Impacted in pelvis: cesarean section + removal of tumour.

Ovarian Cancer

- Malignancies, including germ cell tumours, low-grade ovarian cancers, and invasive epithelial ovarian cancers, comprise 3% of ovarian masses during pregnancy, for an incidence of 1 in 5000 pregnancies
- Most women with ovarian cancer present with stage I disease during pregnancy
- Rare → detected incidentally (likely to be early stage tumours)
- Germ cell tumours may cause endocrine dysfunction, especially virilization
- Management:
  - Germ cell and low malignant tumours → treated conservatively with unilateral oophorectomy or adnexectomy with staging
  - Invasive epithelial cancers → carry the worst prognosis
    - Optimal debulking surgery followed by chemotherapy
  - All chemo-agents are teratogenic in 1st trimester.

Rupture of Ovarian Cyst

Investigations

- Hemoglobin is reduced (depends upon the extent of bleed)
- Ultrasonography → to detect the presence of fluid in the cul-de-sac.

Management and Prognosis

- Surgical
- Conserve as much ovarian tissue as possible
- In the absence of malignancy, the prognosis is excellent.

Adnexal Torsion

- Unusual (1 in 1800 pregnancies)
- Pregnancy predisposes to it, with 1 in 5 adnexal torsions occurring during pregnancy because of the greater laxity of the tissue supporting the ovaries and oviducts during pregnancy.

Investigations

- Leukocytosis is common (though it is otherwise also common in pregnancy)
- Ultrasonography → to detect the presence of an ovarian cyst
- Color Doppler → absent ovarian flow in the central ovarian parenchyma
- If the diagnosis is uncertain, diagnostic laparoscopy can be used.

Management

- Surgical
- Preserve as much ovarian tissue as possible
- Adnexal torsion, diagnosed before tissue necrosis, is managed with adnexa-sparing laparoscopic detorsion, followed by progesterone therapy if the corpus luteum is removed
- If the tissue is necrotic or peritonitis has occurred, removal is warranted and unilateral salpingo-oophorectomy is appropriate
- Untwist the pedicle, remove the cyst, and stabilize the ovary
- If a partial torsion is confirmed, conservative management is appropriate.

Prognosis

- Generally good.

Degenerating Myoma/Painful Myoma Syndrome

- Leiomyomas tend to become smaller during pregnancy, and leiomyomas initially < 5 cm in diameter usually involute completely during pregnancy
- *Earlier months: fibroid diagnosed but pregnancy missed*
- *Later months: pregnancy diagnosed but fibroid missed*
- Large leiomyomas can undergo hemorrhagic infarction resulting in the painful myoma syndrome.

Investigations

- Ultrasonography (directly over the area of pain) and MRI are usually diagnostic
- A degenerating myoma has a mixed echodense or echolucent appearance.

Management

- Red degeneration → a self-limited process, therefore conservative management
- Infection has no role to play (Vascular in origin)
- Close monitoring of the patients
- Analgesia with narcotic or anti-inflammatory agents
- If narcotics are ineffective, a short course of indomethacin can provide effective pain relief
- Because indomethacin has fetal effects, including oligohydramnios and partial constriction of the fetal ductus arteriosus, its use is limited to less than 32–34 weeks.

Effects of Fibroid on Pregnancy

- Pregnancy wastage:
  - Recurrent pregnancy loss
  - Spontaneous abortion (especially with submucous fibroid)
    - Distort uterine cavity
    - Poor placentation, if implantation over fibroid
    - Increased uterine contractility
- Uterine incarceration:
  - If placenta posteriorly
  - If placenta of bigger size
- Abruptio (in retroplacental fibroids)
- Malpresentation (breech) → when situated in lower part of uterus below presenting part
- Dystocia → cervical fibroids or those very low in uterine wall
  - Anterior fibroids → good chances of being drawn up out of pelvis after onset of labor (give chance of vaginal delivery)
  - Posterior → get trapped within pelvis
- Premature rupture of membranes
- Uterine rupture (especially after prior myomectomy)
- More frequent cesarean delivery
- Uterine torsion
- Postpartum hemorrhage
- Puerperal sepsis.

Prognosis

- Good.

PRETERM LABOR

Definitions

Preterm Birth

- Birth at <37 completed weeks.

Moderately Preterm Birth

- Birth occurring between 32–37 completed weeks.

Late Preterm Birth

- Birth occurring between 34 and before 37 weeks.

Very Preterm Birth

- Birth at <32 completed weeks.

Early Term Birth

- Occurring between 37 and before 39 weeks.

Imminent Preterm Birth

- Defined as a high likelihood of birth, due to one or both of the following conditions:
  - Active labor with ≥4 cm of cervical dilatation, with or without PPROM
  - Planned preterm birth for fetal or maternal indications.

Risk Factors for Preterm Birth

- Past obstetric history:
  - Previous spontaneous preterm birth (recurrence rate 15–50%)
  - Previous 2nd trimester abortions
  - Use of ART
- Present pregnancy:
  - Antepartum hemorrhage
  - Rupture of membranes
  - Cervical/uterine factors:
    - Cervical insufficiency
    - Uterine anomalies (septate, unicornuate, bicornuate)
    - Fibroids
    - Excisional cervical treatment for CIN
- Fetal/intrauterine factors:
  - Multifetal gestation
  - IUFD
  - Fetal anomaly
  - Polyhydramnios
  - Maternal hypertension, diabetes, IUGR
- Infection:
  - Chorioamnionitis
  - Bacteriuria
  - Periodontal disease
  - Current bacterial vaginosis with a prior preterm birth
  - Gastroenteritis
- Demographic factors:
  - Low socioeconomic status
  - Low level of education
  - Ethnicity (black women)
  - Maternal age < 18 years or > 35 years
- Lifestyle issues:
  - Cigarette smoking
  - Illicit drug use, stress, physical abuse
  - Coitus late in pregnancy (seminal prostaglandins and female orgasm increase uterine contractions, also risk of infection is increased)
- Inadequate prenatal care, low pre-pregnancy weight and poor weight gain in pregnancy
- Iatrogenic:
  - Indicated preterm birth
  - Induction following calculation of wrong dates
- However, many women who deliver preterm do not have any known risk factors.

Pathophysiology of Preterm Labor

Physiological components of initiation of labor:

Ripening of the Cervix

Transformation of a long, firm and stiff structure into soft and easily dilatable structure
How does cervix become soft?

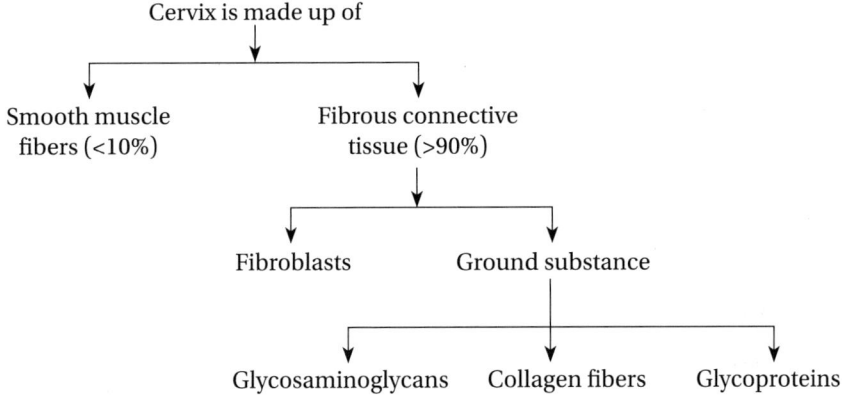

- Before pregnancy, all these elements are tightly aggregated, making cervix a harder structure
- At the end of pregnancy or at the initiation of labor:

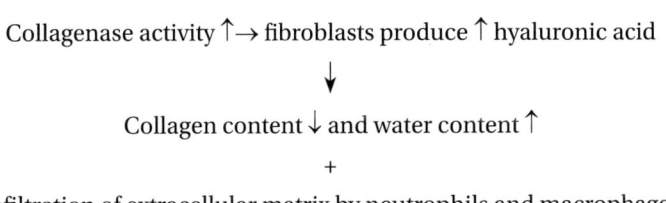

Infiltration of extracellular matrix by neutrophils and macrophages
↓
Production of cytokines, metalloproteinases and prostaglandins
↓
Cervical softening

Stimulation and Activation of Uterine Musculature

- Most of tensile strength of fetal membranes depends upon:
  - Concentration and cross-linkage of collagen
  - Presence of:
    - Elastin
    - Laminin
    - Fetal fibronectin in amnion
      - Cement for fusion of chorioamniotic membrane with decidua
      - This process completes after mid-pregnancy

- Membrane activation is caused by loss of tensile strength of amnion due to alterations in collagen concentration and function,
  - Produced in ↑ amounts in fibroblast layer of amnion in early pregnancy but synthesis decreases after 20 weeks
  - Biochemical marker:
    - Leakage of fetal fibronectin from uterine membrane into cervicovaginal secretions (between 22–37 weeks)
    - It is normally present in cervical and vaginal secretions before 22 weeks and after 37 weeks
    - If present at other times → predictive of preterm labor.

Activation of Fetal Membranes

- Inhibitors of uterine contractions:
  - Progesterone
  - Relaxin
  - Nitric oxide
  - Prostacyclin
- Stimulators of uterine contractions:
  - Estrogen
  - Increase in synthesis of gap junctions
  - Oxytocin
  - Prostaglandin receptors
  - Calcium channels
- Basic elements in uterine contractile system:
  - Actin
  - Myosin
  - ATP
  - Enzyme myosin light chain kinase (MLCK)
  - Calcium

Structural unit of myometrial cell → Myofibril

Contains proteins: Actin, Myosin

Intracellular calcium → calmodulin calcium → MLCK → undergoes phosphorylation → phosphorylated myosin → + Actin → Myometrial contraction

↓ in intracellular calcium → Dephosphorylation of myosin light chain → inactivation of MLCK → myometrial relaxation

Intracellular calcium levels are regulated by two mechanisms:
a. Influx across cell membrane
b. Release from intracellular storage sites (sarcoplasmic reticulum and mitochondria)

Two types of adrenergic receptors are present in uterine membrane:
1. Estrogen →+*alpha receptors →↓ cAMP →+ contraction → release of calcium
2. Progesterone →+ beta receptors →↑ cAMP →-** contraction → relaxation → storage of calcium

Activity of MLCK:
a. Is central to the process
b. Most pharmacological agents for stimulation or inhibition of contraction operate through metabolic pathways that lead to this enzyme.

---

*+ → stimulates
**- → Inhibits

Conditions Causing Premature Activation

- Maternal stress
- Unhealthy and/or morbid condition of the fetus
- Infection:
  - Acute chorioamnionitis
  - Subclinical chorioamnionitis
  - Fetal inflammatory response syndrome (FIRS).

These factors lead to premature initiation of the above mentioned cascade → Premature labor.

CERVICAL LENGTH AND PRETERM LABOR

USG Evaluation of Cervix

Which route?
- TAU
- TLU (translabial/transperineal)
- TVS → preferred

Why not TAU and TLU?

Transabdominal route:
- Full bladder is required to obtain a good image but it results in elongation of cervix by opposing the anterior and posterior lower uterine segments and concealing cervical shortening and masks funneling of internal os
- Fetal parts can obscure the cervix, especially after 20 weeks
- Distance from probe to cervix → degraded image quality (lower frequency transducers are required)
- Maternal obesity.

Translabial route:
- Patient lies on table with hips and knees flexed
- Gloved transducer in sagittal orientation on perineum between labia majora
- As accurate as transabdominal ultrasound in assessing cervical length
- It is more accurate than digital examination
- Should be reserved for only those cases, where TVS is either not acceptable or is unavailable
- Main drawback: gas in rectum can impede visualization of cervix especially external os.

Transvaginal route:
- Most accurate
- More reproducible
- Easier to obtain
- Correlates better with true cervical length.

Technique

- Empty bladder
- Transvaginal probe covered by condom
- Insert probe (in anterior fornix of vagina)
- Sagittal long-axis view obtained of endocervical canal, along its entire length

- Distance from surface of posterior lip to cervical canal should be equal to distance from surface of anterior lip to cervical canal
- There should be no increased echogenicity (suggestive of increased pressure)
- Enlarge image, so that cervix occupies at least 2/3rd of image
- Measure cervical length from internal to external os along endocervical canal
- Ideally, obtain three measurements and record the shortest best measurement in mms
- Apply transfundal pressure for 15 sec and record cervical length again.

Limitations and Pitfalls

- Full bladder → pressure on cervix → mask funneling or opening of internal os
- Too much pressure → mask funneling or opening of internal os and elongates the cervix
- Contraction → may mimic appearance of funneling of internal cervical os.

When to consider LUS contraction?
- When cervical length measures >50 mm
- Cervical canal assumes 'S'-shape
- LUS (either anteriorly or posteriorly or both) are thickened and asymmetric.

Underdeveloped LUS
- Often before 14 weeks, LUS is difficult to distinguish from endocervical canal because gestation sac has not reached a sufficient size to completely expand lower part of uterus. Therefore, measurement of true CL is very difficult before 14 weeks.

Digital Examination – Why Not to Use?

- It is subjective (interobserver variability of 52%)
- Not accurate for evaluating internal os (whole upper ½ of cervix is not measureable by this method) unless there is ≥ 2 cm of cervical dilatation and the entire intracervical canal is examined
- Non specific
- USG CL measurements, on an average, are 11 mm longer than manual estimations.

What to Measure?

1. Cervical length, and
2. Funneling.

Cervical Length (CL)

- From internal os to external os along the endocervical canal.

Observations:
- Short CL is usually straight
- Curved cervix → CL > 25 mm (reassuring finding)
- If AB is >5 mm, then cervical canal is to be measured in 2 steps or else measure as straight line
- Total CL: funnel length + functional CL
- Functional CL: sonographic CL (which we usually take) → if funneling is present, record its 'shape'.

Note: Refer to chapter '3' for diagrams.

Funneling

Four different shapes of funnel:
- "T" shaped
  - Closed normal cervix.
- "Y" shaped
  - Small funnel (<25%)
  - Cervical length ≥ 25 mm
  - May not be clinically significant.
- "V" shaped
  - More significant funnel
  - Closer to external os.
- "U" shaped
  - Funnel of most concern
  - Clinical situation in which more often the cervix can be dilated by manual examination
    - Minimum (< 25% funneling)
      - Common finding
      - Not associated with increase in preterm labor
    - Moderate (25-50%)
      - Almost always, CL is short (25 mm)
    - Severe (>50%)
      - Risk of preterm labor is increased if both short CL and funneling are present, rather short CL alone
- Normal CL:
  - A normal CL is 25-50 mm (lower 10 percent tile and upper 10 percent tile) at 14-30 weeks
- Short CL
  - < 25 mm at these gestational ages
- CL >50 mm is also normal but often reflects a measurement that includes LUS (especially before 16 weeks)
- Best time for measurement of or development of short cervix or funneling is 18-22 weeks. Why?

Between 10–14 Weeks

- Prediction of preterm birth is very low because most females destined to deliver preterm have cervical shortening usually detected ≥16 weeks
- LUS difficult to distinguish from true cervix (in late 1st and early 2nd trimester).

After 30 Weeks

- CL progressively shortens in preparation for term labor, so that CL< 25 mm (15-24 mm) after 30 weeks, can be physiologic and not associated with preterm birth
- In case of RPL- determine between 14-18 weeks (for early intervention)
- Best measure at 14-18 weeks followed by another measurement between 18-22 weeks
- Twins: CL ≤ 25 mm at 24 weeks gestation → best of all predictors of preterm birth in twins (various studies have shown and concluded)
- **Recent advances:** Almost no woman, even the most high risk, have a short CL in 1st trimester, therefore the pressure, the growing gestational sac exerts on cervix will be unlikely to open up even weakest of cervices.

Cervical Length Measurement in Women at Risk of Preterm Birth

Who Can Have a Short Cervix?

- Patients may have a short cervix after:
  - DES exposure in utero
  - Cervical conization
  - LEEP procedure
  - Intrauterine infection/inflammation
  - Decline in progesterone action
  - Idiopathic cervical insufficiency
- Cervical length remains almost constant until the 3rd trimester
- Ranges ≈ 34–38 mm between 24–28 weeks
- Measurement should always exclude funneling and be taken from funnel tip to external os
- Studies have shown that the range of cervical length declines in those who go on to preterm labor, variés from 0.5 mm/week to 8 mm/week.

How Frequently should the Cervical Length be Measured?

- The greatest velocity of cervical length decline mentioned in various studies is 5–8 mm/week
- Interventions should ideally be done when cervical length is 15–25 mm
- Schedule of the next cervical length measurement is estimated, depending on the following factors:
  - Previous history of the patient
  - Initial cervical length
  - Chosen threshold for intervention:
    - For example, if the measured cervical length is 36 mm and the threshold for intervention is 20 mm, then it is reasonable to wait for 2–2.5 weeks or even 3 weeks to reassess cervical length
    - Depending upon the initial cervical length, intervals can be shorter or longer
    - The shorter the interval of time between cervical measurements, the higher is the observational error.

Measures to be Taken to Avoid Preterm Labor

- Routine measurements in at risk women (Asymptomatic women at low risk should be avoided).

Gestational age < 24 weeks and cervical length < 25 mm
- Cervical cerclage preferably.

Gestational age >24 weeks
- Progesterone 100–200 mg daily vaginally
- Reduction of various day to day activities at work, travel, etc.
- Administration of corticosteroids
- Relocation near tertiary care center
- Adequate antenatal visits with ultrasonographic cervical assessments at regular intervals
- Watch for signs and symptoms of preterm labor.

In patients with membrane prolapse at or beyond the external os
- Emergency cerclage may be beneficial as compared to conservative management.

Recent Terminologies

History-indicated Cerclage

- Prophylactic cerclage inserted at 12–14 weeks in an asymptomatic woman on the basis of an indication provided in her history
- Indicated in women with ≥ 3 previous 2nd trimester losses or ≥3 preterm births.

Ultrasound-indicated Cerclage

- Therapeutic cerclage inserted on the basis of short cervical length obtained in ultrasonography, usually performed between 14–24 weeks
- Placed if the diagnosed ultrasound cervical length is ≤ 25 mm and period of gestation is not more than 24 weeks
- Funneling alone, is not an indication to apply this cerclage.

Rescue Cerclage

- Salvage cerclage, inserted in cases of premature cervical dilatation (detected either on ultrasound or on per-speculum examination) and/or with fetal membranes extending beyond the external os
- Cervical dilatation should not be >4 cm.

Transvaginal Cerclage (McDonald)

- A transvaginal purse-string suture placed at the cervicovaginal junction, without bladder mobilization.

High Transvaginal Cerclage (Shirodkar)

- A transvaginal purse-string suture placed following bladder mobilization, to allow insertion above the level of the cardinal ligaments.

Transabdominal Cerclage

- Cerclage at the cervicoisthmic junction placed via laparotomy
- Sole indication – previous failed transvaginal cerclage
- Can be inserted preconceptionally or in early pregnancy but there is increased maternal morbidity, so rarely performed.

Occlusion Cerclage

- Occlusion of the external os by placement of continuous non-absorbable suture in order to retain the mucus plug.

Contraindications to Cervical Cerclage Insertion

- Active preterm labor (≥ 4 cm cervical dilatation)
- Clinical evidence of chorioamnionitis
- Continuing vaginal bleeding
- PPROM

- Evidence of fetal compromise
- Gross congenital anomalies
- IUD.

Risks

- Bleeding during insertion
- Rupture of membranes
- Premature contractions
- Use of anesthesia during removal of cerclage inserted by Shirodkar's technique
- Bucket handle tear if labor sets in, with suture in place.

Recent Advances/Recommendations

- An ultrasound examination for cardiac activity and to rule out gross congenital anomalies, should be performed before placing cerclage
- Prophylactic perioperative tocolysis and antibiotics should be offered to women undergoing cervical cerclage, though not recommended in routine practice
- Higher (closer to internal os) the cerclage is sutured, the most effective is prevention of preterm birth
- Abstinence should not be routinely recommended
- Serial ultrasound monitoring of cervical length post-cerclage is useful for administration of steroids
- Progesterone is not routinely recommended after cerclage
- Usually removed at $36^{+1} - 37^{+0}$ weeks
- Removed at the time of operation in cases of elective cesarean section
- Removed earlier in cases of established preterm labor.

Is There a Role of Cervical Length Measurement Post-cerclage?

- Various studies have shown that cervical length significantly increases post-cerclage but the overall length does not seem to predict preterm birth
- There is some evidence that absent or short cervical length above the cerclage or the appearance of funneling to the level of the cerclage (at 24 to 28 weeks) increases the risk of preterm delivery
- Funneling down to the cerclage has a 50% risk of PPROM
- Progressive shortening may also indicate an increased risk of preterm birth.

How Far is Tocolysis Justified in Preterm Labor?

- There is no clear evidence that preterm labor can be stopped by the use of tocolysis therapy
- They can be considered in those:
  - Who are yet to complete a course of corticosteroids, OR
  - Who are in very preterm labor
  - To transfer the woman to a higher center with neonatal intensive care unit, OR
  - In women with suspected preterm labor who have had an otherwise uncomplicated pregnancy
  - Long-term use of tocolysis or use of multiple tocolytic drugs is not recommended, as it may lead to increase in both maternal and fetal adverse effects
  - There is insufficient data supporting the use of maintenance tocolytic therapy following threatened preterm labor

- Use of a tocolytic drug is not associated with a clear reduction in perinatal or neonatal morbidity or mortality
- Tocolysis is mainly helpful in reducing the number of women delivering within 48 hours up to 7 days
- Nifedipine and atosiban have comparable effectiveness in delaying birth for up to seven days. Compared with ritodrine, nifedipine is associated with improvement in neonatal outcome, although there are no long-term data
- Other uses of tocolysis – in management of intrapartum fetal distress, impaired fetal growth and to facilitate external cephalic version at term.

Drugs for Tocolysis

Beta Agonists (Mainly Ritodrine)

- Has predominantly β_2 receptor effects, relaxing the muscles in uterus, arterioles and bronchi
- Dose: Initially 50 mcg/min increased by 50 mcg every 10 minutes until a max. of 350 mcg/min for 48 hours
- Side effects:

Maternal:
- Tachycardia
- Palpitations
- Tremor
- Nausea or vomiting
- Headache
- Chest discomfort/pain
- Dyspnea
- Hypotension
- Hypokalemia
- Hyperglycemia
- Pulmonary edema though rare but a well-documented complication following aggressive intravenous hydration.

Fetal:
- Tachycardia
- Women are far more likely to stop treatment because of adverse effects
- Contraindicated in tachycardia sensitive maternal cardiac disease and poorly controlled diabetes mellitus.

Calcium Channel Blockers

- Most studies have compared nifedipine with ritodrine. Nifedipine has fewer side effects and there is less need to stop the treatment because of side effects
- Has advantages of oral administration and low cost
- Maternal side effects:
  - Flushing
  - Palpitations
  - Nausea
  - Vomiting
  - Hypotension
  - Dizziness

- Suppression of heart rate, contractility, and left ventricular systolic pressure when used with magnesium sulfate; elevation of hepatic transaminases
- Fetal:
  - No known adverse effects
- Contraindicated in hypotension and preload-dependent cardiac lesions like aortic insufficiency
- To be used with caution in multiple pregnancy and diabetes (because of the risk of pulmonary edema)
- Suggested dosage:
  - Initial 20 mg orally followed by 10–20 mg, three to four times/day and adjusted according to uterine activity for up to 48 hours
- Doses > 60 mg → associated with serious adverse effects (such as headache and hypotension)
- Are associated with very less neonatal RDS, necrotizing enterocolitis and intraventricular hemorrhage when compared to other tocolytic drugs
- Though it crosses the placenta, but long-term effects on child are uncertain.

Isoxsuprine

- Mechansm of action:
  - Peripheral vasodilation by a direct effect on vascular smooth muscle, primarily within skeletal muscle with little effect on cutaneous blood flow
  - Produces uterine relaxation through a direct effect on smooth muscles
- Absorption: from GIT
- Half-life: 1.25 hours
- Onset of action:
  - Oral → 1 hour
  - IV → 10 minutes
- Side effects to the fetus:
  - Crosses the placenta
  - Tachycardia
  - Hypoglycemia
  - Hypocalcemia
  - Ileus
  - Hypotension in the neonate
  - Toxicity is related directly to neonatal blood concentrations of isoxsuprine, which are affected by both gestational age and the interval between administration of isoxsuprine and delivery
- Contraindications:
  - Cardiac disorders
  - Hyperthyroidism
  - Chorioamnionitis
  - Antepartum hemorrhage
  - Intrauterine fetal death
  - Eclampsia and severe preeclampsia
  - Pulmonary hypertension
- Dosage:
  - Oral → 10–20 mg bid/tid
  - IM → 5–10 mg injection 2–3 times/day
  - IV →
    - Infusion is prepared by dilution of the injection in an appropriate quantity of 5% dextrose injection
    - Do not dilute in 0.9% sodium chloride because of the risk of pulmonary edema.

Atosiban

- Oxytocin receptor agonist
- Nausea (main), vomiting, headache, chest pain, dyspnea. Injection site reaction is a documented side effect, making women stop treatment with atosiban
- Diabetes and cardiac disease are not contraindications
- Atosiban when used in women at very early gestations (<26 weeks) may lead to fetal vasopressin receptor blockade, leading to changes in amniotic fluid volume, with resultant alterations to fetal renal and lung development
- Suggested dosage → a three-step procedure:
  - An initial bolus dose of 6.75 mg over 1 minute, followed by
  - An infusion of 18 mg/hour for 3 hours, then
  - 6 mg/hour for up to 45 hours (to a maximum of 330 mg).

Indomethacin

- Indomethacin is a prostaglandin inhibitor that acts by competing with arachidonic acid for cyclooxygenase (COX)
- Prostaglandins are important in the onset and maintenance of labor
  - By enhancing myometrial gap junctions and stimulating calcium intracellular influx as well as its release from the sarcoplasmic reticulum, prostaglandins result in activation of myosin light-chain kinase and muscular contraction
  - Prostaglandin levels increase in the plasma and amniotic fluid of women in labor, and prostaglandin metabolites have also been shown to be higher in women who deliver preterm
- Maternal serum level of prostaglandin $F_{2\alpha}$ metabolite decreases when treated with indomethacin
- Target site of action of indomethacin → cervix and the fetal membranes
- Oral and rectal routes are commonly used
- *Loading Dose:*
  - Rectal suppository: Loading dose of either 50 mg or 100 mg
  - Oral: loading dose of 50 mg
- *Maintenance dose*:
  - Oral route: either 25 mg or 50 mg every 4 to 6 hours for 24 to 48 hours
  - Rectal: 50 mg indomethacin every 6 hours
- Peak maternal plasma concentrations are achieved within 2 hours of initiation of treatment, although rectal administration achieves a peak level somewhat faster than oral administration
- Metabolism:
  - Primarily by the liver, but ~10–20% is excreted unchanged in the urine
- Half-life:
  - In premature infants is at least double (63 hours) that in adult
  - The immature liver accounts for the prolonged half-life in the fetus
- Maternal side effects:
  - Nausea
  - Vomiting
  - Esophageal reflux
  - Gastritis
- Fetal side effects:
  - COX inhibitors cross the placenta → lead to an increased risk of constriction or premature closure of ductus arteriosus, with consequent
    - Pulmonary hypertension
    - Oligohydramnios

- Persistent PDA
- Necrotizing enterocolitis
- Intraventricular hemorrhage
- There is less need to discontinue treatment because of side effects
- Contraindicated in:
  - Platelet dysfunction or bleeding disorder
  - Hepatic dysfunction
  - Gastrointestinal ulcerative disease
  - Renal dysfunction
  - Asthma (in women with hypersensitivity to aspirin).

Rofecoxib

- It has a significant but reversible effect on fetal renal function and the ductus arteriosus but does not decrease the risk of preterm labor before 32 weeks of gestation and increases the risk after treatment is withdrawn at 32 weeks of gestation.

Magnesium Sulfate

- Not very helpful as a tocolytic
- However, according to recent evidence, administration of magnesium sulfate to women at risk of preterm birth before 32 weeks gestation, reduces the severity and risk of cerebral palsy (for this duration of administration, the risk of neonatal depression is very less) when administered for 24 hours.
- Long-term exposure is associated with significant increase in neonatal depression and in fetal, neonatal and infant death
- Contraindicated in myasthenia gravis
- Side effects:
  - Flushing, diaphoresis, nausea, loss of deep tendon reflexes, respiratory depression, and cardiac arrest
  - Suppresses heart rate, contractility and left ventricular systolic pressure when used with calcium channel blockers
  - Produces neuromuscular blockade when used with calcium-channel blockers.

Nitroglycerin

- A nitric oxide donor
- Smooth muscle relaxant
- 10 mg patch releases drug @ 10 mg in 24 hour
- Applied on anterior abdominal wall
- Headache → main and most important side effect.

Terbutaline (Beta Mimetic)

Dose:
- Initially 5 mcg/min for 20 minutes, increasing by 2.5 mcg/min at 20 min intervals until contractions stop, to a maximum of 20 mcg/min
- Followed by 5 mg tds orally for 48 hours.

Contraindications to Tocolysis

Absolute

- Intrauterine fetal demise
- Severe preeclampsia/eclampsia
- Severe anemia
- Advanced cervical dilatation
- Known lethal congenital or chromosomal malformation
- Placental abruption
- Intrauterine infection (chorioamnionitis)
- PPROM (in absence of maternal infection, consider tocolysis only in case of maternal transport or antenatal steroids administration)
- Evidence of fetal compromise or placental insufficiency.

Relative

- Mild hemorrhage due to placenta previa
- Non-reassuring CTG
- IUGR
- Multiple pregnancy.

Corticosteroids in Preterm Labor

- A single course of corticosteroids is recommended for pregnant women between 24^{+0} and 34^{+6} weeks of gestation who are at risk of preterm delivery within 7 days. *Recent evidence suggests the administration of single repeat course of corticosteroids after 7 days who still remain at risk of preterm birth before 34 completed weeks*
- *Benefits*
  Significantly reduces the rates of:
  - Neonatal death
  - RDS
  - Intraventricular hemorrhage
  - Necrotizing enterocolitis
  - Respiratory support
  - Admission to NICU
  - Systemic infections in first 48 hours of life.

An overview and Explanation

- Various studies from Cochrane data have shown that antenatal corticosteroids reduce neonatal death even when infants are born < 24 h after the first dose has been given
- Another study has confirmed that incomplete courses of antenatal corticosteroids are beneficial
- The exact time interval for steroids to become beneficial is unknown
- There is a potential benefit commencing within hours of the first dose
- Safe for the mother but with no additional benefits to the mother
- Antenatal corticosteroids are most effective in reducing RDS up to 7 days after administration of second dose
- Steroids are contraindicated in maternal systemic infections including tuberculosis

- Doses:
  - Betamethasone is the steroid of choice, when available, to be given in a course of two doses of 12 mg administered intramuscularly 24 hr apart
  - An alternative regimen would be four doses of 6 mg dexamethasone intramuscularly every 12 hr
- Both regimens are found to be equally effective for the prevention of RDS
- Two studies have indicated a decreased risk of cystic periventricular leukomalacia (PVL) in premature infants exposed to betamethasone, this association was not found with dexamethasone, particularly when using multiple doses
- A recent study has found that betamethasone is associated with a greater reduction in the risk of death than dexamethasone
- A course of betamethasone is still indicated in patients receiving treatment with hydrocortisone for other causes, because very little hydrocortisone crosses the placenta
- Non-randomized studies in humans suggest that multiple courses of steroids could lead to:
  - Harmful effects on myelination of the fetal brain
  - Reduction in birthweight or effects on brain growth through to adulthood
  - Neurodevelopmental problems in childhood behavior
  - Effects on the hypothalamo-pituitary-adrenal axis with a spectrum from hyperactivity in young life to hypoactivity in adult life.

Recent Advances

- Bed rest and hydration have not been shown to be effective for the prevention of preterm birth and should not be routinely recommended
- The positive predictive value of a positive fetal fibronectin test result or a short cervix alone is poor and should not be used exclusively to direct management in the setting of acute symptoms.

Magnesium Sulfate and Neuroprotection in Preterm Births

Two major complications of CNS occurring in preterm infants are:
- Intraventricular hemorrhage, and
- White matter injury.

Severe Intraventricular Hemorrhage

- Grades 3 and 4 can reliably be detected by ultrasound and occur primarily among babies ≤ 28 weeks' gestation with highest incidence at 24 to 25 weeks.

White Matter Injury

- Peak prevalence at 28 weeks
- MRI is gold standard
- Its severity is associated with adverse motor and cognitive outcomes.

Clinically, the most frequent adverse neurological outcomes associated with preterm birth are cerebral palsy and cognitive impairment. Other adverse outcomes include blindness, deafness, developmental delay, and/or other neurological impairment, learning or motor disabilities.

Cerebral Palsy

- It is a symptom complex of non-progressive motor impairment syndromes secondary to brain injury or anomalies arising in early development
- Can reliably be diagnosed at 2 years of age
- Typical signs:
  - Spasticity
  - Movement disorders
  - Muscle weakness
  - Ataxia
  - Rigidity
- Four main types:
  - Spastic (increased muscle tone)
  - Athetoid or dyskinetic (slow, uncontrolled movements)
  - Ataxic (problems with balance and depth perception)
  - Mixed
- There is no known cure for CP, therefore, preventive care is of utmost importance
- Gestational age at which magnesium sulfate should be administered is from period of viability to $\leq 31^{+6}$ weeks
- During administration of magnesium sulfate, tocolysis should be stopped
- Dosage:
  - For women with *imminent preterm birth*
    - 4g IV loading dose, over 30 minutes, followed by a 1g/hr maintenance infusion until birth or for a maximum of 24 hours, whichever is earlier
  - For *planned preterm birth* for fetal or maternal indications
    - 4g IV loading dose, over 30 minutes, ideally within 4 hrs before birth, followed by a 1g/hr maintenance infusion until birth or for a maximum of 24 hours, whichever is earlier
  - For *threatened preterm labor*
    - Same dosage for a maximum of 24 hours.

Important Points

- Corticosteroids for fetal lung maturity should be administered concurrently (if not given earlier)
- Repeat course of magnesium sulfate is not required
- Delivery should not be delayed for administration of $MgSO_4$
- Signs of magnesium toxicity should be meticulously checked (no requirement of a Foley's catheter for urine output measurement)
- Monitoring of serum magnesium levels is not required
- $MgSO_4$ may be administered before tocolytic drugs have been cleared from the maternal circulation. If nifedipine had been used for tocolysis or hypertension, there is no contraindication to the use of $MgSO_4$ for fetal neuroprotection
- Pediatrician should be kept informed as magnesium can cause hypotonia or apnea in the neonate.

Progesterone in Preventing Preterm Labor

- In women with a history of preterm labor, 17-alpha hydroxyprogesterone 250 mg IM weekly OR progesterone 100 mg daily vaginally should be administered

- In women with short cervix (<15 mm) on TVS detected at 22–26 weeks, progesterone 200 mg daily vaginally
- Therapy should be started after 20 weeks of gestation and stopped when the risk of prematurity is low.

Vaginal progesterone or cervical cerclage. Which is superior?
- Vaginal progesterone is mainly indicated in cases of a sonographic short cervix (<25 mm) with or without a history of preterm birth
- Cervical cerclage is indicated in patients presenting with acute cervical insufficiency and perhaps, in some patients, with a prior history of preterm birth and a sonographic short cervix of <25 mm
- Recent studies (meta-analysis) have proved that they are equally efficacious for the prevention of preterm birth and adverse perinatal outcomes in patients with a short cervix and history of preterm birth.

Characteristics of Preterm Babies

1. Hair:
   - The back has abundant growth of fine hairs called lanugo
   - The hairy area turns bald as gestational age increases
   - There is no difficulty in identifying individual hair fibers.
2. Breast nodule → measures < 5 mm and nipple is small or absent
3. Ear cartilage → external ear is soft and devoid of ear cartilage and hence on folding the external ear, the recoil is poor.
4. External genitalia:
   Males
   - Scrotum is small and does not have rugae
   - Both testes are not descended into the scrotum.
   Females
   - Labia majora are widely separated, not covering the labia minora, resulting in prominent appearance of clitoris.
5. Sole creases → anterior one-third of sole reveals a single deep transverse skin crease. There may be multiple superficial creases.
6. Skin:
   - Shiny
   - Thin
   - Transparent
   - Gelatinous
   - Plethoric
7. Neurologically:
   - Less alert
   - Hypotonic
   - Automatic reflexes → Moro's reflex appear at 28–30 weeks of gestation
   - Grasp reflex → appear around 30 weeks of gestation
   - Glabellar tap → blink response to glabellar tap appears at 29 weeks
   - Rooting and coordinated sucking reflexes → appear at 34 weeks of gestation.
8. Measurements → small in size:
   - Crown heel length is < 47 cm
   - Head circumference is < 33 cm.

9. Head size:
   - Appears large in proportion to the body
   - Sutures are widely separated
   - Fontanelles are smooth and flat.

New Ballard Scoring System

For assessment of gestational age of extremely premature babies and for mature infants. The score is valid until Day 7 of life.
Includes:

Neuromuscular Maturity

- Posture
- Square window
- Arm recoil
- Popliteal angle
- Scarf sign
- Heel to ear.

Physical Maturity

- Skin
- Lanugo
- Plantar surface
- Breast
- Ear/eye
- Genitals (male)
- Genitals (females).

Maturity rating	
Total score (Neuromuscular + Physical)	Weeks
-10	20
-5	22
0	24
5	26
10	28
15	30
20	32
25	34
30	36
35	38
40	40
45	42
50	44

Complications Associated with Preterm Neonates

1. Thermoregulation:
   a. Hypothermia
   b. Hyperthermia
2. Respiratory problems:
   a. Respiratory Distress Syndrome (RDS) or Hyaline Membrane Disease (HMD) → due to surfactant deficiency
   b. Apnea of prematurity
   c. Perinatal depression → in delivery room
   d. Bronchopulmonary dysplasia (BPD) or Chronic lung disease (CLD).
3. Central nervous system:
   a. Perinatal depression
   b. Intraventricular hemorrhage
   c. Periventricular white matter injury.
4. Cardiovascular system:
   a. Patent Ductus Arteriosus (PDA)- may lead to congestive cardiac failure
   b. Hypotension.
5. Metabolic:
   a. Hypoglycemia
   b. Hypocalcemia.
6. Gastrointestinal system:
   a. Necrotizing enterocolitis (NEC)
   b. Regurgitation
   c. Aspiration.
7. Hematologic:
   a. Anemia
   b. Hyperbilirubinemia.
8. Renal system:
   a. Low glomerular filtration rate
   b. Late metabolic acidosis
   c. Inability to handle solute water and acid loads.
9. Ophthalmologic:
   a. Retinopathy of prematurity (ROP).
10. Immunologic:
    Preterm babies are at a greater risk of infection due to deficiencies in both humoral and cellular response.
11. Nutritional:
    a. More prone for anemia
    b. Deficiencies of folic acid and vitamin E
    c. Osteopenia of prematurity.

Pulmonary Surfactant

- Surfactant is a lipoprotein that decreases the surface tension of distal airways and thus maintaining the functional residual capacity (FRC) during expiration
- It increases the lung compliance and hence prevents collapse of alveoli
- Surfactant is produced by type II alveolar cells. It is a heterogeneous mixture of lipids and proteins in which the predominant component is phospholipid dipalmitoyl phosphatidylcholine (DPCC)

- The production of phosphatyl glycerol is inadequate if there is damage to type II alveolar cells due to hypoxia, shock, acidosis, hypothermia or antepartum hemorrhage
- The lack of surfactant due to immaturity of lungs leads to Hyaline Membrane Disease (HMD)
- The incidence of HMD is inversely proportional to the gestational age. Highest incidence is seen in babies born with a gestational age of 26 to 32 weeks
- These babies present with tachypnea, expiratory grunting, flaring of nasal alae, inspiratory retractions, cyanosis shortly after birth
- These symptoms begin at birth or within few hours of birth and show a gradual worsening over next 24-48 hours
- The classical X ray findings show low volume lungs, with a diffuse reticulogranular pattern and air bronchograms
- Gastric aspirate shake test → useful bed side screening test to assess the risk of development of HMD
- The surfactant replacement therapy reduces mortality and morbidity in babies with RDS. It improves oxygenation by resolving atelectases and improves lung compliance
- Surfactant replacement therapy also reduces the duration of ventilatory support, decreases the incidence of pulmonary air leaks (pneumothorax and pulmonary interstitial emphysema) and hence improves survival
- Surfactants are available as human, bovine or porcine origin and synthetic preparations
- Natural surfactants improve survival without bronchopulmonary dysplasia (BPD) and with a lower incidence of air leaks, and they are to be preferred over synthetic surfactants
- Surfactant therapy can be given as prophylactic, early rescue or late rescue therapy:
  - Prophylactic → defined as intubating and administering surfactant within 10–20 minutes after birth, before onset of respiratory distress but definitely after initial resuscitation and stabilization. It is preferably given in preterm babies at < 28 weeks gestation
  - Early rescue → surfactant is administered within 2 hours of birth and is preferably given immediately after onset of respiratory distress. It is given in preterm babies ≥ 34 weeks gestation with respiratory distress
  - Late rescue → defined as surfactant treatment 2 or more hours after birth, administered in preterm babies with established respiratory distress, requiring CPAP or mechanical ventilation
- Preterm infants born at or earlier than 30 weeks gestation have benefited from both prophylactic and rescue surfactant administration
- Infants receiving prophylactic surfactant have had a lower incidence and severity of respiratory distress and also have encountered fewer complications such as pneumothorax, pulmonary interstitial emphysema, bronchopulmonary dysplasia and death
- Therefore, infants who are at a significant risk of RDS should receive prophylactic natural surfactant therapy as soon as they are stable within a few minutes after intubation
- Surfactant is administered intratracheally through an endotracheal tube located in the trachea
- There is no evidence to support the practice of placing the infant in multiple different positions during the administration of surfactant
- Dosage of bovine minced surfactant → 100 mg/kg or 4 mL/kg, natural porcine surfactant - 200 mg/kg or 2.5 mL/kg
- Single or multiple doses of surfactant → depends on the condition of the baby:
  - Infants with RDS who have persistent or recurrent oxygen and ventilatory requirements within the first 72 h of life should have repeated doses of surfactant
- Administering more than three doses has not been shown to have a benefit
- Other than respiratory distress syndrome, surfactant therapy has also been used in meconium aspiration syndrome (MAS), persistent pulmonary hypertension of the newborn (PPHN), pulmonary hemorrhage and neonatal pneumonia.

SUGGESTED READING

1. Agustín Conde-Agudelo, Roberto Romero, Juan Pedro Kusanovic: Nifedipine for the management of preterm labor: A systematic review and metaanalysis. Am J Obstet Gynecol. February 2011;204(2):134.
2. Agustin Conde-Agudelo, Roberto Romero, Kypros Nicolaides, et al. Vaginal progesterone versus cervical cerclage for the prevention of preterm birth in women with a sonographic short cervix, singleton gestation, and previous preterm birth: A systematic review and indirect comparison meta-analysis. Am J Obstet Gynecol. January 2013;208(1):42.
3. Akila Subramaniam, Adi Abramovici, William W Andrews, et al. Antimicrobials for preterm birth prevention: An overview. Infectious Diseases in Obstetrics and Gynecology. 2012.
4. Antenatal corticosteroids to reduce neonatal morbidity and mortality. RCOG Green-top Guideline No. 7. October 2010.
5. Bryan Larsen, Joseph Hwang. Progesterone interactions with the cervix: Translational implications for term and preterm birth. Infectious Diseases in Obstetrics and Gynecology. 2011.
6. Catherine Y Spong, Brian M Mercer, Mary D'Alton, et al: Timing of Indicated Late-Preterm and Early-Term Birth. Obstet Gynecol. 2011 August;118(2 Pt 1):323-33.
7. Dan Farine, William Robert Mundle, Jodie Dodd, et al. The Use of Progesterone for Prevention of Preterm Birth. J Obstet Gynaecol Can 2008;30(1):67-71.
8. Gael Abou-Ghannam, Ihab M Usta, Anwar H Nassar. Indomethacin in Pregnancy: Applications and Safety. Am J Perinatol 2012;29:175-86.
9. Joel D Larma, Jay D Iams. Is Sonographic Assessment of the Cervix Necessary and Helpful? Clin Obstet Gynecol. March 2012;55(1):324-35.
10. Kenneth Lim, Kimberly Butt, et al: Ultrasonographic Cervical Length Assessment in Predicting Preterm Birth in Singleton Pregnancies. J Obstet Gynaecol Can 2011;33(5):486-99.
11. Koucký M, Germanová A, Hájek Z, Pařízek A. Pathophysiology of Preterm Labor. Prague Medical Report. 2009;110(1):13-24.
12. Laura Magee, Diane Sawchuck, et al. Magnesium Sulfate for Fetal Neuroprotection. J Obstet Gynaecol Can 2011;33(5):516-29.
13. Maria Muñoz, Richard P Usatine. Abdominal pain in a pregnant woman. OBG Management. January 2006.
14. Martina Delaney, Anne Roggensack, et al. Guidelines for the Management of Pregnancy at 41+0 to 42+0 Weeks. J Obstet Gynaecol Can 2008;30(9):800-10.
15. Mitchell S Cappell, David Friedel. Abdominal pain during pregnancy. Gastroenterol Clin N Am 2003;32:1-58.
16. Papatsonis, et al. Nifedipine and Ritodrine in the management of preterm labor: A randomized multicenter trial. Obstetrics & Gynecology. August 1997; Vol 90 No 2.
17. Roberto Romero, Kypros Nicolaides, Agustin Conde-Agudelo, et al. Vaginal progesterone in women with an asymptomatic sonographic short cervix in the midtrimester decreases preterm delivery and neonatal morbidity: A systematic review and metaanalysis of individual patient data. Am J Obstet Gynecol. 2012 February; 206(2):124.
18. Tak-yuen Fung: The use of tocolytic therapy in the prevention of preterm labor. The Hong Kong medical diary. March 2009; Vol.14 No.3.
19. Tocolysis for Women in Preterm Labor. RCOG Green-top Guideline No. 1b. February 2011.
20. Tocolytic treatment in pregnancy: Clinical practice guideline. Institute of obstetricians and gynaecologists, Royal College of Physicians of Ireland. Guideline No.22. April 2013.
21. Xavier Miracle, Gian Carlo Di Renzo, AnnStark, et al. Guideline for the use of antenatal corticosteroids for fetal Maturation. J Perinat Med. 2008;36:191-6.

CHAPTER 12

Breech Presentation

Tania G Singh

DEFINITION
- Defined as a fetus in a longitudinal lie with the buttocks or feet closest to the cervix (at the maternal pelvic outlet)
- *Commonest of all the malpresentations.*

INCIDENCE
- 3–4% of all deliveries
- Decreases with advancing gestational age:
  - 22–25% of births prior to 28 weeks gestation
  - 7% of births at 32 weeks gestation
  - 1–3% of births at term
- Fetal abnormalities are observed in:
  - 17% of preterm breech deliveries
  - 9% of term breech deliveries
- Cord prolapse occurs in:
  - 0–2% with frank breech
  - 5–10% with complete breech
  - 10–25% with footling breech
  - 6% in multigravidas
  - 3% in primigravidas
- Nuchal arms (one or both arms are wrapped around the back of the neck) are present in:
  - 0–5% of vaginal breech deliveries
  - 9% of breech extractions
- Fetal head entrapment (results from an incompletely dilated cervix and head that lacks time to mold to the maternal pelvis):
  - 0–8.5% of vaginal breech deliveries
- Perinatal mortality:
  - Increased 2–4 fold with breech presentation, regardless of mode of delivery
  - Commonest causes:
    - Malformations
    - Prematurity
    - Intrauterine demise.

PREDISPOSING FACTORS

- Prematurity (most common cause)
- Uterine malformations (septate; bicornuate uterus)
- Fibroids and cysts
- Polyhydramnios
- Oligohydramnios
- Placenta previa
- Cornual or fundal placement of placenta
- Fetal abnormalities (e.g. CNS malformations—anencephaly, Down's syndrome, hydrocephalus; myotonic dystrophy, neck masses, heart and GIT disorders)
- Multiple gestation
- Multiparity
- Breech presentation in the previous pregnancy
- Stretched and weakened uterine muscle
- Short umbilical cord.

TYPES OF BREECHES

- Frank or extended breech (50-70%)—Hips flexed, knees extended (pike position). Least associated with cord prolapse. Good dilator of the cervix
- Flexed or complete breech (5-10%)—Hips flexed, knees flexed (cannon ball position)
- Footling or incomplete (10-30%)—One or both hips or knees extended, foot presenting
- Kneeling breech—fetus is in a kneeling position, one or both legs extended at the hips and flexed at the knees. This is extremely rare.

DIAGNOSIS

I. Physical examination
   Suspect breech presentation if:
   - On abdominal examination
     - The presenting part,
       - Feels irregular
       - Is not ballotable and
       - A hard round ballotable head is found in the fundus
     - Fetal heart sounds are heard high in the abdomen (usually around or above the umbilicus)
     - Fetal back and irregular parts are felt on sides
   - On pelvic examination:
     - The head is not felt in the pelvis
     - Soft, globular buttocks may be felt
       OR
     - Bony parts like ischial tuberosities, sacrum or heel of foot may be felt
     - Prominence of the heel and less mobile great toe can help identify the foot
     - Thick, formed meconium may be present once the membranes are ruptured
II. Ultrasound:
   - Most reliable method:
     - Confirm type of breech presentation (frank, complete or footling breech)
     - Estimate fetal weight

- Exclude hyperextension of the fetal head
- Exclude placenta previa
- Assess fetal morphology.

Vaginal versus Cesarean Section for Breech Delivery (Past Scenario)

- Vaginal breech deliveries were previously the norm until 1959 when Wright proposed that all breech presentations should be delivered abdominally to reduce perinatal morbidity and mortality.
- Term breech Trial by Mary Hannah, Walter Hannah and Andrew Willian (2000) found cesarean section to produce better outcomes than vaginal breech delivery but did acknowledge that it may be due to the lost skills of operators. Therefore, the recommended mode of delivery is cesarean section. Since then the rate of cesarean birth for the term breech has increased dramatically.
- Important considerations for vaginal breech delivery are size of fetus, presentation, attitude, size of maternal pelvis and parity of the woman.

Case: A primigravida presents at 36 weeks period of gestation, sure of her dates, and also corresponding with 1st trimester USG, with pain abdomen. On examination: vitals are stable. Per abdomen examination reveals a breech fetus with uterine height corresponding to 32 weeks. Per vaginal examination: cervix 1.5 cm dilated, 1.5 cm length, presenting part high up, with bulging membranes. What will be your mode of delivery?
Since this is a case of severe IUGR and preterm labor with breech presentation → the ideal mode of delivery would be by cesarean section. The other indications for the procedure are mentioned below.

Indications for Cesarean Section

- Large baby
- Footling or kneeling breech presentation
- Suspicion of an inadequacy of the pelvis
- Prolonged labor
- Baby with intrauterine growth restriction
- Previous cesarean section
- Oligohydramnios (less amniotic fluid)
- Fetal anomaly incompatible with vaginal delivery
- Preterm labor
- Placenta previa
- Associated other obstetric and medical complications where vaginal birth is contraindicated
- Hyperextended fetal neck in labor (diagnosed on USG)—**Star gaze sign**
- Obstetrician or medical personnel not well trained in vaginal breech delivery
- Delay in descent of the breech any time during the 2nd stage of labor
- Persistent cord presentation.

1. **If you have opted for cesarean section, which manoeuvres can be performed during the procedure? Are there any other complications associated apart from those which are procedure related?**

    Manoeuvres for cesarean delivery
    - Similar to those for vaginal breech delivery, including the *Pinard manoeuvre*, wrapping the hips with a towel for traction, head flexion during traction, rotation and sweeping out of the fetal arms and the *Mauriceau Smellie Veit manoeuvre*

- An entrapped head can still occur during cesarean delivery as the uterus contracts after delivery of the body, even with a lower uterine segment that misleadingly appears adequate prior to uterine incision
  - Entrapped heads occur more commonly with preterm breeches, especially with a low transverse uterine incision
  - As a result, some practitioners opt to perform low vertical uterine incisions for preterm breeches prior to 32 weeks gestation to avoid head entrapment and the kind of difficult vaginal delivery to avoid which cesarean delivery was performed
  - Low vertical incisions usually require extension into the corpus, resulting in cesarean delivery for all future deliveries
  - If a low transverse incision is performed and difficulty is encountered with delivery of the fetal head, the transverse incision can be extended vertically upward (T-incision). Alternatively, the transverse incision can be extended laterally and upward, taking great care to avoid trauma to the uterine arteries
  - A third option is the use of a short-acting uterine relaxant (e.g. nitroglycerin) in an attempt to facilitate delivery.

Complications associated with cesarean section:
- Increased risk of pulmonary embolism
- Infection
- Bleeding
- Damage to bladder and bowel
- Slower recovery
- Longer hospitalization
- Respiratory difficulties for the baby
- Delayed bonding and breastfeeding
- Compromise of future obstetric performance.

Vaginal Breech Delivery

Precautions

- It should be a frank breech and near full-term. Any other type will not dilate the birth canal adequately
- Head of the fetus should be flexed, with the baby's chin on his or her chest
- Mother should have a 'proven' pelvis, means either she should have delivered a child previously that was as big or bigger than breech fetus in index pregnancy or in case of primigravida, mother's pelvis is adequate for the weight/size of the baby at the time of planning labor
- The doctor and other medical personnel should be experienced in attending breech births
- Spontaneous and normally progressing labor
- A healthy and well mother and fetus
- It should take place in a hospital setting where there is well-maintained operation theater for emergency cesarean section
- Epidural analgesia is not routinely recommended.

Types–mainly 3

Spontaneous breech delivery
- It is the natural expulsive action producing:
  - An upward rotation of the baby's back around the symphysis of the mother
  - Simultaneous delivery of the arms and shoulders in that order, and
  - An attitude of extension facilitating the delivery of the head

- No traction or manipulation of the fetus
- Occurs predominantly in very preterm, often previable, deliveries

Assisted breech delivery
- Most common type
- There is:
  - Downward traction in the direction of the birth canal
  - Rotation of the shoulders into an anteroposterior position with delivery of each arm
  - Followed by manual or instrumental delivery of the head

OR

The Bracht manoeuvre
- It is a variant approach to the assisted vaginal breech delivery.

Total breech extraction
- Feet are grasped, and the entire fetus is extracted
- Should be used only for a noncephalic second twin
- Should not be used for a singleton fetus because the cervix may not be adequately dilated to allow passage of the fetal head
- Should not be routinely performed (causes extension of the arms and head)
- Birth injury rate ≈ 25%
- Mortality rate ≈ 10%
- Sometimes performed by less experienced accoucheurs when a foot unexpectedly prolapses through the vagina

Footling breech presentation: Once the feet have delivered, never get tempted to pull the feet. This action may precipitate head entrapment in an incompletely dilated cervix or may precipitate nuchal arms. As long as the fetal heart rate is stable and no physical evidence of a prolapsed cord is evident, management may be expectant while awaiting full cervical dilation.

General Considerations

- Continuous electronic fetal heart monitoring is *preferable* in the 1st stage and *mandatory* in the 2nd stage of labor. Descent of breech and entry of umbilical insertion into the pelvis are commonly associated with an increased incidence of cord compression and variable decelerations
- Fetal membranes should be left intact as long as possible to act as a dilating wedge and to prevent overt cord prolapse
- If there is inadequate progress, proceed for cesarean section
- Induction of labor:
  - Not recommended for breech presentation
  - Oxytocin induction and augmentation—controversial. Concerns that nonphysiologic forceful uterine contractions could result in an incompletely dilated cervix and an entrapped head
  - Oxytocin augmentation is acceptable in cases of uterine dystocia due to epidural analgesia
- Assessing full dilatation in breech presentation is more difficult than in cephalic presentation because the fully dilated cervix does not disappear behind the cephalic crown. Instead, the cervix remains palpable as the fetal trunk descends through it
- Avoid pushing before full dilatation
- Assess for and perform episiotomy, if required, in between contractions. Some routinely perform episiotomy even in multiparas to prevent soft tissue dystocia
- **Hands off until there is reason to assist**
- Anesthesiologist and pediatrician should be informed in advance and be available if and when required

- Thick meconium passage is common as the breech is squeezed through the birth canal. This is usually not associated with meconium aspiration because the meconium passes out of the vagina and does not mix with the amniotic fluid.

Highlights of the Assisted Breech Delivery

Once the buttocks have crowned, maximize maternal bearing down efforts, upright posture and suprapubic pressure
- After crowning, an assistant should exert gentle suprapubic pressure from above to keep the fetal head flexed and facilitate its engagement
- The **Ritgen type manoeuvre** can be applied to take pressure off the perineum during vaginal delivery.

The Original Ritgen Manoeuvre
- Delivery of the head of the fetus by pressure on the perineum while controlling the speed of delivery by pressure with the other hand on the head
- Named after Franz von Ritgen, a German obstetrician
- No downward or outward traction should be exerted on the fetus until the umbilicus is past the perineum.

Delivery of Legs
- Do per vaginal examination and check for the position of the legs
- If the legs are flexed, they will deliver spontaneously with the next contraction
- If the legs are extended, they are delivered by **Pinard's manoeuvre**
  - Flex the knee by applying gentle pressure on the popliteal fossa by index and middle fingers and then hook it down by movement of abduction
- Use a dry towel to wrap around the hips (not the abdomen) to help with gentle downward and outward traction, which is applied in conjunction with maternal expulsive efforts until the scapula and axilla are visible.

Delivery of Arms
- After spontaneous delivery to the fetal umbilicus, expulsive delay despite power from above, with or without nuchal arms may require manoeuvres involving fetal manipulation
- The **Løvset and Bickenbach manoeuvres** are the best described:
  - Only the bony fetal pelvis and legs should be grasped to avoid damage to the fetal adrenal glands, which are disproportionately large
  - Traction on the fetus should be minimized to avoid trapped after-coming fetal parts
  - As a breech fetus transits the pelvis, normal fetal tone and uterine compression keep its head and arms flexed. Fetal manipulation prior to entrance of the elbows and chin into the pelvic inlet can induce extension of fetal limbs and head (**Moro reflex**) resulting in trapped after-coming fetal parts
  - Once the scapula is visible, rotate the infant 90° and gently sweep the anterior arm out of the vagina by pressing on the inner aspect of the arm or elbow
  - Rotate the infant to 180° angle in the reverse direction, and sweep the other arm out of the vagina
  - Once the arms are delivered, rotate the infant back to 90° angle so that the back is anterior

*Delivery of the Fetal Head—**The Most Decisive and Fundamental Step:***
- Should not take >10–15 minutes
- Various manoeuvres can be followed in practice

I. **Burns—Marshall technique**
   - For delivering the head in a breech delivery, if it does not deliver spontaneously:
     - Allow baby's body to hang until you can see the hair at the back of the neck
     - Hold the feet
     - Swing the feet upwards over to the mother's abdomen
     - Free the baby's mouth and pause while you clean it
     - Finish delivery by swinging the baby over the mother's abdomen
II. **Mauriceau-Smellie-Veit manoeuvre or Mauriceau manoeuvre (named after François Mauriceau, William Smellie and Gustav Veit)**
   - An obstetric or emergent medical manoeuvre done by an assistant and an obstetrician to maintain the head in a flexed position to allow its smallest diameter to pass
     - Assistant: applies suprapubic pressure
     - Obstetrician
       Inserts *left hand* in the vagina
         - With the index and middle finger on either side of the maxilla, gently press on it, bringing the neck to a moderate flexion
         - Left hand's palm should rest against the fetal chest
       Right hand
         - Ring and little fingers placed on the baby's right shoulder
         - Middle finger in suboccipital region
         - Index finger on the left shoulder
     - *Aim of the manoeuvre*
       - Neck flexion
       - Traction on the fetus toward the hip/pelvis
       - Suprapubic pressure to allow for delivery of the fetal head
III. Alternatively, **Piper forceps** can be used for head flexion
   - Introduced by Edmond Piper of Philadelphia in 1927. It has long shanks and a perineal curve
   - Piper forceps are specialized forceps used only for the after-coming head of a breech presentation
     - An assistant is needed to hold the fetal body in a horizontal plane
     - The operator gets on one knee to apply the forceps from below
     - Unlike conventional forceps, these are not tailored to the position of the fetal head (i.e. it is a pelvic, and not cephalic, application).
   - *Technique:*
     - The after-coming head must have descended to fill the pelvis and must be in direct occipitoanterior position

       ↓

     - Assistant holds trunk of fetus upwards horizontally, so that it may be out of way as much as possible

       ↓

     - Forceps blades are introduced at 4 o'clock and 8 o'clock position and made to lie against the sides of the head through a short arc

       ↓

- Handles then lie along ventral aspect of fetus, so as to promote flexion

    ↓

- Traction first made downwards and backwards till chin appears, then forceps and fetus are carried upwards towards the mother's abdomen

Advantages
- Very little or no traction is needed for delivery with Piper's forceps
- Controlled delivery of head
- Flexion is well maintained
- Pull is directly applied over fetal head contrary to other manual methods, where it is applied via vertebral column.

Precaution
- During delivery of the head, avoid extreme elevation of the body, which may result in hyperextension of the cervical spine and potential neurologic injury.

Erich Franz Bracht Manoeuvre
- First described in 1935 by a German gynecologist for delivering the frank breech with minimal interference
- Can be used as an alternative to assisted breach delivery mentioned above
    - The breech is allowed to deliver spontaneously to the umbilicus without push or pull
    - The knee-extended legs of the flexed breech are not brought down
    - The body and extended legs are then grasped in both hands, with the fingers around the lower back and the thumbs around the posterior aspect of the thighs, while the upward and anterior rotation of the body is maintained
    - When the anterior rotation is nearly complete, the baby's body is held, not pressed, against the mother's symphysis using only a force equivalent to the weight of that portion of the baby already born
    - The mere maintenance of this position, added to the uterine contractions and, if necessary, gentle suprapubic pressure by an assistant, allows the baby's head to deliver spontaneously in full extension.

Mode of Delivery

- Position of choice → Lithotomy.

Delivery of buttocks
- Engagement → when bitrochanteric diameter enters the pelvic inlet
- Sacrum is in the left anterior quadrant
- Bitrochanteric diameter enters the pelvic brim in the left sacroanterior position
- Further contractions will lead to descent of breech but it is usually slow
- Anterior buttocks reach the pelvic floor and rotate 1/8th of a circle (45°) into the anteroposterior diameter (i.e. forward, downward and towards the midline)
- Anterior hip escapes under the symphysis pubis → lateral flexion occurs → posterior hip rises and sweeps over the perineum
- Buttocks are born.

Delivery of legs
- Restitution occurs to the mother's right → Legs will usually be born with further contractions → Babies with legs extended might require assistance

- When popliteal fossae present at vulva, flex knee by placing index finger in popliteal fossa
- Sweep leg outwards abducting hip slightly
- Repeat manoeuvres with second leg → Second leg is born → Hands off—allow breech to deliver with contractions and maternal effort.

Delivery of arms
- Engagement of shoulders occurs in left oblique diameter of the pelvis
- Anterior shoulder rotates under the symphysis
- Bisacromial diameter turns 1/8th of the circle from left oblique to anteroposterior diameter and escapes under the symphysis pubis → Posterior shoulder sweeps the perineum → Arms will usually be born spontaneously.

Delivery of after-coming head
- When the shoulders are at the outlet, the head is entering the pelvis
- Head enters the pelvic brim with the sagittal suture in the oblique or transverse diameter
- Occiput, which is in the left anterior quadrant of the pelvis, rotates forward, accompanied by simultaneous external rotation of the body
- Maintain flexion of the head
- *No touch*—until nape of neck visible
- Head comes to the outlet with the sagittal suture in the anteroposterior diameter and the occiput comes under the symphysis
- Sacrum rotates towards the pubis to make the back anterior
- When the nape of the neck comes under the symphysis, the chin, mouth, nose, forehead and, finally, the occiput is born by a movement of flexion.

Complications

Fetal Complications

1. Lower Apgar scores, especially at 1 minute:
   - Many advocate obtaining an umbilical cord artery and venous pH for all vaginal breech deliveries to document that neonatal depression is not due to perinatal acidosis
2. Fetal head entrapment:
   - May result from an incompletely dilated cervix and a head that lacks time to mold to the maternal pelvis
   - Occurs in 0–8.5% of vaginal breech deliveries
   - The above percentage is higher with preterm fetuses (< 32 weeks), when the head is larger than the body
   - Dührssen incisions (i.e. 1–3 cervical incisions made to facilitate delivery of the head) may be necessary to relieve cervical entrapment. However, extension of the incision can occur into the lower segment of the uterus, and the operator must be equipped to deal with this complication
   - The **Zavanelli manoeuvre** has also been described, involving replacement of the fetus into the abdominal cavity
     - Fetus that has begun to show is pushed back into the vagina until it can be delivered by cesarean section
     - First described in the 1970s, it is used both for breech presentations and for cases in which the fetus has a cephalic presentation but the shoulders are stuck
     - While success has been reported with this manoeuvre, fetal injury and even fetal death have occurred

3. Nuchal arms (one or both the arms are wrapped around the back of the neck):
   - Present in 0–5% of vaginal breech deliveries and in 9% of breech extractions
   - Nuchal arms may result in neonatal trauma (including brachial plexus injuries) in 25% of the cases
   - Risks may be reduced by avoiding rapid extraction of the baby during delivery of the body
   - To relieve nuchal arms when it is encountered, rotate the fetus so that the face turns towards the maternal symphysis pubis; this reduces the tension holding the arm around the back of the fetal head, allowing for the delivery of the arm
   - Nuchal arms may be reduced by the **Løvset or Bickenbach manoeuvres**
4. Damage to spine or spinal cord:
   Positioning the baby incorrectly while using forceps to deliver the after coming head can damage the spine or spinal cord

   Cervical spine injury
   - Predominantly observed when the fetus has a hyperextended head prior to delivery
   - Complete cervical spine injury can be in the form of transection or nonfunction
5. Cord prolapse:
   - May occur in 7.4% of all breech labors
   - This incidence varies with the type of breech: 0–2% with frank breech, 5–10% with complete breech, and 10–25% with footling breech
   - Cord prolapse occurs twice as often in multiparas (6%) than in primigravidas (3%)
   - Cord prolapse may not always result in severe fetal heart rate decelerations because of the lack of presenting parts to compress the umbilical cord
6. Oxygen deprivation:
   - May occur from either cord prolapse or prolonged compression of the cord during birth, as in head entrapment
   - It may cause permanent neurological damage or death
7. Injury to the brain and skull:
   - This may occur due to the rapid passage of the baby's head through the mother's pelvis
   - More likely to occur in preterm babies
8. Damage to the internal organs:
   - This can occur due to squeezing of the baby's abdomen.

Maternal Complications

1. Tears of the genital tract
2. Complications associated with cesarean section, instrumental deliveries
3. Infection due to manipulations
4. Maternal anxiety.

Factors Leading to Adverse Effects on the Fetal Outcome

- Older mothers
- Footling presentation
- Hyperextended fetal head
- Low birth weight
- Prolonged labor
- Nonexperienced clinician.

Vaginal Versus Cesarean Delivery (Present Scenario)

- After 37 weeks gestation, options for the mode of delivery should be discussed with both the parents explaining the risks in detail
- Prematurity, which is the greatest risk factor associated with intraventricular hemorrhage, should not be misinterpreted for trauma during delivery
- For estimated fetal weight ≥ 3.5 kg, cesarean delivery should be opted for because of the concern for entrapment of the unmolded head in the maternal pelvis, although data to support this practice are limited
- A frank breech presentation is preferred when vaginal delivery is attempted. Complete breeches and footling breeches are still candidates for vaginal delivery, as long as the presenting part is well applied to the cervix and both obstetrical and anesthesia services are readily available in the event of a cord prolapse
- The fetus should show no neck hyperextension on antepartum ultrasound imaging. Flexed or military position is acceptable
- Vaginal breech delivery after one prior cesarean delivery is not contraindicated, though larger studies are not available on it. Studies showing success of vaginal breech delivery with prior one cesarean section are available but simultaneously complications like nuchal arm, brachial plexus injury, uterine dehiscence with subsequent hysterectomy have also been reported in literature.

Primigravida Versus Multiparous

- It had been commonly believed that primigravida with a breech presentation should have a cesarean delivery, although no data (prospective or retrospective) support this view
- The only documented risk related to parity is cord prolapse, which is 2-fold higher in parous women than in primigravid women.

EXTERNAL CEPHALIC VERSION

- Transabdominal manual rotation of a fetus presenting as breech into a cephalic presentation

Historical Considerations

- Initially popular in the 1960s and 1970s, ECV virtually disappeared with time, after reports of fetal deaths following the procedure.

Prerequisites for ECV

1. Written and informed consent (explaining the risks, need for emergency cesarean section or induction of labor, adverse effects of tocolytics)
2. Recent USG (preferably on day of ECV) to confirm the presentation, rule out congenital anamolies, to note placental location and for adequacy of amniotic fluid
3. Performed in the labor room with immediate approach to the operation theater
4. Adequate pelvis
5. Average size baby weight
6. Reassuring NST
7. Adequate amniotic fluid

8. Relaxed uterus
9. Appropriate gestational age
10. Skilled operator
11. Breech should not be engaged
12. Patient should be on IV fluids PREFERABLY but not necessary (NPO, at least 4-6 hours prior to the procedure)
13. Immediate measures for emergency cesarean section (blood availability, OT, anesthetist, pediatrician)
14. No other obstetric or medical complication
15. Some prefer to have an assistant to help turn the fetus, elevate the breech out of the pelvis or to monitor the position of the baby with ultrasonography
16. Excessive force should not be used at any time, as this may increase the risk of fetal trauma
17. No consensus has been reached regarding how many ECV attempts are appropriate at one time.

Period of Gestation

- 35–36 weeks in nulliparous
- From 37 weeks in multiparous.

Candidates for ECV

- Fetus in breech presentation
- Reassuring fetal heart rate tracings
- No contraindications to vaginal delivery at ≥ 36 weeks gestation
- Usually not performed on preterm breeches because:
  - They are more likely to undergo spontaneous version to cephalic presentation
  - They are more likely to revert to breech after successful ECV (approximately 50%)
  - If complications occur, they will result in preterm neonate (iatrogenic prematurity).

Contraindications

Absolute Contraindications

- Inadequate pelvis
- Multiple gestation with a breech-presenting fetus (except in delivery of the 2nd twin)
- Vaginal bleeding (within the past 1 week)
- Major fetal anamoly
- Contraindications to vaginal delivery (e.g. active herpes simplex virus infection, placenta previa)
- Nonreassuring fetal heart rate tracing
- Premature rupture of membranes
- Other obstetric complications (severe preeclampsia, maternal cardiac disease, etc.)
- Cord around the fetal neck.

Relative Contraindications

- Polyhydramnios (associated with spontaneous reversion)
- Oligohydramnios

- Fetal growth restriction
- Small for gestational age fetus with abnormal doppler
- Uterine malformation
- Scarred uterus
- Unstable lie (in cases where induction is not planned).

Controversial Candidates

- Women with prior uterine incisions
- Performing ECV on a woman in active labor.

Procedure

- In delivery room
- Before ECV, foot-end elevation (of bed) to help disengage the breech
- Sprinkle powder over the abdominal wall → mother's skin can get very red and sore
- Scan to confirm breech and position of fetal back
- NST to be performed before and after the procedure
- Tocolytics-β sympathomimetics, slow IV or bolus subcutaneous routes can be used (ritodrine, terbutaline, salbutamol) but not with glyceryl trinitrate, as a patch or sublingually or with nifedipine
- If rhesus negative → anti-D Ig given
- If successful → followed either by induction of labor (keeping in mind the unengaged head and unripe cervix) or the patient can be discharged
- If unsuccessful → can wait (expectant management allows the possibility of spontaneous version) or cesarean section, especially if regional anesthesia given, minimizing the risk of second regional anesthesia.

Success Rate

- Range from 30–80%
- Overall success rate of 25–40% for nulliparas and 60% for multiparous women
- Performance of ECV decreases the cesarean delivery rate by ≈ 50%
- Improved success rates occur with:
    - Multiparity
    - Earlier gestational age
    - Frank (versus complete or footling) breech
    - Transverse lie
    - Thinner patients
    - Posterior placenta
    - Adequate amniotic fluid volume
    - Skill of the practitioner (≈ 30–80% of attempts will be successful, depending on the case selection).

Note:

- As the incidence of breech presentation is only 3–5% of all deliveries, decreasing the cesarean delivery rate for breeches by 50% will have only a marginal impact on the overall cesarean section rate.

Newman score (to predict ECV success)			
	Add 0 points	Add 1 point	Add 2 points
Parity	0	1	>2
Dilatation	>3 cm	1–2 cm	0 cm
EFW	<2500	2500–3500	>3500
Placenta	Anterior	Posterior	Fundal/lateral
Station	> −1	−2	< −3

- *Score < 2* → 0% successful
- *Score > 9* → 100% successful.

Risks

Common Risks

- Alterations in fetal parameters:
  - Fetal bradycardia and subsequent nonreactive NST → both are transient
  - Alterations in umbilical artery and middle cerebral artery waveforms and an increase in amniotic fluid volume:
    - Occurs in ≈ 12–40% of cases
    - Believed to be a vagal response to head compression with ECV
    - Usually resolves within a few minutes after cessation of the ECV attempt
    - Not usually associated with adverse sequelae for the fetus
- Unsuccessful ECV
- 35% report mild-to-moderate discomfort during procedure
- Failure of induction, if induced immediately after ECV with unengaged head and unriped cervix.

Uncommon Risks

- Spontaneous reversion to breech (<5%)
- Dizziness and palpitations from tocolysis (4%)
- High pain score (≈ 5%)
- Fetomaternal hemorrhage (0–5%)
- Cord entanglement (< 1.5%)
- Precipitation of labor
- Premature rupture of membranes — (<1%)
- Abruptio placentae
- Profound fetal bradycardia
- Fractured fetal bones
- Possibility of emergency cesarean section–0.5% (e.g. because of placental abruption following the procedure)
- Small increase in instrumental delivery.

Tocolytics

- Data regarding the benefit of intravenous or subcutaneous beta-mimetics in improving ECV rates are conflicting
- Whether tocolysis should be used routinely or selectively is still unclear.

Regional Anesthesia

Regional analgesia, either epidural or spinal, may be used to facilitate external cephalic version (ECV) success.

Advantages

- When analgesia levels similar to that for cesarean delivery are given, it allows relaxation of the anterior abdominal wall, making palpation and manipulation of the fetal head easier
- Eliminates maternal pain that may cause bearing down and tensing of the abdominal muscles
- After successful ECV, epidural can be removed and the patient sent home to await spontaneous labor or labor is induced (as per indication)
- If ECV is unsuccessful, patient can proceed to cesarean delivery under her current anesthesia, if fetal lung maturity has been documented.

Disadvantages

- Inherent risk of regional analgesia, which is considered small
- Lack of maternal pain could potentially result in excessive force being applied to the fetus without the knowledge of the operator.

Acoustic Stimulation

- Data is scant, though a study conducted, comparing acoustic stimulation prior to ECV with a control group when the fetal spine was in the midline, showed 100% results in shifting of fetus to a spine lateral position after stimulation and 91% had successful ECV.

Amnioinfusion

- Amnioinfusion to facilitate ECV cannot be recommended at this time as studies have not proved its efficacy.

Cesarean Section Rates after Successful Version

Ranges from 0–31% after successful external cephalic version (ECV)

Following factors can be attributed
1. Labor dystocia
2. Increased frequencies of compound presentations after ECV
3. Can revert back to breech
4. Failed induction in women with unripe cervices and unengaged fetal heads
5. Nonreassuring NST after ECV
6. Cephalopelvic disproportion.

Breech Delivery with Hydrocephalic Head

- Most favorable method in case of hydrocephaly because after-coming head is so easily deflated
- Baby delivered till body and arms, the body is then pulled down and transverse incision is made over the highest available cervical spine of fetus
- Straight metal catheter, then introduced into the spinal canal and thrust through the foramen magnum to drain excess cerebrospinal fluid
- Becomes even easier when spina bifida is present
- After deflation, delivery is quickly completed
- When baby can be salvaged, cesarean section is the choice.

1. **What are the risks associated with preterm breech?**
   Risks
   - Intrapartum asphyxia
   - Cord prolapse
   - Entrapment of after-coming head
     - Delivery of the trunk through an incompletely dilated cervix can lead to head entrapment during a preterm breech delivery. Therefore, lateral incisions of the cervix should be considered
   - *Routine cesarean section is not recommended for preterm breech.*

2. **What is Zatuchni-Andros Scoring system or Breech Index Scoring system?**
   It is a prognostic scoring system to decide mode of delivery in breech presentation.

Factor	Score		
	Add 0 points	Add 1 point	Add 2 points
Parity	0	1	2
Gestational age	≥ 39 weeks	37–38 weeks	36–37 weeks
Previous breech > 2.5 kg	0	1	≥2
Estimated fetal weight	> 3.5 kg	3–3.5 kg	< 2kg
Cervical dilatation	2	3	≥ 4
Station of breech	–3 and above	–2	–1 or lower

   Assessment is to be made at the onset of labor
   Total score = 11
   Score 0–3 → LSCS
   Score 4–5 → careful review and to proceed with caution
   Score > 5 → reasonable chance for successful vaginal delivery
   One point should be subtracted for footling breeches, as they are somewhat difficult to manage.

3. **Describe the Westin scoring system.**
   It is used for selecting the mode of delivery in breech.

Parameters	Score		
	0	1	2
Inlet, AP diameter	<11.5	11.5–12	>12
Inlet, Transverse diameter	<12.5	12.5–13	>13
Outlet, AP diameter	<10.5	10.5–11	>11
Outlet, Interspinous diameter	<10	10–10.5	>10.5
Intertuberous diameter	<10	10–11	>11
Sum of outlet	<32.5	32.5–33.5	>33.5
Estimated weight (g)	<1500, >4000	1500–2000	2000–3500
Presentation	Double footling	Complete breech, single footling	Frank
Soft parts	Unripe cervix and rigid pelvic floor	Unripe cervix or rigid pelvic floor	Ripe cervix and relaxed pelvic floor
Previous deliveries	None	Uncomplicated breech	Uncomplicated breech

- Total score = 20
- If all the parameters of the pelvis are included → score of >12 is safe for vaginal delivery
- Score ≤ 12 → indication for cesarean section
- But many parameters are based on pelvimetry, which is not done routinely.

4. **Enumerate the incidence and causes of hyperextended head in breech.**
   Hyperextended neck is defined as an angle of extension > 90° (**'Star-gazing' fetus**)
   - Can be discovered on antepartum radiographs
   - Its persistence is an indication for cesarean section
   - Incidence ≈ 5%.

   Causes
   1. Primary posture
   2. Multiple loops of nuchal cord
   3. Fetal neck masses
   4. Torticollis
   5. Uterine myomas/septa.

   Note:
   - 'Flying fetus' → refers to hyperextended head of fetus in *transverse lie*.

5. **What care should be taken in performing rotation at cervical spine?**
   - Vertebral arteries are susceptible to compromise at this point and excessive rotation (>105°) may result in torsional injury to the cervical spine.

6. **What is Kristellar manoeuvre:**
   - Pressure on the uterine fundus towards the vagina with the aim of expediting vaginal delivery is known as Kristellar manoeuvre.
   - Not of much help in vaginal breech delivery; therefore, should not be applied.

7. **Describe Prague's manoeuvre:**
   - It is a technique used to deliver after-coming head in breech when occiput is posterior (when back of fetus fails to rotate anteriorly).

   Technique
   - Baby is laid with his back on the operator's forearm
   - Index and middle fingers of one hand should be placed on either side of the fetal neck from behind, with the other hand grasping the legs above ankles
   - Assistant uses 2 fingers over facial bones to maintain an attitude of flexion
   - By this, the occiput passes forward over sacral concavity and then over perineum. The fetal larynx serves as a fulcrum in this type of delivery.

8. **Is there any antenatal postural treatment to help spontaneous version?**
   Antenatal postural treatment to help spontaneous version:
   i. Knee chest position (difficult) for 15 minutes every 2 hours of waking for 5 days (**Elkin's manoeuvre**)
   ii. Lying on back with woman's hips elevated well above her shoulders for 20 minutes, 2–3 times/day preferably on an empty stomach at the time of the day when the fetus is active (**Juliet D'Souza treatment**).

9. **Role of ultrasound in breech**
   Ultrasound is a must in breech to confirm:
   a. Presentation
   b. Type of breech

c. Maturity
   d. Fetal well-being assessment
   e. Amount of liquor
   f. Placental site
   g. Hyperextension of head
   h. For uterine anamoly/pelvic tumour.

SUGGESTED READING

1. Andrew Kotaska, Yellowknife NT Savas Menticoglou, et al. Vaginal Delivery of Breech Presentation, SOGC Clinical practice guideline, JOGC. June 2009.
2. Andrew Kotaska. Breech Birth Can Be Safe, But Is it Worth the Effort? J Obstet Gynaecol. Can 2009; 31(6):553-4.
3. André B Lalonde: Vaginal Breech Delivery Guideline: The Time Has Come, J Obstet Gynaecol. Can 2009; 31(6):483-4.
4. Christine L Roberts, Natasha Nassar, Alexandra Barratt, Camille H Raynes-Greenow, et al. Protocol for the evaluation of a decision aid for women with a breech-presenting baby, BMC Pregnancy and Childbirth. 2004;4:26.
5. Dunn PM. Erich Bracht (1882–1969) of Berlin and his "Breech" Manoeuvre, Arch Dis Child Fetal Neonatal. Edn 2003;88:F76-F77.
6. External cephalic version and reducing the incidence of breech presentation: RCOG Guideline No. 20a, 2010.
7. Management of breech presentation: SLCOG National guidelines.
8. The management of breech presentation: RCOG Guideline No. 20b. December 2006.

CHAPTER 13

Cardiac Disease in Pregnancy (Part I)

Tania G Singh

HISTORY

Cardinal Symptoms

- Dyspnea on exertion or breathlessness (including paroxysmal nocturnal dyspnea, orthopnea, platypnea and trepopnea)
- Chest pain
- Cough
- Expectoration
- Hemoptysis
- Palpitations (awareness of heart beat)
- Syncopal attacks
- Dizziness
- Fatigue.

Past History

- Hypertension
- Diabetes milletus
- Coronary artery disease
- Hyperlipidemia
- Obesity
- Recurrent lower respiratory tract infections
- TB/Syphilis/STDs/HIV
- Thyroid/connective tissue disorders
- Smoking/alcohol abuse
- Drug history:
  - Tricyclic antidepressants and β agonists → Tachyarrythmias
  - β blockers and Ca^{2+} channel blockers → bradycardia
  - Vasodilators →↓ in BP → syncopal attacks.

Family History

- Hypertension
- DM
- CAD
- Hyperlipidemia

- Congenital heart disease
- Cardiomyopathies (single family history of sudden death is the single most important indicator of risk).

General Physical Examination

- Build and nutrition
- Nails and conjunctiva (for pallor/icterus) → anemia exacerbate angina and failure
- Clubbing
- Cyanosis
- Lymphadenopathy/thyroid swelling
- Pyrexia
- Edema
- Skin
  - Petechiae ⎫
  - Osler nodes ⎬ Infective endocarditis
  - Janeway lesions ⎭
  - Subcutaneous nodules → rheumatic fever
- CVS examination.

INSPECTION

Central
- Precordium
- Apex impulse
- Pulsations
- Dilated veins over chest wall

Peripheral
JVP
PR
BP
Peripheral signs of wide pulse pressure

Central

Precordium

Anterior aspect of chest which overlies the heart.

Bulging
- Enlarged heart
- Pericardial effusion
- Pleural effusion

Flattened
Fibrosis of lung
Congenital deformity

Apex Impulse

- Lower most and outermost part of cardiac impulse seen
- Normally in 5th left intercostal space just inside mid clavicular line
- Invisible:
  - If lying behind rib → turn patient to left lateral position and see in anterior axillary line
  - Emphysema
  - Pericardial effusion
  - Dextrocardia.

Pulsations

- Juxta apical → ventricular aneurysm
- Left parasternal:

- Right ventricular enlargement
- Left ventricular enlargement
- Aneurysm (localized abnormal dilatation of blood vessel) of aorta
- Epigastric → right ventricular hypertrophy
- In 2nd left intercoastal space
- Suprasternal:
  - Aortic regurgitation
  - Aneurysm of aorta
  - Coarctation of aorta (COA)
- At back → COA
- In neck → Aortic regurgitation (AR)
- On right side of chest → dextrocardia.

Dilated Veins

- SVC and IVC obstruction
- Right sided heart failure.

Scars
- Previous heart surgery.

Peripheral

JVP

Normal
- Fluctuations in right atrial pressure during cardiac cycle generate a pulse which is transmitted backwards into jugular veins
- Best examination: When patient reclines at 45°
- Normal JVP → 5-8 cm from right atrium
- 5 cm → vertically above sternal angle (≈ 8 cm from right atrium)
- We measure JVP for 2 purposes:
  - For inspection of wave forms
  - Estimation of central venous pressure (CVP)

'a' wave—atrial systole (most prominent deflection)
↓
'x' descent interrupted by small 'c' wave, marking tricuspid valve closure
↓
'v' wave—atrial pressure then rises again as atrium fills passively during ventricular systole
↓
'y' descent—decline in atrial pressure as tricuspid valve opens.

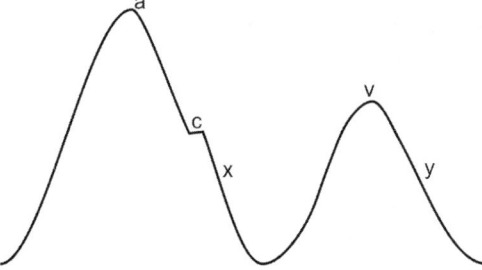

Abnormal

- Absent 'a' wave → atrial fibrillation
- Large 'a' wave → tricuspid stenosis; pulmonic stenosis
    - Cannon 'a' wave → atrial systole against closed tricuspid valve (in complete heart block)
    - Giant 'a' wave → atrial contraction against stenosed tricuspid valve
- Giant 'v' wave → tricuspid regurgitation
- Prominent 'x' and 'y' descents → constrictive pericarditis.

Pulse Rate

- Waveform felt by finger and produced by cardiac systole
- Normal 60-100/min

Tachycardia	Bradycardia
– Emotion	Athlete
– Exertion	Sleep
– Hypovolemia	Hypothermia
– Anemia	Myxedema
– Thyrotoxicosis	Obstructive jaundice

Features of Pulse

Rhythm
- Radial artery
- Regularly irregular:
    - Ventricular bigemini; trigemini
    - Atrial tachyarrythias
- Irregularly irregular:
    - Atrial fibrillation
    - Ectopics

Volume
- Carotid artery
- Pulse pressure (N 30-60 mm Hg) determines pulse volume.

Character
Carotid artery
- Hypokinetic (low volume):
    - Hypovolemia
    - Mitral stenosis
    - Left ventricular failure
- Hyperkinetic (high amplitude with rapid rise):
    - Anemia
    - Mitral regurgitation
    - Aortic regurgitation
    - Ventricular septal defect.

Pulses Parvus et Tardus

- Aortic stenosis (severe).

Bisferiens Pulse

- Brachial or radial artery:
    - Aortic regurgitation
    - Aortic regurgitation with aortic stenosis
    - Hypertrophic obstructive cardiomyopathy (HOCM).

Dicrotic Pulse

- Dilated cardiomyopathy.

Pulse Alternans

- Severe left ventricular dysfunction
- Paroxysmal tachycardia

Pulse Bigeminus

- Pericardial tamponade.

Pulse Paradox

- Pericardial tamponade.

Water Hammer Pulse/Collapsing Pulse/Corrigans Pulse

- Aortic regurgitation
- Patent ductus arteriosus.

Blood Pressure

- Both supine and erect measurements
- Cuff width ≈ 40% the arm circumference
- Auscultation of brachial artery.

Korotkoff Sounds

- Phase 1: first appearance of sounds → systolic pressure
- Phase 2 and 3: increasing loud sounds
- Phase 4: muffling of sounds
- Phase 5: disappearance of sounds

Diastolic BP—Korotkoff 5 is the best. But in conditions where sound remains audible, Korotkoff 4 is taken, as in:
- Aortic regurgitation
- Arterio venous fistula
- Pregnancy.

PALPATION

Apex Beat

Same as apex impulse:
- Heaving apex—left hypertrophy
- Well sustained heave—aortic stenosis
- Ill sustained heave—aortic or mitral regurgitation
- Tapping apex—mitral stenosis (because of loud S_1 and right ventricular enlargement).

Parasternal Heave

- Systolic impulse in left parasternal region commonly seen in right ventricular enlargement is called para sternal heave.

Diastolic Shock (Palpable S_2)

- Loud P_2 (pulmonary component)—pulmonary hypertension
- Loud A_2—systemic hypertension.

Thrill

- Sensation like 'purring' of a cat, that is felt by hand when murmur is palpable
- Its presence → definite evidence of organic heart disease
- Present in systolic lesions
- Absent in regurgitant lesions
- Types:
  Systolic thrill
  - Aortic stenosis
  - Pulmonary stenosis
  - Ventricular septal defect

  Presystolic thrill
  - Mitral stenosis

  Continuous thrill
  - Patent ductus arteriosus.

PERCUSSION

- To determine boundaries of heart
- Right, left and upper borders are percussed
- Lower border cannot be percussed because it can't be distinguished from liver dullness.

Left Border

- Percussion in 4th and 5th intercostal space in mid axillary region and then medially towards left border of heart
- Resonant note of lung becomes dull
- Normally left border is along apex beat
- Outside apex beat in → pericardial effusion.

Upper Border

- Percussion in 2nd and 3rd left intercostal spaces in parasternal line (line between midclavicular and lateral sternal line)
- Normally there is resonant note in 2nd space and dull note in 3rd
- Dull note in 2nd space:
  - Pericardial effusion
  - Pulmonary hypertension
  - Aneurysm of aorta.

Right Border

- Percussion anteriorly in midclavicular line on right side until liver dullness is percussed
- Then percussion is done one space higher from midclavicular line medially to sternal border
- Normally, right border of heart is retrosternal
- Dullness in parasternal region:
  - Pericardial effusion
  - Aneurysm of aorta
  - Right atrial enlargement
  - Dextrocardia.

AUSCULATION

Heart sounds auscultated in all 4 areas of chest:

Mitral Area

- 5th left intercostal space just inside mid clavicular line.

Tricuspid Area

- Lower end of sternum near ensiform cartilage.

Pulmonary Area

- 2nd left intercostal area.

Aortic Area

- 2nd right intercostal area.

Erb's Area

- 3rd left intercostal area.

Heart Sounds

S_1

- Best heard in mitral area
- Single because tricuspid and mitral components occur simultaneously

- Loud in:
  - Mitral stenosis
  - Tricuspid stenosis
- Soft in:
  - Mitral regurgitation
  - Tricuspid regurgitation.

S_2

- Best heard in aortic and pulmonary areas
- Split because aortic valve closes earlier than pulmonary
- Best in pulmonary area (normal A_2–P_2 interval ≈ 30 ms)
- Absent in:
  - Calcific aortic stenosis
  - Emphysema
- Soft in:
  - Calcific pulmonary stenosis
- Loud (A_2) in:
  - Systemic hypertension
  - Aortic aneurysm
- Loud (P_2) in:
  - Pulmonary hypertension.

S_3

- Produced by initial passive filling of ventricles (Ventricular gallop)
- Best heard:
  - At apex
  - In expiration
  - Patient in left lateral position
  - 40-160 ms after A_2
- Causes:
  - Heard in children
  - Adults <40 years
  - Pregnancy
  - Mitral regurgitation
  - Aortic regurgitation
  - Tricuspid regurgitation
  - CHF.

S_4

- Produced by emptying of atrium into non compliant ventricle (Atrial Gallop)
- Causes:
  - Systemic hypertension
  - Aortic stenosis
  - Acute mitral regurgitation
  - Hypertrophic obstructive cardiomyopathy (HOCM).

Murmurs

- Abnormal heart sounds caused by vibration of valves or wall of the heart or great vessels
- May be:
  - Systolic → if between S_1 and S_2
  - Diastolic → if between S_2 and S_1
  - Continuous → throughout systole and diastole.

Grades of Murmur (Levine and Freeman)

Systolic
- Very soft (heard in a quiet room)
- Soft (clearly and definitely audible)
- Moderate
- Loud with thrill
- Very loud with thrill
- Heard even when stethoscope is slightly away from chest wall.

Diastolic
Very soft
Soft
Loud
Loud with thrill

Organic Murmur

Systolic
- Early systolic
  - Acute severe mitral regurgitation
  - Ventricular septal defect.
- Midsystolic (Ejection systolic)

  Aortic cause
  - Aortic stenosis
  - Coarctation of aorta
  - Anemia
  - Thyrotoxicosis.

  Pulmonary cause
  Atrial septal defect
  Ventricular septal defect

- Late systolic
  - Mitral valve prolapse (MVP).
- Holosystolic/Pansystolic
  - Mitral regurgitation
  - Tricuspid regurgitation
  - Ventricular septal defect.

Diastolic
- Early diastolic
  - Aortic regurgitation (*Austin Flint*)
  - Pulmonary regurgitation (*Graham Steell*)
  - Rheumatic fever
  - Infective endocarditis.
- Mid diastolic
  - Mitral stenosis
  - Tricuspid stenosis
  - Carey coombs murmur.

Significant Murmurs

- Any diastolic murmur
- Continuous murmur
- ≥ grade III
- Other signs/symptoms of cardiac disease.

Innocent Murmurs

- Soft systolic murmur without any cardiac abnormality.

Other Sounds

Opening Snap (OS)

- High pitch due to opening of AV valve
- Best heard at lower left sternal border
- Causes:
  - Mitral stenosis
  - Tricuspid stenosis.

Ejection Click

- High pitch, due to opening of semilumar valve
- Causes:
  - Aortic stenosis (valvular)
  - Pulmonary stenosis (valvular).

Pericardial Rub

- Due of sliding of two inflamed layers of pericardium
- Best heard along left sternal border in 3/4th intercostal space with patient bending forward or in knee - elbow position.

QUESTIONS ASKED IN GENERAL

- Dyspnea—Abnormal awareness of breathing occurring either at rest or at very low level of exertion. Major symptom in left heart failure.
- Exertional dyspnea: Exercise →↑ LA pressure → pulmonary congestion → dyspnea.
- Orthopnea: Lying flat →↑ LA pressure → pulmonary congestion → severe dyspnea → use extra pillows or sleep sitting in chair.
- Paroxysmal nocturnal dyspnea: Frank pulmonary edema on lying flat, wakens the patient from sleep with dyspnea and fear of imminent death.
- Dizziness and syncope: By transient hypotension → abrupt cerebral hypoperfusion
  - Other causes → stroke, epilepsy, overdose.
- Types of syncope:
  - Syncope on standing upright (postural hypotension)
  - Vasovagal syncope: caused by autonomic over activity (by emotional/painful stimuli)
  - Carotid sinus syncope.

- Causes of chest pain:
  - MI (constricting)
  - Pericarditis (sharp increase on deep inspiration)
  - Aortic dissection (tearing pain).
- Symptoms specific to various conditions
  - RHD:
    - Fever with sore throat
    - Fleeting joint pains and swelling
    - Involuntary movements (chorea)
    - Nodules under skin (rheumatic nodules).
  - Infective endocarditis:
    - Pyrexia
    - Petechial hemorrhages
    - Pads of finger → tender (Osler nodes)
    - Palpable spleen
    - Phalangeal clubbing
    - Prolonged treatment with increased doses of Penicillin
    - Hemoptysis
    - Hematuria
    - Hemiplegia.
  - CCF
    - Exertional breathlessness
    - Edema of feet, puffiness of face, anasarca
    - Distention of abdomen
    - Pain in right hypochondrium
    - Anorexia
    - Nausea/vomiting.
  - Congenital heart disease
    - Cyanotic spells
    - Squatting episodes.
- Clubbing:
  - Bulbous enlargement of soft parts of terminal phalanges with both transverse and longitudinal curving of nails
  - Swelling is because of:
    - Interstitial edema
    - Dilatation of arterioles and capillaries
  - Grades of clubbing
    - *Grade I* → softening of nail bed
    - *Grade II* → obliteration of angle of nail bed
    - *Grade III* → swelling of subcutaneous tissues over base of nail causing overlying skin to become tense, shiny and wet and increasing curvature of nail → 'parrot beak or drumstick appearance'
    - *Grade IV* → swelling of fingers in all dimensions
  - Clubbing (central)
    - Congenital cyanotic heart disease
      - Not present at birth
      - Develops during infancy → more marked
    - Infective endocarditis

- *Schamrott's sign* → normally when 2 fingers are held together with nails facing each other, a space is seen at level of proximal nail fold. This is lost in cases of clubbing
- Cyanosis:
  - Bluish discoloration of nails due to ↓↓ hemoglobin (>5 mg%) in capillary blood
  - Types:
    - Central
    - Peripheral
    - Cyanosis due to abnormal pigments
    - Mixed.

Central
- Decreased arterial O_2 saturation
- On skin and mucous membrane (tongue, lips, cheeks)
- Pulmonary edema and congenital heart disease.

Peripheral
- Reduced flow of blood to local part
- Skin only
- Physiological during cold exposure
- Mitral stenosis → over "malar area".
- Lymphadenopathy: Inflammatory or non inflammatory enlargement of lymph nodes
- Pyrexia
  - Infective endocarditis (low grade/swinging)
  - After MI (1st 3 days)
- Edema:
  - Subcutaneous edema which pits on digital pressure → CHF
  - Pressure to be applied over a bony prominence (tibia, lateral malleoli, sacrum) to provide effective compression
    - Caused by salt and water retention
    - Effect of gravity on capillary hydrostatic pressure ensures that edema is most prominent around ankles in ambulant patient and over sacrum in bed ridden.
- Petechiae:
  - After 6 weeks occur over conjunctiva, buccal mucosa
  - Most common peripheral sign.
- Osler nodes:
  - Small, tender nodule over fingers, toe, sole.
- Janeway lesions:
  - 1-4 mm non-tender erythematous macules over palms, soles.
- Subcutaneous nodules:
  - Seen in long standing disease
  - Found over extensor surface of joints, shin, occiput and spine
  - Non-tender
  - Patient who has subcutaneous nodules always has carditis.

Heart Disease in Pregnancy

- Rheumatic heart disease
  - Mitral stenosis
  - Mitral regurgitation
  - Aortic stenosis
  - Tricuspid regurgitation
  - Aortic regurgitation

- Congenital heart disease
  - Acyanotic (L to R shunt)
    - ASD
    - PDA
    - VSD
  - Cyanotic (R to L shunt)
    - Fallot's tetralogy
    - Eisenmenger's syndrome
- Other congenital heart lesions
  - COA
  - 1° pulmonary hypertension
  - Marfan's syndrome
- Cardiomyopathies
  - Dilated (congestive)
  - Restrictive
  - Hypertrophic.

Approach to a Pregnant Patient with Cardiac Lesion

Step I: When a patient has come, always keep in mind, certain signs and symptoms that mimic cardiac disease (clinical features):

Symptoms

Physiological	Pathological
Fatigue	Dyspnea on rest
Decreased exercise capacity	Paroxysmal nocturnal dyspnea
Palpitations	Chest pain
Orthopnea	Cough/expectoration
Light headedness	Syncopal attacks
Hyperventilation	Hemoptysis
Breathlessness, Ankle edema — In 30% of normal pregnant women and without ↑ in JVP; does not indicate cardiac disease.	

Signs

Physiological	Pathological
JVP → Mildly distended	Cyanosis
Enlargement of heart with increase in LV volume	S_3/S_4
Ejection fraction → not changed	Diastolic murmur
Apex beat displaced upwards into 4th intercostal space and may reach midclavicular line	Pansystolic murmur
	Continuous murmur
	Atrial flutter or fibrillation
	Harsh basal murmur (with thrill)
	Cardiac enlargement.

Auscultation (normal findings)
- S_1 loud/splitting
- S_2 (may) increase late in pregnancy
- Ejection systolic murmur present (due to hyperkinetic circulation) at 10-12 weeks and disappears postpartum
- Mammary "soufflé" → due to increase blood flow in mammary vessels (may be heard as systolic or continuous murmur)
- Arrhythmias/ectopic beats (both atrial and ventricular) → they only "appear to disappear" on exertion because of tachycardia
- Sinus arrhythmias → pulse irregularity (normal), but PR >100 beats/min., while patient at rest is ABNORMAL.

ECG (normal findings)
- Shift in QRS axis to left or right (because of changes in size and position of heart).

CXR (normal findings)
- Straightening of left upper cardiac border
- Enlarged heart
- Prominent lung markings
- Small pleural effusion in 1st two weeks of postpartum.

Echocardiography (normal findings)
- Increase in LV and RV end diastolic dimensions
- Atrial dilatation
- Small pericardial effusions.

StepII: Decide the functional class—'NYHA classification'
- *Grade I:* No limitations of physical exercise; ordinary activity does not cause undue fatigue, palpitations, dyspnea or angina
- *Grade II:* Slight limitations of physical exercise; ordinary activity results in fatigue, palpitations, dyspnea or angina
- *Grade III:* Marked limitations of physical activity, less than ordinary activity causes symptoms
- *Grade IV:* Inability to carry out physical activity without symptoms.

Step III: Investigations and referral
- Hemogram
- Urine routine and culture
- ECG → in diagnosis of arrhythmias (and not for structural abnormalities)
- 2D echo → investigation of choice
- Other routine investigations
- CXR → not much useful
- Refer to cardiologist.

Step IV: Assess cardiac status (by risk group—"CLARKS maternal mortality risk group") as prognosis depends upon nature and severity of disease

Risk group	*Mortality*
Low risk	0-1%

- ASD
- VSD
- PDA
- Repaired lesions with normal cardiac function

- Mild to moderate pulmonic or tricuspid lesion
- Marfan's syndrome with normal aortic root
- Homograft or bioprosthetic valves
- Bicuspid aortic valve without stenosis.

Intermediate risk   5-15%
- Uncorrected CHD
- Large left to right shunts
- Uncorrected, uncomplicated AS
- Mechanical valve prosthesis
- Severe pulmonic stenosis
- Moderate to severe LV dysfunction
- Previous LV dysfunction, now resolved (e.g. peripartum cardiomyopathy)
- Previous MI.

High risk   25-50%
- Pulmonary hypertension
- Marfan's syndrome with aortic valve involvement
- Cardiomyopathy
- Complicated COA.

Step V: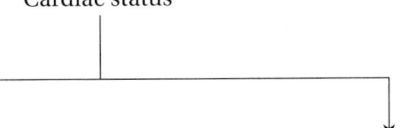

COMPENSATED

- Came for prepregnancy counseling OR
- Is pregnant

Prepregnancy Counseling

- Thorough history of cardiac symptoms including arrhythmias and physical examination
- Explain features of present heart condition/lesion → functional and risk classification
- Should be made aware, that deterioration of NYHA class may occur as pregnancy advances
- Obtain records
- Explain effects of cardiac condition on pregnancy and vice versa
- Adjust medications to avoid adverse fetal effects
- Genetic counseling in cases of heritable lesions
- Need for surgery (valve replacement or repair, if symptomatic prior to pregnancy)/anticoagulation
- Do all baseline investigations (blood tests, exercise tolerance test, ECG, Echocardiography)
- Prenatal visits and need for maternal and fetal testing
- Fetal and neonatal complications (with her specific condition)
- Timing of birth/type of hospital facility required for childbirth
- Pain control and type of anesthesia (during labor and delivery)
- Explain need for cesarean section
- Effective contraception until pregnancy desired.

Other important points to be discussed:
- All potential sources of infection to be looked for:
  - May lie dormant in genital tract
  - Dental roots and caries (dangerous source)
    - No root filling or capping of teeth in cardiac cases, whether pregnant or not
  - UTI
- Anemia → add to complications and failure
- ACE inhibitors → contraindicated in pregnancy
  Side effects
  - Fetal hypotension
  - Anuria
  - Oligohydramnios
  - IUGR
  - Pulmonary hypoplasia
  - Renal tubular dysplasia
  - Hypocalvaria
- Need for diuretics to be reassessed
- Anticoagulants
  - Oral anticoagulants → to be switched over to heparin at ≈ 6 weeks
  - Pregnancy diagnosed → stop warfarin
  - Upto 12th week → Inj. Heparin 5000 IU BD s/c
  - From 12th week up to 36th week → Tab. Warfarin 3 mg daily (at the same time)
  - From 36th week - up to Day 7 postpartum → Heparin
  - Afterwards → give warfarin
- Pregnancy best to be avoided (or if conceived) → terminate (maternal mortality → 30-50%) in following situations:

Absolute indications
- Eisenmenger's syndrome
- 1° pulmonary hypertension
- Cor pulmonale
- Single ventricle
- Marfan's syndrome with dilated aortic root

Terminate in 1st trimester (even for class III and IV patients)—can have permanent sterilization.

Relative indications
- Parous women with grade III/IV
- Grade I or II with previous history of cardiac failure in early months or in between pregnancies.
- Explain them effects of pregnancy on cardiac disease:
  - Maternal mortality may be as high as 15%
  - Dangerous periods in pregnancy ("RULE OF 5")
    - 5th week: When cardiac output begins to increase (physiological changes start)
    - 5 weeks before term → when all changes reach maximum (mainly cardiac output)
    - 5 minutes after delivery
    - **During labor and delivery**
      - Labor: Every uterine contraction injects 300-500 mL of blood from uteroplacental circulation into maternal blood stream increasing cardiac output by 15-20%
      - Simultaneously during 2nd stage → maternal pushing decreases venous return to heart causing a decrease in cardiac output

- These sudden and frequent variations during 2nd stage may be critical.
  - ***Immediately after delivery (of baby and placental separation)***
    - When obstructive effect of pregnant uterus upon return circulation to heart disappears → sudden transfusion of blood from lower extremities and uteroplacental vasculature to systemic circulation → there is ↑ chance of CHF
      a. 5 hours after delivery
      b. 5 days after delivery
- 2 main problems can occur:
  - ↓ PVR with right to left shunting
  - Pulmonary embolization from silent iliofemoral thrombus
  - Especially in patients with:
    - 1° pulmonary hypertension
    - Eisenmenger syndrome
    - AS
    - CHD
- Mortality lowest with RHD and acyanotic heart disease → < 1%
- With cyanotic heart disease → up to 50%. Causes in mother:
  - Cardiac failure mainly after delivery
  - Pulmonary edema
  - Pulmonary embolism
  - Active rheumatic carditis
  - Subacute bacterial endocarditis
  - Rupture of cerebral aneurysm in COA
- Fetal prognosis:
  - Good in RHD (not different from normal patients)
  - Cyanotic → increased mortality (45%). Causes:
    - Abortion
    - IUGR
    - Prematurity
  - Fetal congenital malformation increases by 3-10% if either of parents have congenital lesions, therefore, fetal echo at 20-24 weeks recommended.

Pregnant

- Careful frequent history and physical examination at least once per trimester
- Functional class to be decided during 1st 4 months
- Diet/folic acid/vitamin B complex/calcium
- Bed rest (class II and III) → 12 hours at night and 2 hours during day
- Early part of pregnancy:
  - Class I and II → seen monthly
  - Severe cases → weekly
- More frequent monitoring if:
  - New symptoms develop
  - Changes in functional class
- In case of valvular lesions:
  - Mild valvular disease → monthly till 28-30 weeks, thereafter every 2 weeks or weekly
  - Moderate to severe valvular disease → every 2 weeks until 28-30 weeks, thereafter weekly
  - Hemodynamic changes intensify after the 26th -28th week, which is the most critical period along with the delivery

- Following illnesses avoided and promptly attended to:
  - Anemia → Hemoglobin at least once in each trimester
  - UTI → urine culture in all cases (to exclude asymptomatic bacteriuria)
  - Preeclampsia → very serious
    - Increased burden on heart because of hypertension
    - Increased fluid retention
- Any febrile illness, even in mild cold, patient should take rest
- Any dental procedures → prophylactic antibiotics as follows:

High risk patients
Ampicillin 2 gm IM or IV
+
Gentamycin 1.5 mg/kg (not >120 mg) within 30 min of starting procedure
After 6 hours → ampicillin 1 gm IM or IV or amoxicillin 1 mg per os.

High risk (allergic to Penicillin)
Vancomycin 1 mg over 1-2 hour
+
Gentamycin 1.5 mg/kg

Complete infusion within 30 min of starting procedure.

Moderate risk
Amoxicillin 2 gm per os (1 hour before procedure)
OR
Ampicillin 2 gm IM/IV (within 30 min of starting procedure).

Moderate risk (allergic to Penicillin)
Vancomycin 1 gm IV over 1-2 hour
Complete infusion within 30 min of starting procedure

- Weight gain not to exceed 0.6 kg in any one week
- Watch for earliest signs of failure → particular attention to lung bases
- 3Es
  Elevation of JVP
  Enlarged liver
  Edema of ankles
  } Signs and symptoms of systemic or pulmonary venous congestion
  ↓
  labelled as CHF
- Hydramnios may complicate the picture, therefore bed rest, diuretics, abdominal paracentesis, if required
- Reassessment by cardiologist at 28-32 weeks. Why?
  - In later half of pregnancy, enlarging uterus causes displacement and rotation of heart and to some extent, splints diaphragm
  - Inspite of splinting of diaphragm, vital capacity is not reduced as some compensation is provided by increase in diameter of thoracic cage
  - Therefore, if checked between 28-32 weeks, one can make a reasonable estimate of how heart will behave during labor
- Hospitalization:
  - Class I and II with no other complications → admitted during last fortnight (dangers of transportation avoided)
  - Severe cases (NYHA class III or in failure) → throughout pregnancy
- Diuretics → if intravenous volume expansion is not normal
  - Most common: Chlorthiazide
  - Inhibit Na^+ reabsorption in distal tubule

- Most common side effect:
    - Hypokalemia, therefore give K⁺ retaining agent or increase dietary K⁺
    - Neonatal thrombocytopenia
    - It may decrease plasma volume → placental perfusion and fetal growth are compromised (therefore, serial hematocrit done)
- Prophylactic digitalization:
    - Improves contractility of heart
    - Relieves fatigueability/orthopnea/weakness
    - Avoid ventricular tachycardia and rapid atrial rhythm
- Anticoagulation in case of:
    - CHD
    - Artificial mechanical valve prosthesis
    - Chronic or recurrent arrhythmias
- Fetal echocardiography at 20-24 weeks
- ACE inhibitors are contraindicated
- Inj. Penidure LA_{12} (Benzathine Penicillin) at interval of 3-4 weeks throughout pregnancy to prevent risk of rheumatic fever
- Diagnosis should be made as per the present NYHA class (in case deterioration has occurred)
- A rising pulse rate can be one of the first signs of cardiac decompensation
- Pulse rate is best measured using a stethoscope and auscultating the heart because when the pulse becomes fast, irregular or faint, the radial pulse is often difficult to measure accurately
- BP should be measured using a manual sphygmomanometer in a sitting, not talking, position with appropriately sized cuff placed on the correct arm (for example, the right arm is usually used in women with coarctation of the aorta, 80% of whom will also have a bicuspid aortic valve) at the level of the left atrium
- Auscultation:
    - Murmur may increase by one grade as pregnancy advances because of increase in cardiac output
    - Sudden increase in loudness → suggests development of vegetations from endocarditis
    - Appearance of a new murmur is nearly always significant and requires urgent diagnosis and intervention
    - Lung bases posteriorly should be auscultated at each visit to check for crackles, which can indicate developing pulmonary edema (incipient heart failure)
- Investigations:
  Apart from routine investigations in a cardiac case, others include:
    - Complains of chest pain → check troponin I levels and repeat after 24 hours
    - Suspicion of CAD → Treadmill test, first non-invasive test of choice
    - Suspicion of pulmonary embolism → measure of d-dimer levels → if ↑, anticoagulation
    - Doppler examination of leg vessels → to identify any DVT.

DECOMPENSATED

Conditions which precipitate cardiac failure during pregnancy:
- Anemia
- Infection → pulmonary/urinary or others
- Tachyarrhythmia → atrial fibrillation, atrial flutter
- Rheumatic carditis
- Thyrotoxicosis

- Infective endocarditis
- Preeclampsia
- Exercise or vigorous physical activity

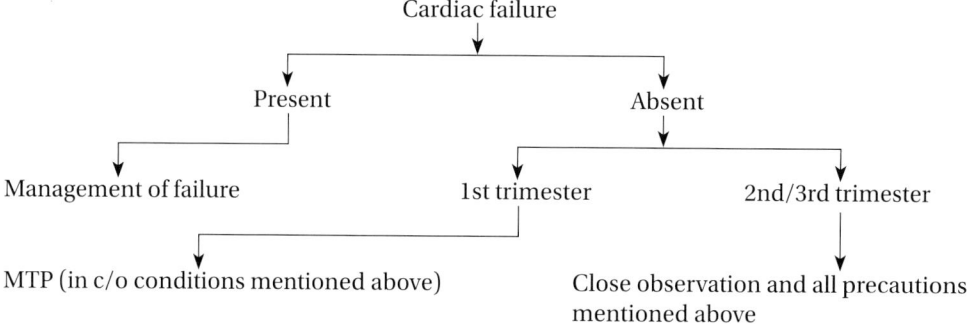

If Mild Failure

- Difficult to distinguish from physiological shortness of breath
- If you are unsure → give mild diuretics
- If improves → continue therapy → improves and transformed into class I → treat as DPD patient with frequent visits
- If no improvements → more intense diuretic → if improves, treat as above
  ↓
- If develops class III/IV or as failure → admit
- Bed rest → essential
  - Risks
    - Venous thrombosis ⎫ Because of ↓ fibrinolytic activity
    - Pulmonary embolization ⎭ and hypercoagulation
  - Therefore, passive leg exercises, prophylactic heparin and pneumatic compression stockings are used
- Salt intake → restrict
- Diuretics → mainstay of therapy
  - Inj. Frusemide 40-80 mg immediately (6-8 hrly)
  - There will be loss of K^+, so as soon as possible change to oral frusemide (20 mg bid)
  - Oral KCl^- can be given
  - Monitor serum K^+ (OD) during IV therapy
- Digitalis:
  - Give to those, who have AF or LV/RV dysfunction
  - To control ventricular rate to 100/min
  - 3 drugs → diltiazem, β blockers, digitalis
  - Diltiazem:
    - Effective
    - Easy to titrate
    - Least toxic
  - In pregnancy, diltiazem and β blockers (may) not be preferred because of the risk of heart block, bradycardia, hypotension and its fetal effects
  - Digitalis:
    - Drug of choice (digoxin most commonly)
    - Given orally

- Rapid onset of action (2 hours)
- Short life
- Loading dose → 0.25 mg IV every 2 hr, up to 1.5 mg
- Maintenance dose → 0.125-0.25 mg daily
- Therapeutic level → 1.0-1.5 ng/mL
- Overdosage can occur easily:
  - Nausea
  - Vomiting
  - PR < 60/min or Pulsus bigemini
  - Cardiac arrhythmias
    o Most serious side effect
    o Antiarrythmic medications
    o Correct hypokalemia
- *Atrial fibrillation:* Patient need to be started on anticoagulants (heparin followed by warfarin)→ dose controlled with INR
  - No obstetric intervention undertaken until failure is not controlled
  - If corrects → need to intervene does not exist
  - If deteriorates:
    - Intubation
    - Ventilation
    - Pulse oximeter
    - ABG analysis
    - Lactic acid levels
  - Prophylactic digoxin → not in failure but are at risk of developing AF as in:
    - Rheumatic mitral valve disease with enlarged left atrium
    - Paroxysmal AF or frequent atrial ectopic beats
  - Diltiazem:
    - Loading dose 0.25 mg/kg IV over 2 min
    - Onset of action 2-7 min
    - Maintenance dose 5-15 mg/ hr infusion(120-360 mg oral in divided doses)
- Vasodilators
  - ↓PVR
  - For maintenance → hydralazine (DOC) → arterial vasodilator (if used in increased doses) →↓↓ BP → alter placental perfusion → fetal distress
  - Acute emergency:
    - Nitroglycerine
      - Predominant effect is on capacitance vessels
      - Reduces pulmonary congestion
    - Dopamine
    - Dobutamine.

If Patient Goes in for Acute Pulmonary Edema

- Propped up position at once
- Inj. Morphine 5 mg IV → repeat every 5-10 min (max. 15 mg)
- O_2 by mask, pulse oximeter and ABG analysis
- Inj. Frusemide 40-80 mg IV (repeat if required)
- Tourniquets can be applied to limbs sufficiently tight (to occlude venous return → decreases output of right heart) → hang legs down

- If exhausted → intubated and ventilated
- Once intubated → if cannot be weaned off the ventilator easily → balloon valvuloplasty or surgery
- If sinus tachycardia → give β blockers
- Basic problem in pulmonary edema—mobilization of fluid from pulmonary interstitial space into alveolar space → impairs gas exchange → O_2 desaturation and retention of CO_2
- Pulmonary edema in pregnancy → 3 main reasons:
  - In management of preterm labor (patients having chorioamniotic infection + β mimetic and glucocorticoid Rx + ↑↑ IV crystalloid solution)
  - Preeclampsia
  - Cardiac disease.

1. **Ideal time to do surgery in a cardiac case.**
   Closed mitral valvotomy
   - 20-24 weeks (in severe MS)
   - Indication:
     - Failure of medical therapy
     - History of pulmonary edema before pregnancy with risk of recurrence in pregnancy
     - Profuse hemoptysis
     - Non-calcified mitral valve
     - No major MR.

   Balloon valvuloplasty
   - 24-28 weeks
   - Risks to patient:
     - Acute MR
     - Procedural tamponade
     - Thromboembolism.

   Open heart surgery
   - Maternal mortality → 1-13%
   - Fetal mortality → 20-33%
   - If fetus has reached viability → can be combined with cesarean section.

2. **What is the place of induction of labor in a cardiac case?**
   Induction of labor—little place
   - Firstly → prolonged Inter Delivery Interval (IDI) → infection and ↑ chances of cesarean section
   - Secondly → patient becomes anxious
   - But if there are obstetric indications—there is no bar to induction
   - Vaginal delivery → safer route
   - Usual method of induction → oxytocin infusion
   - Use double-strength oxytocin but half rate to reduce total volume of fluids given
   - PGE_2 gel: potent vasodilator and causes ↑↑ cardiac output → pulmonary edema especially if associated PIH. Therefore, use with caution.

3. **Tocolytic in case of preterm labor**
   Tocolysis
   - Atosiban → 1st line of management
   - Do not use ritodrine or salbutamol.

Management of Cardiac Patient in Labor

General Measures
- Labor and delivery in lateral decubitus position
- Pulse oximeter
- Adequate pain relief
- Restrict IV fluids to 75 cc/hr
- Antibiotic prophylaxis
- Invasive monitoring, if needed
- Medical therapy, optimization of loading conditions
- Cesarean section as per obstetric conditions
- Oxygen by mask
- Avoid bolus oxytocin and ergot compounds
- Thrombosis prophylaxis
- Prevention of pulmonary edema after delivery.

Treatment Proper

First stage of labor
- Accurate assessment of pelvis because trial of labor is absolutely contraindicated
- Patients with cardiac disease of restrictive variety (e.g. mitral stenosis) are at increased risk of developing failure → therefore extra caution is required
- Labor is fairly easy in majority
  - Inertia is rare
  - Cervix dilates easily because it is softer and more vascular than usual because of venous congestion
- Antibiotics → recommended only for high and moderate risk patients
  - Not recommended in low risk women
- Sedation → IV morphine (2-4 mg) → liberal use
- Pain relief → If patient is not anticoagulated, anesthesia of choice is epidural
- An epidural can be given >12 hours after prophylactic thromboprophylaxis dose or > 24 hours after therapeutic dose or earlier at the discretion of the anesthetist
- IV fluids → ≤ 75 mL/hr
- Pulse oximeter, propped up position, oxygen and IV frusemide for class III and IV
- Class I and II → no serious problem
- Duration of 1st stage → should not be > 8 hours
- Onset of failure in 1st stage → contraindication for interventions like cesarean section.

Second stage of labor
- Episiotomy (for easy delivery)
- Vacuum (better than forceps)
  - Less disturbing to patient
  - Can be used without putting legs in lithotomy position.

Third stage of labor
- Routine use of ergometrine:
  - Barred
  - It will increase the cardiac load by causing additional blood to be squeezed back into circulation and shut down the uterine arteriovenous shunt

- Give oxytocin IV in drip and give frusemide 40 mg IV (to relieve heart of its volumetric load)
- Ergometrine should not be used until 400 mL have been lost
- Immediately after delivery and episiotomy suturing:
  - Patient should be propped up
  - Give morphine
  - O_2 supply
  - Pulse oximeter
- Patient should be brought out from delivery room in trolley with propped up position only.

Place of cesarean section
- Mortality higher 2 or 3 times
- Vaginal delivery is preferred as chances of infection, bleeding, clotting complications, acute shift in blood volume decreases in vaginal delivery
- In class IV and sicker patients—opt for elective cesarean section.

PPH
- Misoprostol 600 mcg/rectally → preferred.

Puerperium

- First 12 hours → most crucial (because right side of heart suffers some overload with diversion of blood that normally would have gone to placenta and uterus)
- Look for signs of pulmonary congestion and edema
- Sedatives for 1st few days → to relieve anxiety and tachycardia
- Bed rest → out of bed in reclining chair
- Any infection → taken seriously
- Visitors restricted to minimum → they interfere with rest; bring respiratory tract infection
- Breastfeeding → contraindicated in class IV and in most cases of class III
- Treat anemia, if present
- Resumption of anticoagulants
- Patients on warfarin are allowed breast feeding (as less drug is secreted in milk)
- These patients are very fertile, therefore:
  - Permanent sterilization
  - Barrier methods
  - Inj. Depot Medroxyprogesterone acetate 150 mg IM 3 monthly
  - Low dose OCPs → in stable patients after 6 months
- Proper counseling → explain the need for valve replacement, if required.

CHAPTER 14

Cardiac Disease in Pregnancy (Part II)

Tania G Singh

Selection of prosthetic valves in women of childbearing age needs to be individualized. There are many types of prosthetic valves but 2 main types are:

Bioprosthetic and Mechanical

Bioprosthetic or Homograft Valves
- There is usually no antenatal complication with a bioprosthetic valve which is well functioning and no other associated cardiac risk factors are present
- Much less thrombogenic
- Do not require anticoagulation
- Better for those in whom close follow up is not possible.

Disadvantages
- Thromboembolism (0.7% per year) → highest in first few months of placement
- Comparatively more risk of thromboembolism when placed in mitral valve position
- Limited life span (≈ 10 years) → needs to be changed earlier than mechanical valves
- Mainly used in aortic region and less frequently in mitral region
- Physiological hematological changes and ↑ wear and tear in pregnancy usually leads to its structural deterioration which may even occur in postpartum period
  - Young age is also a risk factor
  - These patients are usually put on acetylsalicylic acid as chronic maintenance therapy (of concern in 1st trimester)
  - Measures like dental hygiene is required as there is a risk of endocarditis.

Mechanical Valves

- Has 2 leaflets
- Excellent durability
- Much better hemodynamic profile
- A relatively small risk of bleeding and thromboembolic complications with careful anti-coagulation
- Structural deterioration of valve doesn't occur.

Disadvantages
- Thrombogenic (risk more, when placed in mitral valve position)
- Requires lifelong anticoagulation

Section 1: Long Cases

- Stroke, valve thrombosis, myocardial infarction are common during pregnancy if proper anticoagulation is not given.

Antepartum Coagulation

WARFARIN

- Safe during the first 6 weeks
- Stopped from 6-12 weeks
- Restarted at week 12 till 36 weeks (3mg/day; max. upto 5 mg)
- Vitamin K antagonist
- Best results with prosthetic heart valves
- Side effects:
  Warfarin Embryopathy (can be lowered if daily dose is <4 mg/day)
  - Spontaneous abortions
  - Midface and nasal hypoplasia
  - Optic atrophy
  - Hypoplasia of the digits
  - Stippled epiphyses
  - Chondrodysplasia punctata
  - Mental impairment
  - Seizures
  - Hypertelorism
  - Prominence of frontal bone
  - Short stature
  - Scoliosis
  - Deafness
  - Hearing loss
  - Congenital heart disease
  - Microcephaly
  - Minor intracerebral bleeds
  - ↑ risk of fetal intraventricular hemorrhage (especially with forceps delivery).

HEPARIN

- From 6-12 weeks → Inj. Heparin 5000 IU s/c
- Stopped till week 36
- Restarted at 36th week upto 7 days postpartum → to avoid bleeding complications during labor and delivery
- Why at week 36? → because patients with prosthetic valves might go into preterm labor
- Types used:
  - Low molecular weight heparin (LMWH) → dose adjusted
    OR
  - Unfractionated heparin (UFH) → dose adjusted, either by:
    - Intravenously continuous
      OR
    - Subcutaneously
- Add low dose-aspirin.

A. *Unfractionated heparin*
- Does not cross placenta
- Not teratogenic
- Inadequate anticoagulation and lack of monitoring of activated partial thromboplastin time (aPTT) may lead to ↑ in maternal thromboembolism and death.

B. *Continuous IV UFH*
- Offers more consistent anticoagulation
- Recommended in high-risk patients
- Risk of infection, endocarditis and osteoporosis.

C. *Aggressive dose-adjusted subcutaneous unfractionated heparin*
- Given 12 hourly
- aPTT measured 6 hours after dosing (its response usually diminishes in pregnancy owing to ↑ levels of factor VIII and fibrinogen)
- Strict and frequent monitoring is essential.

D. *Low molecular weight heparin*
- Does not cross placenta
- Advantages:
  - Lower incidence of bleeding complications
  - Less osteoporosis
  - Predictable dose response
  - Superior bioavailability
  - Longer half life
  - Lower rate of spontaneous abortion when compared to UFH
- Inadequate dose and lack of anti-Xa levels monitoring may ↑ maternal complications
- Target anti-Xa level 4 hours after dosing is around 1.0 U/mL (usually maintained within a range of 0.6 to 0.7 U/mL), therefore dose adjusted likewise
- Withdrawn 18-24 hours prior to elective delivery to reduce the chance of spinal hematoma during epidural catheter insertion.

DIFFERENT APPROACHES TO ANTICOAGULATION IN PREGNANCY

High Risk Patients (PHV in the Mitral Position, Atrial Fibrillation, History of Thromboembolism, on Anticoagulation)

First 6 Weeks (from LMP)
- Warfarin (INR 2.5-3.5)

6-12 Weeks
- UFH s/c (aPTT >2.5)
  OR
- LMWH (predose anti Xa ≈ 0.7)

  + Acetylsalicylic acid 80-100 mg q.d.

12-36 Week
- Warfarin (INR 2.5-3.5)

36 Week—7 Days Postpartum

- UFH or LMWH.

Low Risk Patients (Second Generation PHV in the Aortic Position)

First 6 Weeks

- Warfarin (INR 2.5-3.0)

6-12 Weeks

- UFH s/c → (aPTT 2.0-3.0)
  OR
- LMWH (predose anti Xa ≈ 0.6)

+ Acetylsalicylic acid 80-100 mg q.d.

13-36 Weeks

- Warfarin (INR 2.5-3.0)

36 Week-7 Days Postpartum

- UFH s/c (mid- interval aPTT 2.0-3.0)
  OR
- LMWH (predose anti Xa ≈ 0.6).

Lab Monitoring

aPTT

- Initially aPTT every 6 hourly, then daily and then weekly.

INR

- Daily → till desired levels obtained on 2 consecutive days
- Then 2-3 times/week × 1-2 week
- Then 4-6 weekly.

Key Points

- If labor starts while on warfarin, vitamin K_1 5-10 mg IV infusion given over a period of 30 minutes to reverse action of warfarin
- Keep FFPs ready (if ↑↑ maternal bleeding)
- Maternal effects of warfarin can be easily reversed with FFPs but takes many hours even with vitamin K_1
- Effects of heparin can be immediately corrected by Protamine sulphate
- Heparin therapy restarted:
  – 6 hours after normal delivery
  – 12 hours after cesarean section
- Warfarin started after 3 days (because warfarin is a procoagulant in initial period and it is therefore essential that the patient is preheparinized before starting warfarin)

- Factors predicting a successful course of pregnancy and labor in patients with prosthetic valves are:
  - Adequate left ventricular function
  - Properly functioning valves
  - Effective anticoagulation
- Antibiotics is mandatory in labor because of increased risk of infective endocarditis.

Conditions Requiring Anticoagulation in Pregnancy

a. Mitral stenosis
b. Atrial fibrillation
c. Deep vein thrombosis
d. Preeclampsia in 3rd month of pregnancy
e. Peripartum cardiomyopathy in 3rd trimester.

Rheumatic Heart Disease

MITRAL STENOSIS (MS)

- In general, 2/3rd of patients are females
- Most common acquired valvular lesion encountered in pregnant women
- Almost always caused by rheumatic fever
- Normal mitral valve orifice 4-6 cm^2
- Has two leaflets—anterior and posterior, which are attached by ≈120 chordae tendinae to two papillary muscles.

Pathophysiology (Altered Anatomy)

- Leaflets: Thickened by fibrous tissue and/or calcific deposits
- Commissures: Fusion results in narrowed orifice (major cause of obstruction)
- Cusps and chordae: Thickened, stiff and shortened.

Severity of Stenosis

- Mild >1.5 cm^2
- Moderate 1-1.5 cm^2
- Severe < 1.0 cm^2
- Symptoms with exercise: ≤ 2.5 cm^2
- Symptoms at rest: ≤ 1.5 cm^2.

Effects on Whole Cardio Pulmonary Circulation Due to Mitral Stenosis

↑ in left atrial pressure → pulmonary venous hypertension → pulmonary artery hypertension → right ventricular hypertrophy → right ventricular dilatation → right ventricular failure
↓
Tricuspid valve ring dilatation → functional tricuspid regurgitation
→ left atrial dilatation → atrial fibrillation
↓
Thrombus formation → systemic embolism

↑↑ in transmitral gradient
↑ blood volume
↑ heart rate
↑ in cardiac output

↑ in blood coming from left atrium to be pumped by restricted valve
↓ in time available for ventricle filling

↓

Poorly tolerated in pregnancy—asymptomatic patients can become symptomatic and even develop pulmonary edema.

Symptoms

- Dyspnea (exertion; at rest)
- Orthopnea and paroxysmal nocturnal dyspnea → because of increase venous return to heart → ↑ pulmonary venous pressure
- Also referred to as *'Cardiac Asthma'*
- ↓ exercise capacity
- Hemoptysis → rupture of pulmonary venous connections
- Pulmonary edema (pink frothy sputum)
    - Occurs in 23% of pregnant patients with mitral stenosis
    - Occurs at a pressure of ≈ 25 mmHg in left atrium and pulmonary capillary bed (transudate can't be cleared by lymphatics)

        ↓

    - Stress on atrial wall → development of arrythmias
- Heart failure, usually progressive, occurs mainly in 2nd or 3rd trimester
- Mortality rate 0-3%
- Fetal morbidity:
    - Prematurity 20-30%
    - Intrauterine growth restriction 5-20%
    - Low birth weight
    - Fetal/neonatal death 1-3%.

On Examination

1. Malar flush with pinched and blue facies
2. Diastolic thrill at cardiac apex
3. Loud S$_1$ → HALLMARK of mitral stenosis
4. S$_2$ → split with loud pulmonary component
5. Mitral opening snap
6. Mid diastolic murmur (rough and rumbling, low pitched)
7. Mitral stenosis with functional tricuspid regurgitation → *Pansystolic murmur* → ↑ with inspiration and ↓ with expiration (*Carvallo's Sign*)
8. Mitral stenosis with pulmonary regurgitation → *Graham Steell murmur*.

Investigation

- Echocardiography: most sensitive and specific.

Management during Pregnancy

- ≤ 1.0 cm^2 → pharmacological management
- ≤ 1.4 cm^2 → expectant management.

Medical Therapy

Mainly two goals → to reduce the heart rate and reduce the left atrial pressure.

Reduction in Heart Rate

- Restriction of physical activity
- β blockers or calcium channel blockers
  - Metoprolol → preferred β blocker
  - Atenolol → IUGR, bradycardia and IUD have been reported
  - Verapamil → preferred over diltiazem
  - Diltiazem → associated with adverse fetal effects
  - Digoxin:
    - Can be used in patients with atrial fibrillation for control of ventricular rate
    - Considered safe
    - Generally well tolerated
    - Few adverse fetal effects.

Reduction of Left Atrial Pressure

1. Diuretics → furosemide (used with caution to avoid uteroplacental hypoperfusion)
2. Amiodarone is contraindicated during pregnancy.

Obstetric Management

1. Prophylactic anticoagulation can be considered in those with severe left atrial dilatation and severe mitral stenosis
2. Hemodynamic monitoring → indicated during labor and delivery in moderate to severe cases
3. Epidural anesthesia is recommended to reduce fluctuations in heart rate and cardiac output
4. Shortening of the 2nd stage of labor and assisted delivery → strongly recommended
5. Cesarean section – only for obstetric indication
6. Pulmonary artery catheter at → ≤ 1 cm².

Role of Percutaneous Balloon Mitral Valvuloplasty (PBMV)

- Indications:
  - Patients refractory to medical therapy
  - NYHA Class III/IV
  - Such cases should get it done before conception
- Most commonly, necessary after the 28th week of pregnancy
- Most patients return to NYHA I/II and remain in that class till the end of pregnancy
- Complications of PBMV:
  - Thromboemboli
  - Stroke
  - Pericardial effusion
  - Atrial arrhythmias
  - New onset mitral regurgitation
  - Severe mitral regurgitation requiring mitral valve repair or replacement is rare
  - Excessive blood loss
  - Uterine contractions

- Precipitous labor
- Unavoidable exposure to ionizing radiation:
  - Adequate pelvic and abdominal shielding necessary
  - Should be avoided in the 1st trimester
  - Must be performed by experienced operators
  - Fluoroscopy should be minimized
  - Procedure should be assisted by echocardiography and Doppler
- No role for prophylactic valvuloplasty in pregnancy
- Recommended over open mitral commissurotomy as maternal and fetal mortality is ≈ 35% with the latter.

MITRAL REGURGITATION (MR)

Etiology

- Mitral valve prolapse and RHD (most common in pregnancy)
- MR without left ventricular dysfunction → well tolerated in pregnancy.

Pathology

- Fibrosis, thickening, calcification → shortening of both leaflets and chordae → improper closure of valve cusps during systole → mitral regurgitation.

During Systole

- Blood goes from left ventricle to left atrium → left atrial blood volume ↑→ left atrium size ↑→ volume of blood returning from left atrium to left ventricle ↑.

During Diastole

- Overfilling of left ventricle → left ventricle hypertrophy and dilatation → left ventricular failure → pulmonary hypertension → failure of right ventricle.

Symptoms

- Asymptomatic for decades
- Fatigue and weakness (early)
  ↓
- Dyspnea on exertion (next)
  ↓
- Palpitations, orthopnea and paroxysmal nocturnal dyspnea (late)
  ↓
- Right heart failure (peripheral edema, tender hepatomegaly, raised JVP (very late).

Auscultation

- S_3 → severe MR
- HOLOSYSTOLIC murmur at the apex → most characteristic finding (systolic murmur of atleast grade III/VI intensity).

Management

1. Preconceptional counseling (valve replacement)
2. Recommended for:
   - Symptomatic patients
   - AF
   - Ejection fraction < 50-60%
   - LV end diastolic dimension > 45-50 mm
   - Pulmonary systolic pressure > 50-60 mm Hg
3. Medical therapy:
   - Asymptomatic
     - Regular penicillin prophylaxis (for rheumatic fever)
     - Antibiotic (for infective endocarditis)
   - Moderate MR and NYHA class II
     - Digoxin therapy
   - Moderately severe and class III
     - Digoxin
     - Diuretics
     - Salt restriction
   - Severe MR and NYHA class IV
     - Vasodilator therapy
4. Surgery:
   - Mitral valve reconstruction (valvuloplasty)
   - Replacement (mechanical or bioprosthetic valve)
5. Afterload reduction:
   - Not indicated in patients with normal or low blood pressure
   - Hydralazine and nitrates are safe and well tolerated
   - ACE inhibitors and angiotensin receptor blockers are highly teratogenic, therefore, contraindicated.

AORTIC STENOSIS (AS)

Etiology

- Congenital bicuspid aortic valve (most common cause in pregnancy)
- Rheumatic aortic valve disease (less common), occurs in combination with mitral valve disease
- Cases with subvalvular and supravalvular AS during pregnancy have been reported

Normal aortic valve area → 2.5 cm^2
Normally there should be NO gradient.

Critical Stenosis

- Valve area < 1 cm^2
- Gradient > 50 mm Hg
- Severe obstruction to left ventricular flow.

Mild AS → < 36 mm Hg
Moderate AS → 36-63 mm Hg
Severe AS → > 63 mm Hg.

Symptoms

- Usually asymptomatic.

Compensated State

- Exertional dyspnea
- Angina
- Syncope.

Decompensated State

- Orthopnea
- PND
- Pulmonary edema

LVF → severe pulmonary hypertension
↓
RVF → systemic venous hypertension/hepatomegaly/AF.

Signs

- Pulsus parvus et tardus (slow rising arterial pulse, best felt in carotids)
- Double apical impulse
- Systolic thrill
- Ejection systolic murmur (at aortic area) → HARSH (related to carotids).

Prognosis

- Mild to moderate AS (valve area >1.0 cm^2) → favorable pregnancy outcomes
- Moderate and severe aortic stenosis can develop:
    - Congestive heart failure (44%)
    - Arrhythmias (25%)
    - Increase cardiac medications (33%)
    - Hospitalization (33%)
    - Maternal mortality → rare
- Fetal complications:
    - IUGR
    - Respiratory distress
    - Prematurity
    - LBW.

Management

- In general, ≤ 60 mm Hg → uncomplicated cases
- Because most cases are congenital in origin → fetal echocardiography is indicated
- Bed rest → because they have fixed stroke volume, any activity will cause →↑ HR →↑ demand on LV
- Pregnant patients with significant AS → very sensitive to loss of preload associated with hemorrhage or epidural induced hypotension

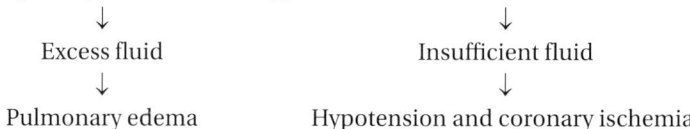

↓ ↓
Excess fluid Insufficient fluid
↓ ↓
Pulmonary edema Hypotension and coronary ischemia.

Preconceptionally

- Severely symptomatic desiring pregnancy → should undergo balloon valvuloplasty or valve replacement.

Antepartum and Intrapartum

- Mainly diuretics
- Refractory to medical management
  - Termination of pregnancy, if early, or
  - Repair of the valve by either percutaneous balloon valvuloplasty (preferred) or valve replacement (↑ fetal mortality)
- Intrapartum hemodynamic monitoring → strongly recommended
- Vaginal delivery with an assisted 2nd stage → preferred
- Epidural (produce no sympathetic blockade) and spinal anesthesia → can be used with caution
- Prolonged induction avoided (induction with favorable cervix preferably)
- Patient can be hydrated over night to achieve a PAWP of 12-15 mm Hg
- Prophylactic antibiotics
- General anesthesia → preferred technique for cesarean section
- C. section → for obstetric indication.

Postpartum

- Strict monitoring for 24-48 hours
- Diuresis → usually spontaneous
- If pulmonary edema → diuretics can be given
- Valve replacement within weeks of delivery because accelerated valve deterioration due to pregnancy is observed.

AORTIC REGURGITATION (AR)

Etiology

1. Congenital bicuspid valve
2. Previous endocarditis
3. RHD
4. Aortic annular dilation

AR without left ventricular dysfunction → usually well tolerated.

Symptoms

- Asymptomatic for decades
- Palpitations → main symptom
- Dyspnea, orthopnea, PND → late
- Angina → very late symptom.

Signs

- Collapsing/Water hammer or Corrigan's pulse (best felt on radial artery when arm is elevated)
- Pulsus bisferiens (double peak pulse)

- Hill's sign → popliteal cuff systolic pressure > brachial cuff systolic pressure by 20mm Hg
- Corrigan's neck sign → prominent carotid pulsations seen in neck
- Dancing brachialis → visible arterial pulsations over brachial artery
- Wide pulse pressure.

Auscultation

- S_3 if LVF
- S_4 if LVH
- Early diastolic murmur
- Austin flint murmur (low pitched, apical diastolic murmur)
- Ejection systolic murmur.

Management

- Rheumatic fever and infective endocarditis prophylaxis
- Role of nifedepine in asymptomatic patients with severe AR and normal LV systolic function → long term treatment helps to ↓ BP and end diastolic volume and ↑ EF → delays surgery
- Diuretics, if required.

Management Proper

- Symptomatic patients:
  - Salt restriction
  - Afterload reduction → hydralazine and nitrates
  - Diuretics
  - Digoxin.
- Asymptomatic patients:
  - Generally do well
  - Should not be considered for prophylactic valve surgery prior to pregnancy.

PULMONIC STENOSIS (PS)

Etiology

- Mostly congenital and valvular
- Can be subvalvular, supravalvular or the result of homograft deterioration as part of a Ross procedure.

Management

- Balloon valvuloplasty is rarely indicated in a pregnant patient with pulmonic stenosis
- Vaginal delivery is usually safe and well tolerated.

DUKE'S CRITERIA

Major Criteria

1. Positive blood cultures (2 separate cultures for usual pathogen, ≥ 2 for less typical pathogens) and

2. Evidence of endocarditis on echo
    - Intracardiac mass on a valve or other site
    - Regurgitant flow near a prosthesis
    - Abscess
    - Partial dehiscence of prosthetic valves
    OR
    - New valve regurgitant flow.

Minor Criteria

1. Fever
2. Embolic vascular signs
3. Immune complex phenomena
    - Glomerulonephritis
    - Arthritis
    - Rheumatoid factor
    - Osler's nodes
    - Roth spots
4. Single positive blood culture
5. Serological evidence of infection
6. Echo signs not meeting the major criteria.

Definite Endocarditis

- 2 major criteria
  OR
- 1 major + 3 minor criteria
  OR
- 5 minor criteria.

Peripartum Cardiomyopathy (PPCM)

OVERVIEW

- Defined in 1971
- Incidence: < 0.1%
- Type of dilated myopathy of unknown origin.

Definition

- An idiopathic cardiomyopathy manifested as heart failure due to left ventricular systolic dysfunction towards the end of pregnancy or in the months after delivery when no other cause of heart failure is found
- PPCM is a diagnosis of exclusion. Exclude other causes of heart failure:
    - Myocardial infarction
    - Sepsis
    - Severe preeclampsia
    - Pulmonary embolism
    - Valvular diseases
    - Other forms of cardiomyopathy.

Definitive Diagnosis

- On echocardiography, identification of new-onset heart failure during a limited period around parturition.

Risk Factors

- Increased maternal age
- Multiparity
- Multiple pregnancy
- Pregnancy complicated by preeclampsia and gestational hypertension
- Young primigravida can also have cardiomyopathy.

Etiology

PPCM is distinguished from other forms of cardiomyopathies by its occurrence during pregnancy.

Factors Implicated in Etiology

1. Viral myocarditis
2. Abnormal immune response:
   - During pregnancy, fetal cells released into the maternal bloodstream are not rejected by the mother because of the natural immune suppression that occurs during pregnancy
   - But after delivery, women lose the increased immunity and if fetal cells reside on cardiac tissue when the fetus is delivered, a pathological autoimmune response can occur, leading to PPCM in the mother after birth
3. Abnormal hemodynamic response:
   - PPCM may be due to exaggerated response of left ventricle (brief and reversible hypertrophy) in response to the physiological changes of pregnancy (↑ in blood volume and cardiac output) during 3rd trimester and early postpartum
4. Apoptosis and inflammation
   ↑ plasma inflammatory cytokines (TNF α; CRP and Fas/Apo-1)
5. ↑ Prolactin → associated with:
   a. ↑ Blood volume
   b. ↓ BP
   c. ↓ angiotensin responsiveness
   d. ↓ in the levels of H_2O, Na^+, K^+
   e. ↑ in circulating erythropoietin and hematocrit levels
6. ↓ Selenium and malnutrition → viral infections, hypertension and hypocalcemia
7. Prolonged tocolysis (β-sympathomimetic drugs for > 4 weeks) → leading to pulmonary edema.

Current Diagnostic Criteria

1. Heart failure developing in last month of pregnancy or 5 months postpartum
2. Absence of preexisting heart disease
3. Indeterminant cause
4. Echocardiographic findings (a, together with b or c; or all of these)
   a. Left ventricular end-diastolic dimension > 2.7 cm/m^2
   b. M-mode fractional shortening < 30%
   c. Left ventricular ejection fraction < 0.45.

Clinical Presentation and Diagnosis

- Occurs mostly in the first 4 months postpartum
- < 10% of cases occur antenatally
- Common symptoms:
  - Dyspnea
  - Cough
  - Orthopnea
  - Hemoptysis
  - Chest pain
  - Paroxysmal nocturnal dyspnea
  - Peripheral edema
  - Neck vein distension
  - Shortness of breath especially on lying flat or at night
  - Fatigue
  - Malaise
  - Palpitations
  - Chest and abdominal discomfort
  - Postural hypotension
  - BP often normal or ↓
  - Tachycardia
- Most affected patients have (NYHA) class III or IV function
- Common signs include:
  - Displacement of the apical impulse
  - S_3 and S_4 gallop
  - Rales
  - Hypoxia
  - Evidence of mitral or tricuspid regurgitation
  - Engorgement of neck veins, pulmonary crepitations, hepatomegaly and pedal edema may also be present.

Differential Diagnosis

- Accelerated hypertension
- Diastolic dysfunction
- Systemic infection
- Pulmonary embolus
- Obstetric complications:
  - Preeclampsia (25% of women will have hypertension)
  - Eclampsia
  - Amniotic fluid embolism.

Diagnosis and Postpartum Monitoring

Investigations

- CBC
- Serum levels of troponin
- KFT with electrolytes

- LFT
- TSH
- Diagnosis confirmation → Levels of B natriuretic peptide and N-terminal pro-B-type natriuretic peptide
- ECG:
  - No particular pathognomonic changes
  - Tracings may be normal
  - Most commonly met:
    - LV hypertrophy
    - ST-T wave abnormalities
    - Dysarrhythmias
- Doppler Echo:
  - Essential for diagnosis
  - Common findings:
    - Globally ↓ contractility
    - ↓ Ejection fraction
    - Thinned out cardiac walls
    - LV enlargement without hypertrophy
- Follow-up Echo:
  - At discharge from the hospital
  - 6 weeks postpartum
  - 6 months postpartum
  - Annually there after
- MRI:
  - Gives accurate measurements of ventricular volumes and helps identify endomyocardial biopsy sites
- Endomyocardial Biopsy:
  - Highly specific
  - Invasive procedure
  - Cannot be used as a first line diagnostic tool
  - Biopsy under MRI guidance improves accuracy
  - Can be followed up with PCR analysis of biopsy DNA extracts for viral assays or immune histochemical staining for autoantibody assays
  - Considered when:
    - Myocarditis is strongly suspected
    - No improvement is seen > 2 weeks of treatment
- Cardiac Protein Assays:
  - Not routinely done.

Management

Compensated peripartum cardiomyopathy

General Measures

- Low-sodium diet: 2 g/day
- Fluid restriction: 2 lit/day
- Light physical activity: if tolerated (e.g. walking).

Antepartum Management

β blocker

Carvedilol
- Starting dose 3.125 mg bid
- Target dose 25 mg twice a day.

Extended-release metoprol
- Starting dose 0.125 mg daily
- Target dose 0.25 mg daily.

Vasodilator

Hydralazine
- Starting dose 10 mg tid
- Target dose 40 mg tid.

Digoxin
- Starting dose 0.125 mg daily
- Target dose 0.25 mg daily
- Monitor serum levels.

Thiazide diuretic
- Hydrochlorothiazide 12.5-50 mg daily
- To be used with caution.

Low-molecular-weight heparin if LVEF < 35%.

Postpartum Management

Angiotensin-converting Enzyme (ACE) Inhibitor

Captopril
- Starting dose 6.25-12.5 mg tid
- Target dose 25-50 mg 3 tid.

Enalapril
- Starting dose 1.25-2.5 mg bid
- Target dose 10 mg bid.

Ramipril
- Starting dose 1.25-2.5 mg bid
- Target dose 5 mg bid.

Lisinopril
- Starting dose 2.5-5 mg daily
- Target dose 25-40 mg daily.

Angiotensin-receptor Blocker (if ACE Inhibitor not Tolerated)

Candesartan
- Starting dose 2 mg daily
- Target dose 32 mg daily.

Valsartan
- Starting dose 40 mg bid
- Target dose 160 mg bid.

Consider nitrates or hydralazine if woman is intolerant to ACE inhibitor and angiotensin-receptor blocker.

Loop Diuretic
Furosemide 20-80 mg (depending upon GFR).

Vasodilator
Hydralazine
- Starting dose 37.5 mg tid or qid
- Target dose 40 mg tid.

Isorbide dinitrate
- Starting dose 20 mg tid
- Target dose 40 mg tid.

Aldosterone Antagonist
Spironolactone
- Starting dose 12.5 mg daily
- Target dose 25-50 mg daily.

Eplerenone
- Starting dose 12.5 mg daily
- Target dose 25-50 mg daily.

β Blocker (As Above)

Warfarin if ejection fraction <35%.

Decompensated heart failure

OVERVIEW

Airway
- Intubation.

Breathing
- Adequate O_2 with continuous pulse oximeter
- ABG every 4-6 h until breathing is stable.

Circulation
- BP monitoring
- Central venous access
- Continuous fetal monitoring in antepartum cases.

Pharmacological Management

Intravenous Loop Diuretic
- Furosemide 20-80 mg depending on GFR (creatinine clearance)
- Reduce preload and treat pulmonary congestion or peripheral edema

- Both hydrochlorothiazide and furosemide are safe during pregnancy and lactation
- However, diuretic-induced dehydration can cause uterine hypoperfusion and maternal metabolic acidosis, so bicarbonate monitoring and management with acetazolamide are needed
- Potassium-sparing diuretic, spironolactone, has been used successfully to treat heart failure but data is scant regarding its safety in pregnancy, therefore use with caution.

Vasodilators

- Hydralazine is safe during pregnancy and is the primary vasodilator drug antepartum
- More severe cases warrant the use of intravenous nitroglycerin starting at 10 to 20 µg/min and continuing up to 200 µg/min
- Nitroprusside is not recommended because of the potential for cyanide toxicity.

Inotropic Agents

- Milrinone: 0.125-0.5 µg/kg/min
- Dobutamine: 2.5-10 µg/kg/min
- Warranted only in cases of severe low output and the patient should be weaned from them as soon as she is hemodynamically stable
- Levosimendan reduces pulmonary capillary wedge pressure and improves cardiac output of peripartum cardiomyopathy patients
- Until adequate safety data are available, levosimendan should be avoided antepartum and lactation should be held
- Since pregnant women are systemically vasoconstricted, vasopressors such as norepinephrine are usually avoided antepartum.

Digoxin

- An inotropic and dromotropic agent
- Safe to use during pregnancy
- The scarcity of available antepartum drug options and the increased hemodynamic loads during late pregnancy make digoxin an easy choice.

β-Blockers

- Crucial for long-term management of systolic dysfunction
- Although safe during pregnancy, $β_1$-selective blockers are preferred over nonselective β-blockers to avoid anti-tocolytic action induced by $β_2$-receptor blockade
- Carvedilol combined with a blockade to restrict peripheral vasoconstriction has been shown to be effective in peripartum cardiomyopathy
- Patients receiving these drugs are weaned from them when ventricular function normalizes, within 6 to 12 months.

Calcium Channel Blockers

- Dihydropyridines, such as amlodipine, have been shown to successfully reduce interleukin-6 levels in heart-failure patients but concomitant uterine hypoperfusion requires cautious use of these agents.

Neurohormonal Blockade

- Angiotensin-modulating agents are considered first-line drugs for heart-failure management
- Angiotensin-converting enzyme inhibitors and angiotensin receptor blockers improve survival but are contraindicated in pregnancy
- Also, since they are secreted in breast milk, breastfeeding must be stopped before commencing therapy.

Other Measures

- Heparin sodium, alone or with oral warfarin (Coumadin) therapy
- ABG every 4-6 h until patient's condition is stable
- Consider endomyocardial biopsy
- If proven viral myocarditis, consider immunosuppressive medications (azathioprine, corticosteroids).

Assist Devices

- Intra-aortic balloon pump
- Left ventricular assist devices
- Extracorporeal membrane oxygenation
- Transplantation.

If a woman remains refractory to therapy, consider suppression of lactation.

Arrhythmia Management

- Atrial fibrillation → most common arrhythmia in patients with peripartum cardiomyopathy
- First line therapy (safe in pregnancy)
    - Quinidine
    - Procainamide
    - Digoxin
- Refractory cases
    - Placement of:
        - Permanent pacemakers
        - Implantable cardioverter defibrillators.

Prognosis

- Recovery is defined as recovery of LVEF to ≥ 0.50
- Usually occurs between 3-6 months postpartum, but might occur as late as 48 months postpartum
- Causes of delayed recovery:
    - Delayed diagnosis
    - Higher NYHA functional class
    - Black ethnicity
    - LV thrombus
    - Multiparity
    - Coexisting medical illnesses
    - High troponin levels at baseline

- Recurrence:
  - High
  - LVEF, once improved, can worsen again.

Congenital Heart Disease (CHD)

OVERVIEW
- Most common birth defects in humans
- Prevalence: 0.8% of all live births.

Preconception Counseling
- Consult cardiologist and obstetrician before pregnancy
- Absolute contraindications of pregnancy should be discussed with patients
- CHD and Maternal Risk in Pregnancy:
  - 30% of all miscarriages are due to CHD
  - Enquire about exposure to teratogens and non-cardiac diagnosis associated with the risk for CHD (Lupus; Phenylketonuria)
  - If mother has CHD, child has a 5-6% risk to be born with CHD
  - If father has CHD, child has a 2-3% risk to be born with CHD
  - 3-5% of CHD are associated with recognizable genetic syndromes, rest seems to be sporadic.

Antenatal Measures
- 1st antenatal visit, as early as possible after conception
- Subsequent visits: every 2-4 weeks until 20 weeks, then every two weeks until 24 weeks, and then weekly thereafter (RCOG 2011).

At each visit ask about the following:
- Shortness of breath (especially at night)
- Exercise tolerance (can patient still climb stairs or walk at her normal pace)
- Palpitations (irregular heart beat)
- Pulse rate and rhythm
- Lung auscultation (for pulmonary edema), auscultate the heart (to detect any changes in murmurs which might indicate a deterioration in the functioning of a valve, or infection of the heart)
- BP, edema, uterine height
- Fetal echo → Indications:
  - Familial or syndromic CHD in parents
  - An abnormal level II ultrasound
  - Presence of polyhydramnios.

Intrapartum and Postpartum Measures
- Natural birth → safest route
- Good pain relief (epidural)
- Cut short 2nd stage (vacuum, forceps)
- C. section only for obstetric indication

- Heparins to prevent deep vein thrombosis
- Contraception.

ACYANOTIC HEART DEFECTS (WITH LEFT TO RIGHT SHUNT)

Atrial Septal Defect (ASD)

- One of the most common congenital defects seen in pregnant women
- Mostly asymptomatic before pregnancy
- In pregnancy: due to volume retention in pregnancy, ↑↑ RV volume overload and enlargement → atrial arrhythmias
- Complications:
  Cardiac
  - Arrhythmias
  - Persistent decline in NYHA functional status

  Obstetric
  Unrepaired cases:
  - Preeclampsia
  - IUD
  - SGA fetus

  Repaired cases:
  - Risk not increased.

Ventricular Septal Defect (VSD)

- Commonly encountered as an isolated defect
- Large defects → significant LV volume overload and heart failure early in life and are generally repaired in childhood
- As a result, most unrepaired defects encountered in the adult population are small
- Complications:
  - Miscarriage
  - Preeclampsia
  - Preterm labor.

Patent Ductus Arteriosus (PDA)

- Tolerate pregnancy well
- If no pulmonary hypertension → surgical management can be undertaken in pregnancy
- Epidural analgesia → better avoided
- Pulmonary hypertension → may even lead to death.

ACYANOTIC HEART DEFECTS (WITHOUT SHUNT)

Congenital Aortic Stenosis

- Common congenital anamoly
- May escape detection in childhood
- Obstruction to aortic outflow → LV hypertrophy and "preload dependence"

- Risk to mother or fetus varies according to severity of lesion
- Most common complications: heart failure and atrial arrhythmias
- Premature delivery and SGA births are common
- In cases of symptomatic, severe aortic stenosis presenting during pregnancy, balloon aortic valvuloplasty in the 2nd trimester is helpful.

Pulmonic Stenosis

- Relatively uncommon
- Many patients remain asymptomatic throughout childhood and early adulthood
- RV outflow obstruction → RV hypertrophy, so patients may be sensitive to the volume overload that occurs during pregnancy and may be expected to have a risk for atrial arrhythmias
- Otherwise pregnancy is well tolerated, even in patients with severe stenosis
- Studies have shown an increased risk of:
  - Miscarriage (19.4%)
  - Preterm birth (16%)
  - CHD among offspring (3.7%).

Coarctation of Aorta

- Results in upper extremity hypertension → difficult to control during pregnancy
- Excessive blood pressure lowering in the upper extremities may result in hypotension distal to obstruction and uterine hypoperfusion. Therefore, hemodynamically significant coarctation should be repaired before pregnancy is intended
- Coarctation may also lead to aortic dissection
- Most common cause of death in pregnancy → aortic rupture
- Elective cesarean section → in unrepaired defect.

CYANOTIC HEART DEFECTS (RIGHT TO LEFT SHUNT)

- Overall maternal mortality with unrepaired cyanotic heart disease → in 2% of cases
- Complications (arrhythmias, heart failure, infective endocarditis) → in 30%
- Patients with chronic cyanosis are at risk for both thrombotic and hemorrhagic complications
- Ensuring proper hydration throughout pregnancy and the use of compression stockings may alleviate thrombotic complications
- Prophylactic anticoagulation is reasonable in the puerperium
- Fetal complications in chronic cyanosis:
  - Spontaneous abortion (50%)
  - Premature delivery (30–50%)
  - SGA birth.

Eisenmenger Syndrome

- Maternal mortality rate is ≈ 40–50%
- Miscarriage rate ≈ 30%
- Patients should be strictly counseled not to become pregnant
- Non hormonal birth control option should be offered
- If pregnancy occurs → elective termination at the earliest.

Tetralogy of Fallot (TOF)

- Most common cyanotic congenital cardiac defect in human
- Consists of:
  - Ventricular septal defect
  - Pulmonary valve stenosis
  - Right ventricular hypertrophy
  - An overriding aorta
- Should ideally be evaluated completely before pregnancy
- Pregnancy should be delayed if pulmonic valve replacement is indicated
- Maximum patients with TOF will have had intracardiac repair already done (consisting of a ventricular septal defect patch and enlargement of the RV infundibulum)
  - Enlargement of RV infundibulum is associated with a high incidence of pulmonic insufficiency, particularly when a transannular patch is used
  - This results in RV volume overload and enlargement → an increased risk of right heart failure and arrhythmias during pregnancy
- General overall risks:
  - Infertility
  - Sub fertility
  - Menstrual disorders
- Maternal risks:
  - Clinically significant arrhythmia
  - Heart failure
  - Deterioration of NYHA class
- Obstetrical complications:
  - Miscarriage
  - Premature rupture of membranes
  - Prolonged 2nd stage of labor
  - PPH
- Fetal risks are highest in patients with severe pulmonary regurgitation and with RV systolic dysfunction:
  - Preterm labor
  - Congenital cardiac defects in the offspring can be found
  - Fetal and neonatal mortality
- Management:
  - The Fontan operation was introduced as a palliative procedure for patients with tricuspid atresia and has since been used extensively to address a range of defects characterized by a single functional ventricle
  - The basic Fontan repair directs systemic venous blood into the pulmonary artery such that it bypasses the right heart. Systemic venous pressures are therefore elevated and equal to mean pulmonary arterial pressure
  - Patients with Fontan physiology are typically sensitive to preload changes and are at risk for edema, ascites, and arrhythmias during pregnancy.

AORTIC DISEASES

Genetic disorders involving the risk of aortic dissection or rupture during pregnancy are:
1. Marfan syndrome
2. The vascular subtype (IV) of Ehlers-Danlos syndrome

3. The Loeys-Dietz syndrome, a recently recognized familial thoracic aortic aneurysm syndrome caused by a mutation in the *tgf-β* gene with autosomal dominant inheritance.

Marfan Syndrome

- Patients with:
  An aortic root diameter of > 4.0 cm
    - Have a 10% risk of dissection during pregnancy
  Normal aortic root diameters
    - Have a risk for dissection of ≈1%
  Diameter > 4.7 cm
    - Should undergo elective surgical repair before pregnancy
- Aortic root diameter < 4.5 cm
    - Early epidural anesthesia and assisted 2nd stage of labor are recommended as there is an increased incidence of dural ectasia in these patients
- Aortic root diameter ≥ 4.5 cm
    - Elective cesarean delivery is recommended.

Loeys-Dietz Syndrome

- Patients appear to be at risk for dissection even in the absence of prior progressive aortic enlargement
- While successful pregnancy and delivery have been reported, the absolute risk remains unclear
- Therefore, considered as a contraindication to pregnancy.

When a fetal cardiac anomaly is suspected, it is mandatory to obtain the following:
1. A full fetal echocardiography to evaluate cardiac structure and function, arterial and venous flow, and rhythm
2. Detailed scanning of the fetal anatomy to look for associated anomalies (particularly the digits and bones)
3. Family history to search for familial syndromes
4. Maternal medical history to identify chronic medical disorders, viral illnesses or teratogenic medications
5. Fetal karyotype
6. Referral to a maternal–fetal medicine specialist, pediatric cardiologist, geneticist, and/or neonatologist to discuss prognosis, obstetric, and neonatal management, and further options
7. Delivery at an institution that can provide neonatal cardiac care, if needed.

Labor Induction

- Oxytocin and artificial rupture of the membranes are indicated when the Bishop score is favorable. A long induction time should be avoided if the cervix is unfavorable
- While there is no absolute contraindication to misoprostol or dinoprostone, there is a theoretical risk of coronary vasospasm and a low risk of arrhythmias
- Dinoprostone also has more profound effects on BP than prostaglandin E_1 and is, therefore contraindicated in active CVD
- Mechanical methods such as a Foley catheter would be preferable to pharmacological agents, particularly in the patient with cyanosis where a drop in systemic vascular resistance and / or BP would be detrimental.

Delivery—Vaginal or Cesarean

- Vaginal delivery is associated with less blood loss and infection risk compared with cesarean delivery, which also increases the risk of venous thrombosis and thromboembolism
- Cesarean delivery is generally reserved for obstetric indications
- Cesarean delivery should be considered for the following:
  - Patient on oral anticoagulants (OACs) in preterm labor
  - Patients with Marfan syndrome and an aortic diameter > 45 mm
  - Patients with acute or chronic aortic dissection
  - Those in acute intractable heart failure
  - In Marfan, patients with an aortic diameter 40–45 mm
  - In women with severe aortic stenosis (AS) and those with severe forms of pulmonary hypertension (including Eisenmenger syndrome), or acute heart failure
  - May be considered in patients with mechanical heart valve prostheses to prevent problems with planned vaginal delivery.

Cardiac Arrest in Pregnancy

Key Interventions

- Start CPR with chest compression (CAB [circulation, airway, breathing] instead of ABC [airway, breathing, circulation])
- Place the woman on hard surface in left lateral position (15°-30° tilt)
- Establish IV access and administer fluids using upper extremity veins
- Consider the possible cause of cardiac arrest to ease targeted management.

Airway and Breathing

- Ventilate with 100% oxygen
- Apply continuous cricoid pressure during ventilation and intubation due to the risk of regurgitation
- Start with two rescue breaths of one second each
- Bag-mask ventilation at a rate of 8-10 breaths/min, during pauses of compressions (synchronization)
- Synchronization between chest compressions and ventilation is not necessary with an advanced airway (endotracheal tube) in place
- Hyperventilation is harmful and should be avoided.

Circulation

- Chest compressions are performed higher than in non-pregnant patients, slightly above the center of the sternum due to the elevated diaphragm and abdominal contents
- "Push fast and hard"! Place the heel of one hand on the center of the chest. Place the other hand on top
- Interlock the fingers and compress the chest at a rate of 100/ min, a depth of 4-5 cm and equal compression : relaxation times
- It is recommended that the CPR operator be changed every 2 minutes

- Incorrectly applied cardiac compressions in pregnant patients may lead to:
  - Liver laceration
  - Uterine rupture
  - Hemothorax
  - Hemopericardium
- A single dose of vasopressin 40 units is an alternative to repeated epinephrine injection
- Amiodarone 300 mg IV has replaced lidocaine for treatment of ventricular arrhythmias.

Defibrillation

- Survival rates are highest with immediate CPR and defibrillation within 3 to 5 minutes of a witnessed pulseless ventricular tachycardia or fibrillation
- Electric cardioversion during pregnancy appears to be safe for the fetus.

Emergency Delivery

- If cardiac arrest is not immediately (4-5 minutes) reversed by basic and advanced life support, emergency hysterotomy (or cesarean delivery, even if fetus is dead) should be performed at >20 pregnancy weeks
- Hysterotomy ideally should be performed no longer than 4-5 minutes after initiation of CPR.

SUGGESTED READING

1. Aleksey Kazmin, Facundo Garcia-Bournissen, Gideon Koren. Risks of Statin Use During Pregnancy: A Systematic Review, J Obstet Gynaecol Can. 2007;29(11):906-8.
2. Anirban Bhattacharyya, Sukhdeep Singh Basra, Priyanka Sen. Peripartum Cardiomyopathy: A Review, Tex Heart Inst J. 2012;39(1):8-16.
3. Cardiac Disease and Pregnancy: Royal College of Obstetricians and Gynaecologists, Good Practice No. 13, June 2011.
4. Chin-Leng Poh, Chi-Hang Lee. Acute Myocardial Infarction in Pregnant Women, Ann Acad Med Singapore. 2010;39:247-53.
5. Farida Mary Jeejeebhoy. Prosthetic heart valves and management during pregnancy, Canadian Family Physician, Vol 55, Feb 2009.
6. Fatoumah Alabdulrazzaq, Gideon Koren. Fetal safety of calcium channel blockers, Canadian Family Physician, Vol 58, July 2012.
7. Gregory AL Davies, William NP Herbert. Acquired Heart Disease in Pregnancy, J Obstet Gynaecol Can. 2007;29(6):507-9.
8. Gregory AL Davies, William NP Herbert. Congenital Heart Disease in Pregnancy, J Obstet Gynaecol Can. 2007;29(5):409-14.
9. Gregory AL Davies, William NP Herbert. Ischemic Heart Disease and Cardiomyopathy in Pregnancy, JOGC, July 2007.
10. Gregory AL Davies, William NP Herbert. Prosthetic Heart Valves and Arrhythmias in Pregnancy, J Obstet Gynaecol Can. 2007;29(8):635-9.
11. Humza T Malika, Amir H Sepehripourb, Alex R Shipolini. Is there a suitable method of anticoagulation in pregnant patients with mechanical prosthetic heart valves? Interactive CardioVascular and Thoracic Surgery. 2012;15:484-8.
12. Ian S Harris. Management of Pregnancy in Patients with Congenital Heart Disease, Prog Cardiovasc Dis. 2011;53(4):305-11.
13. JCS Joint Working Group: Guidelines for Indication and Management of Pregnancy and Delivery in Women With Heart Disease (JCS 2010), Circ J. 2012;76:240-60.

14. Leah Johnson-Coyle, Louise Jensen, Alan Sobey. Peripartum Cardiomyopathy: Review and Practice Guidelines, Am J Crit Care. 2012;21:89-98.
15. PhilippeCharron,MichaelArad,Eloisa Arbustini,etal. Geneticcounselingandtestingincardiomyopathies: a position statement of the European Society of Cardiology Working Group on Myocardial and Pericardial Diseases, European Heart Journal. 2010;31:2715-28.
16. Qi Fu, Benjamin D. Levine: Autonomic Circulatory Control during Pregnancy in Humans, Semin Reprod Med. 2009 July;27(4):330-7.
17. Shobana Chandrasekhar, Christopher R Cook, Charles D Collard. Cardiac Surgery in the Parturient, Anesth Analg. 2009;108:777-85.
18. Sujethra Vasu, K Stergiopoulos. Valvular Heart Disease in Pregnancy, Hellenic J Cardiol. 2009;50:498-510.
19. Tiberiu Ezri, Shmuel Lurie, Carolyn F Weiniger. Cardiopulmonary Resuscitation in the Pregnant Patient—An Update, IMAJ , Vol. 13 May 2011.
20. Vera Regitz-Zagrosek, Carina Blomstrom Lundqvist, et al. ESC Guidelines on the management of cardiovascular diseases during pregnancy, European Heart Journal. 2011;32:3147-97.
21. Vera Regitz-Zagrosek, Ute Seeland, Annette Geibel-Zehender, et al. Cardiovascular Diseases in Pregnancy, Dtsch Arztebl Int. 2011;108(16):267-73.

CHAPTER 15

Pyrexia in Pregnancy

Tania G Singh, Earl Jaspal

MALARIA

Pregnancy associated malaria – also known as **placental malaria**
- P. falciparum - the most dangerous species of malaria and causes the vast majority of deaths worldwide
- In Indian subcontinent, infection with P. vivax is more likely and this can cause a relapsing type of malaria
- P. ovale can also cause relapsing malaria
- P. malariae is unique, owing to late recrudescence after many years.

Epidemiology of Malaria in Pregnancy
- Globally ≥125 million pregnant women per year are at risk of malarial infection
- Pregnancy related malaria causes around 100,000 infant deaths each year, due in large part to low birth weight and around 10,000 maternal deaths
- Sub-Saharan Africa has the largest burden of malarial disease, with over 90% of the world's malaria-related deaths occurring in this region
- Pregnant women are 3 times more likely to develop malaria
- Highest number of cases occurring in 2nd trimester
- Region of central India is exposed to both *P. falciparum* and *P. vivax* species
- In India, *P. falciparum* is responsible for the majority of malaria episodes in pregnant women (≈ 2/3rd) with the remainder due to *P. vivax*.

Causal Agents in Pregnancy

Protozoan parasites:
- P. falciparum (most common; with the 1st pregnancy at a higher risk, irrespective of parity)
- P. vivax
- P. malariae
- P. ovale
- P. knowlesi (extremely rarely).

Factors Affecting Mosquito Breeding
- Temperature
- Humidity
- Rainfall.

Transmission

- By the bite of a sporozoite-bearing female anopheline mosquito.

Human Infection (Route of Transmission)

- On contact (bite) with the human skin → gametocytes in the mosquito fuse and sporozoites develop → sporozoites → transferred from the saliva of the mosquito → into the capillary bed of the host → within hours the parasite migrates to the human liver (pre-erythrocytic development) → liver cell ruptures and merozoite releases → enters the bloodstream → parasite invades the erythrocyte → undergoes asexual reproduction → develop into gametocytes → consumes hemoglobin → alters the red cell membrane → these infected erythrocytes stick inside the small blood vessels of brain, kidneys and other affected organs (resulting in cerebral malaria, renal failure and thrombocytopenia) → with this also adhere the uninfected erythrocytes (resetting) → interfere with microcirculatory flow and metabolism of vital organs.
- Falciparum malaria (most dangerous) - Hallmark in pregnancy → parasites aggregate in the placenta → adhere to chondroitin sulfate A (CSA) on placental proteoglycans causing them to accumulate in the intervillous spaces of the placenta → block the crucial flow of nutrients from mother to fetus.
- P. falciparum → creates immunoglobulin complexes and increased production of tumour necrosis factor. Also these adhered parasites evade host defence mechanisms: splenic processing and filtration → folic acid deficiency and microcytic anemia → at higher risk of developing congestive heart failure, fetal demise and mortality associated with PPH.
- Placental manifestation → maximum in women with highest levels of immunity. How? May not demonstrate symptoms → will not receive treatment → will build a higher placental parasite burden.
 Maternal anemia → stillbirth, intrauterine growth restriction, low-birth-weight neonates →↑ risk for neonatal and newborn death.
 Infected erythrocytes in the placenta → stimulate pancreatic β-cell production of insulin → hyperinsulinemia and hypoglycemia, contributing to the severity of disease during pregnancy.
 Case reports confusing malaria infection with HELLP syndrome demonstrate the overlap in clinical and laboratory findings between the 2 diseases and the importance of proper diagnosis.

Sequestration is not known to occur in the benign malarias due to
- P. vivax
- P. ovale
- P. malariae.

Incubation Period

- From time of insect bite till the development of clinical symptoms → 7-30 days.

In pregnancy, the adverse effects of malaria infection result from:
The systemic infection
- Maternal and fetal mortality
- Miscarriage
- Stillbirth
- Premature birth.

The parasitisation itself
- Fetal growth restriction
- Low birth weight
- Maternal and fetal anemia
- Interaction with HIV
- Susceptibility of the infant to malaria.

The continued public health burden of malaria is due to a combination of factors, including:
- Increasing resistance of malarial parasites to chemotherapy
- Increasing resistance of the Anopheles mosquito vector to insecticides
- Ecologic and climate changes
- Increasing international travel to malaria-endemic areas by nonimmune travellers.

Prevention

Roll Back Malaria (RBM), a supporting agency of WHO, recommends a three prong approach to reduce malaria in pregnancy:
1. Effective case management
2. Insecticide-treated bed nets (ITN)
3. Intermittent presumptive treatment (IPTp) with antimalarial medications:
    - Administration of 2 doses of sulfadoxine-pyrimethamine (ITPp-SP) prophylaxis after 20 weeks of gestation (one during each 2nd and 3rd trimester)
    - Full treatment course of 1.5 gm sulphadoxine and 75 mg pyrimethamine
    - Reduces subclinical malarial load
    - Proven to be very efficacious with very little side effects
    - IPTp can reduce neonatal mortality by > 60%
    - Has a long half life → allows for single dose regimens which can be closely monitored and administered
    - Effective in both clearing parasites from the placenta and preventing new infections of malaria
    - There are concerns about increased resistance to SP treatment, so drug policies should be reevaluated
    - Inexpensive and can be easily delivered to the patients
    - It can be given under direct observation which can guarantee adherence and limit resistance
    - India does have SP in their current drug policy; however, SP is only used as a second line of treatment and is not readily available for pregnant women
    - Further, SP may not be effective in certain states like Assam that have reported SP resistance
    - In this case, use of Artemisinin combination therapy may be considered once the safety profile for pregnancy is established
    - The Indian government has realized the importance of this issue and is currently in the process of expanding and updating their malaria drug policy.

1. **Define complicated and uncomplicated malaria?**

    Classification

    Complicated
    Generally caused by *P. Falciparum*

May manifest as:
- Cerebral malaria
- Hemolysis
- Severe anemia (medical emergency)
- Pulmonary edema
- Acute respiratory distress syndrome
- Thrombocytopenia
- Renal failure
- Cardiovascular collapse

≥ 2% of RBCs are infected (can be even < 2% but severe).

Uncomplicated
< 2% of RBCs are infected with no signs of severity or complications.
Has 2 stages:

Cold stage
- Cold sensation
- Shivering.

Hot stage
- Fever
- Headache
- Sweating
- Seizures (occasionally)
  Symptoms generally last for 6 to 10 hours and occur every 2 to 3 days, depending on the infecting species.

2. **Describe features of complicated malaria**
   Pregnant women with malaria may present with normal symptoms, they may be asymptomatic or may present with flu like symptoms → attribute to the delay in diagnosing →↑ complications.

Features

Clinical
- Fever – intermittent with or without periodicity or continuous
- Chills/rigors
- Headache
- Myalgia
- Arthralgia
- Nausea/vomiting
- Diarrhea
- Cough
- Jaundice
- Perspiration
- Pallor
- Splenomegaly
- Respiratory distress.

Following symptoms may or may not be present, therefore, rule out other causes:
- Running nose, cough and other signs of respiratory infection
- Diarrhea/dysentery

- Burning micturition and/or lower abdominal pain
- Skin rash/infections
- Impaired consciousness/convulsions
- Abscess
- Painful swelling of joints
- Ear discharge
- Lymphadenopathy
- Pulmonary edema
- Shock (BP < 90/60 mm Hg)
- Abnormal bleeding → DIC.

Laboratory
- Hemoglobinuria (without G6PD deficiency)
- Severe anemia (Hemoglobin < 8.0 g/dL)
- Thrombocytopenia
- Hypoglycemia (< 2.2 mmol/L)
- Acidosis (pH < 7.3)
- Renal impairment (oliguria < 0.4 mL/kg body weight/hour or creatinine > 265 µmol/L)
- Hyperlactatemia (correlates with mortality)
- Hyperparasitemia (> 2% parasitized red blood cells)
- 'Algid malaria' - Gram-negative septicemia
- Lumbar puncture to exclude meningitis.

Diagnosis

1. Microscopy:
   - Of thick and thin blood smears (gold standard)
   - The advantages of microscopy are:
     - The sensitivity is high. It is possible to detect malarial parasites at low densities. It also helps to quantify the parasite load
     - It is possible to distinguish the various species of malaria parasite and their different stages
2. Examination of placenta at delivery → to assess the true burden of disease
   Rapid diagnostic tests (RDTs) should be used.

Important Points Regarding RDTs

- Based on detection of circulating parasite antigens or enzymes
- Can detect 1 or more species
- Very helpful in locations where microscopy results may not be available within 24 hours
- May miss low parasitemia
- Relatively insensitive in *P.vivax* malaria
- A positive rapid diagnostic test should be followed by microscopy to quantify the number of infected red blood cells (parasitemia) and to confirm the species and the stage of parasites
- The rapid diagnostic tests should not replace blood films, which should always be prepared, even if they cannot immediately be read
- Produced by different companies, so there may be differences in the contents and in the manner in which the test is done (user's manual should always be consulted before use)
- Results to be read at the specified time

- Expiry date should be properly checked
- Proper storage is important.

In a febrile patient, three negative malaria smears 12–24 hours apart rules out the diagnosis of malaria.

Other important prognostic factors that should be reported on a peripheral blood smear result are:
- The presence and count of mature trophozoites and schizonts of *P. falciparum*
- Finding malaria pigment in more than 5% of the polymorphonuclear leucocytes in the peripheral blood film.

Treatment

Uncomplicated Malaria

Admit in hospital
General recommendations:
- Avoid starting treatment on an empty stomach. The first dose should be given under observation. Dose should be repeated if vomiting occurs within 30 minutes
- For vomiting, metoclopramide can be given even in 1st trimester
- If persistent vomiting, **stop** oral therapy
- The patient should also be examined for concomitant illnesses
- If there is no provision for diagnostic tests but the signs and symptoms are suggestive of malaria, start treatment with chloroquine in full therapeutic dose. It should be considered as **'clinical malaria'**.
    1. *P. falciparum malaria*
        - Oral quinine 600mg tds
        +
        - Oral clindamycin 450 mg tid

        × 7 days (can be taken together)

        In case of persistent vomiting
        - Quinine 10 mg/kg IV in 5% dextrose over 4 hours × 8 hourly
        +
        - Inj. Clindamycin 450 mg IV × 8 hourly
            - When vomiting stops, therapy including quinine and clindamycin to be given orally for complete 7 days.
    2. *For all other species*
        - Tab. Chloroquine in full therapeutic dose of 25 mg/kg divided over 3 days.
    3. *Mixed infections with P. falciparum*
        - Treated as P. falciparum malaria.
    4. *Resistant P. vivax*
        - Treated as P. falciparum malaria.

Relapse

- Relapse rate in India is ≈ 30% (due to the presence of hypnozoites in the liver).
- Prevention of relapse:

In pregnancy
- Tab. Chloroquine 300 mg orally weekly until delivery.

Nonpregnant
- Primaquine at a dose of 0.25 mg/kg daily for 14 days (to be given under supervision)

- Stop immediately if:
  - Dark colored urine
  - Yellow conjunctiva
  - Bluish discoloration of lips
  - Abdominal pain
  - Nausea
  - Vomiting
- Contraindication to primaquine → **Pregnancy** and G6PD deficiency (leads to hemolysis).

Artemisinin Combination Therapy (ACT)

- Consists of an artemisinin derivative + Long acting antimalarial (amodiaquine, lumefantrine, mefloquine or sulfadoxine-pyrimethamine)
- National programme in India → artesunate + sulfadoxine-pyrimethamine
- Presently, Artemether + Lumefantrine fixed dose combination and blister pack of artesunate + mefloquine are also available in India
- Artemisinin derivatives must never be administered as monotherapy for uncomplicated malaria
- These rapidly acting drugs, if used alone, can lead to development of parasite resistance
- ACTs can be given in the 2nd and 3rd trimester of pregnancy.

Complicated (Severe) Malaria

1. Admit in ICU
2. Artesunate (IV)
   - Drug of choice in complicated cases
   - Potent and rapidly-acting blood schizontocide
   - Derived from the leaves of the Chinese herb, Armesia annua
   - Exact mode of action is not clear
   - Excretion: elimination half-life is ≈ 45 min after IV administration
   - Interactions:
     - Antimalarial potentiating action seen with mefloquine, primaquine and tetracycline
     - Additive effect with chloroquine
     - Antagonistic effect with pyrimethamine and sulphonamides
   - Adverse reactions (not common):
     - Transient and reversible reticulocytopenia
     - Drug fever
     - Rash
     - Bradycardia
     - Transient 1st-degree heart block
     - Reversible elevation of serum transaminases
     - Contraindications: hypersensitivity
3. If not available, use IV quinine
4. Severe manifestations can develop in P. falciparum infection over a span of time as short as 12 – 24 hours and may lead to death, if not treated promptly and adequately.

Clinical Features

- Impaired consciousness/coma
- Repeated generalized convulsions

- Renal failure (s. creatinine >3 mg/dL)
- Jaundice (serum bilirubin >3 mg/dL)
- Severe anemia (Hb <5 g/dL)
- Pulmonary edema /acute respiratory distress syndrome
- Hypoglycemia (plasma glucose <40 mg/dL)
- Metabolic acidosis
- Circulatory collapse/shock (Systolic BP < 80 mm Hg)
- Abnormal bleeding and DIC
- Hemoglobinuria
- Hyperthermia (temperature >104° F)
- Hyperparasitemia (>5% parasitized RBCs in low endemic and >10% in hyperendemic areas).

Requirements for Management of Complications

- Parenteral antimalarials, antibiotics, anticonvulsants, antipyretics
- Intravenous infusion equipment and fluids
- Special nursing for patients in coma
- Blood transfusion
- Well-equipped laboratory
- Oxygen.

Treatment

- Parenteral artemisinin derivatives or quinine should be used irrespective of chloroquine sensitivity.

Any Species

Inj. Artesunate
- 2.4 mg/kg IV or IM (after diluting the powder in 5% sodium bicarbonate provided in the pack)
- At '0' hours
  ↓
- At 12 hours
  ↓
- At 24 hours
  ↓
- Then once a day

  OR

Quinine
Loading Dose
- 20 mg/kg IV infusion in 5% dextrose/dextrose saline over a period of 4 hours (infusion rate not to exceed 5mg/kg/hr).

Maintenance Dose
- 10 mg/kg 8 hourly.

Note:

- Loading dose of 20 mg/kg should not be given, if the patient has already received quinine
- Never give bolus injection of quinine

- If parenteral quinine therapy needs to be continued beyond 48 hours:
  - Dose should be reduced to 7 mg/kg 8 hourly OR
  - Dose should be reduced to 12 hourly dosing
- Maximum quinine dose → 1.4 gm
- Recommended treatment in the 1st trimester of pregnancy
- To be avoided in the 2nd and 3rd trimesters, as it is associated with recurrent hypoglycemia
- Once the patient can take oral therapy, the further follow-up treatment should be as below:
  - Quinine 10 mg/kg tid
    +
  - Clindamycin 10 mg/kg body weight bid
  } × 7 days
- Hospitalization with quinine is justified as it has the following significant side effects and patient compliance will be much decreased if treated as outpatient:
  - Cinchonism
  - Tinnitus
  - Headache
  - Nausea
  - Diarrhea
  - Altered auditory acuity
  - Blurred vision.

General Considerations

1. Intravenous preparations should be preferred over intramuscular preparations
2. In 1st trimester of pregnancy, parenteral quinine is the drug of choice. However, if quinine is not available, artemisinin derivatives may be given to save the life of mother
3. In 2nd and 3rd trimester, parenteral artemisinin derivatives are preferred.

Note: *P. vivax can present as severe malaria and should be treated like severe P. falciparum malaria.*

Obstetric Management

- Maintain airway, breathing, circulation
- Prompt management and a strict close watch to avoid complications
- Treat pyrexia with paracetamol, tepid sponging and antimalarials
- Frequent checks on blood sugars to avoid hypoglycemia
- Maintain hydration
- Even acute malaria is not an indication for induction
- Tocolysis and steroid therapy can be considered if no contraindications
- Ultrasound for fetal growth (doppler in cases of IUGR)
- Explain the patient and relatives the risks associated
- NST may show changes like decelerations, fetal tachycardia or bradycardia
- Pediatrician to be kept informed
- Blood should be sent for grouping/cross match/platelet count in severe cases
- Intrapartum malaria can lead to vertical transmission and is an indication for placental histology, placenta, cord and baby's blood group analysis to detect congenital malaria in neonate
- All neonates whose mothers developed malaria in pregnancy should be screened for malaria with standard microscopy of thick and thin blood films at birth and then weekly blood films, for 28 days.

Recurrence in Malaria

- Mostly seen with uncomplicated *P. falciparum*
- Recurrence usually occurs between 4-6 weeks
- Other reported recurrences at:
  - 85 days with quinine
  - 98 days with artesunate
  - 63 days with artemether-lumefantrine
  - 121 days with mefloquine

Therefore, weekly screening by blood film should be advised so that malaria is detected before its symptoms develop.

Prevention from Malaria (Prevention of Bites)

4 ways:
1. Skin repellents
2. Mosquito sprays
3. Insect treated bed nests
4. Clothing and room protection.

Skin Repellents

- 50% DEET (N, N-diethyl-m-toluamide or N,N-diethly-3-methyl-benzamide) – application to exposed areas of arms and legs twice daily is recommended
- Other less effective options, when DEET is not tolerated:
  - PMD (p-methane 3, 8 diol)
  - IR3535 (3-ethylaminopropionate)
  - Picaridin 20% [KBR3023 (2-(2-hydroxyethyl)-1-piperidine carboxylic acid 1-methyl propylester)].

Mosquito Sprays

- Permethrin and pyrethroids sprays.

Insect Treated Bed Nests

- Long lasting pyrethroid-impregnated bed nets offer significant protection
- If the net is not long-lasting it needs reimpregnating every 6 months, starting from the first date on which the net is used after purchase
- Efficacy ≈ 50%.

Clothing

- Clothing that covers the body and forms a barrier from biting mosquitoes will reduce the risk of malaria
- After sunset, long sleeves, long trousers, loose-fitting clothing and socks, regardless of color, protecting from direct bite of the mosquito, are recommended.

Room Protection

- Electrically heated mats that vaporizes synthetic pyrethroids can be used, these are to be changed every night
- Mosquito coils are not very effective.

Malaria Prophylaxis in Pregnancy

- There is no malaria prophylaxis regimen that is 100% protective
- Mefloquine (5 mg/kg once a week) is the recommended drug of choice for prophylaxis in the 2nd and 3rd trimesters for chloroquine-resistant areas. With very few areas in the world free from chloroquine resistance, mefloquine is essentially the only drug considered safe for prophylaxis in pregnant travellers
- The drug does not result in an increased risk of stillbirth or congenital malformation at prophylactic doses.

Dose Regimens for Prophylaxis in Pregnancy

- Tab Mefloquine 250 mg 1 tablet weekly, if chloroquine resistant
- Atovaquone-proguanila 1 tablet daily (250 mg atovaquone + 100 mg proguanil) in cases of chloroquine resistant and mefloquine not tolerated or contraindicated OR mefloquine resistant)
- Proguanila 100 mg 2 tablets daily plus chloroquine 150 mg 2 tablets weekly, if not resistant to chloroquine
- Folic acid supplements (5 mg daily) need to be taken if proguanil is used in those who are pregnant or seeking to become pregnant.

Recent Advances

- Azithromycin—chloroquine is a potential alternative that can replace SP for IPTp, having shown efficacy against P. falciparum among nonpregnant adults in sub-Saharan Africa, Colombia and India, even in the presence of parasite populations saturated with chloroquine-resistance markers
- The combination may be safely administered any time in pregnancy and offers benefits of clearing several STI/RTIs.

Pharmacokinetic measurements in pregnancy suggest that dose adjustments may not be necessary for azithromycin but daily chloroquine dosing needs to be 600 mg for 3 days.

TUBERCULOSIS

History

- Pathology of pulmonary form → established by Dr Richard Morton in 1689
- Name Tuberculosis was given in 1839 by J. L. Schönlein
- Dr. Robert Koch discovered the tuberculosis bacillus in 1882
- Immunization against TB → by Albert Calmette and Camille Guérin in 1906, which was named bacillus of Calmette and Guérin (BCG)
- BCG vaccine → first used on humans in 1921 in France.

Prevalence

- 1/3rd of the world's population is infected with M. tuberculosis
- New infections occur in ≈ 1% of the population each year
- In 2010, there were an estimated 8.8 million new cases globally and 1.5 million associated deaths, mostly occurring in developing countries
- Distribution across the globe is not uniform, occurring mostly in developing countries, also largely due to high rates of HIV infection and the corresponding development of AIDS.

Pathogenesis

About 90% of those infected with M. tuberculosis have asymptomatic, latent TB infections (sometimes called LTBI), with only a 10% lifetime chance that the latent infection will progress to overt, active tuberculous disease.

- Mycobacteria reach the pulmonary alveoli → invade and replicate within endosomes of alveolar macrophages
- Primary site of infection is, either the upper part of the lower lobe or the lower part of the upper lobe → "Ghon focus"
- "Simon focus" when infection occurs via blood stream → typically found in the top of the lung
- TB rarely affects:
  - Heart
  - Skeletal muscles
  - Pancreas
  - Thyroid
- Classified as one of the granulomatous inflammatory diseases:
  - Macrophages, T lymphocytes, B lymphocytes, and fibroblasts aggregate to form granulomas
  - Granuloma prevents dissemination of the mycobacteria
  - Bacteria inside the granuloma can become dormant, resulting in latent infection
  - There is development of abnormal cell death (necrosis) in the center of tubercles
  - To the naked eye, this has the texture of soft, white cheese and is termed 'caseous necrosis'
- Miliary TB: When many foci of infection, all appearing as tiny, white tubercles are present in other tissues of the body→ this has ≈ 30% fatality rate even with treatment.

In many people, the infection waxes and wanes. Tissue destruction and necrosis are often balanced by healing and fibrosis with affected tissue being replaced by scarring and cavities filled with caseous necrotic material.

Transmission

- When people with active pulmonary TB cough, sneeze, speak, sing, or spit, they expel infectious aerosol droplets 0.5 to 5.0 µm in diameter
- A single sneeze can release up to 40,000 droplets
- Each one of these droplets may transmit the disease, since the infectious dose of tuberculosis is very low (inhalation of < 10 bacteria may cause an infection)
- A person with active but untreated tuberculosis may infect 10–15 (or more) other people per year
- Transmission occurs only from people with active TB
- It typically takes 3-4 weeks before the newly infected person becomes infectious enough to transmit the disease to others.

Causative Agent

Mycobacterium tuberculosis
- A small, aerobic, nonmotile, acid fast bacillus
- Has a high lipid content
- Divides every 16-20 hours, which is an extremely slow rate compared with other bacteria, which usually divide in less than an hour
- Has an outer membrane lipid bilayer
- It can withstand weak disinfectants and survive in a dry state for weeks
- In nature, the bacterium can grow only within the cells of a host organism
- Can be cultured in laboratory
- The M. tuberculosis complex (MTBC) includes other TB-causing mycobacteria:
  - M. bovis → use of pasteurized milk has largely eliminated it
  - M. africanum → not widespread
  - M. canetti → rare (mainly in Africa)
  - M. microti → rare, mostly seen in immunodeficient people
  - M. leprae
  - "Non tuberculous mycobacteria" (NTM)
  - M. avium
  - M. kansasii
  - NTM cause neither TB nor leprosy, but they do cause pulmonary diseases that resemble TB.

Risk Factors

- Overcrowding
- Malnutrition
- Illicit drug use
- Prisons and homeless shelters
- Medically underprivileged and resource-poor communities
- High-risk ethnic minorities
- Children in close contact with high-risk category patients, and health care providers serving these patients
- Chronic lung disease is another significant risk factor → with silicosis increasing the risk about 30-fold
- Smoking → 2 fold increase in risk than in nonsmokers
- Alcoholism and diabetes mellitus (threefold increase)
- Corticosteroids and infliximab (an anti-αTNF monoclonal antibody) are becoming increasingly important risk factors, especially in the developed world
- Genetic susceptibility but its overall importance remains undefined.

Signs and Symptoms

- About 5-10% → develop active disease during their lifetime
- If there is HIV coinfection → 30% will develop active disease
- Tuberculosis may infect any part of the body, but most commonly occurs in the lungs (known as pulmonary tuberculosis)
- Extrapulmonary TB may coexist with pulmonary TB as well

- Classic symptoms:
  - Chronic cough with blood-tinged sputum
  - Fever
  - Chills
  - Night sweats
  - Loss of appetite
  - Weight loss (the latter giving rise to the formerly prevalent term "consumption")
  - Fatigue
  - Infection of other organs causes a wide range of symptoms
  - Significant finger clubbing may also occur.

PulmonaryTB

- Active TB → most commonly involves the lungs (in ≈ 90% of cases)
- Symptoms may include:
  - Chest pain
  - A prolonged cough producing sputum
  - Cough may be blood stained
  - In very rare instances, the infection may erode into the pulmonary artery, resulting in massive bleeding (Rasmussen's aneurysm)
- About 25% of people may remain 'asymptomatic'
- Chronic infection may cause extensive scarring in the upper lobes of lungs
- Upper lung lobes → more frequently affected than the lower ones either due to better air flow or due to poor lymph drainage within the upper lungs.

Extrapulmonary TB

- Spread of infection anywhere in the body outside the respiratory organs
- It occurs in ≈15–20% of active cases
- Occurs more commonly in immunosuppressed persons and young children
- In those with HIV, this occurs in > 50% of cases
- Notable infection sites include:
  - Pleura (in tuberculous pleurisy)
  - CNS (intuberculous meningitis)
  - Lymphatic system (in scrofula of the neck)
  - Genitourinary system (in urogenital tuberculosis)
  - Bones and joints (in Pott's disease of the spine)
  - When it spreads to the bones, it is also known as "osseous tuberculosis", a form of osteomyelitis
  - Sometimes, bursting of a tubercular abscess through skin results in tuberculous ulcer (near lymph nodes, may have "wash leather" appearance)
  - A more serious, widespread form of TB is called "disseminated" TB, commonly known as miliary tuberculosis, which makes up ≈ 10% of extrapulmonary cases.

Diagnosis

Active Tuberculosis

Sputum examination
- Any patient presenting with cough for > 2 weeks is a pulmonary TB suspect and is be referred to the RNTCP Designated Microscopy Center

- All TB suspects undergo 2 sputum smear examinations (spot and morning) over two consecutive days
- All specimens are examined by Ziehl-Neelsen staining technique (bright field binocular microscopes) and auramine staining techniques.

Definitive diagnosis
- By identifying M. tuberculosis in a clinical sample (e.g. sputum, pus, or a tissue biopsy)
- However, the difficult culture process for this slow-growing organism can take two to six weeks for blood or sputum culture
- Thus, treatment is often begun before cultures are confirmed.

Latent Tuberculosis

Mantoux test/Tuberculin test/PPD test
- Screening test
- Consists of an intradermal injection of one-tenth of a milliliter (mL) of PPD tuberculin
- The size of induration is measured 48–72 hours later
- A person who has been exposed to the bacteria is expected to mount an immune response in the skin containing the bacterial proteins
- The reaction is read by measuring the diameter of induration (palpable raised, hardened area) across the forearm (perpendicular to the long axis) in millimeters
- If there is no induration, the result should be recorded as "0 mm". Erythema (redness) should not be measured.

Classification of tuberculin reaction

5 mm or more is positive in
- An HIV-positive person
- Persons with recent contacts with a TB patient
- Persons with nodular or fibrotic changes on chest X-ray consistent with old healed TB
- Patients with organ transplants, and other immunosuppressed patients.

10 mm or more is positive in
- Recent arrivals (< five years) from high-prevalence countries
- Injection drug users
- Residents and employees of high-risk congregate settings (e.g., prisons, nursing homes, hospitals, homeless shelters, etc.)
- Mycobacteriology lab. personnel
- Persons with clinical conditions that place them at high risk (e.g., diabetes, prolonged corticosteroid therapy, leukemia, end-stage renal disease, chronic malabsorption syndromes, low body weight, etc.)
- Children < 4 years of age, or children and adolescents exposed to adults in high-risk categories.

15 mm or more is positive in
- Persons with no known risk factors for TB.

Recent Developments

QuantiFERON-TB Gold (QFT-G)
Is an IFN-gamma-release assay that measures the release of interferon after stimulation in vitro by mycobacterium tuberculosis antigens.

- CDC approved it in December 2005
- Quantiferon-TB Gold is FDA-approved
- Recommended in those who are positive to Mantoux test
- The goal of testing for LTBI is to identify individuals who are at increased risk for the development of tuberculosis and therefore, who would benefit from treatment of latent TB infection
- Not affected by immunization or most environmental mycobacteria, so they generate fewer false-positive results
- Affected by M. szulgai, M. marinum and M. kansasii.

Antitubercular Drugs in general - An overview

First line

All first-line anti-tuberculous drug names have a standard three-letter and a single-letter abbreviation:
- Ethambutol is EMB or E,
- Isoniazid is INH or H,
- Pyrazinamide is PZA or Z,
- Rifampicin is RMP or R.

Streptomycin is no longer considered as a first line drug by ATS/IDSA/CDC because of high rates of resistance.
- A prefix denotes the number of months the treatment should be given for
- A subscript denotes intermittent dosing (so 3 means three times a week)
- No subscript means daily dosing
- Most regimens have an initial *high-intensity phase*, followed by a *continuation phase* (also called a consolidation phase or eradication phase): the high-intensity phase is given first, then the continuation phase, the two phases divided by a slash.
  So,
  $2HREZ/4HR_3$
  means isoniazid, rifampicin, ethambutol, pyrazinamide daily for two months, followed by four months of isoniazid and rifampicin given three times a week.

Second Line

- Often used in special conditions like:
  - Resistance to first line therapy
  - Extensively drug-resistant tuberculosis (XDR-TB) or
  - Multidrug-resistant tuberculosis (MDR-TB).
- There are six classes of second-line drugs:
  - Aminoglycosides: e.g., amikacin (AMK), kanamycin (KM)
  - Polypeptides: e.g., capreomycin, viomycin, enviomycin
  - Fluoroquinolones: e.g., ciprofloxacin (CIP), levofloxacin, moxifloxacin (MXF)
  - Thioamides: e.g. ethionamide, prothionamide
  - Cycloserine: e.g., closerin
  - Terizidone.

Third Line

Considered as third line drugs either because they are not very effective (e.g. clarithromycin) or their efficacy has not been proven (e.g., linezolid, R207910).

- Rifabutin
- Macrolides: e.g., clarithromycin (CLR)
- Linezolid (LZD)
- Thioacetazone (T)
- Thioridazine
- Arginine
- Vitamin D
- R207910.

Rifabutin is effective, but is not included in the WHO list because for most developing countries, it is impractically expensive.

The Standard Regimen

- 2HREZ/4HR or 2SHRZ/4HR are the regimens currently recommended
- The WHO also recommend a six-month continuation phase of HR if the patient is still culture positive after 2 months of treatment (approximately 15% of patients with fully sensitive TB) and for those patients who have extensive bilateral cavitation at the start of treatment.

Monitoring DOTS and DOTS-Plus

"DOTS"

- DOTS stands for "Directly Observed Treatment, Short-course" and is a major plank in the WHO Global Plan to Stop TB
- Focuses on five main points of action:
    i. Government commitment to control TB
    ii. Diagnosis based on sputum-smear microscopy tests done on patients who actively report TB symptoms
    iii. Direct observation short-course chemotherapy treatments
    iv. Definite supply of drugs
    v. Standardized reporting and recording of cases and treatment outcomes
- The WHO advises that all TB patients should have at least the first two months of their therapy observed (and preferably the whole of it observed): this means an independent observer watching patients swallow their anti-TB therapy
- DOTS is used with intermittent dosing (thrice weekly or 2HREZ/4HR3)
- Proper treatment has a success rate exceeding 95%.

"DOTS-Plus"

- The WHO extended the DOTS programme in 1998 to include the treatment of MDR-TB (called "DOTS-Plus")
- DOTS-Plus is much more resource-expensive than DOTS, and requires much greater commitment from countries wishing to implement it
- Monthly surveillance until cultures convert to negative is recommended for DOTS-Plus, but not for DOTS
- If cultures are positive or symptoms do not resolve after three months of treatment, it is necessary to re-evaluate the patient for drug-resistant disease or non-adherence to drug regimen
- If cultures do not convert to negative despite three months of therapy, some physicians may consider admitting the patient to hospital so as to closely monitor therapy.

Revised National TB Control Programme (RNTCP)

- 100% Centrally Sponsored Scheme implemented in the entire country, with DOTS strategy, which is WHO recommended
- What role does it play?
  It provides:
  – Diagnosis and treatment facilities
  – Supplies full course of anti TB drugs free of cost
  – Established designated microscopy centres (>1300 across the country) for every one lakh population in the general areas and for every 50,000 population in the tribal, hilly and difficult areas
  – DOT centres > 4,00,000 have been established
  – Monitoring of patients and helping them receive the complete treatment
  – Launched "DOTS Plus" in 2007 for management of drug resistance tuberculosis.

Non-compliance

There are variety of reasons which lead to failure of medication:
- Lack of motivation and discontinuation of drug as symptoms resolve within a few weeks of starting TB
- Lack of regular follow-up
- Lack of regularity of taking the drugs and importance of its completion
- Bulkiness of the tablets → PZA
- Medicines to be taken on an empty stomach (aggravates nausea)
- Side effects caused by specific drugs:
  – Thrombocytopenia → Only caused by RMP and no test dosing required
  – Peripheral neuropathy: INH (Pure sensory neuropathy)
    - Once a peripheral neuropathy has occurred, INH must be stopped and pyridoxine should be given at a dose of 50 mg thrice daily but it will not stop the neuropathy from progressing
    - Therefore, when there is a risk of neuropathy (in cases of DM, malnutrition, pregnancy etc.) pyridoxine 10 mg daily should be given at the start of treatment
  – Vertigo → STM
  – Hepatitis → PZA, RMP, INH (in decreasing order)
  – Rash → PZA, RMP, EMB
  – Itching → RMP
  – Fever → RMP.

Drug-induced hepatitis
- Test dosing must be carried out to determine which drug is responsible
- Liver function tests (LFTs) should be checked at the start of treatment, but, if normal, need not be checked again
- The patient need only be warned of the symptoms of hepatitis
- Elevations in liver transaminases (ALT and AST) are common in the first three weeks of treatment
- If clinically significant hepatitis occurs while on TB treatment, then all the drugs should be stopped until the liver transaminases return to normal
- Fulminant hepatitis is rare.

Prevention

Modes
- Vaccination in infants
- Detection and appropriate treatment of active cases.

Vaccine

- The only currently available vaccine is bacillus Calmette–Guérin (BCG)
- Effective against disseminated disease in childhood
- Confers inconsistent protection against contracting pulmonary TB
- The immunity it induces decreases after about ten years
- A number of new vaccines are currently in development.

Pregnancy and TB

- Pregnancy itself is not a risk factor for TB
- Untreated TB in pregnancy is associated with an increased risk of:
  - Miscarriage
  - Low birth weight
  - Major fetal abnormality (rare)
  - Neonatal TB (rare)
- High doses of RMP (much higher than used in humans) causes neural tube defects in animals, but no such effect has ever been found in humans
- There may be an increased risk of hepatitis in pregnancy and during the puerperium
- It is prudent to advise all women of child-bearing age to avoid getting pregnant until TB treatment is completed
- Aminoglycosides (STM, capreomycin, amikacin) should be used with caution in pregnancy, because they may cause deafness in the unborn child
- Experience in Peru shows that treatment for MDR-TB is not a reason to recommend termination of pregnancy, and that good outcomes are possible.

Difficulties in Diagnosing Tuberculosis in Pregnancy

- Because of the vague, non-specific nature of the symptoms, common to both TB and pregnancy
- Fatigue
- Shortness of breath
- Sweating
- Tiredness
- Most physicians are reluctant to order a chest x-ray for fear of harming the fetus.

Management (CDC)

Active Disease

First 2 months (daily)
- Isoniazid (along with pyridoxal phosphate to obviate peripheral neuropathy caused by isoniazid)
- Rifampicin
- Ethambutol.

For 7 months
- Isoniazid and rifampicin alone , daily or twice weekly.

NOTE: *Streptomycin should not be used because it has been shown to have harmful effects on the fetus. In most cases, pyrazinamide (PZA) is not recommended to be used because its effect on the fetus is unknown.*

Latent Tuberculosis
- The standard treatment is 9 months of isoniazid (300 mg) alone, administered either daily or twice weekly
- Women taking INH should also take pyridoxine (vitamin B_6) supplementation.

Postpartum
- Breastfeeding should not be discouraged for women being treated with the first-line anti-TB drugs because the concentrations of these drugs in breast milk are too small to produce toxicity in the nursing newborn
- Congenital TB (though rare) has morbidity and mortality approaching 50%.

RUBELLA

Other Names
- '3-day measles' or 'German measles'.

Why Called German Measles?
- Rubella is often called "German measles," but it is not related to measles at all
- It got this name because the rash caused by rubella looks like measles and the disease was first discovered in Germany.

Infectious Agent
- Family: Togaviridae (RNA virus)
- Genus: rubivirus and is the only member
- Only natural host → Humans.

Mode of Transmission
- Person-to-person (direct) contact
- By aerosol via respiratory tract
- Transplacental
- Infants with CRS shed virus in their urine and nasopharyngeal secretions.

Clinical Presentation

Incubation period
- ≈ 14-17 days (range of 12–23 days from exposure to clinical illness)
- Period of infection begins from 1 week before and lasts 4 days after the onset of rash
- Infants with Congenital Rubella Syndrome may shed the virus for > 1 year.

Common presentation
- Rash:
  - Nonspecific, maculopapular, transient, generalized or diffuse punctate rash
  - Characteristically begins on the face, becoming generalized and spreads to the trunk and extremities
  - Resolve within 3 days in the same order in which it appeared (face first and then body).

- Lymphadenopathy:
  - Generalized, particularly of the:
    - Posterior auricular
    - Suboccipital
    - Posterior cervical lymph nodes
  - Precedes the rash by 5-10 days.
- As symptoms are non-specific, it may be mistaken for infection due to parvovirus, adenovirus or enterovirus.
- Polyarthralgia/polyarthritis:
  - Transient
  - Involves fingers, hands, wrists, knees, ankles OR
  - Polyarthritis (about 1 week after the rash) occurs symmetrically
  - Pain will last for 1-4 weeks
  - Chronic arthritis rarely develops.
- Rare manifestations:
  - Tenosynovitis
  - Carpal tunnel syndrome
  - Thrombocytopenia
  - Post-infectious encephalitis
  - Myocarditis
  - Hepatitis
  - Hemolytic anemia
  - Hemolytic uremic syndrome.
- ≈ 20-50% of infections are subclinical (without rash or asymptomatic).
- In adults → scarletiniform rash, which may be mildly pruritic, may be preceded by a prodromal period of 1-5-days presenting as:
  - Low-grade fever
  - Malaise
  - Arthralgia
  - Anorexia
  - Mild conjunctivitis/coryza
  - Runny nose
  - Sore throat
  - Lymphadenopathy.

Risks

Congenital rubella syndrome
Can result in following complications:

In utero
- Miscarriage
- Stillbirth and/or
- Fetal infection
- IUGR.

At birth
- Ophthalmological (10-25%):
  - Cataract
  - Pigmentary retinopathy

- Microphthalmos
- Congenital andpigmentary glaucoma.
- Auditory (60-70%):
  - Sensorineural hearing impairment.
- Neurological (10-25%):
  - Behavioral disorders
  - Meningoencephalitis
  - Microcephaly
  - Developmental delay
  - Mental retardation
  - Panencephalitis.
- Cardiac (10-20%):
  - Patent ductus arteriosus
  - Pulmonary artery stenosis
  - Ventricular septal defect.
- Others:
  - Growth retardation
  - Interstitial pneumonitis
  - Radiolucent bone disease
  - Hepatosplenomegaly
  - Thrombocytopenia
  - Characteristic pruritis (blueberry muffin appearance).

Late manifestations
- Diabetes milletus
- Thyroiditis
- Growth hormone deficit
- Behavioural disorder.

Prevention of CRS

- Infant immunization
- Use of the MMR vaccine rather than the monovalent measles vaccine as the immunizing agent in all immunization programs for measles worldwide
- Screening of all pregnant women to confirm seropositivity and to enable postpartum immunization of all women found susceptible on prenatal screening
- Screening for immunity and vaccination, if necessary, of all health care personnel, including students in training
- Immunizing all nonpregnant women
- Fully investigating and reporting every case of possible rubella or CRS
- *Breastfeeding is not a contraindication to immunization.*

Vertical Transmission and Fetal Infection

Maternal blood → placenta → vascular system of fetus → cytopathic damage to blood vessels → spreads to whole body → ischemia in developing organs

Transmission
- 80-85% in 1st trimester
- 25% in late 2nd trimester
- 35% in early 3rd trimester
- 100% at term.

Fetal infection
- 90% before 11 weeks
- 33% at 11-12 weeks
- 11% at 13-14 weeks
- 24% at 15-16 weeks
- 0% after 16 weeks
- Infected infants who appear normal at birth may later show eye, ear or brain damage
- Periconceptual maternal infection does not seem to increase the risk of CRS
- In cases where mother is immunized, chances of congenital rubella are less after maternal reinfection, with practically none after 12 weeks of gestation.

Diagnosis
- Clinical and
- Laboratory evidence (pregnant women only) OR epidemiological evidence.

Clinical evidence
- Acute onset of generalized maculopapular rash
  +
- Temperature > 99°F (37.2°C)
  +
- Arthralgia/arthritis OR lymphadenopathy OR conjunctivitis

The only reliable evidence of acute rubella virus infection is **laboratory diagnosis**
1. Positive serologic test for rubella-specific IgM (most commonly used) by ELISA
2. 4-fold increase in rubella-specific IgG titers between acute and convalescent serum specimens by ELISA
3. Detection of virus either through virus culture or PCR.

Serologic testing:
- Performed within 7-10 days after the onset of the rash
- Repeated after 2-3 weeks.

Viral cultures:
- Drawn from nose, blood, throat, urine or cerebrospinal fluid
- May be positive from 1 week before to 2 weeks after the onset of rash.

Epidemiological evidence
An epidemiological link is established when there is contact between two people involving a plausible mode of transmission at a time when:
- One of them is likely to be infectious (about one week before to at least four days after appearance of rash)
  AND
- The other has an illness which starts within 14 and 23 days after this contact AND
- At least one case in the chain of epidemiologically linked cases (which may involve many cases) is laboratory confirmed.

Maternal evidence
- Isolation of rubella virus
  OR
- Detection of rubella virus by nucleic acid testing

- IgG sero conversion or a significant increase in antibody level or a 4-fold or greater rise in titer to rubella virus. This must be established by the testing of paired sera in parallel
  OR
- Detection of rubella-specific IgM, in the absence of recent rubella vaccination and confirmation of the result in a reference laboratory.

Infant evidence
- Isolation of rubella virus from the infant OR
- Detection of rubella virus, in the infant, by nucleic acid testing OR
- Detection of rubella-specific IgM antibody in the serum of the infant AND confirmation of the result in a reference laboratory
- CVS at 10-12 weeks > Amniotic fluid testing at 14-16 weeks > Fetal blood sampling at 18-20 weeks
- Any fetus presenting with IUGR should be evaluated for congenital viral infections, including rubella
- USG → not informative
- A live infant or still born fetus with ANY of the following compatible defects:
  - Cataracts
  - Congenital glaucoma
  - Congenital heart disease
  - Hearing defects
  - Microcephaly
  - Pigmentary retinopathy
  - Mental retardation
  - Purpura
  - Hepatosplenomegaly
  - Meningoencephalitis
  - Radiolucent bone disease.

Treatment

No specific antibiotic therapy
If there is maternal exposure:
- *Known immune ≥ 12 weeks of gestation*
  - No further testing is necessary
  - CRS has not been reported after maternal reinfection beyond 12 weeks' gestation.
- *Known immune ≤ 12 weeks of gestation*
  - If these women demonstrate a significant rise in rubella IgG antibody titer without detection of IgM antibody, they should be informed that reinfection is likely to have occurred
  - Fetal risk for congenital infection after maternal reinfection during the 1st trimester has been estimated at 8% (95% CI 2–22%)
  - Appropriate counseling should be provided.
- *Non-immune or immunity unknown*
  Gestational age ≤ 16 weeks
  - Acute and convalescent IgG and IgM should be obtained
  - IgM positive → acute infection
  - IgM negative or unavailable → testing of paired acute and convalescent sera for IgG antibody should be performed
  - During a rubella-like illness, the acute specimen should be drawn as soon as possible, followed by a convalescent specimen two to three weeks later if the first IgM specimen was negative

- When there is a suspected exposure, the acute specimen should be drawn immediately, followed by a convalescent specimen 4 to 5 weeks later.

Gestational age between 16 and 20 weeks
- CRS is rare (< 1%)
- May be manifested by sensorineural deafness (often severe) in the newborn
- Provide appropriate counseling to the non-immune pregnant woman.

Gestational age > 20 weeks
- No studies have documented CRS after 20 weeks, hence reassurance.

Diagnostic difficulty-late presentation with unknown immune status
- Diagnostic dilemma → pregnant woman presenting ≥ 5 weeks after exposure to a rash illness or ≥ 4 weeks after onset of a rash
- If IgG antibodies are negative → susceptible to rubella and has no evidence of a recent infection
- If IgG are positive:
  - Previous infection (but date of infection and the risk to the fetus is not known)
  - Low level of antibody suggests more remote infection
  - IgM antibody or repeat IgG antibody levels are to be tested.

Vaccine

- The first live attenuated rubella vaccine was introduced in 1969
- Originally, just one dose of the MMR vaccine was recommended
- In 1989, the American Academy of Family Physicians, the American Academy of Pediatrics, and the Centers for Disease Control and Prevention's Advisory Committee on Immunization Practices, changed the recommendation to two doses:
  - Dose 1 at ages 12-15 months
  - Dose 2 at ages 4-6 years
- A single dose of this vaccine will result in measurable antibody in almost 95% of susceptible persons
- Antibody levels persist for at least 18 years in > 90% of the vaccine recipients
- Primary failure of the rubella vaccine occurs in < 5% of immunizations
- Although reinfection may occur in immunized pregnant women, these reinfections have resulted in only 8% risk of CRS in the 1st trimester of pregnancy
- The rubella vaccine is usually well tolerated
- Side effects of the MMR vaccine are usually mild and include:
  - Fever in 1 out of 6 people
  - Mild rash in 1 out of 20 people
  - Swollen glands in the cheeks or neck in very few people
  - Fever high enough to cause a seizure (jerking or staring) occurs in 1 out of 3,000 people
  - Temporary joint pain and stiffness (mostly in teens and adults)
  - Serious allergic reaction to the MMR vaccine occurs in fewer than 1 in 1 million people
- Contraindications to rubella vaccinations include:
  - Febrile illness
  - Immunodeficiency
  - History of anaphylactic reaction to neomycin
  - Pregnancy
- Rubella vaccine virus (live attenuated) has the potential to cross the placenta and infect the fetus. However, there has been no report of CRS in the offspring of women inadvertently vaccinated during early pregnancy. Therefore, pregnancy termination is not recommended for these patients

- Given the potential risks to the fetus, women are advised not to become pregnant for a period of 28 days after immunization
- Can be given safely to breastfeeding women
- Can be administered with other immune globulin preparations such as Rh-immune globulin.

TOXOPLASMA

- Toxoplasma gondii → an obligate intracellular protozoan parasite
- Belongs to the phylum apicomplexa group [other members of this phylum include known human pathogens such as *Plasmodium* (malaria) and *Cryptosporidium*]
- Replicates in cells and tissues, especially in the brain and eye
- Life style – complex

Animal flesh encysted with *T. gondii*
↓
Ingested by cats (PRIMARY HOST)
↓

Sexual reproduction	*Asexual reproduction*
↓	↓
In digestive epithelium of cats	In mammals and birds (secondary hosts)

↓
1-2 weeks → cats remain asymptomatic
↓
Shed unsporulated (noninfectious) oocysts (up to one million per day) in their feces
↓
After few days to weeks → oocysts start sporulating → become infectious
↓
For many months, can survive:
– In warm and humid conditions (garden, sand box, litter) and remain infectious
– Can remain freezed for up to 18 months in a dark place
Humans, bird, rats, domestic animals become SECONDARY HOST (Lifetime infection)
↓
Sporozoites are released by oocysts → change into tachyzoites
↓
Tachyzoites (during acute infection) enter immuncompetent host
↓
Remain there for a week → change into bradyzoites → forms cysts in tissues (during latent infection)
↓
But till this time, secondary host remains asymptomatic
↓
When immunosuppression occurs → these organisms reactivates and causes symptoms.

Note: Most important is to save the fetus from getting infected and acquiring *congenital toxoplasmosis and its sequelae*, which can be done by the following measures:

I. **Primary prevention**
   Avoid the following sources of infection:
   - Raw and uncooked meat (30-63% of seroconversions occur during pregnancy)
   - Unwashed fruits and vegetables (from soil)
   - Exposure to oocyst-infected cat litter (indoor cats are less dangerous unless fed by raw meat)
   - Tropical regions (infection is highest in areas of world having hot, humid climates and lower altitudes)
   - Drinking contaminated water
   - Gardening without gloves
   - Placenta (in utero)
   - Blood transfusions and organ transplant (rare).

II. **Serological prenatal screening (secondary prevention) as early as possible, followed by antibiotic treatment to prevent transplacental transmission and fetal diagnosis and treatment**

Diagnosis

- Serological testing
- Amniocentesis
- Ultrasound

Serological Testing

IgM antibodies
- Not reliable to make a diagnosis of acute infection
- Titers rise from 5 days to weeks following acute infection
- Reach a maximum after 1 to 2 months
- Decline more rapidly than IgG and become low or even undetectable
- In few cases, may persist for years following the acute infection.

IgG antibodies
- Appear later than IgM
- Usually detectable within 1 to 2 weeks after infection
- Peak reached within 12 weeks to 6 months after acute infection
- Detectable for years after acquired infection
- Usually present throughout life.

Interpretations:

To diagnose
- IgG −ve
- IgM −ve   → Absence of infection or very recent acute infection

- IgG +ve
- IgM −ve   → Old infection (>1 year)

- IgG +ve
- IgM +ve   → Either a recent infection or a false-positive test result

- If acute infection is suspected → repeat the test within 2 to 3 weeks
- A 4-fold rise in IgG antibody titers between tests indicates a recent infection.

To confirm
- Sabin-Feldman dye test → maximum levels after 2 months of infection (> 300 IU/mL)
- IgM indirect fluorescent antibody test.

IgG avidity
- Assists in determining the timing of infection
- Measures the strength of IgG binding to the organism
- Most of the times, avidity shifts from low to high after about 5 months
- If the avidity is high, this suggests that infection has occurred at least 5 months before testing.

Ultrasonography

- Intracranial calcifications
- Ventricular dilatation
- Hepatomegaly
- Ascites
- Placental enlargement.

Amniocentesis

- Organism identified in amniotic fluid by polymerase chain reaction
- Sensitivity 81- 90%
- Specificity 96 - 100%
- Should be offered at ≥ 18 weeks gestation (↑false-positive results before that)
- Should be offered no less than 4 weeks after the time of suspected acute maternal infection.

If mother gets infected, the manifestations can be in the following ways:
- Many remain undiagnosed?
  - > 90% cases are asymptomatic and selflimited except for congenital infection and immuno- compromised patients
  - Recover very quickly.
- Those with symptoms present as follows:
  - Exposure → Incubation period (4-21 days) → symptoms:
    - Low grade fever
    - Malaise
    - Myalgia
    - Lymphadenopathy
      - Cervical
      - Suboccipital
      - Supraclavicular
      - Axillary
      - Inguinal
  - Chorioretinitis → rare in pregnancy
  - If woman presents with weak defence mechanism, the disease has severe manifestations:
    - Severe encephalitis
    - Myocarditis
    - Pneumonitis
    - Hepatitis.

Transmission to fetus
- When mother acquires primary infection in pregnancy → risk of transmission to fetus is very high
- In cases where the mother is a chronic carrier → transmission occurs only if mother's state is immunocompromised
- Infection to the fetus occurs when the placenta is invaded by tachyzoites for a period of 1-4 months
- Infection remains throughout pregnancy → so placenta acts as a reservoir and supplies the organism to the fetus throughout pregnancy.

Vertical transmission
- Overall risk of congenital infection without treatment ranges from 20-50%,
  - 3rd trimester → 60-81% (milder or asymptomatic disease)
  - 2nd trimester → 25% (intermediate severity)
  - 1st trimester → 6-17% (severe disease; results in miscarriage/congenital abnormalities)
- But severity decreases as gestation advances:
  - 60% at 12 weeks
  - 5% - just before delivery.

III. By neonatal screening, followed by antimicrobial treatment of infected newborns to prevent clinical damage.

Congenital Toxoplasmosis

Tetrad described by Sabin in 1942:
- Chorioretinitis
- Hydrocephalus
- Cerebral calcification } Mainly resulting in mental retardation and blindness in infant
- Seizures
- Other signs, symptoms and sequelae in congenital toxoplasmosis patients:
  - Microcephaly
  - Deafness
  - Severe intrauterine growth restriction
  - Skin rash, petechiae
  - Anemia
  - Jaundice
  - Fever
  - Lymphadenopathy
  - Hepatomegaly
  - Splenomegaly
  - Vomiting
  - Diarrhea
  - Cataracts
  - Esinophilia
  - Abnormal bleeding
  - Hypothermia
  - Glaucoma
  - Optic atrophy
  - Microphthalmia
  - Pneumonitis
  - Even death of fetus can occur

- Severe morphological lesions → terminate pregnancy
- Acute maternal infection may even lead to IUFD.

At birth
- >90% of neonates with congenital infection may not show clinical signs at birth
- Severe damage in infancy occurs in only 5% of congenital toxoplasmosis cases
- Intracranial or ocular lesions are observed in 20-30% of cases by 3 years of age
- If no treatment is given, long term sequelae can result in up to 85% of infected children
  - Aqueductal obstruction → cerebral palsy → seizures
  - Hydrocephalus
  - Periaqueductal inflammation
  - Parenchymal calcification
  - Necrosis.

Screening in Pregnancy

- Routine screening is not recommended in pregnancy, where the incidence of toxoplasmosis infection is low
- In whom screening is recommended?
  In immunosuppressed patients } (because of the risk of reactivation and
  HIV-positive cases } toxoplasmosis encephalitis)
  Those with ultrasound findings such as:
  - Hydrocephalus
  - Intracranial calcifications
  - Microcephaly
  - Fetal growth restriction
  - Ascites
  - Hepatosplenomegaly.

Treatment

Only Maternal Infection
- Spiramycin → 1 g (3 million U) orally every 8 hours
- It will be prescribed for the remaining duration of pregnancy if the amniotic fluid PCR is reported negative for T. gondii
- But does not help when fetus is already infected
- Why not reliable in fetal infection?
  - Spiramycin is a macrolide antibiotic that gets concentrated in placenta but does not readily cross the placental barrier and does not reach the fetus in adequate amounts and therefore is not reliable for treatment of fetal infection.

When both are Infected
- The combination of pyrimethamine and sulfadiazine is 8-fold more active than either pyrimethamine or sulfadiazine alone and is regarded as "gold standard" for treating fetal infection
- After 14 weeks of gestation (to avoid teratogenicity)
  - Pyrimethamine 25-100 mg/day + Sulphadiazine 1 gm qid × 3-4 weeks until term
  - Folinic acid 5 mg twice weekly (as these are folate antagonists)

- It produces a reversible, dose related depression of the bone marrow and therefore must be combined with folinic acid
- The combination of pyrimethamine and sulfadiazine results in a significant decrease in disease severity.

Newborn

Overt congenital infection
- Treatment is for 1 year
- First 6 months
  - Pyrimethamine 1 mg/kg/day and sulfadiazine 75 mg/kg/day in two divided doses × 6 months
- Next 6 months
  - Pyrimethamine and sulfadiazine for 1 month is altered with spiramycin 100 mg/kg/day in two divided doses for 1 month
- Give folinic acid along with pyrithemine therapy.

Healthy neonate
- In healthy neonate of mother who definitely had primary toxoplasmosis during pregnancy, give pyrimethamine and sulfadiazine or spiramycin for 1 month.

Outcome of Prenatal Treatment
- Gestational age of acquisition predicts maternal-fetal transmission
- Prenatal treatment delay increases risk of clinical signs in infected children
- Prenatal treatment results in decreased incidence of:
  - Severe infection
  - Cases with mild infection
  - Sequelae at birth
  - Late sequelae
  - Vertical transmission.

CYTOMEGALOVIRUS

- Family: herpesviridae
- Also known as human herpes virus-5 (HHV-5)
- Enveloped double stranded DNA herpes virus
- Infects only humans
- Belongs to the Beta herpes virinae subfamily
- CMV infection is usually harmless
- Once infected with CMV → the virus stays there for life:
  - Primary infection → infection in a previously sero negative person → virus becomes dormant → exists in a latent state → from this it can be reactivated → Recurrent (secondary) infection.

Spread

- Among children in day care centers (most commonly)
- Sexual contact
- Living in overcrowded areas and poor sanitation.

Clinical Manifestations

- Most pregnant women have either no symptoms or have only flu like symptoms:
    - Malaise
    - Persistent fever
    - Myalgia
    - Cervical lymphadenopathy
- Clinically indistinguishable from EBV mononucleosis but with a negative heterophil antibody test
- It is their developing fetuses that may be at risk for congenital CMV disease.

Serious Complications (though not common)

- Interstitial pneumonitis
- Hepatitis
- Meningoencephalitis
- Myocarditis
- Thrombocytopenia.

Congenital CMV

- Cytomegalovirus is the most common cause of intrauterine infection, occurring in 0.2- 2.2% of all live births
- Occurs when the mother suffers a primary infection (or reactivation) during pregnancy
- Mostly infection in 1st half of pregnancy
- Both primary and secondary infection can involve fetus at any time during pregnancy.

Modes of Transmission

- Congenital:
    - Mainly through placenta (manifestations depends on the viral load)
    Perinatal
    - At birth
    - In milk
- Newborn and childhood:
    - Through bodily fluids which are known to contain high titers of virus
        - Saliva ($<10^7$ copies/mL)
        - Urine ($<10^5$ copies/mL)
    - In nursery and day care centers as virus is shed in saliva, urine and respiratory tract for a long time.

Risk of Intrauterine Transmission

- After primary infection → 30-40%
- After secondary infection → 1%.

Disease Manifestations

At birth
- 85-90% → have no signs and symptoms

- 10-15% → present with the following:
  - IUGR/LBW
  - Hyperbilirubinemia
  - Hepatosplenomegaly
  - Thrombocytopenia
  - Petechial rash (similar to "blueberry muffin" rash of congenital rubella syndrome)
  - CNS features (microcephaly/intracranial calcifications) → when infects developing brain tissue
  - After severe brain damage:
    - Cerebellar hypoplasia
    - Aqueductal stenosis
    - Hydrocephalus
- Death occurs in 20-30%.

Sequelae
- In 5-15% (within the 1st few years of life)
- Progressive hearing loss
- Vision impairment
- Mental retardation.

Prenatal Diagnosis

Maternal

When prepregnant immune status is known:
- Appearance of virus specific IgG in the serum in a previously seronegative woman.

When prepregnant immune status is not known:
- Detection of IgM antibodies
- Drawback:
  - IgM can also be detected in 10% of recurrent infections and
  - Can be detected for months after primary infection.

IgG avidity assay
- It can help clear the confusion between primary infection acquired before pregnancy or recurrent infection
- Also determines when the infection has occurred
- Avidity levels are reported in terms of avidity index
- An avidity index of:
  - >60% → highly suggestive of past or secondary infection
  - <30% → highly suggestive of a recent primary infection (duration < 3 months).

Therefore, primary CMV infection acquired during pregnancy will present with:
- CMV-specific IgG antibody in a previously seronegative woman OR
- Detection of specific IgM antibody associated with low IgG avidity.

Fetal

- USG:
  - Helpful but NOT diagnostic
  - May aid in determining the prognosis of the fetus, but does not guarantee the prognosis when following features are not seen:

- IUGR
- Periventricular calcification
- Ventriculomegaly (in mid and late pregnancy)
- Microcephaly
- Ascites/pleural effusion
- Hydrops fetalis
- Oligohydramnios/polyhydramnios
- Hyperechogenic bowel
- Liver calcifications
- Repeat ultrasound examinations every 2-4 weeks, once fetal infection is confirmed, to determine fetal prognosis
- Amniocentesis (Test of choice):
  - High sensitivity and specificity
  - Must be done after 21 weeks period of gestation and at least 5-6 weeks after sero conversion in order to reliably detect CMV
- Viral culture and DNA by PCR in amniotic fluid (to confirm fetal infection):
  - Done either by conventional culture on fibroblasts OR
  - By shell vial technique (detection of virus within 24 hours of amniotic fluid collection).

Neonate

- Within 1st 3 weeks of life, isolation of virus from newborn's:
  - Urine
  - Saliva
  - Tears
  - Rectal swab
  - Isolation of virus.

Screening

- Routine serological screening in pregnancy → NOT recommended
- Should be done:
  - Either before pregnancy
    OR
  - During pregnancy, if:
    - Women develops influenza-like symptoms OR
    - Following detection of sonographic findings that are suggestive of CMV infection which are not explained by any other cause.

Prevention

- Pregnant females who have acquired primary CMV infection → Intravenous CMV hyperimmune globulin (under trials)
- Use of latex condoms helps
- Hygiene especially at centers of infection
  - Avoiding contact with salivarysecretions andurine from young children
  - Careful hand washing after changing diapers and wiping secretions
- Future goals: Development of effective CMV vaccine.

Management

- There is no effective therapy
- Pregnancy termination can be offered once fetal infection is confirmed after weighing the risks and benefits.

Recent Advances

- Phase 2 clinical trials in young mothers done recently have shown that the vaccine developed in 1990s comprising of recombinant cytomegalovirus (CMV) envelope glycoprotein B (gB) with MF59 adjuvant, is found to have efficacy for prevention of CMV infection
- Further studies needed.

HERPES SIMPLEX VIRUS

- Double stranded DNA virus
- Derived from Greek → "creeping" or "latent"
- Family: herpes viridae
- Has 2 strains:
  - HSV-1: causes oropharyngeal infection
  - HSV-2: genital tract infections
- Manifestations in general:

  Herpetic gingivostomatitis:
  - Is often the initial presentation during the first herpes infection
  - It is of greater severity than herpes labialis, which is often the subsequent presentations.

  Herpes labialis:
  - Infection of oral mucosa or abraded skin.

  Herpes genitalis
  - Clusters of inflamed papules and vesicles on the outer surface of the genitals resembling cold sores.

  Herpetic whitlow
  - Painful infection typically affecting the fingers or thumbs, sometimes infecting toes or nail cuticle.

  Herpes gladiatorum
  - Presents as skin ulceration on the face, ears and neck
  - Symptoms include fever, headache, sore throat and swollen glands
  - It occasionally affects the eyes or eyelids.

  Herpes viral encephalitis/meningitis
  - Caused by the retrograde transmission of virus from a peripheral site on the face following HSV-1 reactivation, along the trigeminal nerve axon, to the brain
  - When infecting the brain, the virus shows a preference for the temporal lobe.

  Herpes esophagitis
  - Include painful swallowing (odynophagia) and difficulty swallowing (dysphagia)
  - Mainly occurs in immuno compromised subjects.

Types: 3 groups

- Primary infection: 1st clinical infection with no pre-existing antibodies
- Non primary 1st episode:

- No history of genital tract infection
- HSV1 antibodies present in females who have HSV 2 infection
- HSV2 antibodies present in females with HSV 1 infection
- Recurrent infection:
  - Earlier clinical infection with a positive antibody for the same strain.

Modes of Transmission

- Direct contact → through broken skin or mucosal surface or infected body fluids, during close physical contact, most commonly sexual
- Mother to child transmission
- Recurrent: Genital herpes has a tendency to show recurrent infection as viral particles reside in nerve ganglia and gets reactivated in the same patient → but less severe.

Risk of Transmission to the Neonate

- If genital herpes is acquired near the time of delivery → risk is 30-50%
- Genital herpes acquired during 1st half of pregnancy or in women with history of recurrent herpes →< 1%
- As amount of virus is usually lower during recurrence and recurrent genital herpes is much more common than initial HSV infection during pregnancy, the proportion of neonatal HSV infections is substantial.

Incubation Period

- 2-20 days.

Disease Manifestations

- Genital herpes is a chronic, life-long viral infection
- Two types of HSV have been identified as causing genital herpes: HSV-1 and HSV-2
- Most cases of recurrent genital herpes are caused by HSV-2
- Most persons infected with HSV-2 have not been diagnosed with genital herpes
- Many such persons have mild or unrecognized infections but shed virus intermittently in the genital tract
- As a result, the majority of genital herpes infections are transmitted by persons unaware that they have the infection or who are asymptomatic when transmission occurs.

Prodromal Stage

- Paresthesia
- Tingling sensations
- Neuralgia (pain where lumbosacral nerves innervate the skin)
- Flu like symptoms

This is followed by:

- Eruption of painful vesicles over external genitalia → these when rupture → forms small ulcers which coalesce together → form encrustations and heal without scarring.

In these stages, the following can occur:

- Tender inguinal lymphadenopathy with urinary retention
- Extragenital manifestation → encephalitis/meningitis.

Entire Duration

- 2-4 weeks.

Diagnosis

- Clinical (as mentioned above but should be confirmed with laboratory testing)
- Virological tests:
  - Culture (less sensitive)
  - HSV DNA PCR:
    - More sensitive
    - PCR is the test of choice for detecting HSV in spinal fluid for diagnosis of HSV infection of the CNS
  - Failure to detect HSV by culture or PCR does not indicate an absence of HSV infection because viral shedding is intermittent
- Type specific serology testing glycoprotein G specific assays:
  - Type-specific antibodies to HSV develop during the first several weeks after infection and persist indefinitely
  - Distinguish HSV 1 infection from HSV 2 infection
  - Sensitivity for the detection of HSV-2 antibody vary between 80-98%
  - Specificity ≥ 96%
- *IgM testing for HSV is not useful because the IgM tests are not type-specific and might be positive during recurrent episodes of herpes.*

Management

Mother

- Analgesics and topical anesthetics
- If there is urinary retention: indwelling catheter
- The safety of systemic acyclovir, valacyclovir and famciclovir therapy in pregnant women has not been definitively established
- Available data do not indicate an increased risk for major birth defects compared with the general population in women treated with acyclovir during the 1st trimester
- *1st clinical episode or severe recurrent herpes*
  - Oral acyclovir 200 mg 5 times/day × 5 days OR
  - Oral acyclovir 400 mg 3 times/day × 5 days
  - Category 'C' drug
  - Safe in 1st trimester
- *In systemic infection (severe HSV infection)*
  - Inj. Acyclovir 5-10 mg/kg body weight 8th hourly × 7 days
- Valcyclovir:
  - 1000 mg bid × 7-14 days (category B drug)
  - Prodrug of acyclovir
  - 100% converted to acyclovir in the body
  - Advantages: Higher levels of acyclovir with less frequent dosing
- Famciclovir:
  - 250 mg tid × 7-14 days
  - Category B drug

- Gets completely changed to penciclovir after absorption
- Longer intracellular half life than acyclovir.

Mode of Delivery

- Vaginal delivery is best avoided in patient with active genital herpes (which can be primary or recurrent)
- Women without symptoms or signs of genital herpes or its prodrome can deliver vaginally
- Although cesarean section does not completely eliminate the risk for HSV transmission to the infant, women with recurrent genital herpetic lesions at the onset of labor should be delivered by cesarean section to prevent neonatal HSV infection
- Acyclovir treatment late in pregnancy reduces the frequency of cesarean sections among women who have recurrent genital herpes by diminishing the frequency of recurrences at term
- The effect of antiviral therapy late in pregnancy on the incidence of neonatal herpes is not known.

Prevention of Neonatal Herpes

- By preventing acquisition of genital HSV infection during late pregnancy
- Proper counseling of the pregnant woman:
    - Abstain from intercourse during the 3rd trimester with partners known or suspected of having genital herpes
    - Abstain from receptive oral sex during the 3rd trimester with partners known or suspected to have orolabial herpes
- Mother with HSV → screened for other STDs
- Cesarean section → if active genital herpes
- After birth: hygiene and protecting the baby from vesicles
- Breast feeding allowed → if no vesicles present on breast
- Cultures of mucosal surfaces and administration of prophylactic acyclovir might be considered before the development of clinical signs of neonatal herpes.

Neonatal Infection

Can manifests as:
- In 45%, localized infection of skin, eye and mouth disease → mild disease
- In 30% → progress to encephalitis
- In 25% → meningitis, chorio retinitis, mental retardation, microcephaly, seizures.

Treatment of Newborn
- Infection to skin and mucosa
    - Inj. Acyclovir 20 mg/kg IV 8th hourly × 14 days
- Infection for disseminated and CNS disease
    - Inj. Acyclovir 20 mg/kg IV 8th hourly × 21 days.

CHORIOAMNIONITIS

Definition

- An acute intraamniotic inflammation of the membranes and chorion of the placenta.

Routes of Spread

- Ascending polymicrobial bacterial infection secondary to membrane rupture (most common route)
- With intact membranes, in case of infection with genital mycoplasmas (ureaplasma species and mycoplasma hominis) found in the lower genital tract of > 70% of women
- Hematogeneous spread mainly with Listeria monocytogenes (rare).

Types

Clinical Chorioamnionitis

- When characteristic clinical signs or clinical intraamniotic infection is present.

Histological Chorioamnionitis

- More common diagnosis
- Pathology found on microscopic examination of the placenta
- Presented as either sub-clinical chorioamnionitis or clinical chorioamnionitis
- Funisitis → when umbilical cord is also infected.

Microbiologic Type

- Microbes are cultured from appropriately collected amniotic fluid or chorioamnion.

Incidence

Complicates:
- 40-70% of preterm births with PROM
- 1-13% of term births
- 12% of primary cesarean births at term.

Risk Factors

- Prolonged rupture of membranes
- Prolonged labor
- Nulliparity
- Multiple and repeated vaginal examinations
- Meconium-stained amniotic fluid
- Colonization with group B streptococcus
- Bacterial vaginosis
- Sexually transmissible genital infections
- Vaginal colonization with ureaplasma
- Smoking, alcohol or drug abuse
- Immuno-compromised states
- Epidural anesthesia.

Together with preterm labor, PPROM frequently is the consequence of sub-clinical chorioamanionitis.

Causative Agents

Genital mycoplasmas
- Ureaplasma urealyticum (in 47% of cases)
- Mycoplasma hominis (in 30% of cases).

Ascending infection
- Anerobes
  - Gardnerella vaginalis (25%)
  - Bacteroides (30%)
- Aerobes
  - Group B streptococcus (15%)
  - Gram-negative rods including Escherichia coli (8%).

Hematogenous route
- Listeria monocytogenes.

Pathogenesis

Retrograde or ascending infection from cervix and vagina
↓
Hematogenous/Transplacental passage → **Chorioamnionitis** ← Iatrogenic route (amniocentesis/CVS)
↑
Anterograde infection from peritoneum via fallopian tubes
↓
Release of proinflammatory and inhibitory cytokines and chemokines in the maternal and fetal compartments

Maternal infection 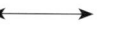 *Fetal infection*

- Clinical chorioamnionitis
- Prostaglandin release
- Ripening of the cervix
- Membrane injury
- Preterm/term labor

Sepsis
Cerebral white matter injury
Cerebral palsy
Other short/long-term neurological deficits.

Clinical Signs and Symptoms

- Maternal fever:
  - Most important clinical sign
  - >100.4°F persisting > 1 h or any fever ≥ 101°F
  - Present in 95-100% of cases
- Maternal tachycardia (>100/min):
  - Present in 50-80% of cases
- Fetal tachycardia (>160/min):
  - Present in 40-70% of cases
- Uterine fundal tenderness ⎫ Present in
- Purulent or foul amniotic fluid ⎭ 4-25% of cases.

NOTE: *Maternal fever, tachycardia and fetal tachycardia should be measured every 4 hourly.*
How chorioamnionitis is misdiagnosed in presence of epidural anesthesia?
- Fundal tenderness may not be appreciable in presence of epidural anesthesia
- May induce maternal and/or fetal tachycardia
- Epidural fever (fever in presence of epidural analgesia) especially when given in nullipara with prolonged labor creates a dilemma in the diagnosis (as low parity and prolonged labor are major risk factors for chorioamnionitis).

Diagnosis

Clinically
- Presence of fever > 100.4 °F along with two any other signs (mentioned above).

Laboratory Tests
- Maternal leucocytosis (WBC >12,000/mm³ or >15,000/mm³) in *presence* of clinical chorioamnionitis
- ↑ levels of the following, when present along with PPROM or preterm labor, carries a higher risk:
  - C-reactive protein
  - Lipopolysacharide binding protein
  - Soluble intercellular adhesion molecule 1
  - Interleukin 6.

Amniotic Fluid Testing
- Obtained by amniocentesis
- Culture of amniotic fluid → Gold standard
- Drawbacks:
  - Invasive procedure, therefore cannot be done when patient is in labor, hence limited value
  - Results may not be available for up to 3 days.

Placenta and Umbilical Cord Testing (Histologic chorioamnionitis)

Depends either on:
- Number of polymorphonuclear leukocytes/HPF OR
- Staging/grading which involves documentation of:
  - Polymorphonuclear leukocyte location
  - Density
  - Degeneration to estimate intensity and progression of chorioamnionitis
- Funisitis
  - Leukocyte infiltration of the umbilical vessel wall or Wharton's jelly.

Note:
- Even if amniotic fluid culture is negative, placental pathology should be performed in suspected cases
- Presence of funisitis makes the diagnosis even stronger as it represents a fetal response to infection
- While chorioamnionitis is present in nearly all cases of funisitis, funisitis is present in only up to 60% of cases of chorioamnionitis.

Complications

Maternal

Common complications
- Cesarean delivery
- Endomyometritis
- Wound infection
- Pelvic abscess
- Bacteremia
- Postpartum hemorrhage.

Rare complications
- Septic shock
- DIC
- Adult respiratory distress syndrome
- Maternal death.

Fetal

Fetal Inflammatory Response Syndrome (FIRS) may cause the following:
- Preterm labor
- Prematurity
- IUD.

Neonatal and Long Term Sequelae

- Perinatal death
- Respiratory distress
- Early onset neonatal sepsis
- Septic shock
- Pneumonia
- Intraventricular hemorrhage
- Cerebral white matter damage
- Cerebral palsy.

Management

Prevention

- Expectant management of preterm premature rupture of membranes → constitutes 70% of cases of clinical chorioamnionitis.

Antibiotics

- Ampicillin 2g IV (or Erythromycin 250 mg orally) 6th hourly
- Gentamicin IV every 8th hourly
- In cases of cesarean section:
    - Clindamycin OR metronidazole IV every 8 hourly
    - Single IV additional dose of antibiotics after delivery has a < 5% failure rate
- Further oral antibiotic treatment is not beneficial in most cases.

Amoxicillin/Co-amoxiclav should not be used as it may lead to increase in incidence of necrotizing enterocolitis.

Antipyretics

- Acetaminophen.

ACUTE PYELONEPHRITIS

Overview

- Acute pyelonephritis is infection of the kidney and the pelvic ureter
- A serious systemic illness affecting 1-2% of all pregnancies and the most common non-obstetric cause of hospital admission during pregnancy
- Without treatment it can cause preterm labor and maternal septicemia
- Recurrent pyelonephritis → a cause of IUGR and IUD
- Recurrence → ≈ 2-3% and it can recur during the same pregnancy.

Presentation

- Occurs beyond 16 weeks
- Usually bilateral, if unilateral, present more on right side
- Lower urinary tract symptoms (e.g., frequency, urgency, dysuria)
- Upper urinary tract symptoms (e.g., flank pain)
- Constitutional symptoms (e.g., fever, chills, malaise)
- Gastrointestinal symptoms (e.g., nausea, vomiting, anorexia, abdominal pain).

Signs and symptoms

- Fever (temperature > 100.4°F [38.0°C])
- Tachycardia
- Hypotension
- Costo vertebral angle tenderness
- Possible abdominal or suprapubic tenderness.

Investigations

- Same as in acute cystitis
- Urine culture growing ≥ 10^5 colony-forming units/mL of urine.

Management

- Hospitalization
- Indications for admissions include:
  - Severe distress (septicemia)
  - Dehydration
  - Poor oral food tolerance
  - Maternal and fetal complications
  - Where intravenous antibiotic is necessary
- IV Hydration

- Vitals charting (PR, BP, temperature, urine output)
- Antibiotics
  - Ampicillin
  - Gentamycin
  - Cefazolin or ceftriaxone.

SUGGESTED READING

1. Alessandra G Commodaro, Rubens N Belfort, Luiz Vicente Rizzo et al: Ocular toxoplasmosis - an update and review of the literature. Mem Inst Oswaldo Cruz, Rio de Janeiro. March 2009;104(2):345-50.
2. Caroline Paquet, Mark H. Yudin et al: Toxoplasmosis in Pregnancy: Prevention, Screening, and Treatment. J Obstet Gynaecol Can 2013;35(1 eSuppl A):S1-S7.
3. Clara Thompson, Richard Whitley: Neonatal Herpes Simplex Virus Infections: Where are we now? Adv Exp Med Biol. 2011;697:221-30.
4. David W. Kimberlin, Jill Baley: Guidance on Management of Asymptomatic Neonates Born to Women With Active Genital Herpes Lesions. Pediatrics 2013;131:e635-e646.
5. Deborah Money, Marc Steben et al: Guidelines for the Management of Herpes Simplex Virus in Pregnancy. J Obstet Gynaecol Can 2008;30(6):514-19.
6. Di Mario S, Basevi V, Gagliotti C et al: Prenatal education for congenital toxoplasmosis (Review). The Cochrane Library 2013, Issue 2.
7. Elena Anzivino, Daniela Fioriti, Monica Mischitelli et al: Herpes simplex virus infection in pregnancy and in neonate: status of art of epidemiology, diagnosis, therapy and prevention. Virology Journal 2009;6:40.
8. F Peyron: When are we going to celebrate the centenary of the discovery of efficient treatment for congenital toxoplasmosis? Mem Inst Oswaldo Cruz, Rio de Janeiro March 2009; Vol. 104(2):316-19.
9. Fabiana Maria Ruiz Lopes-Mori, Regina Mitsuka-Breganó, Jaqueline Dario Capobiango et al: Programs for control of congenital toxoplasmosis. Rev Assoc Med Bras 2011;57(5):581-6.
10. GC Khilnani: Tuberculosis and Pregnancy. Indian J Chest Dis Allied Sci 2004;46:105-11
11. Gianluca Straface,1 Alessia Selmin, 1 Vincenzo Zanardo et al: Herpes Simplex Virus Infection in Pregnancy. Infectious Diseases in Obstetrics and Gynecology 2012.
12. Guidelines for diagnosis and treatment of malaria. National institute of malaria research, Government of India. 2009.
13. Herpes simplex in pregnancy: Clinical Guidelines. King Edward Memorial Hospital Review Perth Western Australia OGCCU. November 2001.
14. Jana N, Barik S, Arora N. Tuberculosis in pregnancy—a major maternal and perinatal challenge. BJOG 2011;118:1145-6.
15. Lawrence Corey, Anna Wald: Maternal and Neonatal HSV Infections. N Engl J Med. October 1 2009;361(14):1376-85.
16. Lorraine Dontigny, Marc-Yvon Arsenault, Marie-Jocelyne Martel et al: Rubella in Pregnancy. J Obstet Gynaecol Can 2008;30(2):152-8.
17. Malaria in Pregnancy: Intermittent Preventive Treatment A cost-effective intervention for preventing maternal and newborn mortality. IS global, Barcelona institute of global health February 2013.
18. Management of genital herpes in pregnancy. RCOG Green-top Guideline No. 30. September 2007.
19. Mark R. Schleiss: Cytomegalovirus Vaccine Development. Curr Top Microbiol Immunol. 2008;325:361-382.
20. Maxim C-J Cheeran, James R. Lokensgard, Mark R. Schleiss: Neuropathogenesis of Congenital Cytomegalovirus Infection: Disease Mechanisms and Prospects for Intervention. Clinical Microbiology Reviews. Jan. 2009. p. 99-126.
21. Peng Zhou, Zhaoguo Chen, Hai-Long Li et al: Toxoplasma gondii infection in humans in China. Parasites & Vectors 2011;4:165.
22. Peyron F, Wallon M, Liou C et al: Treatments for toxoplasmosis in pregnancy (Review). The Cochrane Library 2010, Issue 1.
23. Pooja Dewan, Piyush Gupta: Burden of Congenital Rubella Syndrome (CRS) in India: A Systematic Review. Indian Pediatrics May 16, 2012; Volume 49.

24. Rima McLeod, Francois Kieffer, Mari Sautter et al: Why prevent, diagnose and treat congenital toxoplasmosis? Mem Inst Oswaldo Cruz. 2009;104(2):320-44.
25. Robert F. Pass: Development and Evidence for Efficacy of CMV Glycoprotein B Vaccine with MF59 Adjuvant. J Clin Virol. December 2009;46(Suppl 4): S73-S76.
26. Rubella in pregnancy: Clinical Guidelines. OGCCU. King Edward Memorial Hospital Perth Western Australia September 2011.
27. So-Hee Kang, Angela Chua-Gocheco, Pina Bozzo et al: Safety of antiviral medication for the treatment of herpes during pregnancy Canadian Family Physician. April 2011: Vol 57.
28. Stuart P. Adler: Screening for Cytomegalovirus during Pregnancy. Infectious Diseases in Obstetrics and Gynecology 2011.
29. The diagnosis and treatment of malaria in pregnancy. RCOG April 2010.
30. VK Arora, Rajnish Gupta: Tuberculosis and pregnancy. Ind J Tub, 2003, 50, 13.
31. Women and Tuberculosis: Taking a look at a neglected issue. Advocacy to Control TB Internationally. 2010.
32. Yoav Yinon, Dan Farine et al: Cytomegalovirus Infection in Pregnancy. J Obstet Gynaecol Can 2010; 32(4):348-54.

CHAPTER 16

Postpartum Hemorrhage

Tania G Singh

1. **What is PPH (after vaginal and abdominal delivery?**
   Any loss > 500 mL after vaginal and >1000 mL after cesarean section is termed PPH within 24 hours of the birth of the baby. For Asian women, 300 mL as cut off has been suggested because of lower BMI.

2. **What is primary and secondary PPH?**
   Primary PPH
   Loss of:
   - 500 mL of blood from genital tract at vaginal delivery
   - >1000 mL at cesarean section
   - 1500 mL at cesarean hysterectomy.

   } Within first 24 hours after delivery.

   OR
   - 10% drop in hematocrit.

   OR
   - Need for blood transfusion in first 24 hours after delivery.

   Secondary PPH
   - If excessive blood loss occurs after 24 hours but within 12 weeks after delivery.

3. **What is major and minor PPH?**
   PPH can be:
   - *Minor* (500–1000 mL) or
   - *Major* (more than 1000 mL)

   Major could be divided into:
   - Moderate (1000–2000 mL) or
   - Severe (more than 2000 mL).

4. **Do you know any other definition of PPH?**
   PPH can be subdivided into:
   - *3rd stage hemorrhage* – when bleeding occurs before expulsion of placenta
   - *True PPH* – which occurs after expulsion of placenta.

5. **What is *significant primary PPH***
   - Resulting in blood loss of ≥ 1500 mL, when physiological compensatory mechanisms begin to fail.

6. **What is acute PPH and acute severe PPH?**
   - *Acute PPH:* blood loss >500 mL within 24 hours of delivery
   - *Acute severe PPH:* blood loss >1000 mL within 24 hours of delivery.

- In estimating percentage of blood loss, consideration should be given to body weight and the original hemoglobin (approximate blood volume equals weight in kilograms divided by 12 expressed as liters).

7. **How does iron deficiency anemia lead to PPH?**
   - In iron deficiency anemia, there is depletion of uterine myoglobin levels necessary for muscle action, leading to uterine atony.

8. **Incidence of PPH**
   - Incidence of PPH: 2% of all women who give birth
   - Maternal mortality following PPH: 25-30% (especially in Africa and Asia).

9. **Etiology of PPH**
   1. *Factors affecting 'Tone'*
      - Polyhydramnios ⎫
      - Multiple gestation ⎬ Overdistension of uterus
      - Big baby ⎭
      - Prolonged rupture of membranes } Intraamniotic infection
      - Placenta previa ⎫
      - Uterine anamoly ⎬ Uterine distortion (functional or anatomical)
      - Fibroid uterus ⎭
      - Multigravida ⎫
      - Prolonged labor (>12 hours) ⎬ Uterine exhaustion
      - Obstructed labor ⎪
      - Rapid labor ⎭
      - Previous PPH ⎫
      - Asian ethnicity ⎪
      - Obesity (BMI >35) ⎬ Others
      - Anemia (<9 g/dl) ⎪
      - Age > 40 years. ⎭
   2. *Factors affecting 'Tissue'*
      - Retained products
      - Abnormal placenta
      - Retained cotyledon or succenturiate lobe
      - Retained blood clots.
   3. *Factors leading to 'Trauma'*
      - Operative vaginal delivery ⎫ Cervical, vaginal or
      - Precipitous delivery ⎭ perineal lacerations
      - Extension, lacerations at cesarean section } Malposition, deep engagement
      - Emergency or elective cesarean section
      - Uterine rupture } Previous uterine surgery
      - Uterine inversion.
   4. *Factors affecting coagulation ('Thrombin')*
      - Pre-existing stages:
        – Hemophilia A
        – von Willebrand's disease
      - Acquired in pregnancy
        – ITP
        – Thrombocytopenia with preeclampsia
        – DIC

- Preeclampsia
- IUD
- Severe infection (fever, prolonged rupture of membranes)
- Abruption
- Amniotic fluid embolism
- Therapeutic anti coagulation (history of blood clot).
  NOTE:
- Episiotomy contributes 154 mL to average blood loss
- Increased risk of PPH due to prolonged labor
  - Stage 1 – 1.5 times ↑ risk
  - Stage 2 – 1.5 times ↑ risk
  - Stage 3 – 6.2 times ↑ risk (if >17 min)
    - At 10 min – 2 times ↑ risk
    - At 20 min – 4 times ↑ risk
    - At 30 min – 6 times ↑ risk.

10. **How much time does it take for the patient to die in PPH?**
    Time to death:
    - For PPH – 2 hours
    - For APH – 12 hours
    - For uterine rupture – 24 hours.

11. **How will you diagnose PPH? OR measurement of postpartum blood loss?**
    Two methods (ways):
    1. Quantitative methods
    2. Clinical signs and symptoms of hypovolemia (much more important than any other visual method).

	Class	Symptoms & signs	BP	Blood loss	Percent blood loss	Therapy
Stages of shock or hemorrhage						
None	I	Palpitations, Dizziness, Mild thirst	SBP normal	≈ 750 mL (500-1000 mL)	10-15%	–
Mild	II	Tachycardia (100 beats/min), Minimal tachypnea, Minimal pallor, Extremities cool (anxious/ restless), Sweating	Slight fall (80-100 mmHg)	1000-1500 mL	15-25%	Crystalloids
Moderate	III	PR>100 <120, Pallor ++, Tachypnea, Oliguria	Marked fall 70-80 mmHg	1500-2000 mL	25-35%	Transfusion
Severe	IV	Collapse, Air hunger, Marked pallor, Anuria, PR>120	Profound fall (50- 70 mmHg)	>2000 mL	>40%	Massive transfusion

Quantitative methods

Older methods
1. Visual assessment
2. Direct collection of blood into bed pan/basin/sponges/plastic bag
3. Determination of changes in hematocrit and hemoglobin
4. Gravimetric methods: weighing of materials such as soaked pads on a scale and subtracting the known weights of these materials to determine blood loss (gauze, pads, sponges)
5. Plasma volume changes (blood volume estimation by dye- dilution or radio isotope dilution techniques)
6. Acid Hematin method
7. Measurement of tagged erythrocytes.

Recent methods: BRASS – V Drape
- It is a plastic, caliberated blood collection drape
- Developed by NICHD funded global network UMKC at JNMC/UIC collaborative team, specifically to measure postpartum blood loss
- Can objectively measure blood loss, has shown that visual estimate is 33% less than the drape estimate
- Very good tool for referral, for quantification of blood loss in home settings
- Helps in early referral of patients delivered at home by midwives.

12. **Normal blood changes in pregnancy**
    Blood changes

    Hemoglobin concentration and hematocrit
    - Slightly reduced → whole blood viscosity ↓
    - Hemoglobin concentration at term 12.5 gm/dL
    - The disproportionate increase in plasma and RBC volume produces a state of hemodilution during pregnancy.

    Blood volume
    - Markedly raised (40-45%)
    - Begins to ↑ during 1st trimester, expands most rapidly during 2nd trimester and rises at a much slower rate in 3rd trimester to reach a plateau during last several weeks of pregnancy.

    Plasma volume and erythropoietin
    - Increases to extent of 1.25 liters
    - By 12th week, expands by about 15%
    - Erythrocytes → 450 mL
    - Moderate erythroid hyperplasia is seen in bone marrow
    - Plasma erythropoietin levels peak early during 3rd trimester and correspond to maximal erythrocyte production.

    Coagulation

Pregnancy is a hypercoagulable state	
Non pregnant	Pregnancy
Fibrinogen 200-400 mg%	300-600mg% (↑ by 50%)
Factor VII	↑ 10 times by term
Factor VIII	↑ 2 times by term
Factor IX and X	Increases
Factor XI	↓ by 60%
Factor XIII	↓ by 50%
Platelets (life span 9-12 days)	Width and volume ↑; ↓ platelet concentration due to hemodilution →↑ no. of younger and larger platelets
Fibrinolytic system	Depressed till 60 min after delivery of placenta (due to effect of placentally derived plasminogen activator inhibitor [Type 2])
Serum D dimer	Increases
Clotting time	NO CHANGE
Thromboxane A_2	↑↑ in mid pregnancy → it induces platelet aggregation.

13. **Summarize blood flow in maternal and fetal circulation**

    Maternal circulation
    - Volume of blood in mature placenta: 500 mL
    - Volume of blood in intervillous spaces: 150 mL
    - Volume of blood in villi system: 350 mL
    - Blood flow in intervillous space: 500-600 mL/min (completely replaced 3-4 times/min)
    - Pressure in intervillous space:
        - During uterine contraction: 30-50 mmHg
        - During uterine relaxation: 10-15 mmHg
    - Pressure in supplying uterine artery: 70-80 mmHg
    - Pressure in draining uterine vein: 8 mmHg.

    Fetal circulation
    - Fetal blood flow through placenta: 400 mL/min
    - Pressure in umbilical artery: 60mmHg
    - Pressure in umbilical vein: 10mmHg
    - Fetal capillary pressure in villi: 20-40mmHg

	Umbilical artery	Umbilical vein
O_2 saturation	50-60%	70-80%
PO_2	20-25mmHg	30-40mmHg

14. **Why does placenta separate after birth of baby?**
    - Contraction and relaxation of uterus reduces size of placental area which brings about separation of placenta because it is a relatively rigid and inelastic structure.

15. **Signs of placental separation**
    Signs:
    1. Fresh gush of blood through introitus
    2. Apparent lengthening of cord
    3. Contraction of uterus with fundus rising abdominally.

16. **Describe mechanism of control of blood loss after delivery of placenta**
    - Oblique muscle fibers of myometrium contract strongly following placental delivery to compress the maternal spiral arteries (by obliterating their lumina)
    - Therefore, myometrial fibers are referred to as "living ligatures".
17. **What is normal range of blood loss in Stage 3 of labor?**
    - 100-250 mL.
18. **Name 2 factors which can promote uterine atony in Stage 3?**
    Two factors:
    1. Full bladder
    2. Retained placental membranes and cotyledons.
19. **Describe placenta at term**
    Term placenta
    1. Circular disc
    2. Diameter 15-20 cm
    3. Thickness 2.5 cm at center
    4. Towards edge → thins off
    5. Spongy feel
    6. Weight ≈ 500 gm
    7. Proportion with weight of baby = 1.6
    8. Occupies: 30% of uterine wall.

    Fetal surface
    1. Covered by smooth and glistening amnion
    2. Umbilical cord attached at or near its center
    3. Branches of umbilical vessels are visible beneath amnion as they radiate from insertion of cord
    4. Amnion can be peeled off from underlying chorion except at insertion of cord
    5. At term, ≈ 4/5th is of fetal origin.

    Maternal surface
    1. Rough and spongy
    2. Maternal blood gives it a dull red color
    3. Thin, greyish, shaggy layer may be visible (remnant of decidua basalis → compact and spongy layer)
    4. 15-20 lobes or cotyledons (limited by fissures)
    5. Each fissure is occupied by decidual septum
    6. Many small greyish spots are visible (due to deposition of calcium in degenerated areas/of no clinical significance)
    7. ≈1/5th of total placenta
    8. Only decidua basalis and blood in intervillous space are of maternal origin.

    Margin
    - Limited by fused basal and chorionic plates (placenta is a specialized part of chorion).

    Attachment
    - To upper part of body of uterus encroaching to fundus adjacent to anterior or posterior wall with equal frequency
    - To uterine wall is effective:
        – Due to encroaching villi connecting chorionic plate with basal plate and also
        – By fused decidua capsularis and vera with chorion leave at margin.

Separation
- Line of separation is through decidua spongiosum.

20. **Do all PPHs have a cause?**
    In 2/3rd of cases with PPH, there is no antecedent risk factor.

21. **What precautions can be taken antenatally and during labor to prevent PPH?**
    Antenatal prophylaxis:
    - Frequent ANCs to detect early, any complication arising in high risk cases and timely referral to higher centers for management and delivery

    Avoidable risk factors:
    - Teenage pregnancy (< 20 years)
    - Pregnancy at > 40 years
    - Anemia
      - Iron and folate supplementation in pregnancy
      - Recheck Hb at 32-34 weeks
      - Hb should be ≥ 11g% at onset of labor
      - Hb ≤ 8g% → should be referred to higher center for delivery, where there is facility of blood transfusion
    - Prolonged labor
    - Chorioamnionitis/pyrexia in labor
    - Obstructed labor
    - Retained placenta
    - Patients in following categories should have blood cross-matched on admission for delivery:
      - History of PPH in previous pregnancy
      - Antepartum hemorrhage
      - Previous cesarean section
      - Hemoglobin <10 gm/dL
      - Intrauterine death
      - Fetal distress
    - At risk women, should deliver in the hospital:
      - Those mentioned above and
      - Parity > 5
      - BMI > 35
      - Where estimated weight of the baby is ≥ 4 kg
    - Monitoring 1st stage of labor with partograph (to prevent prolonged labor)
    - In cases of previous cesarean section:
      - Placental site should be determined before, by USG to rule out placenta percreta, accreta
      - MRI can be offered where facilities exist (to look for bladder invasion etc.)
      - Blood and all blood products should be kept ready before surgery
    - Cautious use of oxytocin and misoprostol in multigravidae
    - Injudicious use of oxytocin and misoprotol for induction of labor; using excessive doses and continuing these drugs in the presence of adequate uterine activity can lead to uterine rupture
    - Also inappropriate use of oxytocin for augmentation when there are already signs of CPD or a malpresentation can lead to uterine rupture
    - Management of 2nd stage is important:
      - Deliver baby's trunk slowly in order to allow little time for uterine retraction
      - Prefilled syringe with synto or ergometrine – keep ready in 2nd stage
    - Constant watch on blood loss after 2nd stage

- Start thinking when 250 mL mark in the collecting drape is reached and be prepared to act when loss ≈ 450 mL (don't wait for 500 mL mark)
- In case of cesarean section, 5 IU by slow IV injection can be given to facilitate contraction of uterus
- Following this, oxytocin infusion 10 IU in one liter fluid can be commenced.

22. **How do you prevent atonic PPH at the time of delivery?**
    By AMTSL (Active management of third stage of labor)
    AMTSL: intervention to facilitate delivery of placenta by enhancing uterine contraction and retraction to prevent atonic PPH
    Components: Confirm the absence of additional baby/babies by per abdominal examination
    1. *Immediate administration of utero tonic agent*
        - Enhances uterine contraction and relaxation
        - Hastens separation and delivery of placenta
        - Decreases duration of 3rd stage
        - Minimize blood loss (reduces the risk of PPH by 60%)
        - Main intervention in AMTSL:
            – 10U oxytocin IM or IV within 1-3 min of delivery of anterior shoulder
            – Intravenous infusion of oxytocin (20 to 40 IU in 1000 mL, 150 mL per hour) is an acceptable alternative
            – Carbetocin, 100 mcg given as an IV bolus over 1 minute, should be used instead of continuous oxytocin infusion in elective cesarean section for the prevention of PPH and to decrease the need for therapeutic uterotonics.

    Why oxytocin?
    - Uterotonic of choice
    - Effective 2-3 min after injection
    - Minimal side effects
    - Can be given in all females
    - Recommended uterotonic for prevention of PPH after cesarean section.

    When oxytocin is not available?
    - Misoprostol (600-800 µg), though not as effective as oxytocin (10 IU IV) but it may be used when the latter is not available or bleeding does not respond to oxytocin, especially in cases of home delivery or other community settings
    - Injectables:
        – Ergometrine or methylergometrine
        – Syntometrine (ergometrine-oxytocin) has more side effects like nausea, vomiting, elevation of BP.

    2. *Delayed cord clamping*
        - After 1-3min, (not earlier than first 60 seconds) or after cessation of cord pulsation
        - Facilitates transfer of 80-100 mL blood → helps neonate receive additional blood which increases hemoglobin up to 6 months and lesser need for iron therapy
        - Is of particular help in cases of preterm neonate by providing an additional 30% blood volume and reducing the need for transfusion and reduce intraventricular hemorrhage.

        Early cord clamping: defined as cord clamping immediately or within the first 60 seconds after birth. Not recommended routinely unless following situations arise:
        - When baby needs to be resuscitated immediately
        - If there is tight cord around neck
        - If there is postpartum hemorrhage, placenta previa or vasa previa

- Rh −ve (to prevent antibody transfer from mother to baby)
- In diabetic mothers

Results in decrease in 20-40 mL/kg of blood, which is equivalent to 30-35 mg of iron.

3. ***Controlled cord traction (CCT)***
   - Prevents inversion of uterus
   - This intervention is **now** regarded as **optional** in settings where skilled birth attendants are available and is **contraindicated** in settings where skilled attendants are not present at birth
   - Recommended method for removal of placenta after cesarean section.

   Procedure:
   - Clamp cord close to perineum (after pulsation stops)
   - Keep slight tension on cord and await a strong uterine contraction (2-3min)
   - Place the other hand over suprapubic region and apply upward counter traction (without waiting for signs of placental separation) – discontinue CCT, if:
     - Placenta does not descend within 30-40 sec
     - Wait for next uterine contraction and repeat CCT
     - When uterus becomes rounded or cord lengthens, very gently pull downwards on the cord to deliver the placenta (turn the placenta so that membranes are twisted into a rope).

4. ***Uterine massage***
   - Sustained uterine massage is not recommended as a prevention for PPH in women who have received prophylactic oxytocin
   - Abdominal palpation to determine uterine tonus is recommended for all women
   - Uterus can be palpated every time vitals are being monitored while patient is kept under observation after delivery (for minimum 2 hours).

   NOTE:
   - Examination of placenta to check for its completeness after every delivery is MUST
   - Early latching of the baby to the breast and the mother massaging her own uterus can also assist in reducing PPH.

23. **What is expectant management? What is the advantage of AMTSL over it?**

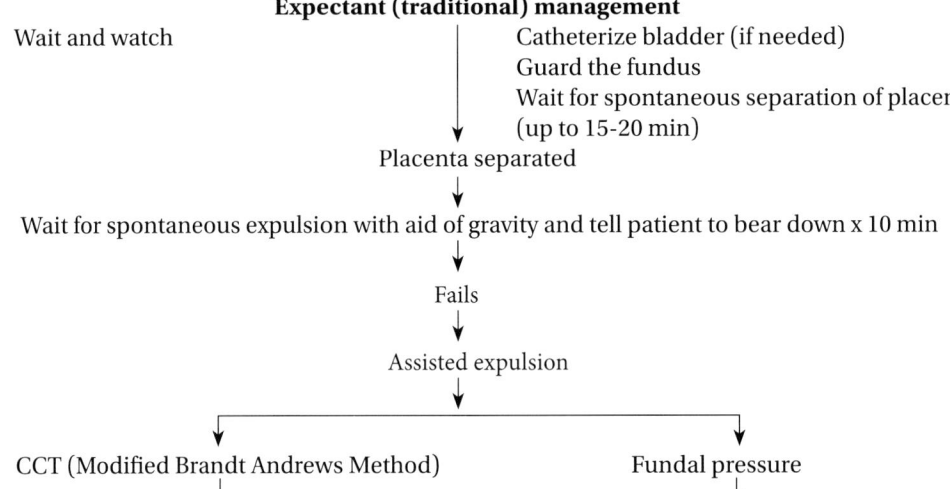

Advantages of AMTSL over it
There is reduced:
1. Duration of 3rd stage of labor
2. Need for therapeutic uterotonics
3. PPH
4. Retained placenta
5. Acute inversion of uterus
6. Need for blood transfusion and manual removal of placenta.

24. **How will you examine placenta/membranes/cord?**
    Examination
    Placenta – placed in tray → washed with running water (to remove blood clots)

    Maternal surface (1st inspected)
    - Greyish
    - Cotyledons placed closely
    - Any gap → missing cotyledons

    Membranes
    - Amnion – shiny
    - Chorion – shaggy
    - No. of vessels – 2 arteries and 1 vein
    - Oval gap in chorion with torn ends of blood vessels:
      – Running up to margin of the gap → missing succenturiate lobe
      – Explore uterus urgently (if something missing).

25. **How do you refer a case of PPH?**
    Referral
    1. Arrange for rapid transport and refer to a center where blood transfusion and emergency obstetric care is available
    2. Establish two wide bore IV cannulas ($\approx \leq 18$ G)
    3. Start resuscitation with NS/RL
    4. Catheterize the patient and foot end elevation
    5. Keep patient warm
    6. Bimanual or aortic compression of uterus during transport
    7. If possible, transfer the patient with intrauterine condom catheter which acts as uterine tamponade and arrests hemorrhage
    8. Ensure adequate donors and attenders accompany the patient
    9. Inform the case and especially blood group of patient, if known, to referral hospital.

26. **What are the immediate and delayed consequences of PPH?**

Immediate	*Delayed*
1. Hypovolemic shock	Anemia
2. ARF	Sheehan's syndrome
3. DIC	
4. Puerperal sepsis	
5. Failure of lactation	
6. Thrombophlebitis → Embolism.	

27. **Protocol for management of PPH**
    Initial assessment
    1. Quick history
    2. Check vital signs

3. Brief examination
4. Documentation of every move is very important
5. Relatives should be kept informed of the situation, consented and possibly reassured.

Initial intervention
a. Airway and Resuscitation
   - Call for help
   - Maintain airway and breathing
   - Oxygen by mask at 10-15 liters/min
   - Endotracheal intubation if SPO_2 is not satisfactory
   - Secure two IV lines with 16/18 G (14 G – orange, preferably)
   - Collect 15-20 mL blood for investigations:
     - CBC:
       - Hemoglobin
       - PCV
       - TLC
       - DLC
       - ESR
     - Blood group and type
     - Platelet count
     - Coagulation profile including fibrinogen:
       - Prothrombin time
       - Thrombin time
       - Partial thromboplastin time
       - INR
     - Renal function test with electrolytes
     - Liver function test
     - Cross matched blood (minimum 4 units) - if unavailable, 'O negative' blood can be transfused
   - Flat position
   - Foot end elevation
   - Infuse rapid warm fluids
     - 2L of Normal saline fast, followed by 200 mL/hr [3.5 liters of warm crystalloid; Hartman's solution (2lit)] and/or colloid (1-2/lit)
     - Salt solutions replace blood loss at the ratio of 3:1
     - Volume expanders replace blood loss at 1:1 ratio (albumin, hetastarch, dextran)
   - Do not infuse 5% dextrose
   - Catheterize and monitor urine output
   - Remove wet clothes and keep patient warm
   - Arrange and transfuse blood and blood products
   - Strict monitoring and charting of vitals (PR, BP, RR, Temp) every 15 minutes.
b. Arrest hemorrhage simultaneously
   Find out the cause:
   Atonic
   - Retained placenta
   - Uterine inversion

Traumatic
- Vaginal lacerations
- Colporrhexis
- Cervical tears
- Vaginal or cervical hematoma
- Broad ligament hematoma
- Rupture uterus

Combined

DIC
- Primary
  - PPH
- Secondary
  - Retained bits
  - Amniotic fluid embolism
  - Abruption placenta.

Initial goals to be achieved

Vitals
- Systolic BP >90 mm Hg
- Urine output ≥ 30 mL/hr
- Review laboratory reports and treat as required

Hematology
- Hemoglobin > 8gm%
- Platelet count > 75000
- Prothrombin (PT) < 1.5 x mean control
- Activated prothrombin time (aPTT) < 1.5 x mean control
- Fibrinogen > 1.0 mg%.

Second assessment: after 30- 40 min

c. *Review lab reports*

Parameters	Lab value	Intervention	Units
Hemoglobin	< 7gm%	Packed RBCs (300mL) No cold blood transfusion	4U 3U FFP 1 amp of calcium gluconate
PT aPTT	>1.5 times	FFP (250mL)	4 U
INR	> 2		
Fibrinogen	< 100mg%	Cryoprecipitate (15mL)	4U
Platelets	< 50000	Platelets (50mL)	Aim is to achieve minimum 50000

NOTE: When the blood loss reaches about 4.5 liters (80% of blood volume) and large volumes of replacement fluids have been given, there will be clotting factor defects and blood components should be given. Up to 1 liter of fresh frozen plasma (FFP) and 10 units of cryoprecipitate (two packs) may be given empirically in the face of relentless bleeding, while awaiting the results of coagulation studies.

Goals achieved
SBP >90 mmHg
UOP ≥ 30mL/hr } Maintain with NS 1.5-2mL/kg/hr
PO$_2$ >90%

Goals not achieved

1. Start inotropic support – Dopamine 5 µ gm/kg/min, ↑ up to 8 µ gm/kg/min, if no response:
2. Insert CVP line (3-4 mm H$_2$O)
3. Send Arterial Blood Gas analysis:
   - If systolic BP <90 mm Hg after 20 mins, inform anesthetist
   - Add dobutamine 5 µ gm/kg/min, ↑ up to 10 µ gm/kg/min
   - Review ABG reports and correction as required.

If atonic, line of management to control bleeding:

Medical
- Inj. Oxytocin
- Inj. Methergin
- Inj. PGF$_{2\alpha}$
- Tab. Misoprostol

Nonsurgical
Bimanual compression of uterus
Intrauterine packing
Intrauterine tamponade (condom catheter)

Conservative surgery
- B- Lynch
- Stepwise uterine artery devascularization
- Bilateral internal iliac artery ligation

Peripartum hysterectomy
Uterine artery embolization

	Medical line of management			
	Oxytocin	*Ergometrine*	*15 methyl PGF$_{2\alpha}$*	*Misoprostol*
Mode of action	Stimulation of upper segment	Stimulation of α adrenergic receptors Stimulation of both upper and lower segment Results in sustained myometrial contraction	Smooth muscle stimulant	Methyl ester of prostaglandin E$_1$ Binds to myometrial prostanoid receptors (derivatives of prostanoic acid; acts as local hormones).
Side effects	Hypotension if rapid IV bolus Water intoxication in higher doses, manifesting as headache, vomiting, drowsiness and convulsions	Nausea, vomiting, dizziness Sudden increase in BP due to vasoconstrictive effect Larger and longer doses can interfere with lactation	Diarrhea, nausea, vomiting pyrexia, dystonia, bronchospasm, systemic hypertension	Shivering, pyrexia (more common with oral administration and when the dose exceeds 600µg), abdominal pain.

Contd...

Contd...

	Oxytocin	Ergometrine	15 methyl PGF$_{2a}$	Misoprostol
Contraindications	Hypersensitivity to drug	As it also acts on the vascular smooth muscle, it is not suitable for those with hypertension, migraine, heart disease and peripheral vascular disease such as Raynaund's syndrome, women taking certain drugs (e.g. proteases for HIV infection), in cases of retained placenta	Cardiac and pulmonary disease (Bronchial asthma)	Hypersensitivity to prostaglandins.
Storage	At 15-30°C, stable only for 1 month Refrigeration (2-8°C) prolongs shelf life	2-8°C	2-8°C	At room temperature.
Dose and route	Infusion IV infuse 20 units in 1 liter @ 60 drops/min Push 5U IV 10 U IM	IM/IV 0.2 mg slowly	IM 0.25 mg or intramyometrially (use a tuberculin syringe)	600 μg orally 800-1000 μg rectally 1000-1200 μg in life threatening events. Sublingual administration results in the most rapid onset of effects and the highest peak concentration. Onset is slower but duration is longer with vaginal and rectal routes.
Continuing dose	IV 20 units in 1 L @ 40 drops/min	Repeated 0.2 mg IM after 15 min	0.25mg every 15 min	Repeat 1 dose
Maximum dose	60U. Not > 3 liters	5 doses (1mg)	Max. 2 mg (8 doses)	2000 μg
Other features	Onset of action: After IM route: 3-7 min After IV route: immediate onset Half life: 3 min	Onset of action: Within 2 to 5 minutes Lasts up to 3 hours Plasma half-life ≈ 30 minutes	Peak of action Intramyometrial: within 5 minutes Intramuscular: Peak within 15 minutes	Cheap and effective Routes: oral, sublingual, vaginal and rectal. Does not require refrigeration. Very good to use in low resource settings.

Carbetocin

- Long acting synthetic oxytocin analogue
- Rapid onset of action, within 2 minutes
- Pharmacokinetics of both IM and IV route is almost the same
- Recommendation:
  - 100 μg of the drug is given as IM or an IV bolus over 1 minute, should be used instead of continuous oxytocin infusion in elective cesarean section for the prevention of PPH and to decrease the need for therapeutic uterotonics
  - For women delivering vaginally with 1 risk factor for PPH, carbetocin 100 μg IM decreases the need for uterine massage to prevent PPH when compared with continuous infusion of oxytocin.

Oxytocin in Uniject

What is Uniject?
- Injection device, increasingly being used nowadays for coverage of immunizations and therapeutics
- Has been used successfully for use in tetanus toxoid and hepatitis B vaccinations
- Features:
  - Single dose
  - Prefilled
  - Non reusable
  - Easy to use
  - Compact size.

How Will it Solve the Purpose in PPH?

- Oxytocin as a drug in Uniject will ensure ready format, accurate, premeasured dose in non reusable, sterile device with minimal preparation and minimum waste, making oxytocin safe for use in measures like AMSTL
- Will greatly improve the ability of midwives and other medical personnel as prefilled dose is kept ready for use within 1 minute of the delivery of the baby
- There will be no need to search for vial, syringe or needles and break ampules or measure correct dose in life threatening emergency situations
- Ideal for use in emergency situations and remote locations
- As oxytocin is a heat-sensitive drug, it has been suggested to include a time-temperature indicator (TTI) as part of oxytocinin Uniject products
- This will help in safe transport and storage of the drug and increase its field utility
- Can be used in home settings even by less trained midwives
- Needles will not be reused which is still done in many underdeveloped countries
- Oxytocin abuse will not be done in laboring patients to augment labor.

Nonsurgical Methods

Uterine Massage and Bimanual Compression

Principle: The first-line approach to mechanical hemostasis → this in itself might control bleeding significantly by assisting the uterus to use its anatomical and physiological properties such as the cross-over interlinked network of myometrial fibers for vascular compression and bleeding control

Technique: With left hand, separate labia → whole right hand is introduced in vagina in cone shaped fashion → clenched into a fist → back of hand directed posteriorly and knuckles in anterior fornix → apply pressure on the lower segment

Left hand → placed over uterus externally making it anteverted
↓
Squeeze firmly between two hands → till tone is regained
↓
Release compression and look for bleeding. If it fails, then
↓

Compression of Aorta

Fist placed at level of umbilicus and push downwards towards spine
↓
This obliterates femoral pulse but does not alter systolic BP
↓

Uterine Tamponade

a. *Tight intrauterine packing*
   5 metres long strip of gauze, 8 cm wide folded twice → soak in antiseptic cream → give GA → place gauze into fundal area, without leaving any empty space in upper portion → fundus made steady through abdominal wall (by other hand)
   ↓
   Pack rest of cavity → separately pack vagina
   ↓
   Place abdominal binder → give antibiotics and remove plug after 24 hours.

   Action:
   - Stimulate uterus to contract
   - Direct hemostatic pressure on open uterine sinuses

b. *Insertion of Sengstaken Blakemore tube ("Tamponade Test")*
   ↓
   Insert into uterine cavity via cervix (under USG guidance → optional)
   ↓
   Inflate balloon with 200 mL NS
   ↓
   Palpable per abdomen → if no/min. bleeding present → test positive
   ↓
   If bleeding continues → test negative → proceed for laparotomy.

1. Originally designed for management of esophageal varices
2. 3 way catheter tube with stomach and esophageal balloon components
3. Bleeding is expected to stop in 4-6 hours
4. Deflate first → watch for bleeding → then remove
5. Remove the balloon during day time in presence of senior staff.

Disadvantages:
1. Not designed for PPH and does not easily adapt to shape of uterine cavity
2. It contains latex.

c. *Hydrostatic condom catheter*

↓

Sterile rubber catheter fitted with a condom → outer end connected to saline set

↓

Inserted in uterus → inflated with 250-500 mL NS (according to need)

↓

After bleeding stops → outer end of catheter folded and tied with thread

↓

Vaginal cavity packed with roller gauze and sanitary pads (hemorrhage arrested within 15 min)
Approach is from Bangladesh.

d. *Bakri balloon*
e. *Urological Rusch balloon*
   - Larger capacity
   - Ease of use
   - Low cost.

Surgical Methods

Management of Retained Placenta

- A retained placenta is diagnosed if the placenta has not been delivered after 30 minutes following the delivery of the baby
- It increases the risk of PPH 8 to 12 fold
- Steps:

Step I: Vaginal examination (to see whether the placenta has separated or not)

Placenta palpable in the vagina or lower segment of the uterus

Yes	No
↓	↓
Already separated	Not separated
↓	↓
Pull the umbilical cord gently with one hand. Push the fundus of the uterus upwards with the other hand (i.e. the Brandt-Andrews method) and deliver the placenta.	If only the umbilical cord is felt then the placenta is still in upper uterine segment → retained placenta.

Step II: Start IV infusion with 20 units oxytocin (to ensure that the uterus is well contracted) and is run throughout the procedure.

Step III: Management in operation theatre
Spinal anesthesia can only be given if following are present:
- Patient is well resuscitated
- Normal blood pressure and pulse rate
- No active bleeding.

Preliminaries:
- Gloves with long sleeves
- Lithotomy position
- Bladder empty

Technique:

Right hand is inserted in the uterus and placental edge is identified
↓
Turn dorsum of your hand against the uterine wall
↓
Peel the placenta off the uterine wall in a slicing manner till it is completely removed
↓
Simultaneously, the other hand is placed on the abdominal wall to stabilize the uterus
↓
Grab the placenta and take it out from the uterus
↓
Check for completeness
↓
If cotyledons or any piece is missing, the uterus must again be explored manually or a gentle sharp curette is done, preferably with Baum's curette
↓
Gently massage the uterus so that it is well contracted
↓
Insert an Auvard or Sims speculum and observe for a few minutes for any bleeding or tears
↓
Observation for a minimum of 4 hours
↓
Continue IV infusion with 20 units of oxytocin
↓
Oral broad spectrum antibiotics for 5 days is indicated.

Umbilical Vein Injection of Oxytocin (Pipingas Technique)

- Another method to facilitate removal of placenta (but no added advantage)
- Attempt only in the following situation:
  - Patient hemodynamically stable and
  - There is delay in accessing operation theatre.

Technique:

Cut the clamped umbilical cord about 5 cm outside the introitus
↓
Insert a number 10 infant nasogastric feeding tube through the umbilical vein (the biggest of the three vessels seen on the cut surface of the umbilicus)
↓
When resistance is encountered, indicating that it has reached the placenta, the tube is withdrawn 5 cm, to ensure that the tip is in the umbilical vein and not in a placental branch
↓
Inject a mixture of 50 units of oxytocin and 30 mL of sterile water through the feeding tube

The tube can be removed and the cord again clamped
↓
Controlled cord traction can be attempted or alternatively can wait for 30 minutes for placenta to deliver
↓
If placenta cannot be delivered → manual removal of the placenta in theatre must be done.

Tears (Cervical, Vaginal or Perineal)

- After every delivery, gently splay the vagina open using the fingers of both hands
- Slight ooze is normal after vaginal delivery
- But anything more than an ooze must be thoroughly explored and sutured
- Examine for tears higher up in the vagina and cervical tears.

Preliminaries:
- Good light source
- Lithotomy poles
- A cervical suturing pack that includes a vaginal retractor, 2 Sims speculum and 2 sponge holders
- An assistant.

Technique:
- Lithotomy position
- Sims speculum and vaginal wall retractor introduced
- Explore upper 2/3rd of the vagina for tears
- Inspect the upper half of vagina and cervix.

Inspection of vagina
- Insert Sims speculum posteriorly into the vagina and elevate anterior vaginal wall with the retractor
- Vaginal tears that involve the muscle layers below the vaginal epithelium need to be sutured.

Inspection of cervix
- Hold the cervix with one sponge holder at 12 o' clock and the other one at 3 o'clock position
- The portion between the two holders is inspected for a cervical tear
- The sponge holder at 12 o'clock is now released and attached to the cervix at 6 o'clock position
- Again inspect the portion between the two holders
- Continue step by step until the whole circumference of the cervix has been inspected.

Suturing
- Once a cervical tear has been identified, sponge holder is placed on either side of it
- Try to locate the apex of the tear by applying gentle downward traction → if seen → start suturing from above the apex with continuous sutures using chromic 0 in a round bodied needle
- Do NOT pull with force (apex may be too high up)
- If apex is still not reached, shift the patient to operation theatre → explore again → still not visualized and patient is continuously bleeding → proceed with laparotomy

- Lloyd-Davis position – lithotomy position with the legs angled slightly downwards at about 30°

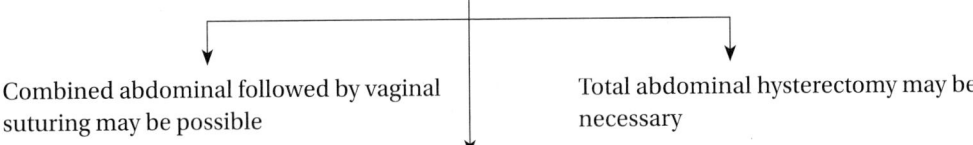

Combined abdominal followed by vaginal suturing may be possible

Total abdominal hysterectomy may be necessary

If there is no uterine bleeding and vaginal tears have been sutured → gently pack the vagina → if soaked and bleeding is confirmed to be from repaired tears → balloon tamponade can be placed in the vagina followed by insertion of a Foley's catheter
- When PPH occurs during cesarean section and the incision is open, B lynch sutures is the best selection
- When it is closed, Hayman and Pereira sutures can be better opted for (but can even be placed when incision is open).

B Lynch Sutures

- B lynch suture, now known as Brace suture technique, was first described by Christopher B-Lynch and colleagues during the management of a patient with a massive postpartum hemorrhage in November 1989, who refused hysterectomy.

Principle

- The suture aims to exert continuous vertical compression on the vascular system.

Technique

Preliminaries:
Surgeon (right handed) stands on right side of the patient → laparotomy performed → lower segment transverse incision is made or cesarean section sutures reopened.

28. **Why is the cavity opened?**
    a. To explore the uterine cavity once again for any remaining bits of placenta, to remove if any large clots are present, to exclude abnormal placentation or decidual tears, which would otherwise not be possible
    b. Hysterotomy ensures that the correct application of the suture provides maximum and even distribution of the compressive effect during and after application of the B-Lynch suture
    c. Blind application of the suture and the possibility of obliteration of the cervical and/ or uterine cavities that may lead to clot retention, infected debris, pyometra, sepsis and morbidity is avoided.

Test to check its efficacy:
- Position of the patient: Lloyd Davies or semi-lithotomy position (frog leg)
- Position of the assistant: Between the patient's legs, intermittently swabing the vagina to determine the presence and extent of the bleeding.

Method:
- Bladder peritoneum is reflected inferiorly to a level below the cervix
- Uterus → exteriorized
- Bimanual compression → performed

- Uterine compression → place one hand posteriorly with the ends of the fingers at the level of the cervix and the other hand anteriorly just below the bladder reflection

  ↓

- If the bleeding stops on applying such compression, there is a good chance that application of the B-Lynch suture will work and stop the bleeding

  ↓

- Even in the presence of coagulopathy, bimanual compression will control diffuse bleeding points (after which management of coagulopathy can be undertaken).

Suture application:
- Uterus remains exteriorized until application of suture is complete → assistant holds the uterus and maintains compression throughout the suture placement.

Sequence of suture placement
- First stitch → 3 cm below the transverse incision on left side → goes through the uterine cavity → emerges 3 cm above the upper incision margin → ≈ 4 cm from the lateral border of the uterus
- Next step → suture is now carried vertically upto the top of the fundus → on reaching the top of the fundus, its distance should be ≈ 4cm from the left uterine cornu → then the suture is moved to the posterior surface of the uterus.

NOTE:
- Proper placement of the suture should be done by maintaining effective compression of the uterus, which will NOT allow the suture to slip laterally and will avoid uterine trauma
- Next placement → the point of entry of the suture into the uterine cavity is on the horizontal plane at the level of the uterine incision at the insertion of the uterosacral ligament
- The suture now lies horizontally on the cavity side of the posterior uterine wall → it passes through the posterior uterine wall → top of the fundus → comes onto the anterior wall (with 4 cm difference from the uterine cornu) → pierces the anterior uterine wall exactly in the same manner as for the first suture (3cm above the upper lip of the transverse incision and 4 cm from the lateral wall) → enters the cavity and then out again through 3 cm below the lower incision margin.

NOTE: Two vital points to always keep in mind while applying brace sutures:
1. Maintain effective compression throughout the procedure
2. Progressive, uniform tension is to be maintained after each suture is placed (of course not too much that can break the suture).

The two ends of the suture are put under tension and a double throw knot is placed for security to maintain tension after the lower segment incision has been closed by either the one- or two-layer method.

NOTE: There is no hard and fast rule. Out of the two, tying the knot or closing the suture first, any step can be performed first according to surgeon's choice

In case the knot is tied first, it is essential that the corners of the incision be identified and stay sutures placed before the knot is tied. This ensures that, when the lower segment is closed, the angles of the incision do not escape it. No bleeders should remain unsecured.

Closure and After Effects

- Abdomen can be closed without waiting
- Assistant standing between the legs swabs the vagina again and can confirm that bleeding has stopped

- Maximum effect of suture tension lasts for only about 24–48 h
- Involution starts in the 1st postoperative week after delivery. By this time sutures must have lost some of their tensile strength but there is no need to worry as bleeding must have stopped by then
  In case of placenta accreta, increta, percreta → a figure of eight; transverse compression or longitudinal sutures in addition can be applied.

Prophylactic Application and Future Fertility after B- Lynch Sutures

- Can be done in cases where signs/risks of imminent PPH develops
- Fertility is preserved.

Drawbacks

- More time consuming
- Incidences of postpartum uterine/myometrial necrosis have been reported in the literature.

Hayman Sutures

- In 2002, Hayman et al. proposed a simplified approach to uterine compression sutures that involved slight modifications of the B-Lynch technique
- Lower uterine segment or uterine cavity is not opened, therefore, a good option when PPH occurs following vaginal delivery
- Faster, easier and less traumatic to atonic bleeding uterus.

Method

- Two to four longitudinal sutures are placed, starting at the anterior wall from below the bladder reflection → then taken to the posterior wall of the uterus at the same level → knots placed at the fundus are tied by the 3 throws technique to avoid the sutures sliding off the side of the uterus
- Continuous compression of the uterus is required as in B Lynch sutures
- Horizontal cervico-isthmic sutures can also be placed, if needed, to control bleeding from lower uterine segment.

Drawbacks

- Concerns on the potential risks of cavity occlusion and infections (hematometra, pyometra and uterine necrosis) have been raised as the cavity cannot be explored directly under vision
- Unequal application of tension may lead to slippage of suture
- Occlusion of the cervical lumen is a potential complication when additional horizontal compression sutures are required
- No feed-back data on fertility outcome
- Data on safety and efficacy is limited.

Pereira Sutures

- Pereira et al. described a technique in which a series of transverse and longitudinal stitches of a delayed absorbable multifilament suture are placed around the uterus
- Sutures are placed via a series of bites into the subserosal myometrium without entering the uterine cavity

- Two or three rows of these sutures are placed in each direction to completely envelope and compress the uterus
- The longitudinal sutures begin and end at the level of the transverse suture which is closest to the cervix
- The knot for the transverse sutures is placed on the anterior uterine wall
- Avoid damage to blood vessels and the ureters when placing the transverse sutures.

Cho Sutures

- These are multiple full-thickness square sutures, used to approximate the anterior and posterior uterine walls
- Disadvantages:
  - Time consuming
  - Involution may be delayed
  - Uterine cavity cannot be explored – retained products may lead to hematometra and pyometra, especially in cases where there was intrauterine infection antepartum (e.g. chorioamnionitis)
  - In future, it may lead to development of uterine synechiae. Use of delayed absorbable suture (1-0 dexon polyglycolic acid suture) have been quoted as one of the reasons
  - Effect on future fertility → data scant.

U Type Sutures

- The U-type suture was described by Hackethal et al.
- The needle is inserted at the ventral uterine wall, led through the posterior wall, and then passed back to the ventral wall where the thread was joined with a flat double knot
- Advantages:
  - Relatively easy to perform
  - Does not distort the uterine shape
  - Does not form closed space inside the uterus.

Stepwise Devascularization

Uterine Artery Ligation

- First described by Waters in 1952
- Bilateral ligation of the uterine vessels (O'Leary stitch) to control PPH has become a first-line procedure for controlling uterine bleeding at laparotomy
- Is primarily indicated when bleeding is due to laceration of the uterine or ovarian artery, but can also temporarily decrease bleeding from other etiologies
- Although it will not control bleeding from uterine atony or placenta accreta, it may decrease blood loss while other interventions are being attempted
- It involves a low abdominal approach like in Pfannenstiel incision
- The uterus is exteriorized and pulled upward to facilitate identification and ligature of uterine vessels,
  - Preferably as it emerges from crossing over the ureter or
  - As it approaches the uterine wall to penetrate and establish its division
- This could be carried out unilaterally or bilaterally about 2 cm from the uterine angle at cesarean section or where the lower segment is opened after conservative surgery for postpartum hemorrhage has failed

- An absorbable suture is placed 2 cm below the bladder reflection on both sides of the uterus avoiding the ureters
- This technique occludes the ascending branch of uterine vessels
- Reported success rate of 80-96%
- Major risk:
  - Injury to the ureter
- Advantages:
  - Technique is comparatively easier
  - Has fewer complications
  - Uterine arteries are more readily accessible
  - There is less risk to major adjacent vessels and the ureter

↓

- Devascularization of the independent branches of the hypogastric artery, that descend to the cervix and vagina can be achieved by independent ligation sutures applied bilaterally to the cervix and/or vagina

↓

- If this does not control bleeding, the vessels of the utero-ovarian arcade are similarly ligated just distal to the cornua by passing a suture ligature through the myometrium just medial to the vessels, then back through the broad ligament just lateral to the vessels, and then tying to compress the vessels

↓

- Unilateral or bilateral ligature of the internal iliac artery needs a special and detailed mention.

Hypogastric Artery Ligation

Knowledge of the anatomic distribution of blood supply to the pelvis as well as implementing the appropriate preventive measures at the occurrence of postpartum hemorrhage can significantly minimize life threatening morbidities.

Arterial Supply of the Pelvis

Ovarian Artery

Course of the artery:
- Arise from aorta, just below the level of renal artery → passes downwards → crosses ureter and then external iliac artery → infundibulo pelvic fold

Branches:
- To ovaries
- Outer part of fallopian tubes
- Branches to cornu
- Branches to round ligament
- Branch to ureter.

Anastomosis:
- With terminal part of uterine artery.

Internal Iliac Artery

- One of the bifurcations of common iliac artery
- 2 cm in length
- Ureter lies anterior
- Internal iliac vein posterior.

Branches:
Posterior division
Has a parietal branch which gives off the following arteries:
- Iliolumbar
- Lateral sacral
- Superior gluteal

Anterior division (supplies pelvic viscera)
- Gives off parietal and a visceral branch.

Divisions of parietal branch
- Inferior gluteal
- Obturator
- Internal pudendal.

Divisions of visceral branch
- Superior vesical
- Uterine
- Vaginal (Inferior vesical)
- Middle rectal.

Uterine Artery

- Arises from → anterior trunk of internal iliac artery

Course:

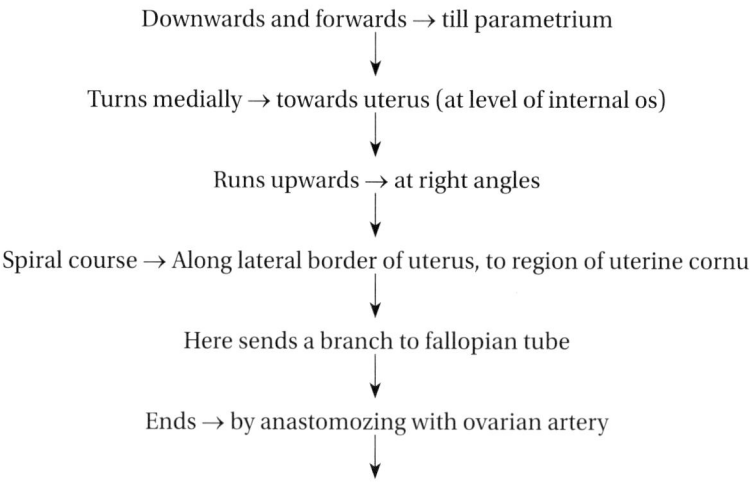

Downwards and forwards → till parametrium
↓
Turns medially → towards uterus (at level of internal os)
↓
Runs upwards → at right angles
↓
Spiral course → Along lateral border of uterus, to region of uterine cornu
↓
Here sends a branch to fallopian tube
↓
Ends → by anastomozing with ovarian artery
↓
During its vertical course, sends branches which run transversely → pass into myometrium (arcuate arteries)

At right angle to it → radial arteries

Reach basal layers of endometrium → basal arteries

From these are derived → Terminal spiral and straight arterioles of endometrium
Tortuosity lost → when uterus enlarges during pregnancy
Least vascular part of uterus → Is in midline.

Vaginal Artery

Arises before uterine artery passes vertically upwards (ascending branch) at level of internal os
↓   (descending branch)
Passes downwards through parametrium
↓
Reaches vagina → in region of lateral fornix

Importance: Has a central role in total abdominal hysterectomy, if not separately clamped and tied → ↑ hemorrhage

In some cases, does not arise from uterine artery, but arises from hypogastric artery.

Arcuate artery supplying cervix → circular artery of cervix
↓
vaginal artery → anterior and posterior Azygous artery of vagina

Branches of uterine artery
- Ureteric artery
- Descending vaginal → unite to form → anterior and posterior azygous artery of vagina
- Circular artery of cervix
- Arcuate → radial artery → basal artery → spiral and straight arterioles of functional layer of endometrium
- Anastomosis with ovarian artery.

Relation to ureter is important
- Crosses above ureter in parametrium → gives off ureteric branch
- Artery runs transversely while ureter runs almost anteroposteriorly through ureteric canal of parametrium.

Middle Sacral Artery

- Single artery which arises from terminal aorta
- Descends → in middle of lumbar vertebra and sacrum to tip of coccyx.

Ligation of Hypogastric Artery

Done first by Sir Howard Kelly in 1890s for uterine cancer.

Principle

1. Pulse pressure in artery just distal to point of ligation is ↓↓ (77%) on same side
2. If both are ligated, pulse pressure decreases by 85%
3. This allows blood clots to form at site of bleeding from damaged vessels
4. Blood flow in vessels distal to point of ligation decreases by only 48%.

Which Division to Ligate, Where and Why?

Anterior division of hypogastric artery distal to posterior parietal branch:
- Flow can still occur distal to point of ligation but only by reversed flow in middle hemorrhoidal arteries
- Ligation converts arterial system into venous system → stable clot formation → hemostasis
- If ligated proximal: flow can still occur distal to point of ligation by reversed flow through iliolumbar and lateral sacral collateral artery.

Collateral Circulation: 3 Main Arterial Groups

a. Those vessels that communicate with branches from aorta	
From aorta	Hypogastric branch
Middle sacral artery	Lateral sacral and iliolumbar
Lumbar artery	Iliolumbar
Inferior mesenteric artery	Superior, Middle and inferior hemorrhoidal artery
b. From external iliac artery	
Inferior epigastric gives obturator artery	With hypogastric directly
Medial and lateral femoral	Obturator and superior gluteal
Iliolumbar	Superior gluteal
c. From femoral artery	
Medial and lateral femoral artery	Inferior gluteal.

Indications of IIAL

1. Uterine atony
2. Uterine rupture
3. Placenta accreta, increta and percreta
4. Radical hysterectomy
5. 1° or 2° PPH
6. Anticipated operative bleeding
7. Others – in combination with other uterine saving procedures of PPH.

Procedure

Approaches:
1. Transperitoneal (mainly followed by obstetricians)
2. Extraperitoneal.

Transperitoneal Approach

Steps:
- Laparotomy
- Viscera packed in a usual manner
- Identify the round ligament and the fallopian tube
- Make a 5cm incision on the peritoneum between the fallopian tube and the round ligament
- The incision results in the formation of a medial and a lateral peritoneal flap
- The ureter is always beneath the medial flap and may be visualized and reflected easily
- The ureter normally crosses the common iliac artery from lateral to medial at a point just proximal to the bifurcation
- Open and enter the retroperitoneal space bluntly with fingers in the direction of the vessels, not across them to avoid unnecessary trauma
- Directly one will be over the division artery with little dissection
- The bifurcation feels like an inverted Y
- Pass the mixter or an aneurysm needle or other fine right angled forceps, from lateral to medial, about 3-4 cm away from the division beneath the internal iliac artery with non-absorbable or absorbable sutures. This prevents injury to external iliac vein (posterior division is avoided)
- Ligate the vessel with 3 knots
- Palpate the femoral artery for pulsations, to ensure the correct vessel ligation
- Ensure perfect hemostasis
- Keep the drain for 12-24 hours
- Close the abdomen as usual.

Other Intraperitoneal Route

- The broad ligament is opened and traced upward until at the level of bifurcation of common iliac artery parallel to the sacroiliac curvature
- The ureter is commonly on the medial leaf of the broad ligament after crossing the bifurcation of common iliac artery
- The vascular sheath needs to be cleared for better visualization and recognition, minimising inadvertent ligature and venous injury
- The internal iliac branches off medio-inferiorly after the bifurcation of common iliac artery
- By using a right angle forceps to isolate this vessel, an absorbable ligature is placed 1 to 2 cm below the bifurcation
- Following this, a distal pulse at femoral artery is checked to ensure its patency
- The same procedure is repeated on the contralateral side.

Extraperitoneal Approach

- A 10-15cm skin incision, parallel to the course of external oblique muscle in a line 3-5 cm medial to the anterior superior iliac spine
- Dissection of fat and subcutaneous tissues
- Peritoneum reflected medially, together with the ureter
- Ligation carried out as described above
- Closure like as in herniorrhaphy.

Complications

1. External iliac vein injury
2. Internal iliac vein laceration/injury
3. Limbs ischemia
4. Ligation of wrong structure like ureter, external/common iliac artery
5. External iliac arterial spasm and thrombosis
6. Gluteal claudication, further bleeding and possible ureteric and nerve injury.

Advantages

- Reproductive function- SECURED
    - Not affected due to good collaterals
    - Menses return normally
    - Pregnancy occurs and reach term and without IUGR → indicates adequate blood supply after ligation
- Less operative time in experienced hands
- Associated with less postoperative morbidity than the other alternative option i.e hysterectomy.

Disadvantages

- If bilateral ligation is done → selective arterial catheterization and embolization of peripheral bleeding arterial branches in pelvis → v.v. difficult.

If PPH has occurred after cesarean section, though basic management remains the same but few important steps should be kept in mind:

- *Atonic uterus*
    - Oxytocics, B lynch compression suture
- *Lateral tears into broad ligament*
    - Bilateral and stepwise uterine artery devascularization
- *Tears down lower segment of uterus*
    - Hemostatic sutures, ensure get apex of tear, check ureteric path if tear goes lateral
- *Bleeding from placental bed*
    - Individual hemostatic sutures and uterine artery ligation, balloon tamponade
- *If morbidly adherent placenta*
    - Use of Baum's curette
- Note:
    - Proceed straight to hysterectomy if placenta percreta, ruptured uterus which is irreparable, or when above conservative measures are unsuccessful.

Hysterectomy (subtotal/total)

- Hysterectomy is the last resort, but should not be delayed in women who require prompt control of uterine hemorrhage to prevent death
- Peripartum hysterectomy has a morbidity rate of 30-40%
- Complications include:
    - Ureteric and bladder injury
    - Persistent bleeding requiring reexploration
    - Pneumonia
    - Urinary fistula

- Can be performed either as total or subtotal hysterectomy
- A total hysterectomy reduces risk of cervical stump malignancy but requires longer operating time and has higher rate of urinary tract injuries
- A subtotal hysterectomy is faster and safer but regular cervical screening is mandatory.

Surgical Principles

Various anatomical and surgical changes in pregnancy create potential surgical difficulties:
- Uterine and ovarian vessels are engorged and distended
- Adjacent pelvic tissues are edematous and friable
- In case of uterine rupture, Green Armytage clamps or sponge forceps can be used to compress bleeding edges of torn uterine muscle
- Structures of adnexa on each side are pulled laterally and clamps applied straight adjacent to top sides of uterus to include all structures → to control blood flow to uterus from ovarian arteries
- Vascular pedicles are thick and edematous and should be double clamped
- If cervix, lower uterine segment and paracolpos are not involved, subtotal hysterectomy can be done
- If the above structures are involved, total abdominal hysterectomy is done
- Avoid ureters by placing all clamps medial to those used to secure uterines.

Post-laparotomy Inspection

- After completion of laparotomy, the operative field should be inspected carefully for hemostasis
- Microvascular bleeding usually can be controlled using topic hemostatic agent.

Inspection of the Bladder

- When injury to the bladder is suspected, 200 mL of saline mixed with 5 mL of indigo carmine can be infused into the bladder through Foleys catheter
- Integrity of the bladder is confirmed by failure of the colored fluid to leak through the serosa.

Inspection of the Ureters

- Ureters should generally be identified before abdominal closure either by:
  - Transillumination through the broad ligament OR
  - Direct visual identification during retroperitoneal dissection
  - It courses horizontally along the peritoneum 1 to 5 cm dorsal to the ovarian vessels
  - Can be identified readily as it passes ventral to the bifurcation of the common iliac artery
- The ureters should be inspected to confirm that they are not damaged
- Their integrity can be assessed by injecting two ampules (10 mL) of indigo carmine intravenously
  - A ureter that has been severed will release blue urine into the pelvis in 10-15 minutes
  - If a ureter has been ligated, cystoscopy or direct visualization of the ureters through a cystotomy will demonstrate that urine is only passing through one of the two ureteral orifices
  - Passage of a ureteral stent can also be employed to localize the site of obstruction.

Uterine Inversion

- Uterine inversion is defined as 'the turning inside out of the fundus into the uterine cavity'
- A serious complication causing severe postpartum hemorrhage and shock.

Classification

Depending upon severity of the condition
- First degree (incomplete): The fundus reaches the internal os but not beyond that
- Second degree (incomplete): The inverted fundus extends through the cervical ring but remains within the vagina
- Third degree (complete): The inverted fundus extends down to the introitus (i.e. the uterus, cervix and vagina are inverted and are visible)
- Fourth (total): The vagina is also inverted.

According to timing of the event
- Acute: Occurs within 24 hours of birth
- Subacute: Occurs after 24 hours, within 4 weeks
- Chronic: Occurs after 4 weeks, rare.

Pathophysiology

There are three possible events:
1. A portion of uterine wall prolapses through the dilated cervix or indents forward
2. Relaxation of part of the uterine wall
3. Simultaneous downward traction on the fundus leading to inversion of the uterus.

Causes and Risk Factors

These include:
- Mismanagement of the third stage
  - Premature or excessive cord traction during AMTSL
  - Use of fundal pressure when the uterus is atonic during placental delivery
- Abnormally adherent placenta
- Spontaneous inversion of unknown etiology
- Short umbilical cord
- Sudden emptying of a distended uterus
- Nulliparity
- Fundal placement of the placenta
- Antepartum use of magnesium sulphate (rare).

Diagnosis

Signs
- Lump in the vagina
- Abdominal tenderness
- Absence of uterine fundus on abdominal palpation
- Polypoidal red mass in the vagina with placenta attached.

Symptoms
- Severe abdominal pain
- Sudden cardio vascular collapse
  - Shock out of proportion to visible blood loss → clue to high index of suspicion
  - Initially is due to the parasympathetic effect caused by traction of the ligaments supporting the uterus, and hypotension with inadequate tissue perfusion, i.e. initially it may be neurogenic with signs of bradycardia and hypotension but with time PPH will set in
- Postpartum hemorrhage (94%) with or without shock.

Differential Diagnosis

- Uterovaginal prolapse
- Fibroid polyp
- Postpartum collapse
- Severe uterine atony
- Neurogenic collapse
- Coagulopathy
- Retained placenta without inversion.

Management

Call for help
Resuscitation and simultaneous manual replacement.

Resuscitation

- 1st line of management
- Shock out of proportion to the amount of blood loss
- Continuous active resuscitation should commence immediately.

Placenta Adherent

- Should be LEFT IN SITU, until uterine replacement is complete.

Correcting the Inversion

Step I. Manual replacement **(Johnson Manoeuvre)**
- Relaxation of uterus (may be required)
- With the palm of the hand, push the fundus of the uterus along the direction of the vagina towards the posterior fornix
- Then lift the uterus towards the umbilicus and return to its normal position
- Maintain the hand in situ until a firm contraction is palpated.

Step II. **O' Sullivan's hydrostatic method**
- Reinversion of the uterus by infusing warm saline (through a catheter) into the vagina.

NOTE: *Uterine rupture should be excluded prior to performing hydrostatic reduction of the uterus.*
If above attempts fail:

Step III. Take patient to **operation theatre**
- Replacement of the uterus is done under general anesthesia
- Re-attempt both manual and hydrostatic methods → If fails, proceed to laparotomy
- A constriction ring will be seen through which the uterus has inverted downwards
- Try to 'peel it back' with gentle traction using Allis tissue forceps placed on the round ligaments of the uterus just inside the dimple where the fundus disappears.

If this fails:

Step IV. **Cut the constriction ring** (about a 0.5 cm incision) **posteriorly**
- The uterus can then be pulled up ('popped backwards')
- The uterus will appear to have a classical incision on the posterior surface that needs to be repaired
- Remove placenta only after uterus is replaced.

Following the Procedure
- Oxytocin infusion to keep the uterus well contracted
- Antibiotics.

Intraoperative Cell Salvage
Has no role in obstetrics at present (the process whereby blood shed during an operation is collected, filtered and washed to produce autologous red blood cells for transfusion to the patient), though it reduces the need for blood transfusion by 39% and absolute risk reduction by 23%.

Why not used in obstetrics?
- Lack of training and equipment
- Fear about safety of use
- Difficulty in effective removal of amniotic fluid
- Another difficulty is the degree of contamination with fetal red cells with potential maternal sensitization
- It may be useful for those who refuse blood transfusion or those where massive blood loss is anticipated (placenta percreta or accreta)
- For women who are RhD negative, to prevent sensitization, the standard dose of anti-D should be given and a Kleihauer test taken, 1 hour after cell salvage has finished, to determine whether further anti-D is required.

Role of Recombinant Factor VIIa
- Was developed for the treatment of hemophilia
- In cases of life threatening PPH and in consultation with a hematologist, rFVIIa may be used as an adjuvant to standard pharmacological and surgical treatments
- Dose: 90 micrograms/kg, which may be repeated in the absence of clinical response within 15–30 minutes
- Although there is no clear evidence of thrombosis with the use of rFVIIa in obstetric practice, there have been case reports of thrombosis with the use in cardiac surgery
- Women with PPH are particularly susceptible to defibrination (severe hypofibrinogenemia) and this is particularly relevant to the most severe cases that will be considered for rFVIIa
- rFVIIa will not work if there is no fibrinogen and effectiveness may also be suboptimal with severe thrombocytopenia (less than 20×10^9/L)
- Therefore, fibrinogen should be above 1g/L and platelets > 20×10^9/L before rFVIIa is given
- If there is a suboptimal clinical response to rFVIIa, these should be checked and acted on (with cryoprecipitate, fibrinogen concentrate or platelet transfusion as appropriate) before a second dose is given.

Role of Antifibrinolytic Agents (Tranexamic Acid)
Seldom have any role in PPH. Advised in cases of refractory atonic bleeding or persistent trauma related bleeding
- It is also important that, once the bleeding is arrested and coagulopathy corrected, thromboprophylaxis is administered, as there is a high risk of thrombosis
- Alternatively, pneumatic compression devices can be used, if thromboprophylaxis is contraindicated in cases of thrombocytopenia.

NOTE: Intraumbilical cord injection of misoprostol (800 g) or oxytocin (10 to 30 IU) can be considered as an alternative intervention before manual removal of the placenta.

SUMMARY

Signs/symptoms → PPH → find cause → atonic → oxytocics → uterine tamponade → conservative surgery → peripartum hysterectomy → uterine artery embolization.

IV Fluid Rates			
Amount of fluid	Time period	Drops per cc (type of tubing)	Drops per minute
1 liter	20 minutes	10	Too fast to count
1 liter	20 minutes	20	Too fast to count
1 liter	4 hours	10	40
1 liter	4 hours	20	80
1 liter	6 hours	10	28
1 liter	6 hours	20	56
1 liter	8 hours	10	20
1 liter	8 hours	20	40

In general, the formula to figure out any IV infusion rate is as follows:

$$\frac{\text{Amount of fluid given (cc)}}{\text{Time for infusion to occur (min)}} \times \text{No. of drops per cc} = \text{No. of drops per minute}$$

In order to convert the time period from hours to minutes, multiply the number of hours by 60. This will give the number of minutes over which the IV fluids are to be given.

BLOOD TRANSFUSION

- Blood and blood products has a great demand in obstetrics
- It is very important to get the right blood to the right patient at the right time
- Proper documentation is of utmost importance while transfusing blood.

Preliminaries before Requesting for Blood

- Assess the patient's clinical need for blood
- When it is required
- What is the indication for transfusion
- Inform the patient's relatives about the proposed transfusion and document the same
- Select the blood product and the quantity required
- Complete the blood request form accurately and legibly
- Write the reason for transfusion so that the blood bank can select the most suitable product for compatibility testing
- If the blood is needed urgently, contact the blood bank by telephone.

If the particular blood group or blood product is available:
- Obtain blood sample of the patient for compatibility testing and label it correctly
- Send the blood sample along with the blood request form to the blood bank.

Obtaining Sample for Compatibility Testing

Step I. Patient's identity

Patient conscious	Patient unconscious
↓	↓
Ask the patient to reveal her identity	Enquire the same from her family members
– Name	
– Family name	
– Date of birth	
– Husband's name etc.	

↓

- Note it and tally it with her case file.

Step II. Obtaining the blood sample
- Take the sample in the tube with NO anticoagulant.

Step III. Labelling the sample tube
- Label the tube correctly and accurately with the following information:
  - Patient's given name and family name
  - Patient's hospital registration number
  - Patient's ward
  - Date
  - Signature of the person taking the sample.

Step IV. Always label the sample tube after obtaining the specimen.

Step V. If required blood group is not available, what is the alternative?

	Choice of alternative blood	
Patient's blood group	Alternative blood group (1st choice) [Given as Packed cells]	Alternative blood group (2nd choice) [Given as Packed cells]
O	None	None
A	O	None
B	O	None
AB	A or B	O

Storing Blood Products Prior to Transfusion

Whole Blood and Red Cells

- Should be issued from the blood bank in a cold box or insulated carrier (temperature between 2°C and 6°C)
- In the ward or OT, store it in the refrigerator at 2°C to 6°C until required for transfusion
  - The upper limit of 6°C is essential to minimize the risk of any bacterial contamination
  - The lower limit of 2°C is essential to prevent hemolysis, which can cause fatal bleeding problems or renal failure.

Platelet Concentrates

- Should be issued from the blood bank in a cold box or insulated carrier (temperature between 20°C to 24°C)
- At lower temperatures they lose their blood clotting capability; therefore should never be placed in a refrigerator.

Fresh Frozen Plasma

- Temperature in the blood transport box is maintained between 2°C and 6°C
- If not required for immediate use, should be stored in a refrigerator at a temperature of 2°- 6°C.

Time Limits for Infusion

Whole Blood

- Start - within 30 minutes of removing from refrigerator
- Finish - within 4 hours.

Platelet Concentrates

- Start – as soon as possible after pooling, generally within 4 hours
- Finish –over a period of 30 minutes.

FFP and Cryoprecipitate

- Labile coagulation factors rapidly degrade, therefore, start transfusion as soon as possible
- Complete infusion within 20 minutes.

Administration of Blood Products

Correct IV Set Up

- No solutions other than 0.9% sodium chloride are infused in the same line as the blood
- No medications should be infused in the line
- In the event of a transfusion reaction, the setup should allow for immediate cessation of fluids through the blood tubing and the start of 0.9% sodium chloride so that no additional blood product is infused
- If using a pre-existing IV site, assess the quality of the line by checking for swelling, redness or pain at the infusion site and adequate infusion rates.

Needle Size

- The largest possible catheter should be used
- The smaller the gauge, the slower the flow rate
- If using a smaller gauge catheter, care should be taken to avoid excess pressure.

Compatible Solutions with Blood Products

- *Only 0.9% Sodium Chloride.*

NOTE

- 5% Dextrose in water will cause clumping of red cells and hemolysis
- Lactated Ringer's may cause clotting due to calcium content
- EXCEPTION → IV immunoglobulin (IG)
    - 5% Dextrose in water (D5W) **must** be used when administering IV IG
    - 0.9% Sodium chloride is **NOT** compatible with IV IG.

Filter (for Whole Blood/Red Cells)

- Use a new sterile blood administration set containing an integral 170-200 micron filter
- Change the set at least 12 hourly during blood component infusion
- In a very warm climate change the set more frequently and usually after every four units of blood, if given within a 12 hour period.

Blood Warming

- There is NO evidence that warming blood is beneficial to the patient when infusion is slow
- Keeping the patient warm is more important than warming the infused blood
- Warmed blood is commonly required in:
    - 'Large volume rapid transfusion'
        - 50 mL/kg/hour
        - Exchange transfusion in infants
        - Patients with clinically significant cold agglutinins
- Blood should only be warmed in a blood warmer
- *Blood should never be warmed in a bowl/oven, as this can result in hemolysis of red cells which can prove fatal.*

Receiving the Blood Bag from Blood Bank

Checking the Compatibility Label on the Blood Bag

This blood is compatible with: ....   Blood pack no. ....
- Patient's name:
- Patient's hospital reference number:
- Patient's ward:
- Patient's ABO and Rh D group:
- Date of compatibility test:
- Expiry date:
- Blood group of blood pack:

Return Blood Promptly to Blood Bank if not used

Checking the Blood Pack

The blood pack should always be inspected for signs of deterioration:
Check for:
- Any sign of hemolysis in the plasma (does it appear pink?) indicating that the blood has been contaminated, allowed to freeze or had become too warm
- Look or hemolysis on the line between the red cells and plasma

- Any sign of contamination, such as a change of color in the red cells, which often look darker or purple/black when contaminated
- Any clots, which may mean that:
  - The blood was not mixed properly with the anticoagulant when it was collected OR
  - Might also indicate bacterial contamination due to the utilization of citrate by proliferating bacteria
- Any sign showing that there is a leak in the pack or that it has already been opened.

Do not administer the transfusion if the blood pack appears abnormal or damaged or it has been (or may have been) out of the refrigerator for > 30 minutes
Inform the blood bank immediately.

MONITORING THE TRANSFUSED PATIENT (BLOOD TRANSFUSION NOTES)

General Information

- Patient's name:
- Patient's hospital reference number:
- Patient's ward:
- Patient's ABO and Rh D group:
- Date of compatibility test:
- Expiry date:
- Blood group of blood pack:
- Blood bag number:

Monitoring

When?

- Before starting the transfusion
- As soon as the transfusion is started
- 15 minutes after starting the transfusion
- Afterwards hourly monitoring
- On completion of the transfusion
- 4 hours after completing the transfusion.

How?

Patient's general appearance:
- PR
- BP
- RR
- Temperature
- Fluid intake.

Record

- Time when the transfusion is started
- Time the transfusion is completed
- Volume and type of all products transfused
- Any adverse effects.

Blood Transfusion Reactions

There can be:

Mild Reactions

Signs and symptoms
- Urticaria
- Rash
- Pruritis
- Hypersensitivity.

Management
- Slow down the transfusion
- Administer antihistamine IM.

Moderate Reactions

Signs and symptoms
- Fever
- Rigors
- Urticaria
- Tachycardia
- Pruritis
- Headache
- Mild dyspnea
- Palpitations.

Management
- Stop the transfusion
- Replace the infusion set and keep IV line open with normal saline
- Administer antihistamine IM
- Antipyretic
- Give IV glucocorticoids and bronchodilators, if there are anaphylactic reactions (bronchospasm, stridor)
- Send to the blood bank, the following:
    - Blood bag with infusion set
    - Fresh blood sample from a different vein
    - Request form to release 1 unit of blood again
- When there is clinical improvement, restart infusion with a new blood bag and monitor closely.

Severe Reactions

Signs and symptoms
- Fever
- Rigors
- Headache
- Hypotension (fall in systolic BP by > 20%)
- Tachycardia (rise in heart rate by >20%)
- Respiratory distress
- Chest pain

- Severe dyspnea
- Loin/back pain
- Hemoglobinuria
- Unexplained bleeding (DIC).

Management
- Stop the transfusion IMMEDIATELY
- Start normal saline
- Elevate patient's legs
- High flow oxygen by mask
- Attach pulse oximeter
- Give:
    - Inj. Adrenaline 0.01mg/kg body weight slowly IM
    - Give IV corticosteroids and bronchodilators
    - Give diuretic (Frusemide 1mg/kg body weight)
    - Antipyretic (paracetamol)
- Send to the blood bank, the following:
    - Blood bag with infusion set
    - Fresh blood sample from a different vein
    - Request form to investigate the bag
- Send urine sample for analysis
- Assess for bleeding from puncture sites. If there is clinical or laboratory evidence of DIC, manage with platelets, FFPs, cryoprecipitate
- Inotropes can be started, if hypotension continues even with fluids.

SUGGESTED READING

1. A Hackethal, D Brueggmann, F Oehmke, et al. Uterine compression U-sutures in primary postpartum hemorrhage after Cesarean section: fertility preservation with a simple and effective technique. Human Reproduction. 2008;23(1):74-7.
2. A monograph of the management of postpartum hemorrhage: National department of health, South Africa. 2010.
3. Ali Abdelhamed M Mostfa, Mostafa M Zaitoun. Safety pin suture for management of atonic postpartum hemorrhage. ISRN Obstetrics and Gynecology. 2012.
4. C Solomon, RE Collis, PW Collins. Haemostatic monitoring during postpartum hemorrhage and implications for management. British Journal of Anesthesia. 2012;109(6):851-63.
5. Care of the Postnatal Mother on Ward 6B: Maternal secondary Post Partum Hemorrhage. neonatology clinical guidelinesking edward memorial/princess margaret hospitals perth western australia. July 2009.
6. Dean Leduc, Vyta Senikas, André B. Lalonde, et al. Active management of the third stage of labor: prevention and treatment of postpartum hemorrhage. J Obstet Gynaecol Can 2009;31(10):980-93.
7. Debasmita Mandal, Sarbeswar Mandal, Tapan Kumar Maity, et al. Role of hypogastric artery ligation in pelvic hemorrhage- is still alive. Al Ameen J Med Sci 2013;6(1):12-16.
8. F Ghezzi, A Cromi, S Uccella, et al. The Hayman technique: a simple method to treat postpartum hemorrhage. BJOG 2007;114:362-65.
9. Introducing oxytocin in the Uniject device: An overview for decision makers. PATH September 2008.
10. Marian Knight, William M Callaghan, Cynthia Berg, et al. Trends in postpartum hemorrhage in high resource countries: a review and recommendations from the International postpartum hemorrhage collaborative group. BMC Pregnancy and Childbirth 2009;9:55.
11. MB Bellad. Internal Iliac Artery Ligation (IIAL): An Uterus/Life Saving Procedure. Journal of south asian federation of obstetrics & gynecology. May-Aug 2009;1(2):32-33.
12. Nihal Al Riyami, Dini Hui, Elaine Herer, et al. Uterine compression sutures as an effective treatment for postpartum hemorrhage: Case Series. Am J Perinatol Rep 2011;1:47-52

13. NL Sloan, J Durocher, T Aldrich, J Blum, et al. What measured blood loss tells us about postpartum bleeding: a systematic review. BJOG 2010;117:788-800.
14. Pili Ferrer, Ian Roberts, Emma Sydenham, et al. Anti-fibrinolytic agents in post-partum hemorrhage: a systematic review. BMC Pregnancy and Childbirth. 2009;9:29.
15. Prevention of Postpartum Hemorrhage Initiative. Tackling the Biggest Maternal Killer: How the Prevention of Postpartum Hemorrhage Initiative Strengthened Efforts Around the World. Washington, DC. PATH 2009.
16. Preventionand management ofpostpartumhemorrhage. RCOG Green-top Guideline No. 52. May 2009.
17. Primary postpartum hemorrhage: Queensland Maternity and Neonatal Clinical Guideline. November 2012.
18. Robert L Barbieri. A stitch in time: The B-Lynch, Hayman, Pereira uterine compression sutures. OBG Management. December 2012;24(12).
19. Supplement: PPH: Queensland Maternity and Neonatal Clinical Guideline. 2010.
20. WHO recommendations for the prevention and treatment of postpartum hemorrhage. World Health Organization 2012.

CHAPTER 17

Puerperium

Tania G Singh, Earl Jaspal

NORMAL PUERPERIUM

"Postnatal" - used for all issues pertaining to the mother and the baby after birth.

Postnatal period begins immediately after the birth of the baby with delivery of placenta and extends up to six weeks (42 days) after birth.

However, some organs may only return to their pre pregnant state weeks or even months after the 6 weeks have elapsed (e.g. the ureters). Other organs never regain their pre pregnant state (e.g. the perineum).

Immediate Postnatal Period

- Refers to the time immediately after birth of the baby till first 24 hours.

Early Postnatal Period

- Refers to a period from day 2 to day 7.

Late Postnatal Period

- Period from Days 8 through 42.

POSTPARTUM CARE

Hospital Care

Immediately after labor, the woman is in a state of physical fatigue such that in many cases, slight shivering, muscular tremors and chattering of teeth occur for about 10–15 minutes.

First 24 hours

After vaginal delivery

1. Vitals/Blood loss:
   Every 15 minutes in first hour,
   at 2 hours, then after 6 hours of birth.
2. Voiding:
   Within first 6 hours.

After cesarean section

Every 15 minutes in first hour, at 2 hours,
then 4 hourly × 24 hours.

Catheter for first 24 hours
Urine should not be concentrated and
should not be <min 30 mL/hr.

3. Abdominal and vaginal examination:
   Due each time with vitals
   Fundus firm, central, +/- 1 finger above /below umbilicus
   Perineal heating.

   Due each time with vitals
   Same.

4. Oral intake:
   Ensure adequate hydration
   Within half hour after delivery of placenta.

   Sips of water after 6 hours and subsequent feeds depending on that.

5. Ambulation:
   Immediately after delivery.

   Encourage ambulation within 12-24 hours. Start leg movements after 6 hours of surgery.

6. Breast feeding:
   Immediately after delivery
   Then × 2 hrly

   In the first hour after surgery
   Then × 2 hrly.

- Breasts should be soft and colostrum can be expressed
- Nipples intact, may appear flat or inverted but protrude well on latching, with minimal tenderness.

Subsequently (in the hospital)

Abdomen/Fundus

- Fundus firm/central, descending ≈ 1-1.5 cm/day
- Not palpable after 7-10 days
- Pre pregnant state at 6 weeks.

Abdominal Wound

- Fundus may be tender but improving
- Scar should be well approximated and free of inflammation
- Little or no drainage
- Dressing should be clean, dry and intact
- Incision swelling decreases
- No signs of gaping
- No signs of infection
- Dressing should be changed at 24-48 hours and waterproof dressing should be provided so as to encourage the patient to take bath
- Patient may experience numbness around incision after a week
- Patient should take a lateral position while getting up from bed.

Breasts and Feeds

- After 24-48 hours, breasts feel firmer, colostrum more easily expressed
- Frequent breastfeeding prevents engorgement
- Well supported brassiere should be worn (not restricting the feed)
- Teach the mother, signs of proper latching.

Attachment and position
Indicators of good position and attachment:
- Less areola visible underneath the chin than above the nipple
- Chin touching the breast, with both the upper and lower lip turned out (everted)

- With the nose free and at the level of the nipple
- Mouth is wide open
- The baby is swallowing
- Baby's head and body in straight line and supported.

Signs of successful milk transfer
The baby has:
- Audible swallowing
- Sustained rhythmic suck and swallowing with occasional pauses
- Relaxed arms and hands
- Moist mouth
- Satisfaction after feeding
- Regular soaked/heavy nappies.

Mother
- Feels no breast or nipple pain
- Experiences her breast softening
- May experience uterine discomfort
- Experiences no compression of the nipple at the end of the feed
- Feels relaxed and sleepy
- Feels thirsty (due to release of oxytocin with suckling).

Various positions
- Sitting position:
  - Baby's head on her forearm on same side
  - Neck slightly extended
  - Baby's ear, shoulder and hip in one line.
- Lateral position:
  - On her side between trunk and arm.

In non-breastfeeding Women

- Breasts soft, colostrum may be present
- Wear supportive bra within 6 hours of birth
- To be worn continuously until lactation is suppressed, about 5–10 days
- Use of anti-inflammatory agents
- Application of cold treatments, such as gel packs, cold packs or cold cabbage leaves for comfort
- Avoid stimulation of the breasts such as heat, pumping etc. until lactation is suppressed
- Medication to aid suppression
- Small amounts of milk may be produced for up to a month postpartum
- Breasts will start to become softer as lactation is suppressed
- Resumption of menstrual periods → as soon as 6–8 weeks
- Contraception use.

Other Measures

Mother
- Adequate rest for mother
- Assess:
  - Fundal height
  - Uterine contraction and retraction

- Vaginal bleeding, including per vaginal examination to look for any hematoma development
    - Blood loss measurement for first 2 hours
- Keep the mother warm
- Breathing and pelvic floor exercises should be taught before discharge
- Ensure extra care if woman had any antepartum or intrapartum complications
- If patient is not able to void urine, use measures to help void:
    - Ambulation
    - Oral analgesia
    - Squeeze bottle with warm water
    - Running water
    - Hands in water
    - Blow bubbles through a straw
    - Sitz bath
    - Shower
    - Teach contraction and relaxation of pelvic floor
- Assess lochia:
    - Amount
    - Clots
    - Color
    - Odor
    - Stage of involution
    - Change pad every 4 hourly
    - Usually subsides by 4 weeks (changes from lochia rubra to lochia serosa, then to alba)
    - It should not be foul smelling
- Perineal care:
    - Wipe the perineum and remove the pad from front to back → this avoids dragging infection from the anal area to the vaginal area
    - Do not use tampons after delivery → cause of infection
    - Sitz bath ideally after every bowel movement:
        - Sitting in shallow water, only deep enough to cover the hips and buttocks
        - Take at least three 20 minute sitz baths every day for the first 7 days
        - Cold sitz bath can decrease swelling at the perineum
          After the first two to three days, warm sitz baths will improve blood flow to the perineum
    - Wash the perineum with warm water
        - Eases urination
        - Relieves pain
        - Pat dry
    - Avoid constipation by eating foods rich in fibre and drinking plenty of oral fluids
    - Kegels exercises: *No one can tell that you are doing Kegels and you can do them anywhere.*
        - Squeeze the perineal muscles as if you are trying to stop the flow of urine
        - Hold for 5-10 sec and then relax
        - Do this exercise 10 times/day in sets of 10 repetitions
        - Do at least 10 Kegel exercises every time you urinate and at least 100 Kegels each day
    - Analgesics.

Baby

- Ensure thermal protection immediately after birth and subsequently
- Educate the mother the importance of burping after each feed → method, its clinical relevance, the risks of not doing it

- Teach mother to observe for danger signs in the baby
- Skin-to-skin contact, massaging a baby's feet or tickling behind baby's ears should be used to wake the baby while feeding
- Assessment of baby by pediatrician before discharge
- Pediatrician should be informed if baby doesn't pass meconium in first 24 hours
- Neonates developing jaundice within first 24 hours should be urgently evaluated
- Anti D to the mother if mother is Rh negative and baby's blood group is positive
- Baby vaccination (MMR)
- A hearing screen of the neonate should be completed prior to discharge.

Care at Home (Advice on Discharge)

- Woman should be counselled properly at the time of discharge (it should not be a 5 minutes discussion)
- Woman should be made aware of the following:

Breasts and Feeds

- Proper and exclusive breast feeding every 2 hourly on alternate breasts
- Importance of colostrum
- Avoid formula milk
- Importance of demand feed
- Use of well supported brassiere
- Awareness and use of breast pumps
- How to relieve engorgement and hand express breast milk
- A woman who decides to feed her baby formula milk should be taught:
  - How to make feeds using correct, measured quantities of formula and water
  - How to clean/sterilize feeding bottles and teats
  - How to store formula milk
  - Pack of powdered milk once opened should not be used for > 3 weeks or as directed
  - Milk should be prepared by 'No touch' technique
- A woman should be reassured that brief discomfort at the start of breast feeds in the first few days is not uncommon, but this should not persist
- Advice on how to store and freeze the expressed breast milk
- Feeding patterns:
  - Variable feeding pattern, for the first few days (takes small feeds in the beginning which increases as the milk supply comes in)
  - Generally feeds every 2–3 hours
  - Offer 2nd breast if baby does not appear satisfied with the first.

Other Measures

- Iron/folic acid and calcium × 2-3 months
- Adequate sleep (though becomes impossible with breastfeeding)
- Avoid strenuous exercise for first 6-8 weeks
- Add 300 calories more to the diet
- Proper hygiene, especially hand washing
- Good nutritious food (high fibre, protein diet, foods rich in vitamins)
- Give information about the physiological process of recovery after birth and that some health problems are common, with advice to report in particular if the following occurs:

a. *Signs and symptoms of PPH:* sudden and profuse blood loss or persistent increased blood loss; faintness; dizziness; palpitations; tachycardia.
b. *Signs and symptoms of infection:* fever; chills; rigors; abdominal pain and/or offensive or purulent vaginal discharge.
c. *Signs and symptoms of thromboembolism:* unilateral calf pain; redness or swelling of calves; shortness of breath or chest pain.
d. *Signs and symptoms of preeclampsia:* headaches accompanied by one or more of the symptoms of visual disturbances, nausea, vomiting, feeling faint.
e. *Signs and symptoms of breast problems:* engorgement, swelling, redness, tenderness, signs of infection, any malodorous discharge from nipples.
- Women who have had an epidural or spinal anesthesia should be advised to report any severe headache, particularly when sitting or standing
- Information on physiological jaundice, that it normally occurs around 3-4 days after birth; reasons for monitoring it and how to monitor should be taught.
- Hearing screen, if not done before discharge should be done within 4 weeks of delivery
- Coitus:
  - Median interval between delivery and intercourse: 5 weeks (1~12 weeks)
  - Coitus may be resumed based on the patient's desire and comfort
  - Breastfeeding causes a prolonged period of suppressed estrogen production leading to vaginal atrophy and dryness with a resulting dyspareunia.

Contraception

- Safe sex practices
- Counsel on birth spacing
- Family planning.

For breastfeeding women:
- LAM: For no more than 6 months postpartum, still amenorrheic;
- POPs/DMPA: after 6 weeks
- Condoms, spermicide, female sterilization within 7 days or delay till 6 weeks, IUD within 48 hours or delay for 4 weeks

For non-breastfeeding women:
- Immediate postpartum: condoms, progestogen only pills (POPs), progestogen-only injection implants, spermicides
- Female sterilization within 7 days or delay for 6 weeks, IUD within 48 hours or delay till 4 weeks;
- After 3 weeks: Combined oral contraceptives, combined injectables, diaphragm, fertility awareness methods.

Examinations and Assessments at First Postnatal Visit (Usually After 1 week)

- Vitals
- Examination of breasts (look for signs of engorgement or any other infection)
- Ask mother how the baby is feeding
- If nipple pain persists even after proper positioning and attachment, consider evaluation for thrush → guide about relevant health practices and antifungal practices
- Look for anemia
- Abdominal wound in case of cesarean section (inadequate repair, wound breakdown or non-healing should be further evaluated)

- Assessment of perineum for signs of pain or swelling (episiotomy site; lochia)
- Management of mild headaches and back pain
- If constipation continues → high fibre, increased amounts of fluids or if severe—a mild laxative should be offered (especially in cases where the woman had hemorrhoids antenatally)
- If the woman is feeling unhappy, having anxiety, fear, depression, exhaustion and easily crying, assess for postpartum depression. Check for gender issues (related to having a girl child) that may result in harm or emotional trauma for the mother
- Advice regarding the time of resumption of sexual intercourse and about possible dyspareunia
- A water-based lubricant gel to help ease discomfort during intercourse may be advised
- Information regarding ceasing of vaginal bleeding by all means at 6 weeks and report if the same doesn't occur
- A woman with involuntary leakage of a small volume of urine, pelvic floor exercises should be taught again
- The woman should be reminded of the danger signs, especially of secondary PPH
- If painful nappy rash persists, it is usually caused by thrush (Candida albicans) and antifungal treatment should be considered
- If jaundice first develops after 7 days or remains jaundiced after 14 days in an otherwise healthy baby and a cause has not already been identified, it should be evaluated
- Again lay stress on proper nutrition, fluid intake, supplements and that this is not a time to diet
- Refrain from smoking and alcohol while breastfeeding.

Physiological Changes Occurring in Puerperium

Uterus

- Grows at least ten times bigger than its usual size during pregnancy
- Weight changes of uterus:
    - 1000 g immediately after birth (excluding the fetus, placenta, membrane and amniotic fluid)
    - 500 g 1 week after birth
    - 300 g 2 weeks after birth
    - 50-100 g 6 weeks after birth
- Immediately after delivery → palpated at or near the woman's umbilicus (20-22 weeks size)
- At the end of 1st week → ≈ 12 weeks size
- At the end of 2nd week → fundus of uterus no longer palpable above the symphysis pubis
- At 6 weeks → shrinks to its non-pregnant size (slightly larger than the nulliparous one)
- Total number of muscle cells does not decrease → individual cells decrease markedly in size
- Separation of the placenta and membrane involves the spongy layer → decidua basalis remains in the uterus
- Consistency → firm and non tender.

Endometrium

- The remaining decidua becomes differentiated into 2 layers within 2 or 3 days after delivery
    - Superficial layer: become necrotic, sloughed in the lochia
    - Basal layer: remains intact, source of new endometrium
- By 7th day, it is restored throughout the uterus, except at the placental site
- Regenerates rapidly by 14-16 days.

Uterine Vessels

- Caliber of extrauterine vessels: decrease to equal size of pre pregnant state after delivery
- Blood vessels within puerperal uterus: obliterated by hyaline change, replaced by smaller vessels.

Placental Site Involution

- Complete extrusion of placental site takes up to 6 weeks
- Immediately after delivery → palm size
- By the end of 2nd week → 3-4 cm in diameter
- Placental site → normally consists of many thrombosed vessels within hours of delivery → ultimately undergo organization of thrombus
- Placental site exfoliation → as the consequence of sloughing of infarcted and necrotic superficial tissues followed by a reparative process.

Lochia

- Vaginal discharge during the post partum period
- The term comes from a Greek word that means "relating to childbirth"
- Consists of blood, sloughed-off tissue from endometrium and bacteria
- Color changes:
  - Bright red **(lochia rubra)** for the first few days (2-4 days) → look like a heavy menstrual bleeding → come out intermittently in small gushes or flow more evenly → more watery, dark brown subsequently
  - Pale yellowish in color/straw colored/pale pinkish (lochia serosa) for ≈ 10-14 days, gradually decreases in amount
  - White **(lochia alba)** - maintains for 2-3 weeks
- Each woman has her own pattern, the process generally taking four to five weeks, though a small number of women continue to have scant lochia or intermittent spotting for a few more weeks.

Cervix

- Immediately after the delivery → the muscular walls of the cervix are relaxed, thin and stretched, may be swollen or bruised
- Within first 24 hours → cervix usually narrows and regains its normal muscular consistency
- Returns to its normal state by 4 weeks
- External os:
  - Circular nulliparous os becomes slit like
  - Permits 1-2 fingers by 24 hours after the delivery
  - By the end of the first post natal week, narrows to one finger width
- As the os narrows, the cervix thickens and a canal reforms
- Bilateral depression at the site of lacerations remain as permanent changes that characterize the parous cervix.

Return of Menstruation and Ovulation

- If not breastfeeding → usually return within 6-8 weeks
- Lactating woman → first period may occur between 2-18 months after delivery

- Ovulation:
  - As early as 36-42 days (5-6 weeks) after delivery
  - Delayed resumption of ovulation with breast feeding but early ovulation is not precluded by persistent feeding
  - Lactation → pregnancy can occur with lactation.

Vagina

- Immediately after delivery, vagina is → large, smooth walled, edematous and congested
- Small vaginal tears, which are very common, usually heal in 7 to 10 days
- Rugae reappear by the 3rd week
- Vagina and vaginal outlet gradually diminishes in size but rarely returns to nulliparous dimensions
- Vaginal outlet relaxes because of extensive laceration and overstretching during delivery
- Resolution of the increased vascularity and edema occurs by 3 weeks
- Vaginal epithelium appears atrophic and is restored by 6-10th week
- There may be small degree of utero vaginal prolapse after parturition → teach pelvic floor exercises.
Surgery is postponed for a later date, if ↑ prolapse.

Vulva

- Congestion and swelling of the vagina and vulva disappears by 2-3 weeks
- Tears and/or an episiotomy usually heal easily, if properly sutured.

Perineum

- Swelling completely disappears within 1-2 weeks
- The voluntary muscles of the pelvic floor and pelvic supports gradually regain their tone during the puerperium but may not return, depending on the extent of injury
- Tearing or overstretching of the musculature or fascia at the time of delivery predispose to genital hernias.

Abdominal Wall

- The abdominal wall is flaccid, loose, wrinkled and divarication of the abdominal muscles occurs
- Striae gravidarum, where present, do not disappear but do tend to become less red in time
- Returning to its original tone greatly depends upon the amount of exercise the woman does as she returns to her full fitness
- Overdistention of the abdominal wall during pregnancy may result in rupture of the elastic fibers, persistent striae, and diastases of the recti muscles
- Involution of the abdominal musculature may require 6-7 weeks and vigorous exercises are not recommended until after that time.

Temperature

- Fever is usually normal
- There may be a slight rise during the first day (reactionary rise) but should not exceed 38°C
- Drops within 24 hours and not accompanied by increased pulse rate.

AfterPains

- After expulsion of fetus and placenta the uterus contracts to regain its normal size, weight and site, this is called involution of uterus
- Primiparas → puerperal uterus tends to remain tonically contracted
- Multiparas → contracts vigorously at interval → afterpain
- Infant suckles → oxytocin release from posterior lobe of pituitary gland → uterine contraction → afterpain
- Characteristic of afterpain:
    - Occur during the 1st 2-3 days of puerperium
    - Abdominal pains (like cramps) and back pain
    - Strong, regular, and coordinated
    - The intensity, frequency and regularity of contraction decreases after the 1st postpartum day, usually becoming mild after the 3rd day.

Cardiovascular System

- Blood volume returns to non-pregnant levels by the 10th day
- Cardiac output ↑ (immediately after delivery) → slowly declines → reach late pregnancy levels within first 2 days postpartum → becomes normal at 2-6 weeks.

Gastrointestinal Tract

- Thirst is common
- Appetite varies from anorexia to ravenous hunger
- There may be flatulence
- Many patients are constipated as a result of:
    - Decreased tone of the bowel during pregnancy
    - Decreased food intake during labor
    - Enema given during labor
    - Less fluid intake in puerperium
- Constipation is common in the presence of an episiotomy or painful hemorrhoids.

Urinary Tract

- Retention of urine is common and may result from decreased tone of the bladder in pregnancy and edema of the urethra following delivery or reflexly from perineal trauma
- Painful and/or difficult micturition may lead to complete urinary retention or retention with overflow incontinence. A full bladder will interfere with uterine contraction
- Puerperal diuresis → physiological reversal of pregnancy-induced increase in extracellular water
    - Usually occurs between 2nd and 5th day
    - In edematous patients, may start immediately after delivery
- Puerperal bladder → source of UTI??
    - Increased capacity
    - Relative insensitivity to intravesical fluid pressure
    - Over distention
    - Incomplete emptying
    - Excessive residual urine
    - Prolonged catheterization

- Stress incontinence, occurring on laughing or coughing may become worse initially but tends to improve with time and with pelvic floor exercises
- Normal micturition → by 3 months
- Dilated renal pelvis and ureters → return to pre pregnant state by 2-8 weeks
- Normal bladder function is likely to be temporarily impaired when a patient has been given epidural analgesia. Complete retention of urine or retention with overflow may occur.

Hematologic Changes

- Hemoglobin concentration ↑ during the first postpartum days
- Several clotting factors (fibrinogen) ↑ on the first few days.

Skin

- There is a tendency to sweating
- The increased pigmentation of the face, abdominal wall and vulva lightens but the areolae may remain darker than they were before pregnancy
- With the onset of diuresis, the general puffiness and any edema disappear in a few days.

Body Weight

- Uterine evacuation and normal blood loss → 4-6 kgs immediately after delivery
- Further decrease through diuresis → 2-3 kgs over subsequent weeks.

Lactation

Colostrum

- The deep lemon-yellow colored liquid secreted initially by the breasts
- Expressed from the nipples by the 2nd postpartum day
- Contains more minerals and protein - globulin
- Less sugar and fat
- Antibodies especially IgA
- Persists for ≈ 5 days
- Gradual conversion to mature milk during the subsequent 4 weeks
- First 3–4 days it will appear thin and watery and will taste very sweet;
- Later, the milk will be thicker and creamier.

Milk

- 600 mL/day
- The onset of copious milk production, otherwise known as stage II of lactogenesis, occurs within the first four days postpartum
- Milk transfer to the nursing infant starts at a relatively low volume of < 100 mL on day one, increasing 36 hours later to reach 500 mL/day by day four
- Major proteins → including α-lactalbumin, β-lactoglobulin and casein
- Also contains interleukin -6, epidermal growth factor
- Human milk quenches the baby's thirst and hunger and provides the proteins, sugar, minerals, and antibodies that the baby needs.

Nursing

- Even though the milk supply at first appears insufficient, it becomes adequate if suckling is continued

- Nursing accelerates uterine involution: repeated stimulation of nipples release oxytocin → contracts uterine muscle
- Milk leakages, engorgement and breast pain peak at 3 to 5 days postpartum→ support with
  - Well-fitting brassiere
  - Ice packs
  - Oral analgesics
  - Frequent breast feeding and feed on demand.

Baby Friendly Hospital Initiative

- Also known as Baby Friendly Initiative (BFI)
- Launched by WHO and UNICEF in 1991
- Adopted worldwide following the adoption of the Innocenti Declaration on breastfeeding promotion in 1990
- It is a global effort to enable mothers to breastfeed their babies.

Aims at

- Improving the care of pregnant women, mothers and newborns
- Increasing the numbers of babies who are exclusively breastfed worldwide, a goal which the WHO estimates could contribute to avoiding over a million child deaths each year.

Criteria for a Hospital's Baby Friendly Accreditation

1. A written breastfeeding policy that is routinely communicated to all health care staff
2. Train all health care staff in skills necessary to implement this policy
3. Inform all pregnant women about the benefits and management of breastfeeding
4. Help mothers initiate breastfeeding within one half-hour of birth
5. Show mothers how to breastfeed and maintain lactation, even if they should be separated from their infants
6. Give newborn infants no food or drink other than breastmilk, not even sips of water, unless medically indicated
7. Practice rooming in → allow mothers and infants to remain together 24 hours a day
8. Encourage breastfeeding on demand
9. Give no artificial teats or pacifiers or soothers to breastfeeding infants
10. Foster the establishment of breastfeeding support groups and refer mothers to them on discharge from the hospital or clinic.
    The program also restricts use by the hospital of free formula or other infant care aids provided by formula companies
    Since the program's inception, approximately 15,000 facilities in more than 152 countries have been inspected and accredited as "Baby-Friendly".

Benefits

Child
Less likely to suffer from:
- Non specific gastroenteritis
- Asthma
- Eczema (atopic dermatitis)
- Respiratory and middle ear infections (acute)

- Sudden Infant Death Syndrome (SIDS)
- UTI up to 7 months of age
- Necrotizing enterocolitis (found mainly in premature infants)
- Increased immunity ($\approx$ 0.25-0.5 grams/day of secretory IgA antibodies pass to the baby via the milk, targeting the microorganisms in baby's intestines)
- Breast milk contains several anti-infective factors such as bile salt stimulated lipase (protecting against amebic infections) and lactoferrin (which binds to iron and inhibits the growth of intestinal bacteria)
- Increased intelligence
- Cold and flu resistance
- Decreased risk of:
  - Childhood leukemia
  - Both type I and II diabetes
  - Dental problems
  - Obesity later in life
  - Autism
  - Cardiovascular diseases in adult life (lower cholesterol and C-reactive protein)
  - Developing psychological disorders, particularly in adopted children
- Exclusive breastfeeding reduces the risk of HIV transmission from mother to child, or death from not being breastfed, when screened donor milk is not available
- Some evidence suggest a negative correlation between breastfeeding and carotid intima-media thickness, a recognised risk factor for atherosclerosis, but the data is inconclusive.

Mother
- Cost effective
- Helps in uterine involution
- Reduces postpartum bleeding
- Releases oxytocin and prolactin
- Helps the mother in returning to her pre pregnancy weight
- Delay in fertility
- Early skin to skin contact (kangaroo care)–enables early latch on and a successful breastfeeding, reduces cry, improves mother to infant interaction and keeps baby warm
- Lowers risk of developing:
  - Breast cancer
  - Ovarian cancer
  - Endometrial cancer
  - Hip fractures in later life
  - Coronary artery disease (if lactation was >24 months)
  - Metabolic syndrome
  - Diabetic mothers require less insulin.

Environment
- Preservation of natural resources
- Decreased waste production.

Recommendation

WHO: Exclusive breastfeeding for the first six months of life, after which "infants should receive nutritionally adequate and safe complementary foods" while breastfeeding continues up to two years of age or beyond.

AAP (American Academy of Pediatrics): Exclusive breastfeeding for the first six months of life. "Breastfeeding should be continued for at least the first year of life and beyond for as long as mutually desired by mother and child".

Reasons when Mothers Cannot Produce Enough Breast Milk

- An improper latch
- Not nursing or pumping enough to meet supply
- Certain medications (including estrogen-containing hormonal contraceptives)
- Illness
- Dehydration
- Sheehan's syndrome, also known as postpartum hypopituitarism, though rare, is associated with prolactin deficiency. This syndrome may require hormone replacement.

Ways to Increase Milk Secretion

- The amount of milk produced depends on how often the mother is nursing and/or pumping; the more she does, the more milk is produced
- It is very helpful to nurse on demand
- If pumping, it is helpful to have an electric high-grade pump so that all of the milk ducts are stimulated
- Domperidone and Reglan may also be used.

Breast Milk

Production

Under the influence of hormones prolactin and oxytocin, at first colostrum is produced.
What is colostrum?
- Also known as beestings, bisnings or first milk
- A thin yellowish fluid, a form of milk produced by the mammary glands in late pregnancy
- Rich in proteins and antibodies, lower in fat than ordinary milk
- As newborns have very immature digestive systems, colostrum delivers its nutrients in a very concentrated low-volume form
- It has a mild laxative effect → encourages passing baby's first stool,which is called meconium → clearing excess bilirubin,which is produced in large quantities at birth due to blood volume reduction
- Contains:
    - Lymphocytes
    - Antibodies (IgA, IgG, and IgM) → provide passive immunity
    - Lactoferrin
    - Lysozyme
    - Lactoperoxidase
    - Complement
    - Proline-rich polypeptides (PRP)
    - Cytokines including interleukins, tumour necrosis factor, chemokines and others
    - Growth factors (stimulate development of gut):
        - Insulin-like growth factors I and II
        - Transforming growth factors alpha, beta 1 and beta 2
        - Fibroblast growth factors

- Epidermal growth factor
- Granulocyte-macrophage-stimulating growth factor
- Platelet-derived growth factor
- Vascular endothelial growth factor
- Colony-stimulating factor-1
- Very rich in:
  - Proteins
  - Vitamin A
  - Sodium chloride
- Contains lower amounts of:
  - Carbohydrates
  - Lipids
  - Potassium
- The most pertinent bioactive components in colostrum are growth factors and antimicrobial factors.

Composition

The exact composition of breastmilk varies from day to day, depending on food consumption and environment, meaning that the ratio of water to fat fluctuates.

Proteins (g/100 mL)
- Total–1.1%
- Casein 0.4–0.3
- α-lactalbumin–0.3
- Lactoferrin (apo-lactoferrin)–0.2
- IgA – 0.1
- IgG –0.001
- lysozyme – 0.05
- Serum albumin—0.05
- β-lactoglobulin - - -
- In an acidic environment such as the stomach, alpha-lactalbumin unfolds into a different form and binds oleic acid to form a complex called HAMLET that kills tumour cells → thought to contribute to the protection of breastfed babies against cancer.

Carbohydrates (g/100 mL)
- Total-7.1%
- Lactose-7
- Oligosaccharides-0.5.

Fats (g/100 mL)
- Total-4.2-4.5%
- Fatty acids - length 8C (%)-traces
- Polyunsaturated fatty acids (%)-14
- The fat fraction contains:
  - Specific triglycerides of palmitic and oleic acid (O-P-O triglycerides)
  - Large quantity of lipids with transbonds
    - Vaccenic acid
    - Conjugated linoleic acid (CLA) accounting for up to 6% of the human milk fat.

Minerals (g/100 mL)
- Total-0.2%
- Calcium-0.03
- Phosphorus-0.014
- Sodium-0.015
- Potassium-0.055
- Chlorine-0.043.

Unique Qualities of Breast Milk

- Level of Immunoglobulin A (IgA) remains high from day 10 until at least 7.5 months post-partum
- Non-protein nitrogen-containing compounds, making up 25% of the milk's nitrogen, include:
    - Urea
    - Uric acid
    - Creatine
    - Creatinine
    - Amino acids
    - Nucleotides
- Breast milk has circadian variations; some of the nucleotides are more commonly produced during the night, others during the day
- Studies have found out that breast milk which was once thought to be sterile, is more similar to cultured yogurt
- Contains:
    - ≈ 600 different species of beneficial bacteria
    - 140 types of oligosaccharides (long chains of complex sugars), a unique sugar found nowhere else in nature
        - As these sugars vary by blood type, not every mother produces the same ones
        - These sugars are meant to feed the beneficial bacteria that live in the intestine and help to fight infections
    - Endo-cannabinoids, which may act as an appetite stimulant and regulator
    - Vitamins, digestive enzymes and hormones
    - Less iron than formula milk, as iron is an essential nutrient for survival of pathogens inside the host
        - At around 4-6 months of age, the internal iron supplies of the infant, held in the hepatic cells of the liver, is exhausted, hence this is the time that complementary feeding is introduced
    - A higher proportion of cholesterol than almost any other food
    - Over 50% of its calories as fat, much of it is saturated fat
        - Both cholesterol and saturated fat are essential for growth in babies and children, especially the development of the brain
    - Strong antibodies and antitoxins that many people believe promote healing and better overall health
- The first milk ingested by the infant (foremilk) has a lower fat content, which steadily increases as the hindmilk comes in promoting satiety
- Lacks sterile and antiseptic properties.

Comparison with Other Milks

Cow's milk differ from human milk in the following ways:
- Is thicker and less sweet than human milk
- Contains very little iron, retinol, vitamin E, vitamin C, vitamin D, unsaturated fats or essential fatty acids

- Contains too much protein, sodium, potassium, phosphorus and chloride which may put a strain on an infant's immature kidneys
- The proteins, fats and calcium in whole cow's milk are more difficult for an infant to digest and absorb than the ones in breastmilk
- A significant minority of infants are allergic to one or more of the constituents of cow's milk, most often the cow's milk proteins.

Breast Milk of Diabetic Mother

Different from non diabetic women by following ways:
- Contains ↑ levels of glucose and insulin
- ↓ polyunsaturated fatty acids
- Language delay has been observed in their infants.

CONTRACEPTION

- Not needed in the first 3 weeks postpartum.

Progestin Only Contraceptives

- Mini-pills, depot medroxyprogesterone, levonorgestrel implant
- Do not affect the quality and increase the volume of milk very slightly
- Contraceptives of choice for breastfeeding women.

Estrogen-progestin Contraceptives

- Reduce the quantity and quality of breastmilk
- Puerperal women have predisposition to venous thrombosis → increased by combination contraceptive pills → low dose pills are preferred if used in lactating women.

Contraindications to Breastfeeding

Mother

- Have active, untreated tuberculosis
- On medications, contraindicated during breastfeeding
- Are undergoing breast cancer treatment
- Cytomegalovirus and hepatitis B virus are excreted in milk
- Women with active herpes simplex virus
- Do not control alcohol use
- Have HIV infection (relative contraindication).

Baby

- Phenylketonuria (PKU)
- Classic galactosemia
- Other inborn errors of metabolism (e.g. Maple Syrup Urine Disease).

Drugs Secretion in Milk

- Most drugs given to the mother are secreted in breastmilk
- But amount of drug ingested by the infant is typically small (do not exceed 2% of the total ingested dose).

Care of the Breasts and Nipples

- Dried milk is likely to accumulate and irritate the nipples → cleaning of areola with water and mild soap is helpful before and after nursing.

Basic Principles of Storing Breast Milk

- Wash hands before all procedures
- Store the milk in clean tightly sealed containers (infant feeding bottle with solid caps, bottles with screw caps or hard plastic containers with tight caps)
- Ordinary plastic carrying bags (which can easily leak or spill) are not to be used
- Clean the container with hot, soap water
- Container should be labelled with date
- Never mix fresh and already frozen milk
- Do not save milk from a used bottle for use at another feeding
- Use the oldest milk first.

Storage of Fresh and Thawed Human Milk

FreshMilk

- *Table*
    - Room temperature (up to 25°-26°C)
    - For 6-8 hours
    - Should be covered
    - Keep as cool as possible (preferably in fridge).
- *Insulated bag*
    - From 15°C to 4°C
    - For 24 hours
    - Load with ice packs.
- *Refrigerator*
    - At ≤ 4°C
    - For 5 days
    - Store milk in the main body of the refrigerator (at the back for minimal handling).
- *Freezer*
    - At -15°C (for 2 weeks), in single door fridge
    - At -18°C (for 3-6 months), if separate doors.
- *Deep freezer*
    - At -20°C (for 6-12 months)
    - Storage for longer durations can result in degradation of some lipids, leading to poor quality.

Thawed Milk

- *Frozen milk, thawed in fridge*
    - At room temperature (≤ 26°C) → can be kept for ≤ 4 hours
    - In refrigerator (at 4°C) → can be kept for 24 hours
    - DO NOT REFREEZE.
- *Frozen milk thawed in warm water*
    - At room temperature → till completion of feed
    - In refrigerator → ≤ 4 hours (ideally to be consumed within 1 hour)
    - DO NOT REFREEZE.

Thawing Breast Milk

- Freezed milk can be thawed by keeping it either in refrigerator or in a bowl of warm water.

DO NOT use microwave. Why?
- Milk may not be heated evenly, which may destroy it
- Excess heat (high temperature or longer duration or both) can lead to:
  - Explosion of bottles
  - Destroys the nutrient quality.

Recommendations to a Nursing Mother while Travelling

If Mother is Travelling along the Child

- Do not stop or supplement breastfeeding while travelling
- Feed frequent which will maintain adequate milk supply
- Try to maintain skin to skin contact as much as possible
- Sling or soft infant carrier can be used to ease carrying the child for longer durations.

If Mother is Travelling without the Child

Plans for the baby
- Begin storing breastmilk for a reasonable period of time before separation
- Try to feed the baby with bottle or spoon, if never fed before.

Plans for the mother
- Separation for a week or so does not pose a major problem
- Regularly express her milk (every 2-3 hours) manually or using breast pump
- Electric breast pumps are allowed on board during air travel and are considered personal.

Weaning from Breast

Exclusive breastfeeding is recommended for the first six months of life and continued breastfeeding with complementary foods for up to two years and beyond (no upper limit has been defined) according to WHO.
- The term "weaning" comes from the Anglo-Saxon word "wenian" meaning "to become accustomed to something different"
- It is a natural, inevitable stage in a child's development
- It is a complex process involving nutritional, immunological, biochemical and psychological adjustments
- Weaning may mean the complete cessation of breastfeeding (an "abrupt" or "final" wean) or, a gradual process of introducing complementary foods to the infant's diet while continuing to breastfeed
- The first introduction of foods other than breast milk marks, by definition, the beginning of weaning
- The most common reason mothers give for weaning is a perceived insufficiency in milk supply.
- Women who breastfeed for longer than three months most often cite return to work as their reason for weaning.

Gradual weaning (infant-led weaning)
- When infant starts eating other food products while still on breastfeeding.

Planned weaning (mother-led weaning)
- A planned wean occurs when the mother decides to stop exclusive breastfeeding without receiving infant's cues about readiness for this change
- Reasons include:
  - Not having enough milk or concerns about the baby's growth
  - Painful feedings or mastitis
  - Returning to work
  - A new pregnancy
  - Eruption of baby's first teeth.

Refusal to Breastfeed: "Nursing Strikes"

Gradual weaning should not be confused with a "nursing strike". Nursing strikes are temporary and can result from any number of causes, including the onset of menses, a change in the mother's diet, soap or deodorant, teething, or infant illness. An infant's sudden refusal to nurse can occur at any time and may lead to complete weaning. The mother might interpret this as a rejection of breastfeeding and stop offering the breast. Simple steps to manage a nursing strike include:
- Making feeding time special and quiet; minimizing distractions
- Increasing the amount of cuddling and soothing of the baby
- Offering the breast when the infant is very sleepy or just waking up
- Offering the breast frequently using different nursing positions, alternating sides or nursing in different rooms.

Abrupt or emergency weaning
- Prolonged and unplanned separation of mother and infant
- Severe maternal illness
- Absolute contraindicated drugs: antimetabolites, therapeutic doses of radiopharmaceuticals and most drugs of abuse.

Effects on Mother and Infant
- Discomfort, especially if it occurs during the early postpartum period when her milk production is high
- Take analgesics
- Express just enough milk that her breasts feel comfortable
- Cold gel packs, cold cabbage leaves or breast massage are reported to relieve engorgement (though not supported by evidence)
- A comfortable and supportive bra can help to reduce discomfort
- Binding the breasts, which will lead to more discomfort and can cause blocked milk ducts, is not recommended
- There is no need for fluid restriction
- Whenever possible, weaning should be a gradual process. An abrupt wean is traumatic for the infant, uncomfortable for the mother and may result in blocked ducts, mastitis or breast abscesses.

Other Measures while Breastfeeding
- Supplement with vitamin D, for the first six months of life
- Breastfeeding for up to two years and beyond with appropriate nutritional guidance
- Introduce iron-fortified foods in the form of meat, fish or iron-fortified cereals as first foods, to avoid iron deficiency

- Advice slow, progressive, natural weaning whenever possible
- Inform and support breastfeeding mothers while ensuring adequate nutrition for their babies, regardless of the timing of weaning
- Inhibition of lactation:
  - When the baby is not put to the breasts, lactation ceases on its own in due course of time
  - Expressing milk relieves of the engorged breasts
  - Well fitted brassieres
  - Analgesics
  - Cabergolin 0.5 mg 2 stat (drug of choice) single dose
  - DO NOT use breast binders.

BREAST PUMPS

- Medical devices for extracting (expressing) breast milk
- Regulated by the FDA.

Uses

- Maintain or increase a woman's milk supply
- Relieves engorged breasts and plugged milk ducts
- Pull out flat or inverted nipples
- To express and store breast milk while on work, travelling or otherwise
- Can be used as a supplement to breastfeeding
- Some pumps are designed to mimic the suckling of a nursing baby.

Types of Breast Pumps

All breast pumps consist of a few basic parts:

Breast Shield

- Cone-shaped cup that fits over the nipple and the areola.

Pump

- Creates the gentle vacuum that expresses milk
- The pump may be attached to the breast-shield or have plastic tubing to connect the pump to the breast-shield.

Milk Container

- A detachable container that fits below the breast-shield and collects milk as it is pumped
- The container is typically a reusable bottle or disposable bag that can be used to store the milk or be attached to a nipple and used for feeding a baby.

Types of Breast Pumps

3 basic types:
- Manual pumps
- Battery-powered pumps
- Electric pumps.

Pumping Types

2 different pumping types: single and double

Single
- Extracts milk from one breast at a time
- Most manual and battery powered pumps are single pumps.

Double
- Can be used to extract milk from both breasts simultaneously
- Some electric pumps are double pumps.

General Tips for using a Breast Pump

1. Wash hands with soap scrubbing for 10-15 sec and dry
2. Need not wash your breasts each time, unless cream or ointment is applied on it
3. Assemble Your Pump
4. Position the nipple in the center of the opening in breast shield (no pinching, pulling or irritation)
5. Method of pumping:
   - Amount of milk produced is different for everyone
   - Atypical pumping session lasts about 10-15 minutes per breast, but pump only as long as it is comfortable
   - Milk may not flow immediately after starting
   - When it does flow, milk should be collected in the container attached to your pump
   - Make sure there is no leakage or if it leaks, stop and reassemble
   - Break the vacuum seal by inserting a finger between the breast and the breast-shield
   - Remove the bottle or bag of collected milk
   - If it is for storage, label it with the date and time
6. Clean with soap and warm water (even boiling the parts may not give it complete sterilization)
7. Microwave sterilizers are available for breast pump parts, but these sterilizers do not meet the FDA definition of sterilization.

Factors Influencing Breastfeeding/Milk Production

Though the following hormones act in concert to stimulate the growth and development of milk secretion by mammary glands but there are certain other factors influencing milk production:

Hormones
- Progesterone
- Estrogen
- Placental lactogen
- Prolactin (very important for lactation)
- Cortisol
- Insulin.

Suckling
- Helps in triggering a rise in prolactin, which usually falls after delivery.

Factors having Positive Impact

Those influenced by prolactin *(Milk Secretion Reflex)*:
- The first feed
- Feeding according to need (night feeds, demand feeds)

- Baby behavioral states
- Proper attachment.

Those influenced by oxytocin *(Milk Ejection Reflex):*
- Rooming in - Thought, sight and sound of baby
- Skin to skin contact (SSC).

Factors which may Negatively Impact
- Use of dummies/pacifiers.

The First Feed
- Putting the baby to breasts within the first one to two hours
- Baby will usually demonstrate the following sequentially:
  - Opens eyes, quietly looks around and searches for mother's nipple
  - Uncurls fists and makes grasping movements towards nipple
  - Makes small 'licking' movements
  - Demonstrates 'rooting' behavior which may include:
    - Opening mouth
    - Turning head towards the nipple
    - Rubbing chin into breast
    - Attempting to self attach
- It is important that the breastfeed is not interrupted until baby indicates satiety by:
  - Spontaneously detaching from the nipple without further rooting behavior
  - Falling asleep at the breast.

Baby Behavioral States
Babies typically exhibit the following behavioral states:
- Birth–2 hours: quiet alert (best time to feed)
- 2–20 hours: light and deep sleep (infrequent feeding)
- After 20 hours: continuum of sleep–wake behaviors (frequent feeding).

Feeding According to Need
Advantages:

Mother
- Increases the rate of successfully establishing lactation
- Reduces the incidence of breast engorgement
- Establishes a supply and demand pattern.

Baby
- Increases breastfeeding duration
- Decreases the incidence and severity of physiological jaundice.

Proper Positioning
- Discussed earlier.

Rooming in

Rooming in (Kangaroo Mother Care), where mother and baby remain together 24 hours a day, helps in Milk Ejection ('letdown') Reflex (MER).

Milk Ejection Reflex
- Stimulates neurohypophysis to liberate oxytocin
- Contraction of myoepithelial cells in the alveoli → expulsion of milk into milk ducts → milk expression from lactating breast
- Occurs a number of times during a feed
- Different mothers will react differently to this reflex:
  - Will only be aware of the initial MER and may not be able to sense subsequent milk ejections
  - May experience a sensation of warmth or tingling in their breasts
  - May experience 'afterbirth'/abdominal pain or discomfort during MER
  - May be unaware of the milk letdown
- Changes in the baby's sucking pattern throughout the feed will indicate that MER is occurring.

Benefits of Rooming in:
- Unrestricted breastfeeding access
- Increases breastfeeding duration
- Mother becomes familiar with the baby's feeding patterns
- Promotes relaxation and sleep
- Reduces the risk of SIDS.

Skin to Skin Contact

Benefits:

Mother
- Stimulates release of oxytocin which:
  - Minimises blood loss
  - Decreases anxiety
  - Promotes mother baby emotional attachment
- May prevent or alleviate breastfeeding problems (engorgement, sore nipples).

Baby
- Maintains body temperature
- Decreases length of crying time
- Increases interaction with mother
- Promotes innate behaviors that assist in establishing breastfeeding
- Increases the duration of breastfeeding
- Maintains normal blood glucose levels.

Dummy (pacifier) use

- Associated with shortened breastfeeding duration
- May contribute to breastfeeding difficulty
- Not recommended in the healthy, term breastfed baby until breastfeeding is well established
- At sleeping time, their use has been associated with a reduced incidence of SIDS in both breastfed infants and those fed infant formula
- Frequent use may negatively impact upon breastfeeding which may reduce milk supply and slow baby's weight gain.

Feeding Frequency

- The initiation of lactation is hormonally driven
- Storage capacity of breasts impacts upon the length and frequency of breast feeds:

- Range from 80 mL to as much as 600 mL but this cannot be determined by visual assessment
- Large breasts may contain increased adipose tissue, rather than mammary tissue
- The baby of a mother with a smaller storage capacity will feed more frequently than a baby of a mother with a larger storage capacity to receive the same amount of milk in a day
- Most healthy babies will feed between 8-12 times in a 24-hour period
- Total length of time at each breast does not correlate with amount of milk transferred.

Sucking Patterns

Non Nutritive Sucking

- Rapid and shallow
- 2 sucks/sec
- Infrequent swallows
- Occurs with periods of slow milk flow:
  - At the beginning of a feed
  - Prior to a milk ejection.

Nutritive Sucking

- Deeper and slower
- Approximately 1 suck/sec
- Swallows after every 1 or 2 sucks
- Occurs with periods of rapid milk flow:
  - After a milk ejection.

Is the baby sufficiently fed? How do you know?

- Hunger signals like increased alertness and rooting indicate when feeding is required
- Baby becomes calm and comes off the breast when satisfied
- Feeding times on either breast should not be limited; the baby will dictate when he has had enough
- Simply observe the baby's bowel and urinary habits:
  - Dark meconium in the first few days changes to yellow stool
  - The more breastmilk the baby drinks, the lighter the stool becomes
  - Normal breast milk stool characteristics:
    - Pasty to watery
    - Little odor
    - Occasionally contains curds
  - Adequately fed baby has 2-3 substantial yellow stools by D3, which increases in frequency thereafter
  - Small infrequent brown stool may indicate inadequate hydration
  - With 2-3 wet diapers in the 1st three days, and at least 6 soaking wet diapers/day thereafter, gives assurance of adequate feeding
- Postnatal weight change
  - A newborn loses between 5-7% of birth weight within the first week but regains this after the first ten days
  - A baby who is fed more frequently and on demand has less weight loss
  - Weight of baby at 3 months of age should be twice its weight at birth
  - There should be increase in height and head circumference.

Certain Facts

- Most chronic illnesses are compatible with breastfeeding, unless the medications used by the mother are known to cause harm to the infant
- In case of GI or respiratory infection, it is recommended to provide continued and increased breastfeeding as it will provide the necessary secretory antibodies and anti-inflammatory agents to hasten recovery
- If the child is hospitalized and is not able to take direct feeds, mother should provide expressed breast milk
- Woman should continue breastfeeding on the affected side, if suffering from breast pain and swelling due to blocked ducts or mastitis
- Candida infections of the nipple are also compatible with breastfeeding
- Ideally, nursing mothers can take medications immediately after breastfeeding, several hours before the next feed or as a single daily dose at bedtime. Drugs compatible with breastfeeding:
  - Penicillins
  - Many topical agents
  - Analgesics
  - Anti-hypertensives
  - Anti-epileptics
  - Anxiolytics
  - Anti-depressant drugs
- Radiation, cytotoxic therapy, recreational drugs, heavy alcohol and smoking are incompatible
- Though weaning is recommended after 6 months of age, many women begin weaning their babies between 4-6 months of age and earlier still, if they need to resume work
- The weaning age 'should be directed by the child rather than the parent', when the child shows dissatisfaction with milk alone, and obvious interest in other foods
- But beyond six months, further delay increases risk of iron deficiency and first complementary foods should be iron-rich
- Supplement daily vitamin D of 10 μg (400 IU) for breastfed infant.

Domperidone or metoclopramide –Which is a better galactogogue?

Domperidone has replaced Metoclopramide as the galactogogue of choice:
- A peripheral dopamine-receptor antagonist
- Uses:
  - In the treatment of dyspepsia
  - Reflux esophagitis
  - Nausea and vomiting
- Side effects:
  - Anxiety
  - Depression
  - Increase in prolactin levels
- Mechanism of action:
  - Works on peripheral dopamine receptors in the GI wall and CTZ centre of the brainstem
  - Its effects on prolactin secretion occurs at the pituitary level (outside the blood-brain barrier)
- Other properties:
  - Less lipid soluble
  - Larger molecular weight
  - Highly protein bound (93%), as compared to metochlopramide
  - Less medication crossing through into breastmilk

- Because domperidone crosses less freely into breastmilk (almost negligible as compared to metoclopramide) the possible risks to the infant are also reduced
- A randomized, double—blind placebo-controlled trial (approved by AAP) have shown an increase in milk volume of 44.5% in domperidone group with a steady increase in milk volume commencing 48 hours after initiation until D7. The rise in prolactin levels increased from 12.9 μ/L measured at baseline to 119.3 μ/L of a randomly sampled blood test on day 5. The serum prolactin levels returned to baseline 3 days after treatment was ceased
- Dose
  - 10-20 mg, orally, 3-4 times/day for 10-14 days. Can be extended up to 8 weeks.

Precautions

1. Reduce the dose in maternal renal or hepatic conditions
2. Avoided with antacids and antisecretory agents
3. Medications that inhibit the cytochrome P_{450} enzyme system (e.g. azole antifungals, macrolide antibiotics, HIV protease inhibitors, and nefazodone) may increase domperidone levels
4. Rare adverse effects include headache, dizziness, abdominal cramps, dry mouth, drowsiness and allergic reactions.

Recommendations

- It should only be given if the mother has been expressing at least 6 times in 24 hours for at least 3 days.

ABNORMAL PUERPERIUM

Puerperal Sepsis

Any bacterial infection of the genital tract occurring after the birth of the baby with the signs and symptoms presenting usually after the first 24 hours except in cases where the woman had prolonged rupture of membranes or a prolonged labor without prophylactic antibiotics. In these cases, disease may become evident earlier.

Puerperal fever—also known as "Childbed fever".
1. **What is the most common site of sepsis in puerperium?**
A. Genital tract especially the uterus, resulting in endometritis.

Risk factors according to the day of occurrence postpartum
- Day 0: atelectasis, risk factors include general anesthesia, cigarette smoking, and obstructive lung disease
- Day 1-2: urinary tract infections, risk factors include multiple catheterization during labor, multiple vaginal examinations during labor, and untreated bacteriuria
- Day 2-3: endometritis (the most common cause), risk factors include emergency cesarean section, prolonged membrane rupture, prolonged labor, and multiple vaginal examinations during labor
- Day 4-5: wound infection, risk factors include emergency cesarean section, prolonged membrane rupture, prolonged labor, and multiple vaginal examination during labor
- Day 5-6: septic pelvic thrombophlebitis, risk factors include emergency cesarean section, prolonged membrane rupture, prolonged labor, and diffuse difficult vaginal delivery
- D 7-21: mastitis, risk factors include nipple trauma from breastfeeding.

Causes of Fever in Postpartum Period

Complete history and detailed clinical examination is of utmost importance in obtaining the cause of fever.

Common Causes

Infectious Causes

1. Puerperal sepsis, depending on how far it has spread, may present as:
   - Localized infection of a wound (cesarean section scar), laceration or episiotomy
   - Infection of laceration or episiotomy which has spread to the underlying soft tissue
   - Metritis
   - Salpingitis
   - Parametritis
   - Generalized peritonitis
   - Septic thrombophlebitis
   - Tubo-ovarian abscess
   - Broad ligament abscess
   - Abscess in Pouch of Douglas
   - Abscesses in other sites in the abdomen or chest
   - Septicemia
   - Septic shock may complicate septicemia
2. Breast infection such as mastitis or, at a later stage, breast abscess
3. Urinary tract infection
4. Respiratory tract infections
   - Pneumonia
   - Bronchitis
   - Malaria
   - Typhoid
   - Pharyngitis
6. Thromboembolic disorders (superficial thrombophlebitis and/or deep vein thrombosis)
7. Gastroenteritis/Hepatitis
8. Any skin infection.

NonInfectious Causes

Low-grade temperature elevations are very common in the early postpartum period, particularly in the first 24 hours

Causes
- Dehydration
- Tissue trauma
- Breast engorgement

Although fever occurring in the first 24 hours after delivery has generally been regarded as unrelated to infection, a temperature of 38°C or higher within the first 24 hours, should alert to the possibility of puerperal sepsis.

Rare Causes

1. Pulmonary tuberculosis
2. Bacterial meningitis.

Very Rare Cause

- Spinal abscess.

Causal Agents

Most common bacteria (usually >1 bacteria may be involved):
- Streptococcus pyogenes (group A β hemolytic streptococci)
- Staphylococci aureus
- Escherichia coli (*E. coli*)
- Clostridium tetani
- Clostridium welchii
- MRSA (methicillin resistant staph. aureus)
- Chlamydia
- Gonococci (bacteria which cause sexually transmitted diseases).

Bacteria can be further classified into:
1. *Endogenous*
    - Bacteria normally present in genital tract (usually the vagina and the rectum)
    - Types: streptococci, staphylococci, E. coli, clostridium welchii etc.
    - Can cause infection in the following ways:
        - Ascending infection from vagina to uterus (even when clean delivery is conducted)
        - From bruised, lacerated or dead tissue (e.g. after a traumatic delivery or following obstructed labor)
        - Prolonged rupture of membranes.
2. *Exogenous*
    - Travel from outside the genital tract
    - Types: streptococci, staphylococci, clostridium tetani etc.
    - Causes:
        - Unclean hands and unsterile instruments
        - Droplet infection
        - Any foreign substance inserted into the vagina (e.g. herbs, oil, cloth)
        - By sexual activity.

Why women catch infection easily after delivery??

Mainly because of the favorable environment provided by placental site in the uterus:
I. It is large, warm, dark and moist → allows bacteria to grow very quickly, making an ideal medium to culture
II. Has rich blood supply and direct connection with the main venous circulation → septicemia can be caused easily, which can lead to death
III. Easily approachable to both endogenous and exogenous microorganisms.

2. Which group of women is at increased risk of developing infection postpartum?
A. Those at risk are:
   Women carrying any source of infection in the antepartum or intrapartum period
   1. Vaginal discharge
   2. Inadequate or no immunization with tetanus toxoid
   3. Prolonged spontaneous rupture of membranes without chorioamnionitis
   4. Chorioamnionitis
   5. History of pelvic infections

6. Repeated pelvic infections during labor
7. Retained products of conception
8. Wound hematoma
9. Poor standards of hygiene
10. Manipulations high in the birth canal
11. Presence of dead tissue in the birth canal (due to prolonged retention of dead fetus, retained fragments of placenta or membranes, shedding of dead tissue from vaginal wall following obstructed labor)
12. Prolonged/obstructed labor
13. PPH.

Women who underwent any procedure
1. Cesarean section
2. Traumatic vaginal delivery
3. Instrumental vaginal delivery
4. Cervical cerclage
5. Amniocentesis or other invasive procedures.

Immunocompromized states
1. Pre-existing anemia and malnutrition
2. DM/GDM
3. Patients on immunosuppressive drugs.

Others
1. Obesity
2. Family member having severe communicable disease
3. Lack of transportation for taking the woman to a higher center
4. Great distance from a woman's home to a health facility
5. Cultural factors which lead to delay in seeking medical care
6. Lack of health education, danger signs of infection or lack of birth and emergency preparation plan.

Infection can extend beyond the uterus
- To involve the fallopian tubes and ovaries, to the pelvic cellular tissue, causing **parametritis**
- To the pelvic peritoneum, causing **peritonitis**
- Into the blood stream, causing **septicemia.**

Signs and symptoms
- Pyrexia ≥ 38°C
- Chills
- General malaise
- Lower abdominal pain
- Uterine tenderness
- Subinvolution of the uterus
- Purulent, foul-smelling lochia
- Light vaginal bleeding
- Shock.

Sites of infection
1. Placental site (most common site)
2. Abdominal and perineal wounds following surgery
3. Lacerations of the genital tract e.g. cervix, vagina and perineum.

Management

Following measures are taken promptly after complete history and physical examination has ruled out causes other than genital infection:
- IV fluids
- Send investigations:
  - CBC
  - Urine routine and culture
  - High vaginal swab
  - Endocervical swab
  - Blood culture
  - If chest signs are present → CXR
  - CT/MRI → if DVT is doubted
- Bed rest
- Ampicillin 2 g IV every 6 hours ⎫
- Gentamicin 5 mg/kg body weight IV every 24 hours ⎬ Preliminary medications until culture report is available
- Metronidazole 500 mg IV every 8 hours ⎭
- Antipyretics/tepid sponging
- Perineal care
- Vitals, intake output charting meticulously
- Tetanus toxoid → if possibility that woman was exposed to tetanus and there is no evidence of vaccination
- Suspect retained placental bits if:
  - Uterus is soft and bulky
  - Excessive lochia
  - Foul-smelling
  - Contain blood clots
- Digital exploration of the uterus to remove clots and large pieces of placental tissue
- Ovum forceps or a large curette may be used, if required
- Kind, sensitive approach towards patient and relatives.

Other causes may be:

Mastitis

History

- Rapid onset in a breastfeeding infant
- Breast engorgement
- Cracked nipple which has allowed bacteria to enter through the broken skin
- Difficulty in fixing the baby to the breast, leading to nipple damage
- Bruising of the breast tissues due to rough handling
- Baby may have signs of skin or eye infections.

Symptoms and Signs

- Breast pain and tenderness
- Reddened, wedge-shaped area visible on breast
- Can occur at any time but typically 3–4 weeks after delivery
- There may be inflammation preceded by engorgement
- Usually only one breast is affected.

Tests/Investigations

Send breast milk for culture and sensitivity, by collection of hand expressed midstream clean catch sample in sterile container.

Important: Start broad spectrum antibiotics without delay if:
- No response to antibiotics within 2 days
- Mastitis recurs
- In cases of hospital acquired mastitis
- In severe cases.

Management

- Mothers should continue breastfeeding
- It is best to begin suckling on uninvolved breast → this will allow let down to commence before moving to tender breast
- Correct attachment and positioning
- Penicillin and cephalosporin
- Cloxacillin 500 mg qid for 1-3 days
- When symptoms subside, 250 mg qid
- Total for 10-14 days
- Erythromycin is given to women who are penicillin sensitive
- MRSA → vancomycin.

Complications

1. Breast abscess
2. Necrotizing fasciitis.

Urinary Tract Infection

- Cystitis
- Severe pyelonephritis.

History

Common risk factors
- Recurrence of UTI present antepartum
- Traumatic vaginal delivery
- Catheterization during labor or prolonged catheterization after cesarean section
- Poor vulval hygiene
- Anemia.

Symptoms and Signs

Cystitis:
- Increased frequency of micturition
- Dysuria (i.e. pain or burning on micturition)
- Slight rise in temperature.

Pyelonephritis:
More serious condition
- Dysuria
- Spiking fever
- Chills and general malaise

- Increased frequency and urgency of micturition
- Abdominal pain.

There may also be:
- Retropubic/suprapubic pain
- Loin pain/tenderness
- Tenderness in rib cage
- Anorexia
- Nausea/vomiting.

Tests and investigations

- Obtain a clean-catch, midstream specimen of urine and send for culture and sensitivity.

Management

1. Cephalosporins and co-amoxiclav
2. Resistant stains, carbapenems may be required
3. If severe, intravenous antimicrobials.

Thromboembolic Disorders

Includes superficial and deep vein thrombosis.

Superficial thrombophlebitis	Deep vein thrombosis
More common in	
Older	>35 years
Obese	High parity
High parity	Obesity
History of varicose veins	Cesarean section
Veins used for IV infusion	Trauma to the legs
	Immobility
	Dehydration and exhaustion
	Smoking
	Use of estrogen
	Previous h/o thromboembolism
Symptoms and signs	
May have fever	Spiking fever, despite antibiotics
Red, inflamed, tender area over the vein	Calf pain may be present, or thigh or abdominal pain
Vein feels firm on palpation from the clot lying within it	Edema and changes in leg color and temperature may also occur
	Pain in leg increased on walking
	Tender mass extending from uterine cornua on either side may be palpable
Obvious on clinical examination	More difficult to diagnose clinically
	Pain in the calf of the leg, especially when walking, is a suspicious symptom of deep vein thrombosis, in particular when accompanied by the above risk factors
Real time ultrasound	-Do-
Ascending phlebography	DVT can lead to pulmonary embolism.
Isotope venography	

Management of DVT or SVT

Prophylactic treatment:
- Early ambulation
- Avoidance of pressure on the thighs and calves
- Sitting position with knee flexed
- Encouragement of circulatory exercises, leg and deep breathing exercises.

If the condition has already occurred:
- Antibiotic is the mainstay of treatment in cases of septic pelvic thrombophlebitis, secondary to infection from placental site
- Fever may persist even after antibiotics
- Use of anticoagulants – not indicated.

Respiratory Tract Infections

May be acute or chronic:

Acute

- Bronchitis
- Pneumonia
- Pleurisy.

Chronic

- Pulmonary tuberculosis
- Chronic bronchitis.

Signs and Symptoms Suggestive of RTI

- Fever
- Tachycardia
- Tachypnea
- Dyspnea
- Chills and rigors
- Cough with/without expectoration
- Chest pain
- Consolidation
- Congested throat
- Rhonchi/wheeze
- Tonsillar exudate
- Hemoptysis (pneumococcal pneumonia)
- Cervical lymphadenopathy.

Investigations

1. Complete blood count
2. Peripheral smear for malarial parasite
3. Widal test (if fever for > 5 days)
4. Blood culture

5. Chest X ray
6. Sputum for culture, Mantoux or Heaf test, if required.

Treatment

1. β lactam antibiotic
2. Macrolides.

Skin and Soft Tissue Infections

Source of infection:
- Site of insertion of IV cannula
- Injection sites
- Cesarean or episiotomy wound site
- Drain, if used during cesarean section.

Management

1. IV cannula sites should be examined twice daily for any signs of infection
2. Daily dressing of abdominal wound
3. Swab for culture/sensitivity from wound site
4. Patient should be advised to lie flat on abdomen several times a day (to expel any accumulated collection)
5. Soaked dressing should be changed without delay
6. Appropriate IV antibiotics after culture report.

Gastroenteritis (uncommon infection in puerperium)

Causal Agents

1. Salmonella
2. Campylobacter
3. C. difficile
   - Diarrhea and vomiting may be features of toxic shock syndrome
   - Managed symptomatically unless features of bacteremia present.

Spinal Abscess

Very rare complication after regional anesthesia.

Causal Agents

1. Staph aureus
2. Streptococci
3. Gram negative rods
   - Complication - neural compression → permanent damage to spinal cord or chorda equina.

Subinvolution of Uterus

- An arrest or retardation of involution, the process by which the puerperal uterus is normally restored to its original proportions
- Cause: retention of placental fragments, pelvic infection

- Accompanied by prolongation of lochial discharge and irregular or excessive uterine bleeding and sometimes by profuse hemorrhage
- Bimanual examination: uterus is larger and softer than normal for the particular period of puerperium.

Treatment

- Ergonovine or methylergonovine (Methergine)
- Oral antibiotics: usually effective in metritis.

Secondary/Late PPH

When excessive blood loss occurs after 24 hours but within 12 weeks after delivery (RCOG 2011).

Cause

- Abnormal involution of placental site (most often)
- Retention of a portion of the placenta:
  - Usually undergo necrosis with deposition of fibrin
  - Forms a placental polyp.

Investigations

Must include the following:
- High and low vaginal swabs
- Blood cultures, if pyrexial
- Full blood count
- C-reactive protein
- Pelvic ultrasound (to exclude the presence of retained products of conception).

Management

- Intravenous oxytocin, ergonovine, methylergonovine
- Prostaglandins
- Curettage (to be done by senior obstetrician as there are high chances of perforation)
- When antibiotics are clinically indicated, a combination of ampicillin (clindamycin if penicillin allergic) and metronidazole is appropriate
- In cases of endomyometritis (tender uterus) or overt sepsis, the addition of gentamicin is recommended
- Breastfeeding is not contraindicated
- Once improved, there is no need for extended oral antibiotic therapy.

BREAST COMPLICATIONS

Breast Engorgement

Tenderness, Warmth, Throbbing (May Extend to Armpits)

- Skin on breast may be taut, shiny, and transparent
- May look red
- Milk NOT flowing
- Bilateral nipples may be flat
- Breast(s) hard, edematous, painful

- Fever may occur
- May be areolar or peripheral
- Can occur at any time during breastfeeding
- Due to exaggerated normal venous and lymphatic engorgement of breasts.

Interventions

- Gentle massage
- Manual expression of breast milk to soften the areola before each feed
- Anti-inflammatory agents
- Analgesics
- Application of warm compresses, shower or breast soak before breastfeeding
- Application of cold treatments, such as gel packs, cold packs or ice application after breastfeeding
- Review of positioning and attachment
- Evaluation for ankyloglossia (tongue tie) should be made if breastfeeding problems persist even after this.

Nipple Pain (Bleeding/Cracked/Bruised Nipples)

Cracks can be

- Straight across the tip of nipple (caused by excessive dryness)
- Star shaped cracks
- Cracks at the base of the nipple (caused by biting).

Interventions

- Assess infant feeding (especially for position and latch)
- Apply expressed breast milk to nipple
- Start feeding with least affected nipple (if nipple pain)
  - Only interrupt breastfeeding if feeding intolerable
  - If baby unable to feed effectively, initiate regular hand expression in the first 24 hours and expression and pumping thereafter
- Every effort should be made to heal the cracks as they are portal of entry for pyogenic bacteria → topical medication or nipple shield.

Flat Nipple

- Nipple embedded in the breast
- Treatment:
  - Compress the breast and the areola between 2 fingers to provide as much nipple to infant as possible
  - Breast shell.

Inverted Nipple

- Inversion of nipple when gentle pressure is applied over it
- Treatment:
  - Nipple shield
  - Manual expression
  - Daily attempts should be made during the last few months of pregnancy to draw the nipple out, using traction with fingers.

Lump in Axilla

- Extra breast tissue in the axilla
- Normal variation, medical intervention not required.

Engorgement in Axillary Region

- Anti-inflammatory agents
- Comfort measure → application of cold.

Plugged Duct

- Usually 1 breast involved
- Localized hot, tender spot
- May be white spot on nipple
- May be a palpable lump (plugged duct).

Interventions

- Shower or warm compress to breast before breastfeeding
- Frequent feeding
- Massage behind the plug toward the nipple, prior to and during feeding
- Vary positions for feeding
- Ice and anti-inflammatory agents
- Avoid missing feeds.

Mastitis

- Parenchymatous infection of mammary glands → leading to cellulitis
- Almost always from nursing infant's nose and throat → the organism enters the breast through the nipple at the site of a fissure or abrasion
- Can occur at any time but usually 1week postpartum
- Sudden onset of intense pain
- Usually in 1 breast (may be both)
- Most common organism – staph. aureus
- Breast may feel hot, appear red or have red streaks and/or be swollen, hard, tender
- Marked engorgement → inflammation → chills or actual rigor (the first sign of inflammation), fever, tachycardia → FLU like symptoms.

Interventions

- Support/rest/adequate fluids
- Continue frequent breastfeeding → milk from affected breast is safe for infant
- Correct attachment and positioning
- If too tender, manual expression or breast pump
- Gentle massage on any firm area
- Shower or warm compresses to affected area, prior to feeds
- After feeds – cool compresses
- Analgesic

- Antibiotics may be indicated if not resolved in 24 hours
  - Penicillin or cephalosporin
  - Cloxacillin 500 mg qid for 1-3 days
  - When symptoms subside 250 mg qid for a total of 10-14 days.

Nipple infection (Candida)
- Sore burning nipples
- Sore all the time but worse when feeding
- Deep burning/shooting pain
- Itchy, flaky nipples
- Tiny blisters
- Deep pink/bright red nipples/areola
- Mother may have recently been on antibiotics or has a yeast infection (infant may have signs of candida in mouth or perineal area).

Interventions
- Differentiate from poor latch
- Frequent hand washing and washing of all items that touch breast and infants mouth
- Antifungal treatment for both mother and infant may be prescribed
- If using breast pads, change when they become wet
- Avoid use of soother.

Breast Abscess
- Localized collection of pus within the breast
- Usually occurs as a complication of mastitis
- Caused by group B streptococcus
- 3 types:
  - Subareolar
    - Unilocular cavities located superficially near the nipples
    - 23%
    - Favorable prognosis
  - Intramammary unilocular
    - Solitary locus of pus deep inside the tissue and distant from nipple
    - 12%
  - Intramammary multilocular
    - 65%
    - Require a longer treatment
    - High recurrence
- Treatment:
  - Incision and drainage under general anesthesia followed by postoperative dressing
  - Small/central abscess—circumareolar skin incision at areolar border
  - Large/peripheral abscess—radial incision
  - Incision should be made corresponding to skin lines for a good cosmetic result
  - USG guided needle aspiration (less invasive) under local anesthesia (80-90% success rate)
  - Multiple abscesses require several incisions and a finger should be inserted to break up the walls of the locules

- Resulting cavity is loosely packed with gauze, which should be replaced at the end of 24 hours by a smaller pack
- Breastfeeding through uninvolved breast.

OBSTETRICAL PARALYSIS

- Pressure on branches of lumbosacral plexus during labor
- Patient complains of intense neuralgia or cramp like pains on extending down one or both legs as soon as the fetal head begins to descend the pelvis
- Nerve involvement:
  - External popliteal n.
  - Femoral n.
  - Obturator n.
  - Sciatic n.
- Muscles involved → gluteus.

PSYCHOLOGICAL DISORDERS

Postpartum blues (transient depression)

- Fairly common
- The emotional letdown that follows the excitement and fears that most women experience during pregnancy and delivery
- The discomforts of the early puerperium
- Fatigue from loss of sleep during labor and postpartum in most hospital settings
- Anxiety over her capabilities for caring for her infant after leaving the hospital
- Fears that she has become less attractive
- Self-limited and usually remits after 5~7 days.

Postpartum Depression

- More depressive
- Negative thinking, loss of libido, feeling of worthlessness
- Severe depression occurs in 6% of women
- Recurrence in future pregnancies is seen in 25-50%
- Supportive care
- Selective serotonin reuptake inhibitors can be used even in breastfeeding mothers
- Progesterone may not help.

Postpartum Psychosis

- Severe form of depression
- Occurs in merely 0.2% of cases
- Patients become dangerous to self and to the newborn
- Patients live in unreal, imaginary world
- Treatment:
  - Hospitalization
  - Case to be reviewed by a psychiatrist
  - Anti psychotics.

SUGGESTED READING

1. ABM Clinical Protocol #10. Breastfeeding the Late Preterm Infant (340/7 to 366/7 Weeks Gestation). Breastfeeding Medicine. 2011;6(3).
2. ABM Clinical Protocol #17. Guidelines for Breastfeeding Infants with Cleft Lip, Cleft Palate or Cleft Lip and Palate. Breastfeeding Medicine 2007;2(4).
3. ABM Clinical Protocol #20: Engorgement: Breastfeeding Medicine. 2009;4(2).
4. ABM Clinical Protocol #24. Allergic Proctocolitis in the Exclusively Breastfed Infant. Breastfeeding Medicine2011;6(6).
5. ABM Clinical Protocol #25. Recommendations for Preprocedural Fasting for the Breastfed Infant: "NPO" Guidelines. BreastfeedingMedicine 2012;7(3).
6. ABM Clinical Protocol #3: Hospital Guidelines for the Use of Supplementary Feedings in the Healthy Term Breastfed Neonate. Breastfeeding Medicine. 2009;4(3).
7. ABM Clinical Protocol #6. Guideline on Co-Sleeping and Breastfeeding. Breastfeeding Medicine. 2008;3(1).
8. Acceptable medical reasons for use of breast-milk substitutes. World Health Organization 2009.
9. Alex Stagnaro-Green. Approach to the Patient with Postpartum Thyroiditis. J Clin Endocrinol Metab. February 2012;97(2):334-42.
10. Anne Chevalier McKechnie1, Anne Eglash. Nipple Shields: A Review of the Literature. Breastfeeding Medicine 2010;5(6).
11. Anne Rowan-Legg, et al. Ankyloglossia and breastfeeding. Canadian Paediatric Society 2013.
12. Bacterial Sepsis following Pregnancy: RCOG Green-top Guideline No. 64b. April 2012.
13. Becker GE, Cooney F, Smith HA. Methods of milk expression for lactating women (Review). The Cochrane Library 2011, Issue 12.
14. Breastfeeding initiation. Queensland Maternity and Neonatal Clinical Guideline. October 2010.
15. Breastfeeding Multiples: British Columbia Reproductive Care Program. January 2007.
16. Brian Symon. Feeding in the first year of life. Australian Family Physician. April 2012;41(4).
17. Carol E Blenning, Heather Paladine. An Approach to the Postpartum Office Visit. Am Fam Physician 2005; 72:2491-6, 2497-8.
18. Chongsomchai C, Lumbiganon P, Laopaiboon M. Prophylactic antibiotics for manual removal of retained placenta in vaginal birth (Review). The Cochrane Library 2011, Issue 6.
19. Donor milk banks: the operation of donor milk bank services. NICE clinical guideline 93. February 2010.
20. Ewa Piejko. The postpartum visit. Why wait 6 weeks? Australian Family Physician. September 2006;35(9).
21. Formula feeds. RCN guidances for nurses caring for infants and mothers. Royal College of nursing. 2007.
22. French L, Smaill FM. Antibiotic regimens for endometritis after delivery (Review). The Cochrane Library 2012, Issue 8.
23. Guideline: vitamin A supplementation in postpartum women. World Health Organization 2011.
24. Hay-Smith J. Therapeutic ultrasound for postpartum perineal pain and dyspareunia (Review). The Cochrane Library 2009, Issue 4.
25. Infant and young child feeding: model chapter for textbooks for medical students and allied health professionals. World Health Organization 2009.
26. Jaafar SH, Jahanfar S, Angolkar M, Ho JJ. Effect of restricted pacifier use in breastfeeding term infants for increasing duration of breastfeeding (Review). The Cochrane Library 2012, Issue 7.
27. Jaafar SH, Lee KS, Ho JJ. Separate care for new mother and infant versus rooming-in for increasing the duration of breastfeeding (Review). The Cochrane Library 2012, Issue 9.
28. Katie L Mason, David M Aronoff. Postpartum Group A Streptococcus Sepsis and Maternal Immunology. Am J Reprod Immunol. February 2012;67(2):91-100.
29. KramerMS, Kakuma R. Optimal duration of exclusive breastfeeding (Review). The Cochrane Library 2012, Issue 8.
30. Lumbiganon P, Martis R, Laopaiboon M, et al. Antenatal breastfeeding education for increasing breastfeeding duration (Review). The Cochrane Library 2012, Issue 9.
31. Management of Breastfeeding for Healthy Full-Term Infants: MOH nursing clinical practice guidelines. Ministry of Health, Singapore. Dec 2002.
32. Management of Puerperal Sepsis: SLCOG National Guidelines.

33. Managing puerperal sepsis. Education material for teachers of midwifery. World Health Organization 2008.
34. Mattar CN, Fok D, Chong YS. Common concerns regarding breastfeeding in a family practice setting. Singapore Med J 2008;49(4):272.
35. Moore ER, Anderson GC, Bergman N, et al. Early skin-to-skin contact for mothers and their healthy newborn infants (Review). The Cochrane Library 2012, Issue 5.
36. NE MacDonald. Maternal infectious diseases, antimicrobial therapy or immunizations: Very few contraindications to breastfeeding. Paediatr Child Health 2006;11(8):489-91.
37. Nina R O'Connor: Infant Formula. Am Fam Physician. 2009;79(7):565-70.
38. Perinatal Services BC. Health Promotion Guideline. Breastfeeding Healthy Term Infants. May 2012.
39. Perinatal Services BC: Obstetrics Guideline 20. Postpartum Nursing Care Pathway. March 2011.
40. Ran D Goldman. Pacifier use in the first month of life. Canadian Family Physician. May 2013; Vol 59
41. Report of the expert consultation on the optimal duration of exclusive breastfeeding. World Health Organization, 2002.
42. S Balasubramanian, R Ganesh. Vitamin D deficiency in exclusively breast-fed infants. Indian J Med Res. March 2008;127:250-5.
43. Samuli Rautava, W Allan Walker. Academy of Breastfeeding Medicine Founder's lecture 2008: Breastfeeding—An Extrauterine Link Between Mother and Child. Breastfeeding Medicine 2009; Volume 4, Number 1.
44. WHO multicentre growth reference study group: Breastfeeding in theWHO Multicentre Growth Reference Study. Acta Pædiatrica, 2006;Suppl 450:16-26.
45. WHO Technical Consultation on Postpartum and Postnatal Care. World Health Organization 2010.

SECTION 2

Short Cases

SECTION OUTLINES

- **Post-term Pregnancy**
  Tania G Singh, Earl Jaspal
- **Convulsions in Pregnancy**
  Tania G Singh
- **Rh Negative Pregnancy**
  Tania G Singh, Earl Jaspal
- **Jaundice in Pregnancy**
  Tania G Singh, Earl Jaspal
- **HIV in Pregnancy**
  Tania G Singh, Earl Jaspal
- **Thyroid Disorders in Pregnancy**
  Tania G Singh, Earl Jaspal

CHAPTER 18

Post-term Pregnancy

Tania G Singh, Earl Jaspal

DEFINITION

Post-term pregnancy refers to a pregnancy that has $\geq 42^{0/7}$ weeks of gestation or ≥ 294 days from the first day of LMP or ≥ 14 days when added in EDD
Postterm, postmaturity, prolonged pregnancy, postdated pregnancy, protracted pregnancy – all refer to postmature birth.

Incidence

- 3-12% (overall)
- By LMP: 7.5%
- By USG: 2.6%
- By LMP + USG: 1.1%
- Previous 1 post-term: 27%
- Previous 2 post-term: 39%.

Factors Influencing its Prevalence

1. Routine early ultrasound assessment of gestational age significantly reduces the rate of interventions at a later stage i.e. inaccurate dating (most frequent cause)
2. Rate of spontaneous preterm births reduces its incidence
3. Prevalence of primigravid women (who are more likely to deliver post term)
4. Prevalence of women with pregnancy complications (who are less likely to deliver post term)
5. Local practice patterns of terminating pregnancy at a certain gestational age.

Risk Factors

1. Primiparity
2. Prior post-term pregnancy
3. Male gender of fetus
4. Genetic factors (mainly maternal) but few studies suggest that risk decreases to 15.4% when 2nd child has a different father, indicating the role of paternal genes in length of gestation
5. Placental sulfatase deficiency → decreased synthesis of placental estrogens → necessary for development of gap junctions and increased expression of oxytocin and prostaglandin receptors in myometrial cells
6. Obesity (appears to increase the risk of pregnancies progressing beyond 41 or 42 weeks of gestation)

7. Fetal anencephaly → lack of development of fetal hypothalamus →↓ production of CRH and ↓ stimulation of pituitary-adrenal-placental axis necessary for initiation of parturition
8. Maternal age > 30 years
9. Placental senescence.

Role of LMP and USG in Calculation of Gestational Age in Post Term pregnancy

Although LMP is used to calculate EDD, but it can make the accuracy of gestational age determination unreliable because of:
- Irregular cycles
- Hormonal contraception stopped just prior to conception
- Conception in lactational amenorrhea
- 1st trimester bleeding
- Cycles > 28 days (especially oligomenorrhea), T_2 USG will not be powerful enough to redate pregnancy. Therefore, regularity and length of cycles must be taken into account
- Inconsistent ovulation times (delayed ovulation)
- On USG, the gestational age calculated by fetal biometry must take into account the range of possibilities as below:
  Range
  CRL +/- 3-5 days
  At 12-20 weeks - 7-10 days
  At 20-30 weeks - 2 weeks
  After 30 weeks- 3 weeks
- An agreed EDD should be made as early as possible in pregnancy
- Gestational age of the earliest USG should be taken, when LMP is not known
- If the difference is greater than the above mentioned ranges, then also the earliest USG is to be considered
- If correct gestational age cannot be determined, elective induction is to be planned at 39 weeks, provided:
  – 36 weeks have elapsed since documentation of positive hCG OR
  – 20 weeks have passed from documentation of FHS by stethoscope or fetoscope OR
  – 30 weeks by Doppler OR
  – Gestation is established using CRL OR by USG performed before 20 weeks of gestation consistent with patient's LMP.

Physiological Changes Associated with Post Term Pregnancy

Following are the changes which, without any pathology will occur in post-term pregnancies
1. Placental changes
2. Changes in amniotic fluid
3. Cord problems
4. Meconium
5. Postmaturity dysmaturity syndrome.

Placental Changes

Grannum B. Hobin's grading
- It is the grading of placenta on ultrasound
- Depends on placental senescence and morphological changes

	Grading system	
Grades	Period of gestation	Features
'0'	<18 weeks	• Placenta homogenous • Smooth chorionic plate • Uniform echogenicity
'I'	18-29 weeks	• Occasional parenchymal calcification • Chorionic plate shows subtle undulations • Echogenic densities (hyper-echoic areas) appear randomly throughout placenta except at basal layer
'II'	>30 weeks	• Occasional basal calcification • Near term: indentations on chorionic plate are marked • Echogenisities (Hyper-echoic areas) in basal layer • Comma-like densities → from chorionic plate into substance of placenta
'III'	>39 weeks	• Significant basal calcification • Indentations → more marked → look like cotyledons • Increased confluency of comma-like densities that become inter-cotyledonary septations • Center portion of cotyledons become echo free (fall out areas) • An early progression to grade III is a matter of concern and is sometimes associated with placental insufficiency

Structural changes in placenta after 37 weeks
- Infarcts
- Calcification
- Thinning
- Shortening of chorionic villi
- Fibrinoid necrosis
- Slow degeneration of vessels in decidua.

a. Hemorrhagic infarcts
   - More common at borders of placenta
   - Term placenta – 10-25%
   - Post term placenta – 60-90%.

b. Calcium deposits or 'white infarcts' in
   - Post term placenta – 10 gm/100 gm of dry tissue weight
   - Term placenta – 2-3 gm/100gm of dry tissue weight.

c. Other changes:
   - Appearance of syncytial knots
   - Few langhan's cells
   - Decrease in stroma
   - Appearance of Nitabuch's layer
     – It is where trophoblasts meets the decidua
     – It limits further invasion of decidua by trophoblasts
   - Rohr's stria – inconsistent deposition of fibrin at bottom of intervillous space.

Amniotic Fluid Changes

Functions
- Amniotic fluid is "inhaled" and "exhaled" by the fetus – essential for the development of lungs
- Swallowed amniotic fluid also forms urine and contributes to the formation of meconium
- Amniotic fluid protects the developing fetus by cushioning against blows to the mother's abdomen
- Allowing for easier fetal movements
- Promotes muscular and skeletal development.

How does it change with advancing gestational age?

Appearance
- During the first two trimesters
  - Clear and yellow
- During the third trimester
  - Becomes colorless
- Approximately from 33rd-34th week onwards
  - Cloudiness and flocculation occur, at first very slowly, after the 36th -37th week steadily faster
- At term
  - Moderately cloudy and contains a moderate number of flakes of vernix
  - Increased number of lamellar bodies released from fetal lungs
  - L/S ratio $\approx \geq 4:1$
  - Color → greenish or yellowish (when meconium)
- The appearance of the amniotic fluid depending on the degree of cloudiness and on the number of flakes, has been expressed by means of a score system, the so called *"Macroscore"*.

Quantity and Constituents
- Completely surrounds the embryo after the 4th week of pregnancy
- Main constituents are:

1st trimester:
- Water and electrolytes only.

2nd trimester:
- Water and electrolytes (99%) together with
- Glucose
- Lipids from the fetal lungs
- Proteins with bactericide properties
- Flaked-off fetal epithelium cells (they make a prenatal diagnosis of the infantile karyotype possible)
- Normally has a pH of 7.0 to 7.5.

Quantity Changes
- 20 mL in the 7th week
- 400 mL at 20th week
- 600 mL in the 25th week
- 800 mL at 28th week
- 1000 mL in the 30th-34th week

- 800 mL at birth
- 400 mL in 42nd week
- 250 mL at 43 weeks
- 160 mL at 44 weeks
- From the 5th month onwards, the fetus also begins to drink amniotic fluid (400 mL/day)
- Near to the end of pregnancy the amniotic fluid is replaced every 3 hours
- If at 40 weeks, it is < 400 mL → fetal compromise
- With each increasing week → there is 33% decrease in amniotic fluid.

Cord

- Cord compression due to oligohydramnios → Wharton's jelly decreases
- Decreased oxygen saturation in umbilical vein as age advances.

Meconium

- Usually appears from 20th week
- At term: uniformly distributed throughout gut up to rectum → presence of intestinal peristalsis
- Composition:
  - Lanugo, hair, epithelial cells from fetal skin (swallowed with liquor)
  - Mucus, intestinal epithelial cells (exfoliated), intestinal juices
- Color
  - Greenish black color is due to bile pigments especially biliverdin.

Causes of Meconium-Stained Amniotic Fluid (MSAF)

Under normal circumstances
- The passage of meconium from the fetus into the amnion is prevented by the lack of intestinal peristalsis, which is caused by several factors, including:
  - Low motilin levels
  - Tonic contraction of the anal sphincter
  - A terminal cap of viscous meconium
- MSAF may be a natural phenomenon that neither indicates nor causes fetal distress but simply reflects a post-term fetus with a mature gastrointestinal tract in which motilin levels have risen
- Vagal stimulation produced by cord or head compression may also be associated with the passage of meconium in the absence of fetal distress.

In conditions of stress
- Meconium passage may occur, with resultant fetal hypoxia and acidosis producing relaxation of the anal sphincter
- Term and post-term fetuses are more likely to pass meconium in response to such a stress than a preterm fetus
- Passage of meconium into the amniotic fluid may increase the risk of intra-amniotic infection and subsequent meconium aspiration syndrome.

Meconium aspiration syndrome (MAS)

- Approximately 13% of all live births are complicated by meconium-stained amniotic fluid (MSAF)
- Fortunately, only 5% of neonates born through MSAF develop MAS
- MAS is defined as respiratory distress in an infant born through MSAF whose symptoms cannot be explained otherwise.

Severity criteria to define MAS by Cleary and Wiswell
- Mild MAS is disease that requires less than 40% oxygen for less than 48 hours
- Moderate MAS is disease that requires more than 40% oxygen for more than 48 hours with no air leak
- Severe MAS is disease that requires assisted ventilation for more than 48 hours and is often associated with persistent pulmonary hypertension.

Cause of meconium aspiration
- Unclear why some infants born through MSAF develop an aspiration syndrome whereas others do not
- Aspiration of meconium may occur
  - In utero
    OR
  - After delivery with the first few breaths
- Chronic fetal hypoxia and acidosis → lead to fetal gasping → in utero aspiration of meconium, which presents as more severe disease at birth or may even lead to an IUD
- In contrast, the vigorous infant who aspirates meconium-stained fluid from the nasopharynx at birth usually develops mild to moderate disease.

Mechanisms of meconium injury
- Mechanical obstruction of airways
- Chemical pneumonitis
- Vasoconstriction of pulmonary vessels
- Inactivation of surfactant.

Postmaturity Dysmaturity Syndrome

Needs a special mention

Synonyms
- Ballantyne's Syndrome
- Runge's syndrome
- Clifford's syndrome
- Dysmaturity syndrome
- Placental dysfunction syndrome
- Postmaturity syndrome
- Prenatal dystrophy syndrome
- Prolonged gestation syndrome.

Short History

Why named Ballantyne syndrome?
- The Scottish obstetrician Ballantyne (1902) was the first to call attention to dysmaturity
- He described the dry, parched skin, the long nails, the paucity of the amniotic fluid, the presence of meconium in amniotic fluid, and the advanced ossification in the skull
- He found the weight and length of these children to be nearly always above average.

Why named Runge syndrome?
- Runge (1939-1948) gave a detailed description of dysmature child

- He called attention to the fact that in some women who eventually are delivered of dysmature children, the amount of amniotic fluid and concomitantly the circumference of the abdomen decreases successively before delivery
- He considered this to be a sign of placental insufficiency.

Why named Clifford syndrome?
- Clifford in 1945, introduced the term "Placental dysfunction syndrome"
- He classified the appearances of infants into different stages:

Stage 1
- Skin
  - Cracked
  - Parchment-like
  - Peeling present
- Arms and legs → thin
- Infants → more awake and alert than usual
- May have respiratory distress and a tendency to vomit
- The bones of the skull are harder than is ordinarily found.

Stage 2
- All above features but in a very marked degree
- In addition,
  - Trunk → thin
  - Meconium staining of the liquor (greenish skin, nails, umbilicus).

Stage 3
- Trunk and extremities are strikingly thin
- A pronounced dystrophic appearance
- The skin peels off in large flakes
- The nails and the skin are yellowish in color.

Fetal and Neonatal Risks in Post Term Pregnancy

Fetal risks

1. Perinatal mortality (defined as stillbirths + early neonatal deaths) at 42 weeks is twice that at 40 weeks and 4 fold at 43 weeks
2. Meconium aspiration syndrome- refers to respiratory compromise with tachypnea, cyanosis and reduced pulmonary compliance in newborns → chemical pneumonitis
3. Placental insufficiency → calcium deposition on walls of blood vessels and protein deposition on surface of placenta
4. Fetal distress
5. Low umbilical artery pH levels at delivery
6. Neonatal academia
7. Low Apgar scores
8. Macrosomia and subsequent prolonged labor, CPD, shoulder dystocia, birth injury (orthopedic or neurological)

9. Dysmaturity (postmaturity) syndrome in about 20% of infants with characteristics of chronic IUGR from uteroplacental insufficiency. These pregnancies are at increased risk of:
   - Oligohydramnios
   - Umbilical cord compression
   - Nonreassuring CTG (both ante and intrapartum)
   - Meconium
   - Short term neonatal complications – hypoglycemia, seizures, respiratory insufficiency)
10. Neonatal encephalopathy
11. Intermittent Positive Pressure Ventilation (IPPV with intubation)
12. Cerebral palsy if delivered ≥ 42 weeks (recent study concluded)
13. Increased risk of death within first year of life.

Maternal Risks

1. Increase in labor dystocia (9-12%)
2. Increase in severe perineal injury (3rd and 4th degree perineal tears) related to macrosomia
3. Operative vaginal delivery
4. Increase in number of labor inductions with unfavorable cervices
5. Increase in rate of cesarean section by 2 folds → increased risks of endometritis, hemorrhage, thromboembolic disease
6. Intrauterine infections
7. Postpartum hemorrhage
8. Anxiety and frustration of carrying a pregnancy more for 1-2 weeks beyond due date.

Management of Post-term Pregnancy

Preventive Measures

- Rule out wrong dates
- USG, preferably in 1st trimester or as early as possible in pregnancy
- Routine 18-22 weeks pregnancy ultrasound to confirm dates and rule out fetal anamolies
- Sweeping of membranes → should be offered from 38-41 weeks after explaining risks and benefits.

Place of Induction of Labor (IOL)

- IOL is typically recommended when the risks to the fetus by continuing pregnancy are greater than those faced by the neonate after birth (selective IOL)
- Medical expert consensus favors IOL around 38+0 to 39+0 weeks of gestation for women with significant perinatal complications of pregnancy
- At term, low risk women should be counselled about the risks and benefits of an IOL at 41+0 to 41+3 weeks of gestation compared with expectant management
- When determining timing of delivery, consider:
  – Identifying perinatal complications of pregnancy, e.g. preeclampsia, gestational diabetes, intrauterine growth restriction
  – Results of antepartum fetal surveillance
  – Favourability of the cervix
  – Gestational age
  – Maternal preference and risks if the woman chooses expectant management.

Case: A $G_2P_1L_1$, booked patient, who was lost for follow up after 30 weeks period of gestation, visits the outpatient department at 41 weeks 2 days. She has no complaints. All routine investigations were normal till 7th month of pregnancy. Her previous delivery was also postdated according to the patient for which labor was not induced. How will you manage this case if she is not willing for induction even after explaining all the above mentioned consequences?

What are the various methods for induction of labor? What are the risks and benefits of induction?

Management Proper

During pregnancy

Step I. Establish appropriate gestational age
Step II. Ensure fetal maturity
Step III. Rule out other obstetric complications → if present → terminate pregnancy
Step IV. Discussion with patient explaining risks and benefits of induction and expectant management
Step V. Offer induction at 40 completed weeks in all healthy uncomplicated pregnancies, as the present evidence reveals a decrease in perinatal mortality without increased risk of cesarean section during this period
Step VI. If willing for induction → induce
Step VII. If patient has opted for expectant management, monitor with:

- Daily fetal kick count by the mother
- Biweekly modified BPP (NST and AFI assessment)
- BPP weekly (though Modified BPP is as sensitive as full BPP)
- Doppler → role in post-term pregnancy is not supported by evidence
- Terminate at 42 weeks

Remember: Regardless of BPP score, oligohydramnios is an independent risk factor for perinatal mortality. Therefore, should never be overlooked.

Intrapartum

- Left lateral position
- Watch for the following complications:

Meconium
- ↑ uteroplacental insufficiency (also contributed by ↓ liquor) → hypoxia in labor → activation of vagal stimulation
- Recent studies contradict the use of saline amnioinfusion and aggressive naso/oropharyngeal suctioning at perineum to decrease the risk of meconium aspiration
- Early ARM in active phase may help.

Macrosomia
- Maternal and fetal birth trauma → one should be prepared to manage shoulder dystocia
- Arrest of 1st and 2nd stage of labor.

Nonreassuring CTG
- Continuous CTG monitoring
- Should not lead to acidosis
- In cases of equivocal tracings → fetal scalp stimulation and/or fetal scalp blood sampling may provide reassurance
- Neonatologist → at the time of delivery.

INDUCTION OF LABOR (IOL)

Definition

- Artificial initiation of uterine contractions prior to their spontaneous onset, any time after fetal viability, with or without ruptured membranes by a method that aims at vaginal delivery
- Indicated only when it is agreed that the mother or fetus will benefit from a higher probability of healthy outcome than if birth is delayed.

Indications

Obstetric Indications

- Routinely at 41 weeks (40 weeks + 7 days) in an otherwise uncomplicated pregnancy
- Post term or prolonged pregnancy/postmaturity
- Preeclampsia/eclampsia
- IUD in present pregnancy
- Previous unexplained IUD
- Significant IUGR
- Non reassuring fetal surveillance
- Prelabor rupture of membranes at term
- Rh-isoimmunization (moderately or severely affected cases), where pregnancy has already reached 34th week
- Malformed fetus
- Severe hydramnios producing increased pressure symptoms.

Medical Conditions

- Chronic nephritis
- Hypertension- gestational or chronic
- Type I DM
- Significant pulmonary disease.

Contraindications

Absolute

1. Previous classical/Inverted T incision
2. Previous hysterotomy/Myomectomy (entering endometrial cavity)
3. Previous uterine rupture
4. Presence of placenta praevia (major degree/vasa praevia)
5. Transverse lie
6. Cord presentation and prolapse
7. Pelvic structural deformity/CPD
8. Active genital herpes/HIV
9. Where a tumour occupies pelvis/invasive carcinoma cervix.

Relative

1. Severe IUGR
2. Malpresentation

3. Breech presentation
4. Maternal heart disease
5. Multiple pregnancy
6. Abnormal NST
7. Suspected fetal macrosomia.

Extreme Caution

1. Case of previous LSCS
2. Grand multipara (because of risk of precipitate labor).

Risks

1. Increased risk of operative vaginal delivery
2. Cesarean section
3. Excessive uterine activity
4. Abnormal FHR pattern
5. Uterine rupture
6. Prolonged labor due to abnormal uterine action
7. Possibly cord prolapse with AROM
8. Failed induction (prolongation of latent phase beyond 12-18 hours)
9. Prematurity
10. Maternal water intoxication
11. Partial placental detachment and bloody tap
12. Fetal pneumonia (in case of PROM >18 hour without antibiotics).

Factors for Successful Induction

1. Term or post term
2. Bishop score ≥ 6 (state of cervix)
3. Positive oxytocin sensitivity test
4. Parous woman
5. PROM.

Prerequisites for Induction

1. Determine the appropriate indication/any contraindication
2. Confirm gestational age
3. Determine Bishop score
4. Assess for CPD
5. Membrane status (intact or ruptured)
6. Assess fetal health-NST for minimum 20 minutes (facilities should be available)
7. Informed consent
8. During induction-obstetrician must be present.

Cervical Assessment

Modified Bishop Score or Prelabor Scoring or Preinduction Score

- Bishop score is a pre-labor scoring system to assist in predicting whether induction of labor will be required or not

- Components included to calculate the score are (Original Bishop's score)
  - Cervical dilatation
  - Cervical effacement
  - Cervical consistency
  - Cervical position
  - Fetal station.
- According to the Modified Bishop's pre-induction cervical scoring system, effacement has been replaced by cervical length in cm.

Score	0	1	2	3
Dilatation	Closed	1-2	3-4	5
Length	> 4	3-4	1-2	0
Consistency	Firm	Medium	Soft	-
Position	Posterior	Midline	Anterior	-
Station	-3	-2	-1/0	+1, +2

Interpretation

- Total score = 13
- Favorable score = 6-13
- Unfavorable score = 0-5
- A score of ≤ 5 suggests that labor is unlikely to start without induction
- A score of ≥ 9 indicates that labor will most likely commence spontaneously.

Another modification for the Bishop's score is the 'Modifiers'. Points are added or subtracted according to special circumstances as follows:

One point is added for:
- Existence of preeclampsia
- Every previous vaginal delivery.

One point is subtracted for:
- Postdate pregnancy
- Nulliparity (no previous vaginal deliveries)
- PPROM (preterm premature rupture of membranes).

State of cervix is the most important predictor of success of induction.

METHODS OF INDUCTION

Surgical Methods

Sweeping/Stripping of Membranes

- Stripping the membranes off from cervix and lower uterine segment
- Releases phospoholipase A_2 and ↑ production of $PGF_{2\alpha}$
- Finger inserted in internal os is moved circumferentially, when cervix is sufficiently dilated or try to open the cervix or cervical massage, when closed
- Plasma prostaglandin concentrations after sweeping are 10% of those achieved in labor, thus possibly improving labor outcomes

- Maternal morbidity is related mainly to significant discomfort or pain during procedure, bleeding, and contractions not leading to labor within 24 hours
- Generally most efficacious in nulliparous women with unfavorable Bishop scores
- Multiple episodes may be more effective.

Concerns:
- Patient discomfort
- Bleeding
- Accidental rupture of membranes
- Initiation of irregular uterine contractions.

Recommendations
- Routine use of sweeping of membranes at term is not recommended and alone it should not be used as a method of induction
- Along with oxytocin should be used for induction of labor, only when prostaglandins are unavailable or are contraindicated
- Sweeping can be performed prior to inducing labor while assessing cervix.

Amniotomy

- Artificial rupture of membranes
- Alone is not recommended as a method of induction of labor
- Works well, when amniotomy is followed by oxytocin in patients with favorable cervix.

Pharmacological Methods

- Prostaglandins
- Oxytocin
- Mifepristone
- Relaxin.

Prostaglandins

- Derivatives of prostanoic acid
- Prostaglandins are 20 carbon compounds, acts as local hormones
- Half life in peripheral circulation is 1-2 min
- Inactivated in lungs and liver
- Types PGE_2, $PGF_{2\alpha}$, PGE_1, PGI_2
- Prostaglandins used in induction are PGE_2 (Dinoprostone) and PGE_1 (Misoprostol).

Common side effects
- Nausea
- Vomiting
- Diarrhea
- Pyrexia
- Bronchospasm
- Shivering.

Contraindications
- Hypersensitivity to drug
- Glaucoma
- Asthma.

How they act?
Different mechanisms of cervical ripening are involved:
- They alter the extracellular ground substance of cervix
- PGE_2 increases activity of collagenase in cervix
- They cause an increase in elastase, glycosaminoglycan, dermatan sulphate and hyaluronic acid levels in cervix
- Relaxation of smooth muscle of cervix facilitates dilatation.

Dinoprostone (PGE_2)
- Gel
- Tablet
- Inserts

Gel
1. Intracervical
2. Intravaginal

Intracervical Gel
Patient selection (prerequisites)
- Recommended dosage is 0.5 mg
    - Bring gel to room temperature before application, per manufacturer's instructions
    - Monitor FHR and uterine activity continuously, starting 15-30 min before gel introduction and continuing for 30-120 min after gel insertion
- Each prefilled syringe contains 0.5mg of PGE_2 gel
- Gel is inserted under direct vision using a vaginal speculum → introduce the gel into endocervix just below the level of internal os
- Patient to remain recumbent for 30 min before being allowed to ambulate
- Maximum recommended dosage → 1.5 mg of dinoprostone (3 doses) in 24 hours
- May be repeated every 6-8 hours, depending upon the response
- Do not start oxytocin for 6 (intracervical) -12 (intravaginal) hours after placement of last dose, to allow for spontaneous onset of labor and to protect the uterus from hyperstimulation
- Finally prostaglandins allow for an increase in intracellular Ca^{2+} levels, causing contraction of myometrial muscle
- Data suggests that contractions usually start 1 hour after prostaglandin application and peak in first 4 hours.

Drawback
- Expensive drug.

Intravaginal Gel
- Available in prefilled syringes (containing 1 mg and 2 mg)
- The initial dose for dinoprostone (PGE_2) gel is:
    - 2 mg (per vaginally) → nulliparous woman with unfavorable cervix (Bishop score < 4)
    - 1 mg (per vaginally) → multiparous woman
    - 1 mg (per vaginally) → suspected fetal compromise (IUGR)
- Second dose → 1-2 mg PGE_2 may be administered 6 hours later
- Maximum dose in a 12 hour period
    - 4 mg for nulliparous woman with unfavorable cervix
    - 3 mg for all other women.

Intravaginal Tablets
- Recommended dosage: 3 mg into posterior fornix
- Available as 3.0 mg tablet form
- Dose can be repeated 6-8 hours after the first dose
- Maximum total dose → 6 mg for all women.

Dinoprostone vaginal Inserts/Controlled release Prostaglandin
- Consists of a polymer base containing 10 mg of dinoprostone with a polyester retrieval string
- Insert releases 0.3 mg/hr of PGE_2 over a 12 hour period
- Is placed in posterior fornix of vagina
- Removed with:
  - Onset of labor
  - Spontaneous rupture of membranes
  - Excessive uterine activity OR
  - After 12 hours
- Warming before insertion is not required
- Theoretical advantages:
  - Ability of insertion without use of a speculum
  - Slow continuous release of prostaglandin
  - Only one dose being required
  - Ability to use oxytocin 30 minutes after its removal
  - Ability to remove insert, if required.

Manufacturer Indications:
- It should not be used with ruptured membrane
- Manufacturer reports that women treated with it provided no evidence to suggest that the retrieval string was a source of infection to enter reproductive tract
- Patient should remain recumbent for 2 hours.

Technique for Placement
- Patient selection
- Using a small amount of water-miscible lubricant, place the insert into posterior fornix of vagina
- As the device absorbs moisture and swells, it releases dinoprostone at the rate of 0.3 mg/hr for 12 hours
- FHR and uterine activity monitoring continuously for the duration of insert placement and for 15 minutes after its removal should be done.

Misoprostol (PGE_1)
- Was developed as a treatment for NSAIDs induced ulcers but is widely used today in obstetrics
- Misoprostol was first used for induction of labor with a dead fetus in 1987.

Doses and Routes
Vaginal Misoprostol
- 25 µg per vaginally every 4-6 hourly (maximum of 6 doses).

Oral Misoprostol Solution
- A single misoprostol tablet is dissolved in drinking water so that 1 mL contains 1 µg (e.g. 100 µg tablet in 100 mL water), rather than breaking the tablet into 4 or 8 pieces

- 25 mL of misoprostol solution is then given after every 2 hours
- If no response after 2 hours in nulliparous females → double the dose
- Solution is stable for up to 24 hours at room temperature but should then be discarded.

Oral Misoprostol Tablets
- 50 µg every 4 hourly (maximum of 6 doses) OR 25 µg 2 hourly.

Note:
- These regimens can be used irrespective of:
  - State of membrane (ruptured or intact)
  - Parity
  - State of cervix
  - Period of gestation
- Care is needed in women with favorable cervix and ruptured membranes as they often progress rapidly in labor once induced
- In case of an intrauterine dead or an anomalous fetus, vaginal or oral misoprostol is recommended for induction of labor. Why?
  - For 2 main reasons:
    - Increased uterine contractility leading to fetal distress is no longer a major concern
    - Often induction of labor in women with an anamolous or dead fetus is performed before term, when the uterus may be less responsive to uterotonics than it is at term
  - The following doses are recommended:

Misoprostol regimen (in case of an IUD)		
Period of gestation	Dose	Repetitions
13-17 weeks	Vaginal misoprostol 200 µg every 6-12 hour	Total of 4 doses
18-26 weeks	Vaginal misoprostol 100 µg every 6-12 hours	Total of 4 doses
>26 weeks	Cervix unripe: • 25-50 µg every 4 hourly Cervix ripe (Bishop score ≥ 6): • Oxytocin	Not > 6 doses (of misoprostol)

Monitoring
- Before starting induction, NST for 30 minutes
- Once started, woman must be monitored closely
  - FHR
  - Uterine activity
  - Mother's vitals

  Are continuously monitored for 30 minutes after each dose of misoprostol and every 30 minutes from the onset of uterine contraction
- At the time of each planned misoprostol dose, woman should be clinically reassessed
- If there are 0-1 contractions for every 10 minutes → further dose can be given
- If there are ≥ 3 clinically adequate contractions in every 10 minutes → dose can be withheld till further needed
- An IV oxytocin infusion → not to be commenced
  - < 4 hours after last dose of vaginal misoprostol and
  - 2 hour after last dose of oral misoprostol
- If cervix remains unfavorable after course of misoprostol is completed → alternatives should be sought.

Benefits of misoprostol
- Inexpensive
- Stored at room temperature
- No refrigeration required, therefore easily transported
- Shorter induction to delivery interval
- Lower cesarean section rates.

Pharmacodynamics
Oral route
- Rapidly absorbed
- Peak concentration at 12 minutes
- Half life 30-40 minutes.

Rectal and vaginal route
- Much slower absorption
- Bioavailability of 4-6 hours.

Side effects of misoprostol
- Rapid onset
- Prolonged action
- Shivering, pyrexia, diarrhea
- Total bioavailability >> oral route, therefore, not to be used routinely for induction of labor
- Not recommended for women with previous cesarean section.

Risks and Side Effects of Prostaglandins

Highly effective stimulator of uterine contractions

Uterine hyperstimulation
- Defined as either occurrence of uterine contractions each lasting > 60 seconds, or occurrence of > 4 contractions in 10 minutes, regardless of the state of the fetus
- Occurs only with higher doses of prostaglandins
- With the following doses, rate of hyperstimulation is similar to that with dinoprostone
  - 25 µg vaginal misoprostol every 4–6 hourly OR
  - 50 µg oral misoprostol 4 hourly OR
  - 20-40 µg oral misoprostol solution 4 hourly
- Tocolytics should always be available
  - Betamimetics (terbutaline subcutaneous) are recommended for women with uterine hyperstimulation during induction of labor but are contraindicated in cardiac disease
- If uterine tachysystole, a category III FHR tracing (defined as either a sinusoidal pattern or an absent baseline FHR variability) or any of the following:
  - Recurrent late decelerations OR
  - Recurrent variable decelerations OR
  - Bradycardia

occurs with misoprostol use and there is no response to routine corrective measures (maternal repositioning and supplemental oxygen administration), cesarean delivery should be considered.

Uterine rupture
- Risk
  - 5.6% with misoprostol
  - 0.2% with dinoprostone.

Uterine tachysystole after PGE$_2$
- Intracervical PGE$_2$ gel (0.5 mg) has a 1% rate of uterine tachysystole with associated FHR changes
- Intravaginal PGE$_2$ gel (2-5 mg) or vaginal insert has a 5% rate of tachysystole.

Pain relief after induction of labor
- Simple analgesics by oral route
- Epidural analgesia can be offered.

Oxytocin

- IV oxytocin is used for induction of labor since 1950
- Half life 5-12 min
- In 1st trimester, uterus is almost refractory to oxytocin
- As pregnancy advances, number of oxytocin receptors in uterus increases (by 100 fold at 32 weeks and by 300- fold at onset of labor)
- Oxytocin activates the phospholipase C- inositol pathway and increases intracellular calcium levels, stimulating contractions in myometrial smooth muscle
- Physiology of oxytocin stimulated labor is similar to that of spontaneous labor but sensitivity and response can be different in different patients
- Onset of action starts 3-5 minutes after starting the infusion
- Steady level of oxytocin in plasma is achieved by 40 minutes
- Better response is seen with the following:
  - Lower BMI
  - Greater cervical dilatation (ripe cervix)
  - Increased parity
  - Advanced gestational age
  - After rupture of membranes, especially when cervical dilatation is > 3 cm
- Destroyed rapidly in GIT, therefore, administered parenterally in obstetrics.

Side effects
- Are principally dose related
- Uterine tachysystole or category II or III FHR tracings are the most common side effects
- Uterine tachysystole may result in abruptio placenta or uterine rupture (though uterine rupture is rare even in parous women)
- Water intoxication can occur at higher concentrations of oxytocin infused with large quantities of hypotonic solutions, but is rare in doses used for labor induction
- Hypotension may occur following a rapid IV injection of oxytocin, so is always diluted when used for induction.

Dose
- Commence oxytocin @ 1-2 mU/min (i.e. 6-12 mL/hr of 10 units oxytocin diluted in 1000 mL of an isotonic solution to make an oxytocin concentration of 10 mIU/mL)
- Use minimum dose possible and aim for a maximum of 3-4 contractions in 10 minutes
- Maximum dose → 20 mIU/min

Dose of oxytocin			
Regimen	Starting dose (mIU/min)	Incremental increase (mIU/min)	Dosage interval (min)
Low dose	0.5-2	1-2	15-40
High dose	6	3-6	15-40

Low dose
- Decreased uterine tachysystole
- Reduced FHR changes.

High dose
- Shorter labor duration
- Less chances of chorioamnionitis
- Decreased number of cesarean sections for dystocia
- Increased chances of uterine tachysystole.

Failed induction
- Prolongation of latent phase of labor beyond 12-18 hours despite adequate and appropriate stimulation in absence of cephalo pelvic disproportion.

SUGGESTED READING

1. Arwa Abbas Hussain, Mohammad Yawar Yakoob, Aamer Imdad: Elective induction for pregnancies at or beyond 41 weeks of gestation and its impact on stillbirths: a systematic review with meta-analysis, BMC Public Health 2011;11(Suppl 3):S5.
2. Ellen L Mozurkewich, Julie L Chilimigras, Deborah R Berman: Methods of induction of labour: a systematic Review, BMC Pregnancy and Childbirth 2011;11:84.
3. Gülmezoglu AM, Crowther CA, Middleton P et al: Induction of labour for improving birth outcomes for women at or beyond term (Review), The Cochrane Library 2012, Issue 6.
4. Induction of labor: ACOG Aug 2009.
5. Induction of labor: Clinical management guidelines for obstetrician- gynecologist, ACOG practice bulletin No 107, Aug 2009.
6. Induction of labour: Queensland Maternity and Neonatal Clinical Guideline Supplement, 2010.
7. Jennifer Moore, Lisa Kane Low: Factors That Influence the Practice of Elective Induction of Labor: What Does the Evidence Tell Us? J Perinat Neonatal Nurs. 2012;26(3):242-50.
8. Martina Delaney, Anne Roggensack: Guidelines for the Management of Pregnancy at 41+0 to 42+0 Weeks, J Obstet Gynaecol Can 2008;30(9):800-10.
9. Postterm pregnancy: British columbia reproductive care programme, March 2005.
10. Prolonged pregnancy management Guideline: Clinical Protocols and Guidelines, Maternity, August 2009.
11. Prolonged pregnancy: SA Perinatal Practice Guideline, January 2012.
12. Runa Heimstad: Post-term pregnancy, Norwegian University of Science and Technology, 2007:242.
13. Steven L. Gelfand, Jonathan M. Fanaroff, JD, Michele C. Walsh: Meconium stained fluid: approach to the mother and the baby, Pediatr Clin N Am 51(2004) 655-67.
14. WHO recommendations for induction of labour, 2011.

CHAPTER 19

Convulsions in Pregnancy

Tania G Singh

Case: A booked primigravida, 33 years of age, with 31 weeks period of gestation, is brought to the emergency department in a semiconscious state. According to her husband, she had thrown a fit at home 2 hours back and another fit on the way to the hospital. Each fit lasted for 2-3 minutes. He denied of any such incidents before, nor the patient was taking medications for any medical illness. Both 1st and 2nd trimesters were uneventful. On examination: PR 88/min; BP 126/84 mmHg. Pedal edema present. Per abdomen: uterus 32 weeks period of gestation, relaxed, FHS 132/min regular. What do you think of this patient? How will you make out, whether she really had a fit?

Step I: Assess nature
(Patient's relatives may call it a fit, but it can be)
- Syncope
- Hysteria
- Hyperventilation syndrome

Step II: True convulsions → Typical features

Pseudoconvulsions → Reassurance and support

1. Abrupt onset and offset
2. Brief duration (a few minutes or less)
3. Not provoked by emotional distress or other outside factors
4. Motor activity (if present) is not purposeful
5. Little or no recall for details of attack
6. Postictal confusion and lethargy

Step III: Assess past history of convulsions or is it a first attack
1. Prior history of staring spells, transient loss of contact, childhood seizures
2. Prior history of unexplained nocturnal incontinence, tongue biting or other injury

Step IV:

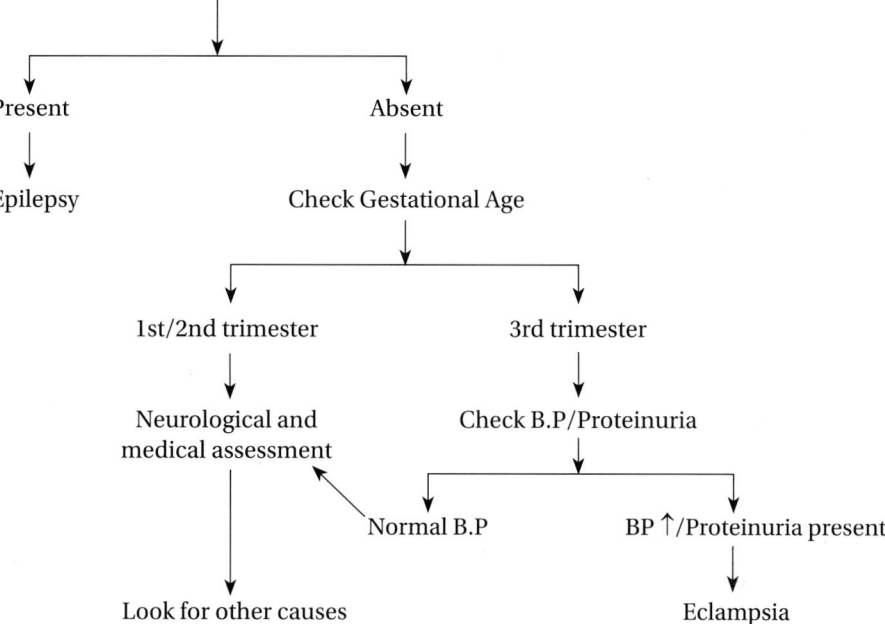

Other Causes

1. Epilepsy
2. Meningitis/encephalitis
3. Tetanus
4. Septicemia
5. Complicated malaria (falciparum)
6. Strychnine poisoning
7. Hysteria
8. Electrolyte imbalance
9. Cerebrovascular accident
10. Mass lesion
11. Cerebral sinus thrombosis
12. Head injury
13. Hypertensive encephalopathy
14. Intracranial tumour.

EPILEPSY

In India there are about 2.73 million women with epilepsy (WWE) and 52% of them are in the reproductive age group.

Characteristics

- B.P – normal
- No proteinuria
- Past history of convulsions

Effects of Epilepsy on Pregnancy and Fetus

1. ↑ risk of IUGR/small for gestational age/oligohydramnios/still births/spontaneous abortions/ anemia/ preterm birth/induced labor/cesarean section/PPH
2. Increased risk of fetal malformations
3. Small head circumference at birth
4. Low Apgar scores
5. All anticonvulsants has adverse effects on fetus:
   - Cleft lip and/or palate
   - Mental retardation
   - Cardiac abnormalities
   - Limb defects
   - Hypoplasia of terminal phalanges
   - NTDs → with sodium valproate
   - Neonatal hemorrhage → anticonvulsants induce vitamin K dependent coagulopathy
   - Offspring developing epilepsy →↑ by 4-fold.

Effects of Pregnancy on Epilepsy

1. The condition may worsen, improve, or be unaffected by pregnancy
2. Frequency of convulsions → unchanged in 50% and ↑ in some
3. Estrogens probably activate seizure foci
4. Increased plasma clearance of anticonvulsant drugs during pregnancy
5. On mother → 3rd trimester bleeding and megaloblastic anemia may be related to anticonvulsant induced folate deficiency.

Antiepileptic Drugs (AED)

There are 3 generations:

First Generation

- Bromide, phenobarbital, phenytoin, carbamazepine, valproate.

Second Generation

- Vigabatrin, lamotrigine, gabapentin, topiramate
- Newer drugs launched from 2000-2007: levetiracetam, pregabaline, zonisamide, stiripentol, rufinamide
- *Note:* The second-generation AEDs did not generally prove to be more effective than the first-generation AEDs but many of them are better tolerated, less prone to drug interactions and have more predictable pharmacokinetics.

Third Generation

- Launched recently
- Eslicarbazepine (2010); Lacosamide (2010); Retigabine (ezogabine) (2011).

Factors which may Alter AED Pharmacokinetics during Pregnancy

- Serum concentrations of AEDs and/or their metabolites that are predominantly eliminated via the kidneys may be reduced as there is 50-80% increase in renal blood flow and GFR in pregnancy
- Increased estrogen levels, lead to accelerated drug glucuronidation
- Reduced serum albumin concentrations → may affect AED protein binding and therefore total plasma clearance
- Increased plasma volume and/or increased total body water may increase the volume of distribution, and thus lead to reduced AED serum concentrations.

Breastfeeding

- All second-generation AEDs pass into breast milk, although to variable degrees
- Serum concentration in infants depends not only on the amount of AED in the breast milk, but also on the metabolic capacity of the child
- Adverse effects are rarely reported and consist mainly of sedation, poor suckling and similar, unspecific symptoms
- Replacement of one or more breast-milk meals with formula milk meals may reduce the AED exposure of the infant.

AEDs of Concern in Pregnancy

Valproic Acid

- When taken during embryogenesis, the risk of malformations increases by > 2.5 times
- Risk is dose dependent (increasing statistically at 600 mg/d) and highest when daily dose is >1000 mg
- Malformations associated with valproic acid:
  - Spina bifida (0.6%)
  - Atrial septal defect (0.5%)
  - Cleft palate (0.3%)
  - Hypospadias (0.7%)
  - Polydactyly (0.2%)
  - Craniosynostosis (0.1%)
- Studies have shown that impaired cognitive function at 3 years of age is more when valproic acid is used as an antiepileptic in utero as compared to other AEDs.

Carbamazepine (CBZ)

- 2- to 10-fold increased risk of NTDs in women with epilepsy taking CBZ; however, the risks associated with CBZ are not as great as those associated with valproic acid
- Unlike valproic acid, CBZ does not appear to have adverse effects on neurobehavioral development.

Lamotrigine (LTG)

- Most commonly used 2nd generation AED
- Initially developed as an antifolate agent but in 1994, lamotrigine was approved by FDA for use as an antiepileptic drug

- The International Union of Pure and Applied Chemistry (IUPAC) name of lamotrigine is 6-(2,3-dichlorophenyl)-1,2,4-triazine-3,5-diamine
- Empirical formula is C9H7C12N5
- Molecular mass is 256.091 g/mol
- Plasma half-life → 15-30 hours
- Mechanism of action: Mainly by decreasing glutamate release
    - LTG → acts on Na^+ channels → inhibits release of glutamate
    - LTG → interferes with neuronal sodium channels → inhibit the release of excitatory amino acids, glutamate and aspartate
- Absorption in GIT, therefore oral administration
- Metabolized by → enzyme uridine- diphosphate glucuronyl transferase 1 A4 → mainly to LTG-N2-glucuronide
- Clearance in pregnancy doubles → serum concentration reduces by 40-60% owing to increased renal blood flow in early pregnancy and estradiol induced glucuronidation in later months → returns to prepregnancy levels by 10-14 days. Therefore, close monitoring required both antepartum and postpartum making it little difficult to prescribe the drug in pregnancy
- Safe dosage in pregnancy → <300 mg/day
- In infants exposed to LTG in utero, LTG concentrations are highest at birth and gradually decrease over time—this is irrespective of whether or not the infant is breastfed
- LTG passes over into breast milk and may accumulate in infants probably due to low glucuronidation capacity reaching the adult level by 2-6 months of age. Though regarded safe, lamotrigine should be used with caution
- Regular monitoring at conception, in each trimester, at the time of delivery and shortly after delivery should be done to avoid seizure precipitation during pregnancy or symptoms of toxicity after birth
- This corresponds with an increase in seizure frequency during the 7th month of gestation. A prophylactic increase in LTG dosage throughout pregnancy has been recommended, although it is difficult to predict how much each patient's dose will need to be increased
- LTG is a dihydrofolate reductase inhibitor and it decreases fetal folate levels. Therefore, folic acid supplementation should be considered for all women of child-bearing potential taking LTG
- *Common side effects*
    - Dizziness
    - Visual disturbances
    - Diplopia
    - Sedation
    - Ataxia
    - Headache
    - Tremor
    - Skin rash
    - Dyspepsia
    - Nausea
    - Stevens-Johnson syndrome and DIC are rare systemic side-effects.

Levetiracetam (LEV)

- Protein binding is very low, therefore, changes in serum albumin hardly affects its serum concentration
- 1/4th of the drug is metabolized in blood by hydrolysis
- 2/3rd – found unchanged in urine

- Clearance increases during pregnancy → serum concentration decreases to 40% due to increased blood flow through kidneys
- Serum levels return to normal within the 1st week after pregnancy
- Excreted in breast milk in good amounts but no adverse effects on the infant has been noticed.

Oxcarbazepine (OXC)

- Almost completely metabolized to its active form monohydroxycarbazepine, which is then eliminated as a glucuronide
- Protein binding of monohydroxycarbazepine is ≈ 40%
- Serum concentrations is reduced to 36% in pregnancy due to increased rate of glucuronidation, induced primarily by raised estradiol levels and to some extent by renal excretion
- Postpartum serum concentrations return to prepregnancy levels within a few weeks
- Passes in breast milk but no adverse effects in the nursing infants are observed.

Topiramate (TPM)

- Only 20-30% is metabolized
- Rest found unchanged in urine. Thus, increased renal blood flow in pregnancy might lead to increased renal clearance of TPM and a decline in its serum concentrations
- Serum concentration is reduced by 30-40% during pregnancy
- Studies indicate an increased risk of major congenital malformations, mainly oral cleft and hypospadias and is also associated with decreased birthweight
- No adverse effects are found in breastfed infants, as very low drug concentrations are found in them.

Gabapentin (GBP) and Pregabalin (PGB)

- GBP and pregabalin are not metabolized, hence, eliminated unchanged by the kidneys
- Their serum concentrations may fall considerably due to increased blood flow in pregnancy
- Very few studies have been done but no increased risk of fetal malformations was found
- Gabapentin crosses the placenta → in the newborn the half-life is 14 hrs, compared with 5-7 hrs in adults, in accordance with immature kidney function in the first weeks of life
- Breastfeeding is safe as no adverse effects are noted.

Zonisamide (ZNS)

- Only 40-50% is protein-bound
- 15-30% appears unchanged in urine
- Serum concentrations affected by increased renal blood flow
- Daily dose ≈ 300mg
- Monotherapy does not lead to malformations
- Crosses breast milk but no adverse effects on fetus noted so far.

Eslicarbazepine (ESL)

- Eslicarbazepine is rapidly converted to the S-enantiomer of monohydroxycarbazepine
- It has recently been launched as a drug of its own and is by some authors considered a third-generation AED in spite of the fact that the racemate of monohydroxycarbazepine is the active metabolite of oxcarbazepine. Only a very small fraction of ESL is biotransformed to oxcarbazepine

- Furthermore, lower serum concentrations of the S-enantiomer seem to be needed, compared with the monohydroxycarbazepine racemate, which may represent an advantage during pregnancy
- Serum concentrations decline in pregnancy
- No reports on ESL and breast feeding have been published so far.

Other AEDs

The use of the other second-generation drugs such as tiagabine, vigabatrin, felbamate, stiripentol and rufinamide, as well as the third-generation drugs retigabine and lacosamide, is at present mainly restricted to add-on treatment in cases of difficult-to control epilepsy or in specific syndromes:
- Vigabatrin: West syndrome;
- Stiripentol: Dravet syndrome;
- Rufinamide: Lennox–Gastaut syndrome

Very scarce data is available of their use in pregnancy.

Lacosamide and Retigabine

- Great part of lacosamide is excreted unchanged in the urine whereas retigabine is cleared from the body via multiple pathways: N-acetylation, renal clearance and glucuronidation (mainly by UGT1A4)
- An increased clearance during pregnancy can be expected for both drugs.

Dosages

1. Phenobarbitone 60-180 mg daily (in 2-3 divided doses)
2. Phenytoin 150-300 mg daily in 2 divided doses
3. Carbamazepine 0.8-1.2 gm daily in divided doses.

During Fits

1. Inj. Diazepam IV 10-20 mg
2. Vitamin K 10 mg daily orally → in last 2 weeks
3. Normal labor and delivery can be anticipated.

Incidence of Malformations

- Highest with valproic acid (10.7%)
- Phenobarbital (7.4%)
- Less with carbamazepine (4.6-5.6%) and least with lamotrigine (2.9%)
- Lamotrigine < carbamazepine < phenobarbital < phenytoin < valproic acid.

Preconceptional Counseling

1. Explain the effects of epilepsy on pregnancy and fetus and vice versa
2. Detailed information to the woman on risks and benefits of AEDs
3. Take AED serum concentrations as reference value. In case of withdrawal of combined hormonal contraceptives in a patient on LTG, consider reduction of the LTG dose in order to avoid an unintended increase in serum levels
4. Instruct the woman to report to the obstetrician as soon as pregnancy is diagnosed
5. Consultation with neurologist

6. Polytherapy → changed to monotherapy (at lowest effective dose)
7. Monotherapy at the lowest effective dose as a starting point may result in vulnerability to potential pregnancy related seizure deterioration. Close monitoring of the pregnant patient, both clinically and by measurement of AED serum concentrations, is generally advisable
8. Folic acid 1 mg daily (for at least 1 month preconceptionally and throughout pregnancy)
9. Importance of prenatal diagnosis → discussed
10. Any change in treatment is done as soon as possible to allow time to assess effects of these changes so that proper adjustments can be made timely.

Management

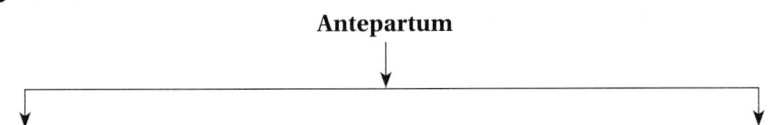

Pregnancy Unplanned
Fetus has already been exposed to current drug, during at least part of most sensitive stage of gestation, prior to mother seeking medical attention

Pregnancy Planned
Change drugs at least 6 months before pregnancy to see for any change

1. Monitor AED serum concentrations as soon as pregnancy is established and then monthly
2. Consider dose increments by 25% when serum concentrations fall below the patient's prepregnancy reference value or according to clinical needs
3. Change in medicine may increase maternal seizures
4. Any change, if done should be under the supervision of neurologist
5. Folic acid 1 mg daily (Recent studies have suggested that folic acid may reduce the number of spontaneous abortions in women using AEDs as well as protect against cognitive impairment in children exposed to AEDs in utero)
6. Risk of seizures is higher in 1st trimester and around delivery time
7. Serum AFP done, ideally at the end of 1st trimester (usually drop towards 4th month of pregnancy)
8. NT scan at 11-13 weeks. At this time acrania, precursor of anencephaly should be recognized on USG
9. Anamoly scan at 18-22 weeks
10. Current guidelines → AED levels to be measured:
    - Before conception (baseline)
    - At beginning of each trimester
    - During last 4 weeks of pregnancy
    - Additional monitoring if any change in seizure frequency

Non protein bound ("free") drug levels should be obtained (remain ≈ constant);
Total levels ↓ during pregnancy because of ↑ blood flow, ↑ hepatic and renal clearance of drug.

Intrapartum

1. IV line
2. Continue taking antiepileptics
3. Maternal exhaustion avoided
4. "Water birth" (laboring in water) → NOT recommended
5. GTCS → associated with hypoxia therefore continuous CTG monitoring in an event of seizure
6. Inj. Lorazepam/Diazepam → recommended to terminate a seizure
7. Be careful, loss of baseline variability of FHR tracing expected for 1 hour after this.

Postpartum

1. Monitor maternal serum concentrations. If high, perform measurements in infant and aim at concentrations below therapeutic levels in infant. Consider restricted breastfeeding, if necessary
2. Maternal plasma levels of AEDs may fluctuate until 8th postpartum week → therefore monitoring is required
3. Gradually reduce the dose, if it has been increased during pregnancy, to avoid overdosing
4. Breastfeeding – NOT contraindicated but feeds may be given before female takes her AED doses with particular attention while using high LTG doses
5. Seizures can occur because of sleep deprivation, therefore adequate sleep is necessary
   (Express breast milk so that partner can give night feeds to the infant)
6. Feeding the baby on floor is recommended (to avoid fall from seizures occurring during feeding)
7. Bathing the baby when alone → should be avoided
8. Proper medicines at regular time
9. Neurologist consultation → MUST.

Contraception

1. Mirena (LNG releasing IUCD) – highly effective and reversible
   Failure rate 1% (1st line contraceptive for patients on enzyme inducing drugs or on lamotrigine)
2. COCP: when COCP is necessary, increase both estrogen and progesterone (> 50 mcg of estrogen) e.g. microgynon 30, 2 tabs daily
3. Barrier methods
4. DMPA 3 monthly.

Enzyme inducing drugs (EI): by inducing hepatic enzymes in cytochrome P-450 system, it increases clearance of contraceptive steroids and increases level of SHBG → ↓ freely circulating progestins
1. Phenobarbital
2. Primidone
3. Phenytoin
4. Carbamazepine
5. Topiramate.

Nonenzyme inducing: Activity of oral contraceptives is not affected
1. VPA (valproic acid)
2. Benzodiazepines
3. Gabapentin
4. Vigabatrin.

1. **What is the current evidence regarding the association between hemorrhagic disease of the newborn and maternal use of hepatic enzyme-inducing antiepileptic drugs (e.g. carbamazepine, phenobarbitone, topiramate)?**
   - The American Academy of Neurology updated its recommendations in April 2009 and concluded that there is inadequate evidence to support the routine use of vitamin K of 10 mg/day orally from 36th week onwards until delivery in women with epilepsy taking AEDs to prevent early first 24 hours hemorrhagic disease of newborn
   - Instead Inj. vitamin K IM should be given to neonates at birth exposed to enzyme inducing AEDs (e.g. carbamazepine, phenobarbitone, topiramate) in utero
   - Use of EI drugs may induce fetal hepatic enzyme activity culminating in vitamin K deficiency and increase risk of neonatal bleeding.

STATUS EPILEPTICUS

Continuous seizure activity that persists for ≥ 30 min or as recurrent seizures that occur without full recovery between attacks.

Causes

1. Withdrawal of anticonvulsant drug
2. Metabolic derangements (electrolyte abnormalities, hypo or hyperglycemia, etc)
3. Eclampsia
4. CVS infection, head trauma.

Management

1. Correct serum hypoglycemia, if present
    - Obtain blood samples for:
        - Glucose
        - Electrolytes
        - AED levels
    - Consult neurologist
    - Rest same as eclampsia management
2. For continuous seizures, Inj. Lorazepam IV 2-8 mg in 2 mg increments → Drug of choice
3. For intermittent seizures, use Inj. Phenytoin 20 mg/kg IV at < 50 mg/min
4. If phenytoin fails, Phenobarbital 20-30 mg/kg IV
5. If both phenytoin and Phenobarbital fail → paraldehyde 3-5 mL deep IM.

Drugs and their Associated Malformations

1. Phenytoin: Fetal Hydantoin syndrome
    - Microcephaly
    - Facial clefts
    - Facial dysmorphism
    - Limb malformation
    - Nail hypoplasia
    - Distal phalangeal hypoplasia.
2. Phenobarbitone:
    - Cleft lip
    - Cleft palate
    - Cardiac malformation.
3. Carbamazepine:
    - Syndrome like fetal Hydantoin.
4. Valproic acid:
    - Face – Heart - Limb Syndrome
    - Lumbosacral spina bifida.

MENINGITIS

- Most common cause: streptococcus pneumonia and N. meningitides
- Pneumococcal meningitis can be associated with seizures
- Hypertension – not associated

- Coma may precede convulsions
- Onset
  - Sudden in pneumococcal meningitis
  - Gradual in tubercular meningitis
  - Meningococcal meningitis occurs in epidemics
  - History of ear infection (otitis media, mastoiditis) or sinusitis in streptococcal and staphylococcal meningitis.

Clinical Features

- Headache ⎫
- Fever   ⎬ 85%
- Neck stiffness ⎭
- Altered mental status (75%) – confusion, drowsiness, coma
- Seizures (40%)
- Nausea/vomiting
- Photophobia.

Signs

1. Resistance to neck flexion
2. Kernig's sign – patient in supine position, hip and knee flexed, pain induced by attempt to extend leg. This movement stretches the sacral nerve roots and there will be pain due to inflamed meninges
3. Brudzinski's sign – passive flexion of neck, so that the chin is on the chest → spontaneous flexion of hip and knees.

Diagnosis

Lumbar puncture for differentiating it mainly from subarachnoid hemorrhage
This will show:
- Increased pressure of cerebrospinal fluid
- The fluid looks cloudy in coccal forms of meningitis but is clear in viral meningitis
- Bacteriological examination reveals the type and cell count of bacteria
- Protein is increased, sugar and chlorides decreased.

Treatment

- Ceftriaxone + vancomycin.

COMPLICATED FALCIPARUM MALARIA

History

- Woman living in endemic area must not have taken antimalarial prophylaxis.

Clinical Signs and Symptoms

- Obtundation
- Delirium
- Coma

- Seizures
- High fever with chills and rigors
- Headache
- Vomiting
- Lethargy
- Joints and muscle ache
- Orthostatic hypotension
- Patient can have jaundice
- Severe malaria – prone to hypoglycemia, pulmonary edema, anemia and coma → patient rapidly deteriorates.

Diagnosis

- Complete blood count
- Peripheral Smear (Giemsa staining).

Treatment

1. Quinine
2. Phenobarbital for seizure control.

TETANUS

Pathology

- C. tetani is a spore-forming, strictly anerobic bacillus
- Spores are prevalent in the environment, particularly in the soil of warm and moist areas and may be carried in the intestinal tracts of humans and animals
- When introduced into necrotic wounds, the spores may convert to toxin producing tetanus bacilli
- The site of entry of C. tetani is in some cases unknown or is no longer visible at the time of symptoms
- Favorable anerobic conditions (dirty, necrotic wounds) → produces tetanospasmin, an extremely potent neurotoxin → blocks inhibitory neurotransmitters in the CNS → muscular stiffness and spasms typical of generalized tetanus
- Can occur at any age leading to ↑ fatality even with modern intensive care
- Majority of tetanus cases are:
  - Birth-associated, following unclean deliveries and poor postnatal hygiene
  - Occur in developing countries among newborn babies
  - Following injuries.

Incubation period - varies between 3 and 21 days (median 7 days, range 0 to > 60 days)
Neonatal tetanus starts 3–14 days after birth.

Symptoms and Signs

In majority of cases, tetanus presents as a generalized spastic disease

Other features:
- Trismus or 'lock jaw' and 'risus sardonicus' (difficulty opening mouth and chewing) → followed by spasm of the back muscles (opisthotonus) and sudden, generalized tonic seizures (tetanospasms)

- Spasms of face, neck, and trunk
- Arched back
- Board-like abdomen
- Spontaneous violent spasms
- Spasm of the glottis may cause sudden death.

Neonatal Tetanus

- Generalized spasms are commonly preceded by inability to suck or feed and excessive crying
- WHO definition of neonatal tetanus:
    - An illness occurring in a child who has the normal ability to suck and cry in the first 2 days of life but who loses this ability between days 3 and 28 of life and becomes rigid and has spasms.

Protection against Tetanus (Vaccines)

- Antibody-dependent
- Can be achieved only through active (tetanus vaccine) or passive (tetanus-specific immunoglobulin) immunization
- Tetanus vaccines are based on tetanus toxoid, a modified neurotoxin → induces protective antitoxin → passes from mother → via placenta → to fetus → prevents neonatal tetanus
- Tetanus toxoid vaccines are available as:
    - Single toxoid (TT)
    - Combined with diphtheria toxoid (DT) OR
    - Low-dose diphtheria toxoid (dT) OR
    - In combination with diphtheria and pertussis vaccines.

Safety from Tetanus

- Tetanus toxoid is considered very safe, even for use in immunodeficient individuals
- A woman is considered protected from tetanus when she has received 2 doses of tetanus toxoid at least 4 weeks apart, and with an interval of at least 4 weeks between the last vaccine dose and pregnancy termination (delivery or abortion). Women who have received a vaccination series (5 injections) more than 10 years before the present pregnancy, should be given a booster.

Tests: Culture of infected tissue.

Treatment

- Wound care, where required, as well as management of the symptoms and complications associated with the disease
- Prompt treatment with antitetanus immunoglobulins and appropriate antibiotics may prevent further progression of the disease but is unlikely to influence existing pathology.

CDC updates 2013

Advisory Committee on Immunization Practices (ACIP), 2012, recommend use of Tdap (Tetanus Toxoid, Reduced Diphtheria Toxoid, and Acellular Pertussis Vaccine) during every pregnancy.

PUERPERAL SEPSIS

Common Risk Factors

- Poor standards of hygiene
- Poor aseptic technique
- Manipulations high in the birth canal
- Presence of dead tissue in the birth canal (due to prolonged retention of dead fetus, retained fragments of placenta or membranes, shedding of dead tissue from vaginal wall following obstructed labor)
- Insertion of unclean hand, instrument or packing into the birth canal (traditional practices should also be examined)
- Pre-existing anemia and malnutrition
- Prolonged labor
- Prolonged rupture of membranes
- Frequent vaginal examinations
- Cesarean section and other operative deliveries
- Unrepaired vaginal or cervical lacerations
- Pre-existing sexually transmitted diseases
- Postpartum hemorrhage
- Not immunized or inadequate immunization with tetanus toxoid
- Diabetes.

Symptoms and Signs

- Fever ≥ 38°C
- Chills and general malaise
- Lower abdominal pain
- Tender uterus
- Subinvolution
- Purulent, foul-smelling lochia

There may also be:
- Light vaginal bleeding
- Shock

In severe infections:
- Joints may become painful and tender
- Woman very ill/delirium
- Coma and fits may occur.

Tests

- Midstream specimen of urine
- Wound swab, e.g. perineal or abdominal
- Blood culture, in the presence of chills or evidence of severe infection.

Treatment

- Broad spectrum antibiotics
- Close monitoring.

ELECTROLYTE IMBALANCE

Hyponatremia (Serum Na$^+$ <135 mmol/L)

Symptoms

- Confusion
- Lethargy
- Disorientation
- If Na$^+$ is <120mmol/L → seizures and coma.

Management

- Hypovolemic hyponatremia:
  - 0.9% NaCl or RL
- Hypervolemic hyponatremia:
  - Treat the underlying disease
  - Na$^+$ restriction
  - Diuretic therapy.

Euvolemic Hyponatremia

Cause
- CVS disease
- Drugs – carbamazepine.

Treatment
- H$_2$O restriction to <1 liter/day (depending upon severity).

Hypocalcemia (Check Calcium Levels)

Symptoms

- Peripheral and perioral paresthesia
- Muscle spasm
- Laryngeal spasm
- Seizures
- Respiratory arrest.

Treatment

- Inj. calcium gluconate.

Hypoglycemia

Glucose: fuel for brain.

Symptoms

At plasma glucose < 45-50 mg/dL

Anatomic
- Palpitation
- Tremor
- Sweating

Neuroglycopenic
- Confusion
- Seizures
- Loss of consciousness

Management

- Oral glucose OR
- 25 gm of 50% sol. IV → followed by constant infusion of 5-10% dextrose.

ECLAMPSIA

Definition

- Occurrence of convulsions or coma unrelated to other cerebral conditions with signs and symptoms of preeclampsia during pregnancy or postpartum
- Eclampsia is a Greek word meaning *'bolt from the blue'* or *'lightening.'*

Incidence

- Accounts for ≈ 10% of direct maternal deaths
- Eclampsia is rare in Europe, with 2-3 cases reported per 10,000 births
- In low- and middle income countries, eclampsia is more common, with the incidence estimated as 16 - 69 cases per 10,000 births
- An estimated 1.5- 8 million women develop preeclampsia worldwide per year, of whom 150,000 may develop eclampsia
- Where the incidence is high, a greater proportion of women with eclampsia have the onset before birth
- In high-income countries, where incidence of eclampsia is lower, a greater proportion of women have postpartum onset.

Risk Factors

Primary prevention of eclampsia → Prevent women from developing pre eclampsia
- Family history
- Little or no antenatal care
- Age < 20 years
- Having had ≥ 4 previous pregnancies
- ≥ 2 signs and symptoms of imminent eclampsia (such as headache, epigastric pain, hyperreflexia, visual disturbances and severe hypertension).

Eclampsia Unpredictable?

- Ideally preeclampsia should precede eclampsia as disease always progresses from mild to severe form. But this is not the case
- Few women have normal blood pressure at the time of their first fit, and some become very sick and may even die without developing eclampsia
- About one-quarter of cases of eclampsia occur without signs or symptoms suggestive of imminent eclampsia, such as headache, proteinuria etc.
- Predicting who is at risk of an eclamptic seizure is difficult as only around 1–2% of those with even severe preeclampsia will have a seizure.

Why Convulsions Occur?

Due to:
- Cerebral vasospasm
- Cerebral hemorrhage
- Cerebral ischemia
- Cerebral edema
- Hypertensive encephalopathy.

Pathology

Cerebral blood flow remains normal when cerebral perfusion pressure ranges between 60-120 mmHg. In this normal range, vasoconstriction of cerebral vessels occur when BP increases and vasodilatation when BP decreases

When this pressure is > 130-150 mmHg → this autoregulatory mechanism fails → vasoconstriction becomes defective → cerebral blood flow increases → segments of vessels become

- Dilated
- Ischemic with increased permeability

⟶ Exudation of plasma
↓
Focal cerebral edema and compression of vessels → ↓ cerebral blood flow.

Organ System Derangements in Eclampsia

CVS

- Generalized vasospasm
- ↓ Peripheral vascular resistance
- ↓ Central venous pressure
- ↓ LVSI
- ↓ Pulmonary wedge pressure.

Hematologic

- ↓ Plasma volume
- ↓ Blood viscosity
- Hemoconcentration
- Coagulopathy.

Renal

- ↓ GFR
- ↓ Renal plasma flow
- ↓ Uric acid clearance.

Hepatic (at autopsy)

- Peripheral necrosis
- Hepatocellular damage
- Subcapsular hematoma.

CNS (at autopsy)
- Cerebral edema
- Cerebral hemorrhage.

Time of Occurrence
- Antepartum – 50% (mostly in 3rd trimester)
- Intrapartum – 10-20%
- Postpartum – 30% (Fits occurring beyond 7 days of delivery rules out eclampsia).

Atypical Eclampsia
Occurring before 20 weeks gestation or > 48 hrs postpartum
At < 20 wks → with (i) Molar pregnancy or hydropic degeneration of placenta
               (ii) Multiple gestation
               (iii) Antiphospholipid antibody syndrome.

Status Eclampticus
- When the fits occur in quick succession
- Management:
  - Inj. Thiopentone sodium 0.5 mg in 20 mL of 5%D IV slowly.

What are Intercurrent (Antenatal) Fits?
- When patient becomes conscious after recovery from convulsions and pregnancy continues beyond 48 hours (Though literature even states the time limit of continuation of pregnancy to be as long as 7-10 days).

How much Fluid is to be given to an Eclamptic Patient?
- Fluid management is extremely important in case of preeclampsia and eclampsia
- In these patients, though there is hypovolemia, the tissues are overloaded and any excess fluid will aggravate tissue overload → pulmonary edema and ARDS
- Ringer lactate – fluid of choice
- Colloids (albumin/hemaccel)
  - Remain in vascular tree
  - Withdraw fluids from interstitial space
  - Use very carefully or else → circulatory overload
- Total fluids → urine output (in previous 24 hours) + 1000 mL (insensible loss through lungs and skin)
- Normally ≤ 2 liters /24 hours, that is ≈ 75-100 mL/hr.

Symptoms and Signs of Impending Eclampsia
1. Headache → persistent occipital or frontal
2. Visual disturbance → blurred vision and photophobia
3. Fundoscopy → marked retinal edema → severe hemorrhages, exudates and papilloedema

4. Restlessness and agitation
5. Epigastric and/or RUQ pain
6. Nausea/vomiting
7. Oliguria (< 400 mL urine in 24 hours)
8. Laboratory evidence of DIC/HELLP syndrome
9. Sudden swelling of face, hands or feet
10. Signs of clonus (≥3 beats)
11. Platelets <1 lakh/mm^3
12. Liver enzymes >70 IU/liter.

Clinical Features

Eclamptic Fit (Grandmal Seizures)

Stage I: Premonitory stage (10-20 sec)
- Eyes roll or stare
- Muscles of face and hand may twitch
- Loss of consciousness.

Stage II: Tonic stage (10-20 sec)
- Muscle – stiff or rigid
- Spasm of diaphragm, breathing stops and cyanosis occurs (1-2 min)
- Back arched
- Teeth clenched
- Eyes bulge.

Stage III: Clonic stage (1-2 min)
- Violent contraction and relaxation of muscles
- Increased salivation and frothing
- Deep, noisy breathing
- Face looks congested and swollen
- Tongue may be bitten.

Stage IV: Coma stage (several minutes to hours)
- Deep unconsciousness
- Breathing – noisy and rapid
- Cyanosis fades but face remains congested and swollen
- Further fits may occur before woman regains consciousness.

Other features:
1. Absence of other neurologic conditions
2. Almost always associated with hypertension and proteinuria
3. Convulsions can occur even with diastolic BP of 90-100 mm Hg
4. Proteinuria → can be as high as 15-20 g/day to even very low amounts
5. Most cases, occurring before or shortly (< 24 hours) after onset of labor → rapid progression to delivery
6. Late postpartum eclampsia: > 48 hours but within 4 weeks postpartum
7. Fits can be 1 or occurring at regular intervals → status epilepticus.

Fetus at the time of fit: Profound hypoxia and lactic academia after convulsions adversely affects the fetus → fetal bradycardia even up to 3-5 min. → may lead to IUFD due to:

- Intrauterine anoxia
- Cerebral hemorrhage
- Prematurity.

Before Moving to the Actual Treatment, MgSO$_4$ Needs a Special Mention

Introduction
- Anticonvulsant of choice for treatment of women with eclampsia
- Was introduced in 1920s as an anticonvulsant, following reports of its use for control of convulsions due to tetanus
- Used as magnesium sulphate heptahydrate (provided as a 50% solution; ≈ 2 mmol magnesium/mL).

Mechanism of Action

Mechanism I:
- Magnesium acts as an N methyl-D-aspartate (NMDA) antagonist and inhibits NMDA receptors, also blocking neuronal damage associated with ischemia
- These receptors when stimulated by neurotransmitters such as glutamate may lead to seizures when neuronal networks are over-activated.

Mechanism II:
- Magnesium sulphate may lead to cerebral vasodilatation, with subsequent reduction of cerebral ischemia.

Mechanism III:
- Magnesium is also a calcium antagonist, and a smooth muscle relaxant. It may therefore affect the cerebral endothelium which forms the blood brain barrier
- Lowering intracellular calcium may limit paracellular transport of vascular contents, such as ions and proteins, effectively decreasing the factors which promote cerebral edema and seizure activity.

Normal Serum Concentrations of Mg^{2+}

- 1.5 to 2.5 mEq/L (1.8 to 3.0 mg/dL)
- 1/3rd to 1/2 → bound to plasma proteins

   MgSO$_4$ reduced the risk of recurrent seizures in eclamptic women by 52% when compared to diazepam and by 67% when compared to phenytoin

   Do not use diazepam, phenytoin, lytic cocktail as an alternative to MgSO$_4$ in the treatment of eclampsia.

MANAGEMENT OF ECLAMPSIA

I. **Emergency care - management of convulsion**
   3 main aims:
   i. Anti hypertensives
   ii. Administration of MgSO$_4$
   iii. Maternal and fetal investigations.

II. **Obstetric management**

Emergency Care

Referral

- If symptoms developed at home:
  - Kept in bed
  - Sedate the patient
  - Transferred to tertiary care center
  - A doctor or mid wife or paramedical worker should accompany the patient and her relatives
  - Inform place of referral by telephone (so that proper arrangements can be made and treatment is not delayed)
  - Semiprone position with mouth gag in situ
  - Give loading dose of $MgSO_4$ at PHC, if possible
  - Nifedepine 10 mg orally, if BP ≥ 160/110 mmHg
  - Maintain IV line with Ringers lactate at a very slow rate.

Step I
On admission

Work with speed → it takes only 4 minutes for permanent brain damage, if the brain is deprived of oxygen

If the woman is anemic, she will withstand lack of oxygen less well

1. Keep the patient in quiet, darkened room
2. Any stimulus (noise, bright light, handling the woman) may precipitate a fit, so external stimuli are reduced to a minimum
3. Sedated, if required but NOT to be left alone
4. To be kept NPO
5. Do not try to stop the convulsion
6. Duration of convulsion - to be noted
7. Minimize risk of aspiration:
   - Lateral decubitus position
   - Vomitus/oral secretion sucked out (suction apparatus should be in easy approach)
8. Oxygenation 8-10 L/min after auscultating lung bases for rales
9. Prevent tongue bite (insert a padded tongue blade between teeth)
10. Prevent maternal injury from fall off the bed. Bed side rails should be padded and elevated
11. Establish 2 IV lines:
    - Draw blood for investigations from one
    - Administer $MgSO_4$ from the other
12. Fluids very slowly at the rate of 75-100 mL/hr
13. Catheterize the patient with Foleys catheter attached to a urometer/ urobag and hourly input/output charting should be maintained
14. If BP ≥ 150/100 mmHg, give IV labetalol (in the following manner)
    '0' hrs

            Inj. Labetelol 20 mg IV (over 2 min)
            ↓

    If BP > 150/100 mm Hg, double the dose every 20 minutes
            ↓

'20 min'
    Inj. Labetelol 40 mg IV
    ↓

'40 min'
    Inj. Labetelol 80 mg IV
    ↓

'60 min'
    Inj. Labetelol 80 mg IV
Total → 220 mg/hr
    OR

'0 hrs'
    Nifedepine 10 mg orally stat
    ↓

'30 min'
    If BP > 150/100, opt 10 mg every 30 min (check BP every 15 min)

Once BP is controlled (≤ 150/100 mm Hg) → maintain with nifedepine 10 mg every 6 hourly till maximum of 120 mg/day

15. Reassure relatives and explain prognosis
16. Monitoring:
    - Pulse rate, BP → pulse oximeter
      – Sudden drop in BP may indicate either abruption or an IUD
    - Respiratory rate and FHS monitored hourly
      – RR should by no way be <12/min which may indicate cerebral hemorrhage
    - Temperature checked every 4 hourly
    - Turn the woman every 2 hourly to avoid hypostatic pneumonia
    - Intermittent chest auscultation
    - Level of consciousness should be noted
    - Urine output hourly (should be min 30 mL/hr or 100 mL in 4 hours)
    - Any signs of twitching or restlessness are to be looked for
    - Sudden cyanosis may indicate cardiac failure
17. Stabilize the patient before delivery
18. Arterial blood gas analysis (ABG), if saturation < 92%
19. P/V → assess cervical status

***NEVER BE IN A HASTE TO DELIVER.

Step II: Investigations
Maternal
1. Hematocrit
2. Urine (albumin/microscopy)
3. 24 hr urine protein
4. Renal function tests (serum creatinine, blood urea, uric acid) with electrolytes
5. Liver function tests
6. Platelet count, if count < 1 lakh/mm^3, send
    - Coagulation profile/serum fibrinogen
    - Peripheral smear
7. *Blood film to rule out malaria (as a part of initial investigation in all patients presenting with a convulsion)*

8. Fundoscopy
9. NST, if > 32 weeks period of gestation (optional)

Fetal
1. USG for:
    - Gestational age
    - Fetal heart rate
    - AFI
    - Lie ⎫ In case immediate
    - Presentation ⎭ delivery is anticipated
    - Placental localization
    - To rule out IUGR and abruption
2. Doppler, if IUGR
3. Cerebral imaging:
    - Woman with neurological deficits
    - Prolonged coma
    - Convulsions < 20 weeks or > 48 hrs after delivery
    - Eclampsia refractory to $MgSO_4$ regimen.

Step III
Control of convulsions → $MgSO_4$ therapy
Many different regimens have been described in the literature. Of note are:
1. Pritchard's Regimen
2. ICMR (Low dose regimen)
3. Continuous IV Magnesium Infusion
4. Zuspan regimen
5. Sibai regimen.

Low dose (ICMR)
Loading dose
IV
6 mL $MgSO_4$ (3 gm)
    +
9 mL DW* → Inj. 15 mL sol (slow over 15 min)
IM
5 gm drug (5 amp) → 10 mL
2.5 gm +2.5 gm in each buttock

Maintenance dose
2.5 gm deep IM in alternate buttock × 4hrly
Total → 20.5 gm
(With 1mL, 2% lidocaine solution).

Pritchard's regimen
Loading dose
IV
8 mL $MgSO_4$ (4gm)
    +
12 mL DW* → Inj. 20 mL sol (slow over 20 min)
IM
10 gm drug → 20 mL
5 gm + 5 gm in each buttock

Maintenance dose
5 gm deep IM in alternate buttock × 4 hrly
Total → 39 gm

Magnesium Infusion (Continuous IV Regimen)

- 4 g loading dose IV over 15-20 minutes [can be repeated at a half dose (2 g) if convulsion recurs] followed by
- Infusion of 1g/hr maintained for 24 hours.

---

*DW = Distilled water

Zuspan Regimen

- Zuspan regime was introduced in 1978
- Loading dose:
  - Inj. $MgSO_4$ 4 gm IV over 15-20 minutes
- Maintenance dose:
  - IV Infusion 1 gm/hr
- Total duration of therapy = 24 hours

OR
- Continue until 24 hours after delivery

OR
- To stop treatment after 12 hours unless there is a specific indication to continue.

Sibai Regimen

- 6 gm $MgSO_4$ over 20 min followed by 2 gm $MgSO_4$ IV infusion.

Overall maternal mortality: **0.4%**

Precautions

1. Do not give nifedepine sublingually
2. DO NOT give nifedepine with $MgSO_4$ → marked hypotension because of synergistic effect of Mg^{2+} ions on Ca^{2+} channel function
3. Side effects: palpitations, flushing, headache, ankle edema, nausea, hypotension
4. Look for signs of magnesium toxicity

Signs	Magnesium levels (mg/dL)
Loss of patellar reflex	10-12
Respiratory arrest	14.6
Paralysis	15.0
Cardiac arrest	30

5. Routine monitoring of magnesium levels is not necessary as it is costly and unnecessary (but may be done in women with impaired renal function →↑ magnesium toxicity)
6. Withhold drug if the following is observed:
   - Loss of patellar reflex
   - Urine output < 100 mL in previous 4 hours
   - Respiratory rate < 16/min
7. Antidote:
   - Inj. Calcium gluconate (10%) 10 mL IV over 3 min
   - May cause bradycardia and arrhythmia.

Management of Recurrent Convulsion

- Convulsion occurring 30 min after loading dose or at any time later
- Once convulsion is ceased, administer 2 gm $MgSO_4$ (4 mL) + 6 mL distilled water (to make a total of 10 mL)
- Give slowly over 5-10 min.

Obstetric Management

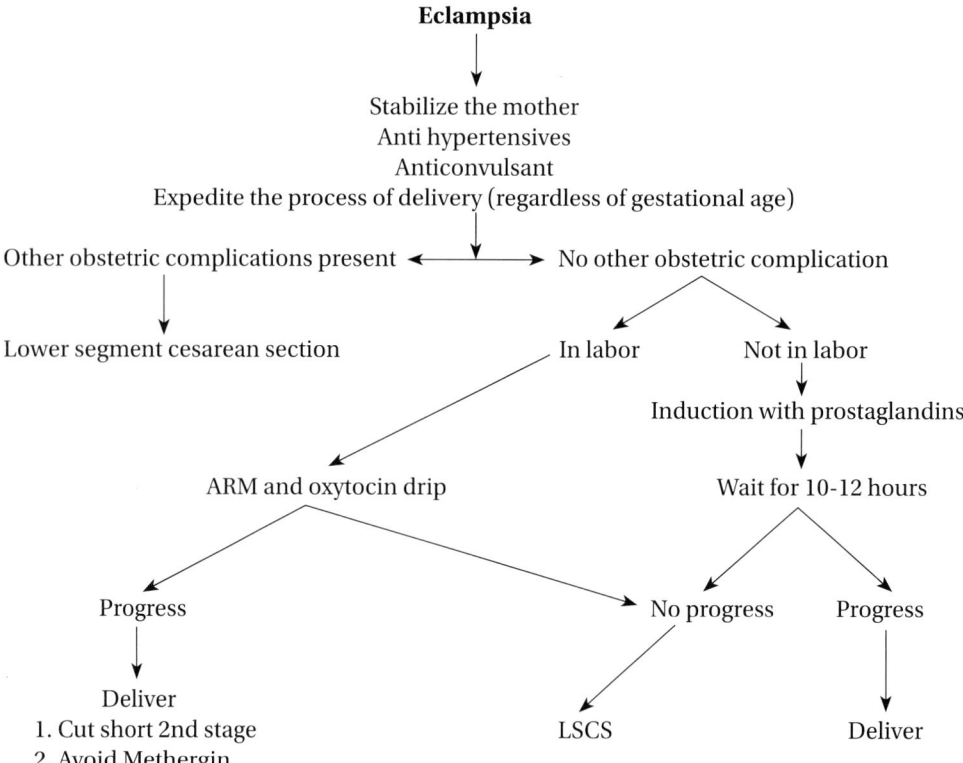

Indications of Cesarean Section

(Carried out under general anesthesia after excluding coagulopathy)
a. Uncontrolled fits despite therapy
b. Unconscious patient
c. Poor prospect of vaginal delivery (unfavorable cervix, non reassuring FHR pattern on NST)
d. Obstetric indication (malpresentation etc.).

Postpartum

- Close observation for 24-48 hours (convulsion can recur)
- Continue antihypertensives, if diastolic BP is >100 mmHg
- Continue anticonvulsant for 24 hours (after delivery or convulsion, whichever is last)
- Monitor urine output carefully for atleast first 24 hours (Do not give extra fluids during this period)
- Allow breastfeeding
- Do not give methyldopa postpartum
- Can give labetalol, nifedepine
- Reassess after 1 week and again at 6 weeks (12 weeks will be too late in a complicated case)
- Contraceptives (barrier, progesterone only pills).

How does Eclampsia Affect the Mother and the Fetus?

Effects on Mother

- Injuries during convulsions:
  - Tongue bite
  - Fractures (due to fall from the bed)
  - Bed sores
- Respiratory problems:
  - Asphyxia
  - Aspiration of vomitus
  - Pulmonary edema (due to leaky blood capillaries)
  - Bronchopneumonia (aspiration, hypostatic, infective)
  - ARDS
  - Embolism
- Visual disturbances:
  - Temporary blindness due to edema of the retina
  - Retinal detachment or occipital lobe ischemia
- Hyperpyrexia
- HELLP syndrome:
  - Hemolysis
  - Elevated liver enzymes
  - Low platelet count
- Disseminated intravascular coagulopathy
- Effects on the brain:
  - Hemorrhage
  - Thrombosis
  - Edema
- Liver necrosis
- Left ventricular failure
- Acute renal failure
- Postpartum:
  - Shock
  - Sepsis
  - Psychosis

Note: Up to 40% of women who develop eclampsia will not have had both hypertension or proteinuria in the week preceding their first seizure.

Effects on Fetus

- Mortality → 30-50%
- Prematurity
- IUGR
- Intrauterine and postnatal asphyxia
- Side effects of all the drugs used
- Admission to NICU.

Which Fetal Complication Occurs Immediately after an Eclamptic Fit?

- Fetal bradycardia

For 3-5 minutes

- Is a common observation
- No need for immediate cesarean section
- It is because of maternal acidosis and hypoxia.

For > 10 minutes

- Evaluate for uterine hyperstimulation or abruption.

Omnious Features Having Worse Prognosis

Eden's criteria: Eclampsia is considered severe if one or more of the following is present:
1. Coma of ≥ 6 hours
2. Temperature 39°C or more
3. Pulse > 120/min
4. Systolic blood pressure > 200 mmHg
5. Respiratory rate > 40/min
6. More than 10 convulsions

More than 2 criteria present → Poor prognosis.

Recurrence

- In subsequent pregnancies:
  - Ecalmpsia in 2% of cases
  - Preeclampsia in 25% of cases
- Eclampsia will recur to daughters of these patients in 3% of cases.

Which are the Other Popular Drugs/Regimens for Managing Convulsions (Though Not used these Days) if MgSO$_4$ is Not Available?

Diazepam

- Benzodiazepine
- First suggested for women with eclampsia in 1960s
- Diazepam binds to a specific site of the - aminobutyric acid A (GABAA) receptor, the major inhibitory neurotransmitter in CNS, which, when activated, decreases neuronal activity
- The anticonvulsant properties of diazepam may be in part or entirely due to binding to voltage-dependent sodium channels
- Use only if magnesium sulphate is unavailable
- To abort convulsion:
  - Inj. Diazepam 10 mg IV slowly over 2 minutes
  - If convulsion recurs, repeat the above dose
- To prevent recurrence:
  - IV infusion with 40 mg diazepam in 500 mL of Ringer lactate (continued for 24 hours)
  - Woman kept sedated but rousable
  - Not to give >100 mg of diazepam in 24 hours
- Onset of action – immediate (rapidly crosses the blood brain barrier)
- Duration of action → 20 - 30 minutes
- Half-life time of elimination → 20 - 50 hours

- Eliminated by the liver enzymes
- Fetal side effects (as it crosses the placenta):
  - Neonatal depression
  - Neonates floppy
  - Hypothermia
- Maternal complications:
  - Minor side effects: drowsiness, confusion, amnesia
  - Maternal depression if > 30 mg of the drug is given over a period of 1 hour
  - Mortality ≈ 5%
- There is NO antidote.

Phenytoin

- Was first used for epilepsy but in 1980s it was introduced for prevention and management of an eclamptic fit
- There are many different regimens suggested for phenytoin
- Loading dose of 1000-1500 mg as a short IV infusion followed by
- Maintenance dose: infusion of half the loading dose for 12 hours
- Given slowly with simultaneous ECG monitoring
- Has no sedative effects
- Side effects:
  - Hypotension
  - Cardiac dys arrhythmias
  - Phlebitis.

Lytic Cocktail

- Described by Krishna Menon (in 1961)
- Lytic cocktail was once standard treatment in India and some other parts of the developing world, but is no longer in widespread use
- Maternal mortality 2.4%
  '0' hours
  - Inj. chlorpromazine 25 mg and Inj. pethidine 100 mg in 20 mL of 5% dextrose IV together with
  - Inj. chlorpromazine 50 mg IM and Inj. pethidine 25 mg IM followed by
  - Alternate IM injection of 25 mg promethazine and 50 mg chlorpromazine at 4 hourly intervals for a period of 24 hours
  - Simultaneously, pethidine drip (100 mg in 500 mL of 10% dextrose) @20-30 drops/min for 24 hours following last fit
  - Not > 300 mg of pethidine and 1000 mL of fluids in 24 hours
  - Reversible with naloxone.

Chlorpromazine

- Antipsychotic agent
- Has CNS depressant effects
- Given as an IM injection
- Onset of action → ≈15 minutes
- Metabolised by the liver and excreted in urine
- Adverse effects:
  - Cardiac arrhythmias
  - Seizures.

Promethazine
- H1 histamine antagonist
- Moderate sedative and antiemetic properties
- IM administration → preferred mode
- IV use has been associated with severe tissue damage
- Onset of action → ≈ 20 minutes (IM route)
- Metabolised by the liver and excreted in urine and faeces as inactive metabolites
- Toxic effects include:
  - Hallucinations
  - Incoordination
  - Seizures.

Pethidine (meperidine)
- An opioid analgesic
- Produces generalised CNS depression
- When given with chlorpromazine and/or promethazine this potentiates its sedative effects
- Metabolised by the liver into active and inactive metabolites
- The active metabolite, normeperidine, has half the analgesic effect and two to three times the CNS effects of pethidine
- Normeperidine can accumulate and in high doses may cause seizures
- When these drugs are combined, as in lytic cocktail, they potentiate and augment each other
- Also a well-documented side effect of chlorpromazine is that it may cause seizures, as may pethidine and promethazine in high doses. This is a serious potential adverse effect for women with eclampsia.

STRYCHNINE POISONING

- Strychnine is a highly toxic, colorless, bitter, crystalline alkaloid used as a pesticide, particularly for killing small vertebrates such as birds and rodents
- Strychnine causes muscular convulsions and eventually death through asphyxia
- The most common source is from the seeds of the Strychnos nux-vomica tree
- Poisoning can occur by inhalation, swallowing or absorption through eyes or mouth
- It produces one of the most dramatic and painful symptoms of any known toxic reaction.

Presentation

- Ten to twenty minutes after exposure, the body's muscles begin to spasm, starting with the head and neck in the form of trismus and risus sardonicus
- Spasms then spread to every muscle in the body, with nearly continuous convulsions, and get worse at the slightest stimulus
- Convulsions then progress, increasing in intensity and frequency until the backbone arches continually
- Convulsions lead to lactic acidosis, hyperthermia and rhabdomyolysis
- These are followed by postictal depression
- Death comes from asphyxiation caused by paralysis of the neural pathways that control breathing, or by exhaustion from the convulsions
- Patient dies within 2–3 hours after exposure.

Treatment

- There is no specific antidote
- Oral application of an activated charcoal infusion which absorbs any poison within the digestive tract that has not yet been absorbed into the blood
- Anticonvulsants such as phenobarbital or diazepam - to control convulsions
- Muscle relaxants such as dantrolene sodium to combat muscle rigidity
- If the patient survives past 24 hours, recovery is probable.

SUGGESTED READING

1. Aleksey Kazmin MD Renee C Wong MB BS Mathew Sermer: Antiepileptic drugs in pregnancy and hemorrhagic disease of the newborn An update, Canadian Family Physician, vol 56: December 2010.
2. Anna G Euser, Marilyn J Cipolla. Magnesium Sulfate for the Treatment of eclampsia: A Brief Review, Stroke. 2009;40:1169-75.
3. Arne Reimers, Eylert Brodtkorb: Second-generation antiepileptic drugs and pregnancy: a guide for clinicians, Expert Rev. Neurother. 12(6), 2012.
4. Duley L, Gülmezoglu AM, Chou D. Magnesium sulphate versus lytic cocktail for eclampsia (Review), Issue 4 The Cochrane Library 2011.
5. Duley L, Gülmezoglu AM, Henderson-Smart DJ, etal. Magnesium sulphate and other anticonvulsants for women with preeclampsia (Review), Issue 11, The Cochrane Library 2010.
6. Duley L, Henderson-Smart DJ, Chou D. Magnesium sulphate versus phenytoin for eclampsia (Review), Issue 10, The Cochrane Library 2010.
7. Duley L, Henderson-Smart DJ, Walker GJA, et al. Magnesium sulphate versus diazepam for eclampsia (Review), Issue 12, The Cochrane Library 2010.
8. Gideon Koren, Alejandro A Nava-Ocampo, Myla E Moretti, et al. Major malformations with valproic acid, Canadian Family Physician, vol 52: April 2006.
9. Janneke Jentink, Maria A Loane, Helen Dolk et al for EUROCAT Antiepileptic Study Working Group: Valproic Acid Monotherapy in Pregnancy and Major Congenital Malformations, N Engl J Med 2010;362:2185-93.
10. Jeremy Matlow Gideon Koren: Is carbamazepine safe to take during pregnancy? Canadian Family Physician, Vol 58: Feb 2012.
11. Managing Eclampsia: World Health Organization 2008.
12. Parvaz Madadi, Shinya: Perinatal exposure to maternal lamotrigine, Canadian Family Physician vol 56: Nov 2010.
13. Prakash, Prabhu LV, Nasar MA, Rai, et al. Lamotrigine in pregnancy: safety profile and the risk of malformations, Singapore Med J 2007;48(10):880.
14. Sanjeev v thomas. Managing epilepsy in pregnancy, Neurology India, vol 59, Issue 1 Jan-Feb 2011
15. WHO recommendations for prevention and treatment of pre eclampsia and eclampsia, WHO 2011.

CHAPTER 20

Rh Negative Pregnancy

Tania G Singh, Earl Jaspal

HISTORY

- Discovery of Rhesus (Rh) blood group by Landsteiner and Weiner – in 1940 and by Levine in 1941
- The first description of hemolytic disease of the newborn (HDN) – in 1609 by Louise Bourgeois, a French midwife, in case of 2 twins – first died of hydrops and second died of kernicterus.

Epidemiology

People RhD negative worldwide:
- West Africa – 5%
- China - virtually no Chinese people are RhD negative
- Vellore, India – 5.5% of blood donors have been found to be RhD negative
- Caucasian population ≈ 15%
- African-Americans - 5–8%
- Asians and Native Americans 1–2%.

Problem in Rh Negative Pregnancy

- Human blood has two <u>main</u> systems: the *ABO system* and the *Rhesus (Rh) system* (both are inherited)
- In Rh system – Rhesus D (Rh D) is the *most* important of all the proteins
- Individuals who are Rh D positive – carry this antigen
- Who are Rh D negative – do not carry this antigen
- Because it is inherited, fetus can get it from either parents
- Rhesus system constitutes 2 more very similar transmembrane proteins called C and E
- Other non Rh groups are Kel, MNS, Kidd. They can also produce red cell antibodies as well.

Understanding The Disease

Angiogenesis in the fetus starts at about 3 weeks of in utero life
↓
Rh antigen is identified in the red cell membrane as early as 38 days after conception
↓
If feto maternal hemorrhage occurs in 1st pregnancy of a mother who is Rh- ve (i.e. she lacks the red blood cell antigen) carrying Rh+ ve fetus, during pregnancy or during labor,

↓

She gets exposed to RhD +ve fetal erythrocytes into her circulation (i.e. she is 'sensitized', a process called "alloimmunization" or "isoimmunization")

↓

The initial response of mother to this D antigen is slow
(sometimes taking as long as 6 months to develop)

↓

That's why 1st pregnancy is usually not affected

↓

But re-exposure to this antigen (in subsequent pregnancies) produces a rapid immunological response (i.e. formation of IgG anti – D antibodies) which usually can be measured in days

↓

These IgG anti-D antibodies cross the placenta → coat D-positive fetal red cells → which are then destroyed and removed from circulation in the fetal spleen (hemolysis).

Note:
- The risk of sensitization is greatest in the first pregnancy and decreases with each subsequent pregnancy. Once sensitization has occurred it is irreversible.

Results of Hemolysis

Before Birth

- Mild to moderate hemolysis → manifest as increased indirect bilirubin (of the fetus) which appears in the amniotic fluid → it is cleared by placenta and is not harmful
- Severe hemolysis → severe anemia → ↑ RBC production by the spleen and liver of the fetus
- Subsequently:

Hepatic circulatory obstruction (portal hypertension)

↓

Placental edema (which interferes with placental perfusion), leading to ascites in fetus

↓

Hepatomegaly, increased placental thickness and polyhydramnios

↓

Progressive liver damage → decreased albumin production results in the development of hydrops fetalis (can be managed with intrauterine transfusions, but this carries a 2% risk of fetal loss) eventually

↓

Fetal heart failure

After Birth

Neonatal liver cannot bear the increased production of bilirubin

↓

Hemolytic disease of the newborn

↓

If not treated (with phototherapy and exchange transfusions) in time → damage of specific areas of the neonatal brain

↓
Kernicterus
↓
Cerebral palsy, deafness, motor and speech delay.

Now Few Questions Must be Disturbing You

Can the development of this cascade be reduced? How?

In 2 circumstances it may be reduced:
1. In cases of ABO incompatibility
   - It may result from the rapid clearance of incompatible red cells thus reducing the overall exposure to D antigen
2. By giving anti D prophylaxis after the 1st pregnancy, if baby is Rh +ve.

When and how can this prophylaxis be given?

When?
- As soon as possible → but always within 72 hours
- If it is not given by this time → within 10-13 days
- Some studies suggest → giving up to 28th day postpartum can also be helpful.

Where?
- Should be administered into the *deltoid muscle*
- Injections into the gluteal region often only reach the subcutaneous tissues and absorption may be delayed
- Women *with bleeding disorder* should receive anti-D Ig via the *subcutaneous or intravenous route*
  Imp: Never forget to mention the administration in the discharge slip which will also help to differentiate between passive (prophylactic) and immune anti-D in many cases
- Women who are already sensitized to RhD should not be given anti-D Ig
- Women who have a weak expression of the RhD blood group (Du) do not form anti-D and therefore do not require prophylaxis
- It should be noted that anti-D Ig does not protect against the development of other antibodies which can also cause hemolytic disease of the newborn
- In cases of IUD or early neonatal death, where no sample can be obtained from the baby, anti-D Ig *should* be administered to a non-sensitized Rh -ve woman.

Which are the other sensitizing events, when and how much anti D is required after them?

When and how much anti-D?

Antepartum, if sensitizing event has occurred:
- Till 12 weeks → 30 µg
  - The total volume of fetal blood at 12 weeks of gestation = 3 mL (FMH 1.5 mL), sufficient dose of IgG anti-D = 30 µg but still better to give 50 µg
- Up to 19^{+6} weeks → 50 µg or 250 IU
- ≥ 20 weeks → 100 µg or 500 IU (neutralises FMH of up to 4 mL).

Sensitizing Events

Abortions
- Spontaneous and incomplete miscarriage after 12 weeks
- Surgical evacuation of uterus, regardless of gestation
- Medical evacuation of uterus, regardless of gestation
- Threatened miscarriage > 12 weeks of gestation
- If bleeding continues intermittently after 12 weeks of gestation, anti-D Ig should be given at 6-weekly intervals
- If there is heavy or repeated bleeding or associated abdominal pain as gestation approaches 12 weeks.

Invasive prenatal diagnostic procedures
- Amniocentesis
- Chorion villus sampling
- Cordocentesis
- Intrauterine transfusion.

Other intrauterine procedures
- Fetal therapy - insertion of shunts
- Multifetal reduction
- Evacuation in case of partial molar pregnancy
- Laser.

Ectopic pregnancy
- Anti-D Ig should be given to all non-sensitized RhD-negative women who have an ectopic pregnancy, regardless of management and period of gestation
- 25% of cases of ruptured tubal ectopic pregnancy are associated with a significant fetomaternal hemorrhage (FMH)
- There is a risk of alloimmunization associated with medical and conservative management and therefore, reasonable to offer anti-D Ig.

Antepartum hemorrhage (abruption/placenta previa)
- When bleeding continues intermittently, anti-D immunoglobulin should be given at 6-week intervals, after assessing volume of fetomaternal hemorrhage.

Others
- External cephalic version of the fetus (including attempted version)
- Any abdominal trauma (direct/indirect, sharp/blunt, open/closed)
- Fetal death
- Non availability of Rh-ve platelets (in cases of severe bleeding)
  - Though each unit of platelets contain < 0.1 mL of red cells, it is prudent to give 50 µg of anti D Ig following every 3 units of platelets
  - Administration should be by subcutaneous route in cases of marked thrombocytopenia (to avoid hematoma formation after IM administration).

Note: When there is concern about the frequency of recurrent bleeding, estimation of FMH using a Kleihauer test can be performed at 2-weekly intervals; if positive, an additional dose of anti-D Ig can be administered (500 IU or greater, depending on the size of the FMH). This dose is given irrespective of the presence or absence of passive anti-D.

Anti D not required
- Complete spontaneous abortion < 12 weeks gestation, provided there is no instrumentation of the uterus.

After each sensitizing event, what is the risk of development of "Alloimmunization"?

The risk of RhD alloimmunization after:
- Spontaneous miscarriage → 1.5–2%
- Induced abortion → 4–5%
- Chorionic villus sampling → 14%
- Amniocentesis → 2–5%

If this prophylaxis is not given, what are the chances of developing antibodies in subsequent pregnancies?

Chance of developing antibodies if Rhesus prophylaxis is not given:
- 1% → after the delivery of the 1st baby
- 7% → after the delivery of the 2nd baby
- 17% → after the delivery of the 3rd baby
- 30% → after the delivery of the 6th baby.

But there are a number of factors which affect the risk of sensitization:
- Blood type of the fetus
- Volume of fetal blood entering the mother's circulation
- Mother's immune response
- ABO compatibility
    - If both mother and fetus are ABO compatible (which is found in 80% of cases), risk is 16%
    - If mother and fetus are ABO incompatible, the risk is only 2%.

What should be the size of fetomaternal hemorrhage so as to cause sensitization?

After 1st pregnancy
- With 1 mL of Rh +ve fetal red blood cells entering maternal circulation → ≈ 15% of Rh –ve women will get sensitized
- With 10 mL of fetal RBCs → 33% will get immunized

This is Primary response and is Dose dependent, detectable after 4 weeks but may take as long as 6 months.

After subsequent pregnancies
- The response will be *Secondary* and requires *only about 0.03mL* of fetal Rh +ve cells to stimulate the immune response within *1-2 weeks.*

How much fetomaternal hemorrhage usually occurs after any uncomplicated labor?

Of all cases of Rh –ve pregnancies, FMH (whole blood) will be:
- Upto1mL in 98%
- > 5 mL in 1.5%
- > 12.5 mL in 1%
- > 25 mL in 0.5%
- ≥ 30 mL in 0.03% of cases.

How can we calculate the dose of anti D in any amount of FMH?

20 µg of Rh Ig is sufficient for 1 mL of <u>fetal cells</u>

OR

2 mL of <u>whole</u> blood

Therefore, if FMH is 30 mL, the dose will be 300 µg of anti D
1 vial = 1 unit = 300 µg = 1500 IU
No. of vials = vol. of FMH / 30

Note: If increased dose (>30 mL) is required, give IV up to 600 µg (3000 IU) 8th hourly till total dose.

How FMH is calculated?

Volume of FMH (whole blood) → % of fetal blood cells × 50
(50 → To account for an estimated maternal blood volume of 5000 mL).

At what period of gestation can fetal red cells be found in maternal circulation? What is the expected amount?

Alloimmunization by the RhD antigen may already be detected at 6 completed weeks of gestation.

Amount of fetal RBCs found in maternal circulation and % of women affected		
	Amount of FMH	% of women affected
1st trimester	0.07 mL	3%
2nd trimester	0.08 mL	12%
3rd trimester	0.13 mL	45% (sensitization is 'silent' secondary to occult FMH)
At the time of detachment of placenta	Already mentioned above	50%

Why anti D is given from 28 weeks onwards? How does it help?

- Antenatal anti-D prophylaxis:
  - Reduces the risk of Rh(D) immunization in the next pregnancy to < 0.4%
  - Is not harmful for the fetus
  - Has a strong immunosuppressive effect (i.e. exposure to D antigen in subsequent pregnancies will cause primary response and NOT secondary)
  - Success rate of postnatal Rh immunoprophylaxis is 98.4 - 99%
  - As the only source of therapeutic anti-D Ig is human plasma, earlier there were concerns about viral and prion transmission from the donors but now it is found to be extremely safe
  - Prophylaxis should be given irrespective of whether anti-D Ig has been given at an earlier gestation (e.g. in case of prenatal diagnosis or vaginal bleeding)
  - FMH occurring after administration of prophylactic dose should be covered with an additional dose of 100µg (unless Kleihauer test indicates a larger dose)
  - The disadvantage of this approach is that approximately 40% of Rh -ve women receive unnecessary antenatal anti-D Ig while carrying an Rh-ve fetus.
- Why administered at 28 weeks?
  - FMH occurring in the first two trimesters, is not big enough so as to cause sensitization
  - Approximately 92% of cases are protected till the beginning of 3rd trimester
  - The overall incidence of sensitization is 1%.
- 2 approaches:
  - Single dose of 300 µg IM at 28 weeks
    OR
  - 2 doses of 100-125 µg, one at 28th week, the other at 34th week.

- What is the rationale behind giving 2 doses?
  - Half-life of anti D IgG is ≈ 24 days (range 11-29 days) and single dose may not provide benefit if delivery occurs beyond 40 weeks
  - But compliance with the two-dose regimen might be poorer than with a single-dose regimen.

Recent Advances

- Studies have proved that both protocols are effective for a period of further 12 weeks from the time of administration
- After 12 weeks, they still show a minimum residual concentration of 25 µg of anti-D IgG (which is given by WHO as a protective level).

Diagnostic Tests

1. Coombs test
2. Amniocentesis to follow severity of the disease
3. USG
4. Doppler sonography
5. Free fetal DNA in maternal serum.

Coombs Test

The Coombs test was first described in 1945 by Cambridge immunologists Robin Coombs (after whom it is named), Arthur Mourant and Rob Race. Historically, it was done in test tubes. Today, it is commonly done using microarray and gel technology.

Also known antiglobulin test (or AGT). Coombs test and AGT refers to two clinical blood tests used in immunohematology and immunology respectively.

Two types:
- Direct Coombs test (DCT, also known as direct antiglobulin test or DAT)
- Indirect Coombs test (also known as indirect antiglobulin test or IAT).

Direct Coombs Test

Use
- Test for autoimmune hemolytic anemia.

Rationale behind the test
- Certain diseases or conditions may contain IgG antibodies in individual's blood
- These can specifically bind to antigens on the RBC surface membrane
- Complement proteins may subsequently bind to the bound antibodies causing RBC destruction
- DCT is used to detect these antibodies or complement proteins that are bound to the surface of red blood cells.

Procedure
- Blood sample is taken → RBCs are washed (removing the patient's own plasma) → then centrifuged and incubated with antihuman globulin (also known as "Coombs reagent")
- If this produces agglutination of RBCs → DCT is positive (a visual indication that antibodies [and/or complement proteins] are bound to the surface of red blood cells)
- A positive Coombs test indicates that an immune mechanism is attacking the patient's own RBCs. This mechanism could be autoimmunity, alloimmunity or a drug-induced immune-mediated mechanism.

Indirect Coombs test

Use
- Prenatal testing of atypical antibodies in pregnant women
- Testing blood prior to a blood transfusion
- Can also be used for antibody identification, RBC phenotyping, and titration studies.

Rationale behind the test
- It detects antibodies against RBCs that are present unbound in the patient's serum.

Procedure
The IAT is a two-stage test.

First stage
- Washed test red blood cells (RBCs) are incubated with a test serum. If the serum contains antibodies to antigens on the RBC surface, the antibodies will bind onto the surface of the RBCs.

Second stage
- The RBCs are washed three or four times with isotonic saline and then incubated with antihuman globulin. If antibodies have bound to RBC surface antigens in the first stage, RBCs will agglutinate when incubated with the antihuman globulin (also known Coombs reagent) in this stage, and the indirect Coombs test will be positive
- Serum is extracted from the blood sample taken from the patient
- Serum is then incubated with RBCs of known antigenicity that is, RBCs with known reference values from other patient's blood samples
- If agglutination occurs, ICT is positive.

Amniotic Fluid Analysis

- Carried out anytime after 18-20 weeks depending upon the previous history or the present titers
- Spectral analysis of amniotic fluid → determines the level of bilirubin (an indirect indicator of degree of fetal hemolysis) that reaches the amniotic fluid primarily by excretion into fetal pulmonary and tracheal secretions and diffusion across the fetal membrane and umbilical cord
- The peak value at 450 nm is subtracted from the baseline (a line drawn between data points at 525 and 375 nm) to determine the delta OD 450 (Δ OD 450)
- Explanation:
  - Using a semi logarithmic plot, the curve of optical density of normal amniotic fluid is almost linear between wavelength of 525 nm and 375 nm
  - Bilirubin causes a shift in spectrophotometric density with a peak of the wavelength at 450 nm.
  - "The amount of shift in optical density from linearity at 450 nm (Δ OD 450) is used to estimate the degree of red cell hemolysis"
  - This shift falls within one of the Liley's zones
- For monitoring fetal disease, amniocentesis is repeated at 10-14 days intervals and continued till delivery
- A rising or plateauing ΔOD 450 value that reaches 80th centile of zone 2 of Liley's curve or a value that enters upper zone of Rh +ve affected zone of Queenan curve, necessitates investigation by fetal blood sampling
- Sensitivity → 88%
- Negative predictive rate → 89%.

Liley's curve (1963)
- Extremely useful
- Tells when intrauterine transfusion is necessary
- Avoids unnecessary premature delivery
- The curve is divided into three zones:
  - Zone I
    - Indicates mild or no disease
    - Fetuses are usually followed with amniocentesis every 3 weeks
    - Delivery at term (labor induced).
  - Zone II
    - Indicates intermediate disease
    - Fetuses are usually followed by amniocentesis every 1-2 weeks
    - Patients in middle of this zone can progress to 36-38 weeks.
  - Zone III
    - Severely affected
    - Either delivered or require intrauterine fetal transfusion.

Queenan Curve for ΔOD_{450} values
- Rh negative (unaffected) zone
- Indeterminate zone
- Rh positive (affected) zone
- Intrauterine death risk.

Advantage over Liley's curve: Can be used in both 2nd and 3rd trimesters whereas Liley's curve can only be plotted in the 3rd trimester

Procedure (if intravascular transfusion is required in the same sitting):
- Abdomen prepped aseptically
- An ultrasound guided, 20-guage, 5-inch spinal needle is then guided into the umbilical vein at the site of placental insertion
- Fetal blood (1 mL) is aspirated for immediate hematocrit, CBC, blood type and Rh factor
- If hematocrit is < 30%, transfusion is indicated
- Prior to transfusion pancuronium bromide may be administered as an IV bolus → suppresses the fetal movements almost instantly
- Transfusion is performed using type O, Rh-negative, CMV, HIV, Hepatitis B and C negative, washed, irradiated packed cells, cross-matched against maternal blood
- Blood is packed to a hematocrit of 75-85%
- The donor blood is infused at 3-5 mL/min
- The volume of blood to be transfused depends on:
  - Pretransfusion fetal hematocrit
  - Estimated fetoplacental blood volume
  - Hematocrit of the donor blood
- Fetoplacental blood volume is first calculated:
  - Volume (in mL) = 1.046 + EFW (gm) × 0.14
- Then volume to be transfused is calculated:

$$\text{Volume transfused (mL)} = \frac{\text{Hematocrit (final)} - \text{Hematocrit (initial)}}{\text{Hematocrit (transfused)}} \times \text{Fetoplacental volume (mL)}$$

- Keep a continuous check on the flow of blood

- Check the hematocrit of the transfused blood at the end of procedure (Target hematocrit = 40-50%)
- 2nd transfusion → not before 10 days
- Subsequent transfusions, depending upon the achieved hematocrit.

Note:
Hematocrit may fall between transfusions due to:
- Fetal growth
- Plasma expansion
- Hemolysis of any remaining Rh + ve cells
- Rate of fall of haematocrit after transfusion ≈ 1%/day.

Limitations and pitfalls of the procedure

There can be a wrong diagnosis in the following situations:
i. Wrong fluid can be withdrawn
   Other fluids can be:
   - Fetal urine when bladder is inadvertently punctured
   - Fetal ascitic fluid
   - Though rarely mistaken, cyst in the ovary can be punctured.
ii. Amniotic fluid can be meconium/blood stained
   - Meconium → causes a peak at 410 nm
   - Blood → causes a peak at 412 nm.
iii. Aspiration of blood instead of amniotic fluid in cases of anterior placenta.

Ultrasonography

Features of prehydropic fetal anemia:
1. Fetal ascites
   - *Showing:* 'Bowel halo sign' → free fluid within peritoneal cavity or visualization of both sides of fetal bowel wall (1st sign)
2. Pericardial effusion
3. Polyhydramnios
4. Placental thickness > 4 cm
5. Dilatation of cardiac chambers
6. Chronic enlargement of spleen and liver
7. Dilatation of umbilical vein
8. Signs of extramedullary erythropoiesis
   - Increase in fetal liver length
   - Enlargement of splenic size.

Doppler Sonography

- Doppler ultrasonography of the middle cerebral artery has also been used to identify fetuses at risk for moderate to severe hemolytic disease
- A noninvasive method
- Gives accurate time of transfusion
- How does it correlate with fetal anemia?
  - ↓ Hemoglobin → ↑ cardiac output → ↓ blood viscosity → ↑ in maximum systolic flow velocity in fetal circulation → reflects fetal anemia → estimated on Doppler.

MCA Doppler Overview

- MCA measurements started as early as 18 weeks' gestation and repeated every 1-2 weeks depending on the trend
- Values after 35 weeks gestation are associated with higher rate of false positive results, after which amniocentesis may be better
- MCA is examined close to its origin in the internal carotid artery
- The angle of the ultrasound beam and the direction of the blood flow should be zero degrees
- The risk of anemia is highest in fetuses with a pre transfusion peak systolic velocity of 2.5 times the median or higher.

Technique

- Anteroposterior axis of fetal head typically lies in transverse plane
- Examiner can use either MCA vessel (anterior or posterior), both give equivalent results
- First locate the anterior wing of sphenoid bone at the base of the skull
- Color or power Doppler, then, is used to locate MCA
- Angle of insonation is maintained as close to 'zero' as possible by positioning the USG transducer on maternal abdomen
- Doppler gate is then placed in proximal MCA because the vessel arises from carotid siphon
- Measurements in more distal aspect of vessel will be inaccurate as reduced peak velocities will be obtained
- Fetus should be in a quiescent state because acceleration of FHR can result in a false elevation in peak velocity especially late in 3rd trimester (after 35 weeks)
- After 35 weeks, amniocentesis is a better modality.

Cell free Fetal DNA Testing

- It's a non invasive procedure
- Not done in routine practice
- Mainly confined for those pregnancies who are at high risk of developing serious complications if not managed properly
- Fetal blood group genotyping is done with the development of cell-free fetal DNA (cffDNA) from maternal plasma
- Diagnostic accuracy → 96-97%.

Can Rh D +ve blood transfused to an Rh D –ve woman? What precautions should be taken?

- Rh + ve blood can be transfused to Rh-ve women
- Dose = 100 μg (500 IU) of anti-D Ig will suppress immunization by 4 mL of Rh +ve RBCs, therefore, appropriate dose need to be calculated
- When <15 mL of RhD-positive blood, 500 IU can be given
- When > 2 units of positive blood have been transfused, an exchange transfusion should be considered to reduce the load of fetal cells in maternal circulation and likewise it will reduce the dose of anti D to be administered
- Immediate transfusion of a single-blood-volume exchange will achieve a 65–70% reduction in RhD-positive cells, and a two-volume exchange → 85–90% reduction
- After exchange transfusion, calculate the residual volume of Rh +ve cells either by flow cytometry or rosette test

- Dose of anti D after transfusion:
  - *IV anti-D Ig* - preparation of choice
  - Achieves adequate plasma levels immediately
  - Is twice as effective as IM dose at clearing red cells
  - 600 IU is adequate for 10 mL of fetal red cells. Based on this, calculate further dose, if and when required
  - Follow up tests for residual Rh +ve fetal cells should be done every 48 hours till no longer detected
  - **Remember:**
    IM preparation is NOT to be given by IV route
- Passive (prophylactic) anti-D Ig, given in large doses, may be detectable for up to 6 months or more and tests for immune anti-D may not be conclusive for 9–12 months.

Will the first RhD +ve fetus be affected?

In following scenarios:

Scenario 1
- If the mother is already sensitized from a previous Rh +ve blood transfusion and adequate anti D cover was not given.

Scenario 2
- In case of an abortion.

Scenario 3
- In cases where sensitization has already occurred in the previous pregnancy but ordinary routine tests could not detect it
  - In the present pregnancy anti-D will appear before 28 weeks' gestation and if there is any sensitizing event, she will give a secondary immune response
  - **Remember:** *once a woman has developed anti-D antibodies she cannot be desensitized.*

In which situations, quantitative tests are done?

I. Circumstances where large FMH is associated:
   - Traumatic deliveries including cesarean section
   - Manual removal of the placenta
   - Stillbirths and fetal deaths
   - Abdominal trauma during the 3rd trimester
   - Twin pregnancies (at delivery)
   - Unexplained hydrops fetalis.

II. Other antepartum indications for testing:
   Urgent
   - Unexpected/unexplained stillbirth (prior to induction of labor)
   - Significant maternal abdominal trauma, with non reassuring NST
   - Sinusoidal fetal heart rate trace in a non-immunized woman
   - Nonimmune hydrops with an abnormally raised MCA PSV
   - Decreased fetal movements after two consecutive nonreactive NSTs unless the first NST has:
     - Very reduced variability
     - A sinusoidal pattern

- Specific clinical signs suggestive of a FMH
- An inactive fetus on ultrasound.

Non urgent
- Women who have undergone an ECV (whether or not this was successful)
- Where the blood group in Rh negative.

III. Postpartum
- Take sample from cord blood at the time of delivery to check:
  - Blood group
  and
  - Direct coombs test (where there is unexplained jaundice) and if +ve, check
  - Bilirubin levels in the newborn

Note: Where the mother has taken anti D at and after 28 weeks, the following observations have been found:
- Rh +ve infant may be born with a positive DAT but have no evidence of hemolysis and
- Mother's blood will show anti-D reactivity, as the half-life of anti-D immunoglobulin in the absence of significant FMH, is ≈ 24 days.

Quantitative tests that can be performed

Kleihauer Acid Elusion Screening Test
- Detects fetal hemoglobin
- Ideally should be performed within 2 hours of delivery (0.5–1.0 mL of venous blood collected in an EDTA vial) but within 72 hours of placental separation
- Is used to identify women with a large FMH (> 6 mL of packed fetal red cells) who may need additional anti-D Ig
- A negative test indicates that one dose of anti-D Ig is sufficient
- For Kleihauer counts > 240 fetal red cells/50 LPF, a repeat Kleihauer Test is required 48 hours after administration of anti-D
- For antepartum Kleihauer tests, the result may stay positive in cases where the fetus is Rh-ve even though one or more doses of anti-D have been given.

Flow Cytometry
Advantages over Kleihauer test
- Results are more accurate and more reproducible
- Particularly helpful in women with high fetal hemoglobin levels
- Most effectively employed in those cases where a Kleihauer screening test indicates a large FMH which requires accurate quantitation and follow-up.

Rosetting Technique
- Quantifies FMH of RhD-positive red cells > 4 mL.

Scope for Future Pregnancies
- If the father is homozygous RhD positive (i.e. has two RhD positive genes), then all future pregnancies will be affected and will require intensive monitoring and intervention, with the possibility of an unsuccessful outcome
- If the father is heterozygous (i.e. has one RhD positive gene and one RhD negative gene), there is still a 50% probability that a given pregnancy will be affected

- As the severity with which the fetus is affected, increases with each RhD positive pregnancy, a successful outcome becomes less likely with each successive pregnancy.

Hemolytic Disease of the Newborn (HDN)

- Hemolytic anemia resulting from the transplacental passage of antibodies created by the mother and directed against fetal red cell antigens inherited from the father
- Antibodies causing the disease are of IgG type
- Associated antibodies:
  - Anti-D, -c, -E, -e, -C, -K and –k antibodies
  - Anti-D, anti-c and anti-K antibodies are most often associated with moderate to severe HDN
- Severity of disease depends on:
  - Certain properties of the antibody
  - Its level in the maternal blood
  - Duration of exposure of the infant to that level of antibody
- Forms in which HDN can manifest:

Mild
- Infant has sensitized red cells → detectable only in laboratory tests
- Mild degree of jaundice, which responds to phototherapy.

Severe
- Significant anemia
- Progressive hyperbilirubinemia
- Thalamus and corpus striatum are particularly sensitive to damage by unconjugated bilirubin. If severe jaundice is not treated by exchange transfusion → kernicterus → results in permanent brain damage → death in 70% of affected infants.

Most severe
- The in utero anemia causes hydrops and intrauterine death.

Management

Intrauterine fetal blood sampling (introduced in the early 1980s)
↓
Identification of fetal Rh D type and hemoglobin level
↓
Intrauterine blood transfusion under direct ultrasonographic guidance before the occurrence of complications

- Overall survival – 86-90%
- Those with hydrops – 55%
- With mild hydrops – 98%.

Future Health Concerns

Can develop the following with time:
- Myopia
- Squint
- Delay in speech and fine motor skills
- Permanent neurodevelopmental problems

- Sensorineural disabilities (mainly associated with prematurity)
  - Nontransient hearing loss
  - Bilateral sensorineural hearing loss
  - Mild conductive hearing loss
  - Permanent hearing deficit
  - Severe bilateral deafness
  - Cerebral palsy of varying degrees of severity.

Antepartum Management of Rh Negative Pregnancy

First Pregnancy (Unaffected with No Previous Sensitizing Events)

Mother Rh −ve

Step I
- Father Rh -ve → nothing to be done

Step II
- Father Rh +ve → ICT (at 28 weeks)

Step III
- Give Anti D 300 µg at 28 weeks

Step IV

After delivery, determine baby's blood group

- If negative → Nothing to be done
- If positive → Consider anti D within 72 hours of delivery
  - If bleeding normal → (300 µg IM)
  - If heavy bleeding → (Calculate FMH and give required dose).

First affected Pregnancy (Sensitized Due to Previous Event but no Severely affected Pregnancy)

Step I
- Check maternal titers (method used should be stated by the lab.)
- An albumin titer of 1:16 is equal to an indirect antiglobulin test (IAT) titer of 1:32 to 1:128
- Titer of > 1:4 → considered sensitized.

Step II
- If titer is ≤ 1:32, repeat antibody titers every 4 weekly till 24 weeks and then every 2 weeks thereafter.

Step III
- If titer is ≥ 1:64 (critical titer, for each lab. it is different) → amniocentesis → fetal RhD status (if facility for fetal genotyping from maternal plasma is not available).

Step IV
- If fetus RhD positive → serial fetal MCA Doppler OR serial amniocentesis for Δ OD_{450} every 1-2 weeks starting at 24 weeks and continued till 35 weeks.

Step Va
- When peak MCA velocity > 1.5 MoM OR Δ OD_{450} falls into:
  - 80th centile of zone 2 OR
  - In zone 3 of Liley's curve OR
  - In upper portion of Queenan Rh positive, affected zone
    ↓
- Cordocentesis, to determine fetal hematocrit
- If < 30% → intrauterine transfusions.

Step Vb
- If pregnancy is followed only with Doppler assessments and values remain normal till 35 weeks, amniocentesis need to be done at 35 weeks for fetal lung maturity and Δ OD_{450} values and further pregnancy managed accordingly.

First Sensitized Pregnancy/Previously affected Pregnancy

- For patients with a previously affected pregnancy, the timing of the initial procedure is determined by past clinical history
- It is usually performed at least 4-8 weeks earlier than the prior gestational age at which significant morbidity occurred in previous pregnancy
- Usually amniocentesis is started at 15 weeks (determine fetal genotype) OR if MCA Doppler is opted, testing should be started at 18 weeks
- In these cases, Queenan's curve is opted
- Rest managed as mentioned above
- Where the titers are extremely high (≥ 256) at < 28 weeks and the fetus does not demonstrate hydrops, but there is a documented history of IUD due to hydrops in the previous pregnancy, IV immune serum globulin might be offered,
  - Dose = 400 mg/kg/day × 5 days
  - Repeat infusions every 15 to 21 days
  - Contraindications to its use:
    - A previous episode of intravenous immunoglobulin-induced anaphylaxis (rare)
    - Selective IgA deficiency.

Exchange Transfusion

Indications

1. To treat hyperbilirubinemia when bilirubin reaches toxic levels such as in Rh incompatibility, ABO incompatibility
2. Severe jaundice with risk of kernicterus not responding to phototherapy lights
3. Neonatal polycythemia
4. Any Total Serum Bilirubin (TSB) >12mg/dL in first 12 hours
5. Cord Hb <10g/dl and/ or Cord TSB >5 mg/dL
6. Severe anemia
7. Septicemia.

Blood Volume Requirement

a. For term neonates → 70-90 mL/kg
b. For preterm neonates → 85-110 mL/kg

Types of Exchange Transfusion (Depending on Volume)

a. Double volume exchange transfusion (DVET)
   - Removes 85-90% of red cells
   - The volume of blood exchanged = 2 × baby's circulating blood volume i.e. total 140-180 mL/kg in term neonates
b. Single volume exchange transfusion
   - Removes 60-75% of red cells
   - The volume of blood to be exchanged = 1 × baby's circulating blood volume.

Which blood product is to be used and when?

a) In emergency situations: O Rh negative blood
b) If ABO incompatibility: O +ve RBCs suspended in AB plasma
c. If Rh incompatibility: Rh negative blood of baby's ABO type
d. In other babies: ABO type of baby cross matched with mother's blood.

What should be the size of aliquot?

- Depends upon the weight of the baby
- The smaller the baby, smaller is the volume of aliquot
- Weight:
  - < 1000 g → 5 mL,
  - 1000 g → 2000 g-10 mL,
  - >2000 g → 15 mL.

Pre Requisites for Exchange Transfusion

- Ensure that the procedure is explained to the parents in their understandable language and a written consent is obtained
- Place the baby under servo controlled open care radiant heat source
- Attach multipara monitors and monitor heart rate, temperature, respiratory rate and oxygen saturation throughout the procedure
- Resuscitation equipment and all medicines should be easily accessible
- Baby should be nil by mouth
- Insert a nasogastric/orogastric tube and aspirate stomach contents
- Collect the following blood samples before starting the procedure:
  - Hemoglobin
  - Hematocrit
  - Blood gases
  - Serum bilirubin
  - Potassium
  - Blood glucose
- Prepare exchange transfusion chart which includes in and out volume, heart rate, respiratory rate, temperature, oxygen saturation, color of baby, medications administered.

Equipment Required

- Protective gowns or plastic aprons
- Protective eye glasses
- Sterile gloves
- Cross matched blood
- Blood administration set
- Umbilical catheters
- IV cannula No. 24
- Exchange transfusion recording sheet
- Sterile drapes
- 3-way stopcock/ taps
- Syringes (assorted sizes as required)
- Blood gas syringes
- Tapes
- Suture material
- Resuscitation equipment
- Inj Calcium gluconate 10%
- Inj Sodium bicarbonate
- Inj Frusemide (20 mg/2 mL)
- Glucose 10%
- Pathology and biochemistry collection tubes
- Alcohol swabs
- Sterile gauze
- Urine drainage bag.

Types of Exchange Transfusion (Depending on Procedure)

- Continuous Exchange - performed by two operators, one infuses blood and the other simultaneously withdraws it. It can be done through the following routes:
  - A UVC and UAC
  - A UVC and a peripheral arterial cannula
  - Peripheral cannula and a UAC
  - Peripheral cannula and a peripheral arterial cannula
- Push-Pull Method (commonly used) can be done through:
  - A single UVC with tip in IVC or right atrium
  - A single UAC with tip in lower aorta.

Procedure for Push and Pull Method

Prerequisite

- Perform six steps of hand washing. Ensure complete aseptic precautions
- Use fresh CPDA blood
- Make sure that blood has been screened for HIV, Hbs Ag, HCV, malaria and syphilis
- Warm the blood to 37°C
- Preheparinize the umbilical catheter
- Cannulate the umbilical vein or umbilical artery depending upon the method used
- Attach the umbilical catheter to 2 three ways stopcock/taps in such a way that its ports are connected to:

- Umbilical catheter
- Cross matched donor blood
- Sterile container for waste
- Syringe (used for push pull technique).

Procedure

The blood is gently withdrawn (out) and the donor blood is slowly injected (in) using push pull technique. The size of aliquot depends on size of the baby. During the procedure, the operating person must call out the volume in and out with each infusion and withdrawal (e.g., "six in - six out"). A qualified nurse should keep recording the number of cycles with each aliquot and also record heart rate, respiratory rate, color of baby and oxygen saturation every 10 minutes. The donor blood bag should be kept moving intermittently to prevent RBCs from settling. If any time during the procedure there is dip in baby's oxygen saturation, change in color of baby, respiratory distress or fall in heart rate to <100 beats/min, the procedure should be withheld immediately till the baby's condition improves. Inj. Calcium gluconate should be given in 1:1 dilution under cardiac monitoring for every 50 mL of exchange while using CPDA blood. After completion, the catheter should be removed gently and umbilical stump should be pressed and dressing should be applied. Whole procedure takes approximately one hour.

Post Exchange Care

- Send blood samples for hemoglobin, hematocrit, serum bilirubin, potassium, calcium, blood sugar and blood gases
- Proper dressing over umbilical stump
- Observe for bleeding
- Monitor heart rate, respiratory rate, color of baby, temperature and oxygen saturation every half hourly for 1st four hours
- Continue phototherapy until serum bilirubin level is in normal range.

Complications

1. Cardiac:
   - Bradycardia
   - Hypo or hypertension
   - Arrhythmias
   - Arrest
   - Shock
   - Volume overload leading to cardiac failure.
2. Hematological:
   - Thrombocytopenia
   - Neutropenia
   - Polycythemia
   - Coagulopathy.
3. Metabolic:
   - Hypocalcemia
   - Hypoglycemia
   - Hyperkalemia
   - Acidosis
   - Hypomagnesemia
   - Hypernatremia.

4. Gastrointestinal:
   - Feed intolerance
   - Necrotizing enterocolitis
   - Perforation of intestine
   - Portal vein thrombosis.
5. Catheter related complications:
   - Air emboli
   - Thrombosis
   - Hemorrhage.
6. Infection:
   - Septicemia (bacterial or viral).

SUGGESTED READING

1. Blood Grouping and Antibody Testing: Clinical Guidelines, OGCCU King Edward Memorial Hospital, Perth Western Australia, January 2008.
2. Davor Brinc, Alan H. Lazarus: Mechanisms of anti-D action in the prevention of hemolytic disease of the fetus and newborn, Hematology 2009.
3. E Austin, S Bates, M de Silva: Guidelines for the Estimation of Fetomaternal Hemorrhage, BCSH FMH Guidelines 2009
4. Giancarlo Maria Liumbruno, Angelo D'Alessandro, Federica Rea: The role of antenatal immunoprophylaxis in the prevention of maternal-foetal anti-Rh(D) alloimmunisation, Blood Transfus 2010;8:8-16.
5. H Pilgrim, M Lloyd-Jones, A Rees: Routine antenatal anti-D prophylaxis for RhD-negative women: a systematic review and economic evaluation, Health Technology Assessment 2009; Vol. 13: No. 10.
6. Karen Fung Kee Fung, Erica Eason: Prevention of Rh alloimmunization, J Obstet Gynaecol Can 2003; 25(9):765-73.
7. Management of alloimmunization during pregnancy: ACOG Aug 2006.
8. Management of Rhesus Negative Mother: SLCOG National Guidelines
9. Marek Lubusky: Prevention of rhd alloimmunization in RhD negative women, Biomed Pap Med Fac Univ Palacky Olomouc Czech Repub. 2010;154(1):3-8.
10. Routine antenatal anti-D prophylaxis for women who are rhesus D negative: NICE technology appraisal guidance 41, August 2008
11. Screening for Rh (D) Incompatibility Recommendations: U.S. Preventive Services Task Force, November 2004.
12. The Use of Anti-D Immunoglobulin for Rhesus D Prophylaxis: RCOG Green-top Guideline No. 22, March 2011.

CHAPTER 21

Jaundice in Pregnancy

Tania G Singh, Earl Jaspal

BILIRUBIN METABOLISM

Old RBCs (after 120 days) get destroyed into globin and heme
↓
Heme is degraded in RE system (especially liver and spleen)
↓ Heme oxygenase
Biliverdin (green)
↓
Bilirubin (red orange)
↓
Binds to albumin in circulation (mostly)
↓
Goes to liver cells
↓
Fate in liver

1. **Uptake of bilirubin by hepatocytes:**
   - Bilirubin dissociates from its carrier albumin and enters hepatocytes.
2. **Conjugation of bilirubin:**
   - In hepatocytes, bilirubin is conjugated with two molecules of glucuronic acid by the enzyme glucuronyl transferase.
3. **Excretion of bilirubin into bile:**
   - Conjugated bilirubin (bilirubin diglucuronide) is transported into bile canalculi and then into bile

↓
Intestines
↓ Intestinal bacteria removes glucuronic acid
Urobilinogen
↓

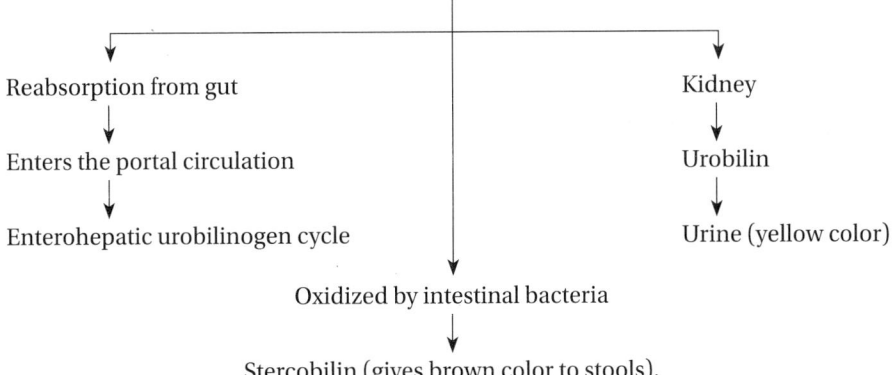

JAUNDICE

- The term jaundice comes from the French word *'jaune'*, meaning 'yellow'
- Also known as icterus
- Yellow discoloration of the skin, the conjunctival membranes over the sclerae and other mucous membranes secondary to hyperbilirubinemia
- Jaundice in itself is NOT a disease, it is a SIGN of an underlying disease
- Normal concentration of bilirubin in blood plasma is <1.2 mg/dL (<25µmol/L)
- A concentration ≥ 2.0-2.5 mg/dL (>50µmol/L) leads to jaundice.

Causes (in General)

Indirect (Unconjugated)

Hemolytic
1. Inherited
   - Spherocytosis
   - G6PD deficiency
   - Sickle cell anemia
2. Acquired
   - Microangiopathic hemolytic anemia
   - Paroxysmal nocturnal hemoglobinuria (PNH).

Ineffective erythropoiesis
1. Cobalamin deficiency
2. Folate deficiency
3. Serum iron deficiency
4. Thalassemia.

Drugs
1. Rifampicin
2. Probenecid.

Inherited
1. Criggler—Najjar (type I and II)
2. Gilbert's syndrome.

Direct (Conjugated)

Inherited
1. Dubin—Johnson syndrome
2. Rotor's syndrome.

VARIOUS FORMS OF JAUNDICE

Parameter	Hemolytic/Prehepatic	Hepatocellular	Obstructive/Post hepatic
Blood			
Hemoglobin	Decreased	Normal	Normal
Total bilirubin	Normal/increased	Increased	-
Unconjugated bilirubin	Much increased	Normal / increased	Normal
Conjugated bilirubin	Normal	Increased	Increased
Alkaline phosphatase	Normal	Normal/ increased	Much increased
Aminotransferase	Normal	Much increased	Normal
Cholesterol	Normal	Normal	Increased
Urine			
Bilirubin	-	Increased	Increased
Urobilinogen	Increased	Increased	Decreased
Stool			
Color	Normal	Normal	Pale
Splenomegaly	Present	Present	Absent

1. **How will you approach to a case of jaundice?**

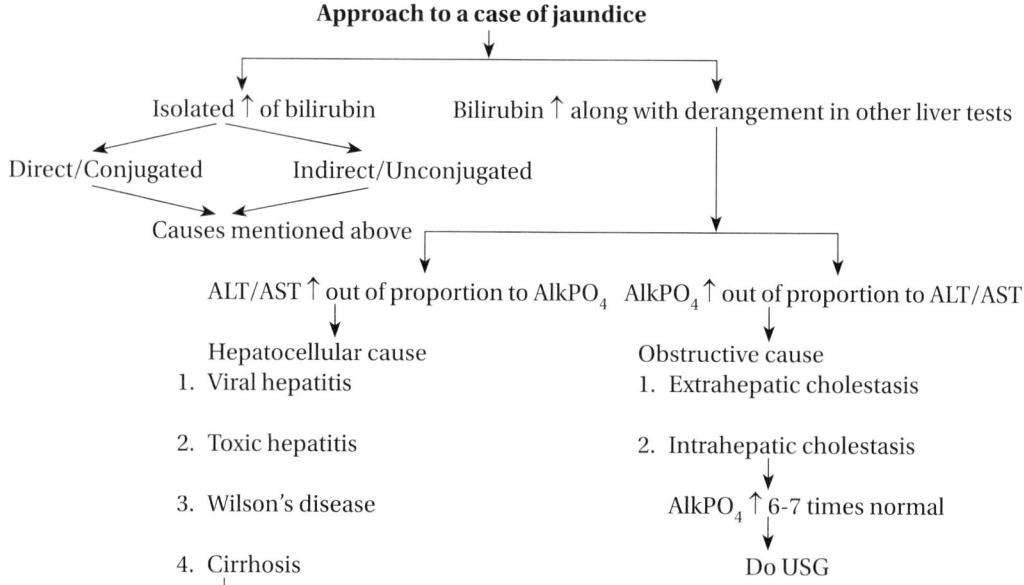

2. What are the causes of jaundice in pregnancy?

Jaundice, though not very common in pregnancy, can be met with the following pregnancy related complications. Other rare causes are not being mentioned.

Different liver diseases causing jaundice in pregnancy

	Hyperemesis gravidarum	Acute hepatitis	ICP	HELLP	AFLP
Trimester	1st and early 2nd	Any	3rd	3rd	3rd Typically between 30th-38th week
Presenting symptoms	Intractable nausea, vomiting, weight loss ≥ 5% Jaundice occurs at a later stage (as a complication)	Fever, jaundice	Pruritis (most severe at night) Most common site: palms and sole) Jaundice (uncommon)	Malaise (90%) Epigastric or RUQ pain (90%) Nausea and vomiting (50%) Jaundice—rare (Total bili > 1.2 mg/dL, mainly unconjugated)	Nausea, vomiting, anorexia, malaise, mid epigastric or right upper abdominal pain, jaundice—characteristic (upto 5-15mg/dL)
AST and ALT	Mild ↑ Mild ↑ in serum bilirubin Low albumin	↑↑↑	Normal to mildly ↑	Moderately ↑	Moderately ↑
Alkaline PO$_4$		Normal to mildly ↑	High	Normal	Normal
LDH				> 600U/L	
Platelets		Normal	Normal	< 1 lakh/mm^3 (Appearance of thrombocytopenia preceeds ↑ in PT, aPTT)	Initially mild or normal (appear after ↑ in PT, aPTT) Others: ↓ fibrinogen and antithrombin Leucocytosis, ↑ creatinine, uric acid, ammonia, ↑ bilirubin
Proteinuria					Absent
Hypertension					Absent
Significant weight gain and generalized edema				+	

Contd...

Contd...

	Hyperemesis gravidarum	Acute hepatitis	ICP	HELLP	AFLP
Incidence	0.3-1.5%		0.1-0.2%	0.1%	0.01%
Fetal complications	LBW; IUGR; IUD	Transmission of infection in HBV and HCV	Prematurity/ IUGR/IUD	IUGR/Prematurity/ IUD/ Preterm delivery, neonatal thrombo-cytopenia, RDS	Premature delivery
Maternal complications	Malnutrition; Fluid and electrolyte imbalance; dehydration; ketoacidosis; hospitalization; weight loss	↑ cases of acute liver failure with HEV	Generally none	Abruptio, eclampsia, subcapsular liver hematoma, liver rupture, DIC, septicemia, multiorgan failure	Acute liver failure

INTRAHEPATIC CHOLESTASIS OF PREGNANCY

Defined as a multifactorial condition characterized by:
- Pruritis without rash
- Abnormal liver function in the absence of other liver disease
- Progression with pregnancy
- Resolves following delivery (within 48 hours).

Diagnosis is made only after excluding other causes.

Epidemiology

- Incidence highest in south America
- Incidence increases:
    - After IVF
    - In twin pregnancies
    - Age ≥ 35 years
- Risk factor → Hepatitis C seropositivity leading to early onset of the condition
- These women have more severe and prolonged emesis and higher rates of drug sensitivities.

CLINICAL FEATURES

Effects on Mother

- PRURITIS (an unpleasant sensation that evokes the desire to scratch) → most common symptom
- After 30 weeks, but may occurs as early as 8 weeks
- Palms of hands and soles of feet → most common sites, but can be generalized in few cases
- Usually presents at night, sometimes causing insomnia
- O/E: excoriation marks on skin (dermatographia artefacta)
- Other skin conditions MUST be excluded like eczema or atopic eruption of pregnancy

- Jaundice → rare
- Anorexia, malaise and abdominal pain may occur
- Rarely → pale stools, dark urine and steatorrhea is seen
- Itch may present either before or after abnormal liver function is detected and usually resolve within 2-8 weeks of delivery.

Effects on Fetus

- Passage of meconium in ≈16 – 58% cases, mostly with ↑↑ maternal s. bile acids
- CTG abnormalities (both ante- and intrapartum)
  - Reduced FHR variability
  - Tachycardia
  - Bradycardia(<100bpm)
- Preterm labor, mainly when fasting serum bile acids > 40micromol/lit
- Sudden IUD, which can be reduced by:
  - Increased fetal monitoring
  - Frequent biochemical testing
  - Pharmacotherapy with ursodeoxycholic acid (UDCA)
  - Delivery at 37-38 weeks gestation.

Investigations

1. Bile acids
2. Liver function test
3. Urine routine and microscopy
4. Ultrasound whole abdomen.

BILE ACIDS

Metabolism

- *Classified as*
  - *Primary*
  - *Secondary*
  - *Tertiary*
- *95% of all bile acids are reabsorbed in terminal ileum and re-enter liver.*

1. Cholic acid (CA) and Chenodeoxycholic acid (CDCA)
   - *Primary* bile acids
   - End products of cholesterol metabolism in liver
   - Conjugate with taurine or glycine (in a ratio of approx. 1:3) → enter bile → transported to terminal ileum and colon → undergo deconjugation and 7α-dehydroxylation to form
   ↓
2. Deoxycholic acid (DCA) and Lithocholic acid (LCA)
   - *Secondary* bile acids
3. UDCA
   - *Tertiary* bile acid
   - Results from bacterial modification followed by hepatic metabolism
   - Only traces found in normal serum.

Bile Acids in Normal Pregnancy

- Minimal rise in total serum bile acids (10-14 µmol/L)
- No change in DCA and CA levels
- CDCA doubles by term
- Ratio of CA: CDCA is between 0.68-1.9 at term.

Bile Acids in ICP

- Serum bile acid levels → most suitable biochemical marker for both the diagnosis and monitoring of ICP
- CA level or the CA:CDCA → most sensitive indicator for early diagnosis
- ↑DCA → impairment of enterohepatic circulation
- Maternal cholestasis →↑ bile acids in the fetal circulation
- Though random bile acid levels are used in routine practice, its significant rise after a meal and fall after fasting should be kept in mind.

LIVER FUNCTION TESTS (LFTs)

In Normal Pregnancy

- ALT, AST and γ-glutamyl transpeptidase is reduced by 20% in later pregnancy
- Total and free bilirubin is also lower during all 3 trimesters
- Conjugated bilirubin is lower in 2nd and 3rd trimester.

LFTs in ICP

- ALT (SGPT) → most sensitive marker (↑ by 2-10 fold)
- ↑ AST (SGOT)
- Bilirubin → usually normal. If raised, it tends to be a conjugated hyperbilirubinemia
- GGT normal or raised
- Alkaline phosphatase may ↑(has limited diagnostic value due to ↑ production by placenta
- Glutathione S-transferase alpha (GSTA) is a phase II detoxification enzyme—considered to be more sensitive and specific marker of hepatic integrity than standard LFT
- Some women will have itching days or weeks before the appearance of abnormal LFT, therefore LFT should be repeated every 1-2 weeks
- LFTs may increase in the first 10 days of the puerperium, therefore should be deferred for atleast 10 days postnatally.

3. **What is Asymptomatic hypercholanemia of pregnancy (AHP)?**

   AHP
   - Raised serum bile acids in the absence of symptoms and other biochemical markers of ICP
   - It has:
     - ↑ CA
     - Unchanged CDCA
   - Affects ≈ 10% of pregnancies
   - 2-3% of patients with AHP during 2nd trimester subsequently develop ICP.

URINE ROUTINE/MICROSCOPY

- ↑ excretion of total bile acids
- 10-100-fold ↑ in CA and CDCA
- ↓ excretion of DCA and LCA.

USG

- Features of cholelithiasis
- In ICP, the intrahepatic bile ducts appear normal
- Fasting and ejection volumes of gallbladder are greater, predisposing these women to formation of gallstones.

4. **Possible etiology of complications.**

   Fetal

   MSAF
   - Bile acids are known to cause an increase in colonic motility → fetal distress and subsequent meconium passage.

   CTG abnormalities
   - ↑ levels of bile acids are responsible.

   Spontaneous preterm labor
   - Myometrium of ICP patients may be more responsive to effects of oxytocin.

   RDS
   Main cause → Bile acid
   - Aspiration
   - Accumulation within fetal circulation
   - Cause severe chemical pneumonitis and pulmonary edema
   - May lead to atelectasis, eosinophilic infiltration and formation of hyaline membrane when injected intra-tracheally (can be reversed by administration of surfactant)
   - Cause a reversal of action of phospholipase A_2 → degradation of phosphatidylcholine and lack of surfactant.

   IUD
   - Presence of meconium containing ↑ levels of bile acids, in almost all cases of ICP associated stillbirths
   - Meconium penetrates deep into placental and umbilical cord tissue in < 3 hrs and can cause vasoconstriction of the placental and umbilical vessels
   - *Bile acids cause vasoconstriction of placental chorionic vessels → IUD.*

   Maternal

   Estrogen and progesterone
   - ICP occurs mainly during the 3rd trimester, when serum concentrations of estrogen and progesterone reach their peak
   - More common in twin gestations.

   Genetic factors
   Evidence suggests their role:
   - This explains familial cases
   - Higher incidence in some ethnic groups
   - High rate of recurrence of ICP in subsequent pregnancies and the susceptibility of affected women to progesterone.

MANAGEMENT OF ICP

Treatment Options

Fetal Monitoring

- Fetal surveillance (CTG, fetal movement count) do not actually prevent IUD.

Elective Delivery

- Few studies report good outcome with induction of labor at 37-38 weeks. There is increased risk of RDS if iatrogenic delivery is anticipated at 37 weeks with either induction of labor or elective cesarean section.

Drugs

Ursodeoxycholic acid
- Naturally occurring hydrophilic bile acid
- Constitutes < 3% of the physiological bile acid pool in humans
- Has antiapoptotic effects and has been shown to reduce the mitochondrial membrane permeability to ions and cytochrome c expression
- UDCA lowers serum levels of ethinyl-estradiol 17β-glucuronide, a major cholestatic metabolite of estrogen
- UDCA 300mg BD show significant reduction in pruritis and LFTs, including bile acids, compared to baseline
- Results in normalization of CA:CDCA and glycine: taurine ratios and a reduction in urinary excretion of sulfated progesterone metabolites
- Does not harm the fetus
- UDCA treatment has been shown to reduce the bile acid level in cord blood, amniotic fluid and colostrum and it reduced cord blood bilirubin levels in one study
- Levels of bile acids in meconium is considerably elevated in ICP and this is not influenced by treatment with UDCA.

Dexamethasone
- Conflicting reports of efficacy and there are concerns over safety
- It inhibits placental estrogen synthesis by reducing secretion of the precursor, dehydroepiandrosterone sulphate, from the fetal adrenal glands
- It has been widely used to promote fetal lung maturity but it crosses the placenta and repeated high doses are associated with decreased birth weight and abnormal neuronal development.

Rifampicin
- Rifampicin has been used with success in liver diseases, including gallstones and primary biliary cirrhosis where it has significantly reduced serum levels of transaminases and total bile acids with improvement of pruritis
- But no studies have been published in context of ICP.

Vitamin K
- No studies to support the use of vitamin K in ICP
- Few clinicians opt to treat women with oral vitamin K to guard against the theoretical risk of fetal antepartum and maternal intra and postpartum hemorrhage.

S-Adenosyl–L-methionine (SAMe)
- SAMe is the principal methyl group donor involved in the synthesis of phosphatidlycholine and therefore it influences the composition and fluidity of hepatic membranes and hence biliary excretion of hormone metabolites
- It reverses estrogen induced impairment of bile flow
- In few studies, SAMe was shown to prevent ethinylestradiol induced elevations in AST/ALT, bile acids and bilirubin
- It reduces pruritis and biochemical parameters but is more efficacious when used together with UDCA
- Some patients have reported problems with peripheral veins following prolonged intravenous administration. No other adverse maternal and fetal effects have been reported and SAMe seems to be well tolerated.

Cholestyramine
- Cholestyramine, an anion exchange resin which acts by binding bile acids in the gut, thereby inhibiting the enterohepatic circulation and increasing fecal excretion of bile acids
- But it has no effect on serum bile acid levels or other biochemical markers of cholestasis
- Further, it may reduce the intestinal absorption of fat soluble vitamins, thus depleting the levels of vitamin K and increasing the risk of hemorrhage for the mother and the fetus.

Guar gum
- It is a dietary fibre that acts in a similar manner to cholestyramine
- RCTs have shown that guar gum is no more effective in improving pruritis or reducing serum bile acids.

Activated charcoal
- Though per oral activated charcoal reduces serum bile acids but fails to improve symptoms.

Menthol
- Topical treatment with aqueous cream with 2% menthol is of value in the relief of pruritis but does not improve biochemical abnormalities.

Prognosis

- Most women have no lasting hepatic damage but ICP recurs in the majority of cases, with variations in intensity in subsequent pregnancies
- Recurrence is less likely following multiple pregnancy
- Women with the history of ICP may also develop symptoms if taking the combined COCs or in second half of menstrual cycle
- Long term follow up studies have shown an increased risk of gallstones, non alcoholic cirrhosis and pancreatitis, Hep C and autoimmune hepatitis.

HEPATITIS

World Hepatitis Day—July 28 every year.
Aims to raise global awareness of hepatitis B and hepatitis C and encourage prevention, diagnosis and treatment. It is one of the only four disease awareness days recognized by the World Health Organization.

Clinical and epidemiologic features of viral hepatitis					
Features	HAV	HBV	HCV	HDV	HEV
Incubation period (days)	15-45	30-180	15-160	30-180	14-60
Age	Children/young adults	Young adults	Any age but more in adults	Any age	Young adults
Transmission					
Fecal-oral	+++	---	---	---	+++
Percutaneous	Unusual	+++	+++	+++	---
Perinatal	---	+++	+	+	+
Sexual	+	++	+	++	---
Clinical					
Severity	Mild	Mild/severe	Moderate	Mild/severe	Mild
Fulminant	0.1%	0.1%-1%	0.1%	5-20%	1-2%
Becomes chronic	No	In 1-10%	In 50-70%	Common	No
Carrier	None	0.1-30%	1.5-3.2%	Variable	None
Cancer	None	Present	Present	Variable	None
Prognosis	Excellent	Worse with age	Moderate	Acute: good Chronic: poor	Good
Prophylaxis	IgG vaccine	HBIG Recombinant vaccine	None	-	Unknown

Hepatitis A

- Picornavirus
- Single stranded, 27 nm, RNA virus
- There is only 1 serotype of the virus
- Clinical symptoms:
  - Incubation period: 2-6 weeks
  - Active disease: usually last for 40-50 days or even longer
  - Symptoms:
    - Fatigue
    - Fever
    - Nausea
    - Appetite loss
    - Jaundice
    - Dark urine
    - Clay-colored feces
- Detection
  - IgM anti-HAV antibodies in the blood → detectable from one to two weeks after the initial infection and persists for up to 14 weeks
  - IgG anti HAV antibodies → after 35-40 days → persist lifelong (indicates that the person is immune)
  - ALT—↑↑ (during acute phase)

- Treatment

  Prophylaxis

  Vaccination
  - Invented by Maurice Hilleman at Merck
  - Protection against the virus in > 95% of cases (for at least fifteen years)
  - 2 types:
    - 1st—contains inactivated Hepatitis A virus
    - 2nd—contains a live but attenuated virus
    - Injectable vaccine:
      - Initial dose provides protection starting two to four weeks after vaccination
      - Second booster dose, given 6-12 months later, provides protection for >15-20 years.

Good hygiene

Proper sanitation.

Treatment proper
- Rest
- Hydration
- Avoid fatty food
- If exposed recently—give immunoprophylaxis
  - IG 0.02 mL/kg IM → single dose (within 2 weeks of exposure)
    +
  - Hep. A (formalin inactivated) virus vaccine
  - Though produced from inactivated virus → safety still not determined
- Breastfeeding is not contraindicated with HAV with proper hygiene.

Hepatitis B

Viral markers in hepatitis B infection
Sequence in which they appear:
HbsAg → HbeAg → Anti HbcAg (IgM) → Anti HbeAg → Disappearance of HbsAg → Appearance of anti HbsAg.

HbsAg

- Comes before ↑ in transaminases and clinical symptoms
- Remain till end of icteric phase (from 2-6 months)
- Indicates that the person is infected
- It may be:
  - Acute disease
  - Chronic disease
  - Carrier state.

HbcAg

- Hidden component of viral core
- Not detectable at all.

HbeAg

- Denotes high infectivity
- Active disease.

Anti HbeAg

- Low infectivity.

Anti HbcAg

- 1st antibody to appear after an acute (or recent) infection
- Persists in serum even during recovery phase
  - When acute, antibody is of IgM type → remains for 6 months
  - When chronic, antibody is of IgG type → lifelong.

Anti HbsAg

- With its appearance, HbsAg antigen disappears from serum
- There is a gap of several weeks
- It means patient is immune (with immunization antibody develops and HbsAg disappears)
- Patient is protected
  - Anti HbsAg means → good immunity and protection against Hep. B
- **Window period:** Period during recovery phase when both of these are negative and diagnosis may be missed if test includes only HbsAg and anti HbsAg.

Hepatitis B Viral DNA

- Refers to a test to detect the presence of Hepatitis B virus DNA in a person's blood
- A positive test means:
  - The virus is multiplying in a person's body and he or she is highly contagious and can pass the virus to others
  - If a person has a chronic Hepatitis B virus infection, the presence of viral DNA means that a person is possibly at increased risk for liver damage
- This test is also used to monitor the effectiveness of drug therapy for chronic Hepatitis B virus infection.

Hepatitis B Infection

The virus

- Has a circular genome of partially double-stranded DNA
- Virus replicates through an RNA intermediate form by reverse transcription, which relates them to retroviruses
- Although replication takes place in the liver, the virus spreads to the blood where viral proteins and antibodies against them are found in infected people
- The hepatitis B virus is 50 to 100 times more infectious than HIV
- Has 4 proteins:
  - Surface protein → HbsAg
  - Core protein → HbcAg and HbeAg
  - DNA polymerase
  - X protein

Risk factors

- Those with HCV or HIV
- Received treatment for STD
- Requires immunosuppressive therapy

- Having multiple sexual partners
- Born in an endemic area but has not received vaccination for hepatitis B during the 1st year of life
- IV drug users
- Pregnant females
- Hepatitis B positive sex partner.

Course of HBV

Depends on age at which infection is acquired:
- Vertical transmission → 90% case of chronic infection
- Horizontal transmission (7-12 months) → 40% case of chronic infection
- 1-3 years → 10-20% case of chronic infection
- Adults → Clear HBV by 6 months
  - Few carry for lifetime in inactive state but there can be acute exacerbations.

Risk of Transmission in Different Trimesters

- Risk of transmission increases as the gestational age increases with maximum risk of exposure when baby comes in contact with the infected maternal blood during delivery
- The risk of transmission of hepatitis B associated with amniocentesis is low
- In utero infection is uncommon, (no more than 5 percent of perinatal HBV infections)
- The following factors may be associated with antepartum infection:
  - HBeAg positive
  - Preterm labor
  - High HBsAg and HBV DNA titers
- Risk of transmission is same for both vaginal and cesarean delivery.

Course and prognosis is NOT altered by pregnancy.

The Vaccine

- Recombinant vaccine (1986)
- Is developed by inserting the HBV gene that codes for the surface protein into a species of yeast called Saccharomyces cerevisiae
- The yeast then produces only the noninfectious surface protein, without any danger of introducing actual viral DNA into the final product.

Available as

- HBV Recombinant (alone)
- HBV in combination with Hemophilus influenzae type b (Hib) vaccine
- HBV in combination with DTaP (Diphtheria-Tetanus-acellular Pertussis) and inactivated polio vaccines
- HBV in combination with hepatitis A (HAV) vaccine.

Response to Vaccination

- Give primary course of 3 doses at 0,1 and 6 months intramuscularly
- Check anti Hbs antibody levels in blood after 1-4 months

- Levels:
  - >100 mIU/mL → full response (seen in 85-90% of cases)
  - Between 10-100 mIU/mL → poor response → give single booster dose now and no further testing is required
  - Levels <10 mIU/mL → no response → check whether having acute or chronic infection (i.e. present or past infection with hepatitis B virus) → again repeat the 3 doses and test levels after 1-4 months → if still no response, either give higher dose of the vaccine or give intradermal injection.

Duration of Protection

- Indefinite and is safe.

Management

General Overview

Acute infection:
- Does not usually require treatment because most adults clear the infection spontaneously
- Early antiviral treatment may be required in <1% of people, whose infection takes a very aggressive course (fulminant hepatitis) or who are immunocompromised.

Chronic infection:
- May be necessary to reduce the risk of cirrhosis and liver cancer
- Candidates for therapy:
  - Those with persistently elevated serum alanine aminotransferase, a marker of liver damage
  - High HBV DNA levels
  - Treatment lasts from six months to a year, depending on medication and genotype
- HBV infection in pregnancy does not increase the risk of maternal or fetal mortality.

Mother

- Routine prenatal screening of all pregnant women is recommended regardless of previous hepatitis B vaccination or previous negative HBsAg test results, at the 1st prenatal visit
- Vaccination, if mother at risk regardless of HBsAg status
- Dose: 3 doses total → at 0, 1 and 6 months
- Management of chronic HBV infection:
  - Telbivudine and tenofovir are pregnancy category B medications, approved by FDA
  - Entecavir, lamivudine and adefovir as category C medications
  - Interferon has been classified as category X
- The advantages of antiviral therapy during pregnancy include:
  - Potent antiviral suppression
  - Relative safety and tolerability in pregnancy
  - Reduction in perinatal HBV transmission
- Disadvantages include:
  - Risk of developing antiviral resistance in the mother depending on the antiviral agent used
  - Contraindication to breastfeeding
  - Risk of hepatitis flares upon discontinuation of therapy [threefold increase in alanine amino transferase (ALT)]
- Acute infection:
  - Hospitalization, if signs of liver decompensation are present

- For HBsAg positive carriers who develop active liver disease during pregnancy, early treatment (starting in the 1st trimester) may be considered
- Tenofovir would be preferable due to overall safety and its very low risk of antiviral resistance
- Chronic infection:
  - Ideally HBV DNA levels and ALT should be measured in all HbsAg positive women at the end of 2nd trimester (28-30 weeks)
  - If ALT and HBV DNA (titers < 10^7 IU/mL) are not high:
    - Vaccination and Immunoglobulin at birth to the baby → monitor maternal postpartum flares (HBV DNA and ALT every 1-2 months × 3) → Check baby for HbsAg and HBs Ab at 9-18 months
  - If high ALT and HBV DNA titers >10^7 IU/mL
    - Consider early treatment with antiviral drugs starting at 32 weeks → discontinue treatment at the time of delivery → vaccination and IG at birth to the baby → monitor maternal flare up postpartum → Check baby for HbsAg and HBs Ab at 9-18 months.

Baby

CDC vaccination schedule for HBV

Maternal status—Positive

- Hepatitis B immunoglobulin (HBIG) and HBV vaccine within 12 hours of birth (WHO recommends the 1st dose be given within 24 hours)
- All 3 doses should be completed by 6 months of age
- Between 9-18 months of age, child should be tested for anti Hbs and HbsAg to look for response and to exclude perinatal infection
- Infants with anti-HBs levels <10 mIU/mL should be revaccinated with a 2nd three-dose vaccine series and then retested for anti-HBs one to two months after completion of the series
- When birth weight of the baby is <2000 gm, give birth dose, but do not count as part of the three-dose series, and give next dose at one month of age (will receive four total doses).

Maternal status—Negative

- First HBV vaccine should be given before hospital discharge in full term infants, and one month after birth or at hospital discharge in pre term infants.

Unknown maternal status

- Infants should receive hepatitis B vaccine within 12 hours of birth, followed by hepatitis B immune globulin as soon as possible (but not later than 7 days after birth) if the mother tests positive for HbsAg.

Breastfeeding is not contraindicated in those chronically infected with hepatitis B if the infant receives HBIG passive prophylaxis and vaccine active prophylaxis, as per American academy of pediatrics recommendations.

But as per WHO guidelines, breastfeeding can be continued even in infants in endemic areas where vaccination may not be readily available, owing to high antiviral properties and other benefits of breastmilk.

Hepatitis C

The Virus

- Size → 55–65 nm
- Enveloped, single-stranded RNA virus

- Genus Hepacivirus
- Family Flaviviridae
- Virus particle consists of a:
  - Core of RNA
  - Surrounded by an icosahedral protective shell of protein
  - Which is further encased in a lipid envelope of cellular origin
- Two viral envelope glycoproteins, E_1 and E_2, are embedded in the lipid envelope.

Risk of Transmission (Cochrane 2010)

- In case of chronic infection → pregnancy is not contraindicated as ≈5% of pregnant women with chronic HCV infection will transmit the virus to their infants
- Rate is 1.7%, if the mother is positive for HCV antibody but is HCV RNA negative
- If mother is an IV drug user or is HIV positive, the risk is as high as 19- 25%
- Currently, there are no specific interventions known to decrease perinatal transmission
- Studies have shown that paternal exposure to ribavirin–interferon alpha 2B has no adverse effects on reproduction and if an unexpected pregnancy occurs while father on treatment, there is NO indication for termination of pregnancy
- Amniocentesis or fetal scalp pH is contraindicated (promotes mixing of fetal and maternal blood)
- Though maximum transmission is during delivery, its mode can be any (vaginal or cesarean) but definitely avoiding prolonged rupture of membranes
- Cesarean section → only for obstetric indications.

Screening

- Routine screening is not recommended
- Screen the following high risk woman so that antiviral therapy can be started in postpartum period:
  - Previous or current IV drug use
  - Being sexual partner of IV drug user
  - Those who received blood transfusions before 1990 in developed countries or at any time in developing countries
  - Patients with unexplained elevated aminotransferase levels
  - Patients who have undergone organ or tissue transplantation from unscreened donors
  - Those who are HIV positive
- Before adolescence, the infection is transmitted almost exclusively by perinatal exposure.

Management

Mother
- Treatment of chronic HCV infection before getting pregnant definitely lowers the risk of transmission but is only indicated in presence of other indications for therapy
- Can be given if the woman is not an IV drug user at present and is ready for effective birth control measures
- There is no safe treatment in pregnancy
- Successful treatment is possible with pegylated interferon and ribavirin but both are contraindicated in pregnancy.

Newborn
If child is born to HCV infected woman
- There is no need to isolate the child in NICU as blood is the main source of transmission (saliva, urine and stool is not harmful)
- Single HCV RNA test (very sensitive and specific but expensive) at 2 months of age can be done, though earlier detection is very unlikely to alter the course of management
  - If test is positive:
    - HCV RNA and aminotransferase levels every six months to determine whether chronic infection or spontaneous clearance will ensue
    - In such cases, Hepatitis B vaccine can also be given at birth or within 1 month and Hepatitis A vaccine at 1 year of age, to avoid concurrent infections with these, which may prove even more fatal
  - If test is negative:
    - Serology should be performed at 12-18 months of age to confirm seroreversion (test of choice)
  - Though not being contagious, children with chronic HCV infection should be followed up, as few of them may develop progressive liver disease and there is a risk of hepatocellular carcinoma
  - Spontaneous clearance will occur in 25% of children
- Breastfeeding is allowed (viral load is low)
- HCV serology is not reliable during infancy because passively transferred maternal IgG antibody may persist for up to 18 months
- But if serology is positive after 18 months of age, it means infection is from the mother
- No vaccine is available.

Hepatitis D

- Hepatitis delta virus
- Single stranded circular RNA virus
- The HDV is a small, spherical virus with a 36 nm diameter
- It has an outer coat containing three HBV envelope proteins (called large, medium, and small hepatitis B surface antigens), and host lipids surrounding an inner nucleocapsid
- Depends upon presence of HBV for replication
- When HBV and HDV both are present → the severity is much increased
- Risk to infant → same as with HBV
- The vaccine for hepatitis B protects against hepatitis D virus because of the latter's dependence on the presence of hepatitis B virus for it to replicate.

Hepatitis E

- Single-stranded RNA icosahedral virus with a 7.5 kilobase genome
- Infection with this virus was first documented in 1955 during an outbreak in New Delhi, India
- Hepatitis E virus infection occurs in non-industrialized nations, usually as an epidemic disease during the monsoon season in central and south Asia and India
- Severity and fatality rate increased → 15-25% especially in 3rd trimester
- Non enveloped single stranded RNA
- Fetus is adversely affected:
  - Abortion
  - Stillbirth
  - Death

- Check IgM anti HEV antibodies
- IG to mother may reduce infection
- Prevention:
  Proper sanitation
  - Proper disposal of human waste
  - Safe drinking water
  - Personal hygiene

  Vaccine
  - A vaccine based on recombinant viral proteins was developed in the 1990s, was tested and appeared to be effective and safe, but development stopped for economical reasons, since hepatitis E is rare in developed countries
  - Recently, a vaccine—called HEV 239 is developed in 2012 and is being sold as 'Hecolin' in China
  - It has already been approved by Chinese Ministry of food and technology
  - Worldwide, it is not available
- Breastfeeding
  - Although anti-HEV antibody and HEV-RNA are present in the colostrum of HEV infected mothers, breast-feeding appears to be safe for these infants, reported by a study done in 2004, but needs further confirmation.

Simplified diagnostic approach in patients presenting with acute hepatitis				
Diagnosis	HbsAg	IgM anti HAV	IgM Anti Hbc	Anti HCV
Acute hep B	+		+	
Chronic hep B	+			
Acute hep A superimposed on chronic hep B	+	+		
Acute hep A and B	+	+	+	
Acute hep A and B (HbsAg below detection threshold)			+	
Acute hep C				+

Case: A 32 yr old woman, at 34 weeks gestation, is feeling unwell since past 24 hours. She has headache and has noticed odd visual symptoms such as wobbling of objects. She has epigastric discomfort and nausea. Her legs are swollen for some weeks but now her hands and face are puffy. Fetal movements are normal, there is no lower abdominal pain and no bleeding or abnormal discharge. She is a booked patient.

BP: 140/85 mmHg;   Hb: 9.3g/dL;   Platelets: 97000/mm^3; ALT 172 IU/L
PR: 98/min   AlkPO$_4$: 238 IU/L;   Bilirubin: 37 µmol/L
Fundus normal/normal patellar reflexes   Albumin 26   Urine albumin: 1+

PA: mild right upper quadrant and epigastric tenderness
Uterus is non tender, SFH 33cm, cephalic presentation
What is your likely diagnosis?

Diagnosis: HELLP
Weinstein named it as HELLP in 1982.

Important Points
- Incidence—0.2-0.9% of all pregnancies and 10-20% of cases with severe preeclampsia
- 2/3rd—antepartum (70%)
  - Peak frequency between 27th – 37th week
  - 10% occur before the 27th week
  - 20% occur after 37th week
- Excessive weight gain and generalized edema precede the syndrome in >50% of cases
- Positive D dimer (subclinical coagulopathy) → Preeclampsia patients at high risk of developing HELLP
- Patients may not have preeclampsia → not necessary for diagnosis of HELLP
- Oozing from operative site → very common
- To reduce risk of hematoma formation → bladder flap left open → subfascial drain x 24-48 hours.

HELLP

Hemolysis →↓ Hb → Microangiopathic hemolytic anemia →↑ LDH

- Liberated hemoglobin is converted to unconjugated bilirubin in the spleen or may be bound in the plasma by haptoglobin
- The hemoglobin-haptoglobin complex is cleared quickly by the liver → low or undetectable haptoglobin levels in the blood
- Low haptoglobin concentration (<1 g/L – < 0.4 g/L) is the preferred marker of hemolysis and can be used for diagnosis
- Therefore, for diagnosis:
  - ↑LDH
  - Presence of unconjugated bilirubin
  - Low or undetectable haptoglobin (more specific indicator)

  Peripheral smear:
  - Schizocytes-fragmented red cells
  - Burr cells → contracted red cells with spicula
  - Echinocytes.

Liver

- Primary target organ
- Periportal or focal parenchymal necrosis
- ↑ AST and ALT → mark liver injury.

Thrombocytopenia

- Vascular endothelial damage and prostacyclin deficiency →↑ platelet agglutination
  - ↑ Thromboxane A_2
    ↓   → Thrombocytopenia (<150·10^9/L)
  - ↑ Platelet aggregation
- Decreased PLT count
- Therefore, thrombocytopenia is due to increased consumption and increased turnover with shorter lifespan.

Clinical Symptoms

- Right upper abdominal (fluctuating, colic like), quadrant or epigastric pain
- Nausea and vomiting
- History of malaise some days before presentation
- Headache in 30-60%
- Visual symptoms in 20%
- Might have unspecific symptoms or subtle signs of preeclampsia or non-specific viral syndrome-like symptoms
- Also characterized by exacerbation during the night and recovery during the day.

Diagnostic Criteria

Mainly 2

I. *Tennessee Classification System by Sibai*
   True or Complete HELLP has been proposed by:
   - Abnormal peripheral blood smear
   - ↑ s. bilirubin (≥ 1.2 mg/100 mL)
   - ↑ LDH (> 600 Units/L)
   - ↓ Platelets (100000/mm^3)
   - ↑ AST (≥ 70 IU/L).
II. *The Mississippi-Triple Class System*

Class 1

- Platelets ≤ 50000/mm^3
- AST or ALT ≥ 70 IU/L
- LDH ≥ 600 IU/L

Class 2

- Platelets ≤ 100000 but ≥ 50000/mm^3
- AST or ALT ≥ 70 IU/L
- LDH ≥ 600 IU/L

Class 3

- Platelets ≤ 1,50000 but ≥ 100000/mm^3
- AST or ALT ≥ 40 IU/L
- LDH ≥ 600 IU/L
- This class is a clinically significant transition stage which has the ability to progress.

5. **How will you classify this patient?**
   Based on number of abnormalities present:
   - When 1 or 2 abnormalities present → partial or incomplete HELLP
   - When all 3 present → full or complete HELLP.

6. **Can HELLP recur in future pregnancy?**
   - Recurrence rate → 2-19%.

7. **What are the general guidelines in treatment of HELLP syndrome?**
   1. Platelet count and LDH levels → Best markers to follow disease progression
   2. Class I/II
      OR   → High dose   - Arrest progression
      Class III with symptoms   parenteral corticosteroids   - Improve biochemical parameters
      of impending eclampsia   - ↓ transfusion rates
   3. Mississippi protocol:
      Dexamethasone IV 10mg BD → antepartum HELLP
      Dexa IV 10 mg (2 doses 12 hourly)
      followed by   → Postpartum
      Dexa IV 5 mg (2 doses 12 hourly)
          +
      Give:
      - IV fluids
      - Antihypertensives
      - Prophylactic anticonvulsants.

      Note: Recently, betamethasone, instead of dexamethasone, has been recommended as a drug of choice for promotion of fetal lung maturation in preterm delivery, as betamethasone is associated with decreased rates of intraventricular hemorrhage and cerebral palsy and is more protective to the brain.

      But there is evidence from randomized controlled trials, that glucocorticoids which do not cross the placenta (such as prednisolone or dexamethasone) induce clinical and biochemical remission of HELLP syndrome and prolong pregnancy. A Cochrane review of the evidence, however, suggests, as yet, there is insufficient data to make one superior to the other.
   4. Termination according to:
      - Gestation
      - Favorability of cervix (Bishop score)
      - Severity of disease.

   Delivery → Definitive treatment

   HELLP per se is NOT an indication for immediate cesarean section:
   1. <30-32 weeks and those with oligohydramnios and/or unfavorable Bishop score:
          ↓
      Cesarean section (give GA)
      - Delay delivery for 6 hours and give aggressive steroid therapy, if possible
      - If not possible to delay and platelet count < 40,000/mm^3 → give 6-10 units platelets before intubation
   2. >32 weeks → Induction and vaginal delivery (continue steroid treatment)
   3. No DIC   - Give 2 doses of steroids
      Absent fetal lung maturity   - Intense monitoring
   4. Pudendal block or epidural anesthesia (platelet count <75,000/mm^3) → contraindicated because of risk of bleeding in these areas
   5. BP should be kept below 155/105 mmHg.

Platelet Therapy for HELLP Syndrome

- If platelet count is >50,000/mm^3 and no active bleeding or platelet dysfunction, prophylactic transfusion is not recommended even prior to cesarean section
- Platelet transfusion is strongly recommended prior to delivery (vaginal or cesarean), when platelet count is <20,000/mm^3

- Steroids can be administered with a platelet count < 50000 mm^3
- No recommendation regarding the usefulness of plasma exchange or plasmapheresis
- Only in women who demonstrate progressive elevation of bilirubin or creatinine for >72 hours after delivery may benefit from plasma exchange with fresh frozen plasma.

Postpartum

- Maternal platelet counts continue to decrease immediately post-partum but start increasing on the third day
- Risk of renal failure and pulmonary edema is significantly increased
- 1/3rd ($\approx$ 30%) cases develop postpartum, mainly within 48 hours (up to 6 days)
- There is conflicting evidence regarding postpartum administration of corticosteroids, with most studies highly advocating its use for speedy recovery (10 mg of dexamethasone every 12 hours) while one randomized trial not supporting.

ACUTE FATTY LIVER OF PREGNANCY

- More common in nulliparas
- More common in those who have male fetus or twins
- $\approx$ 50% → have signs of preeclampsia
- Liver normal or small
- Presence of hypoglycemia and increased prothrombin time (PT) differentiates it from HELLP
- A rare life-threatening complication of pregnancy
- Occurs in 1 in 7000–15000 pregnancies
- Also called hepatic lipidosis of pregnancy
- The disease was first described in 1940 by H.L. Sheehan as an "acute yellow atrophy" of the liver
- Occurs in the third trimester or the immediate period after delivery
- Cause: Disordered metabolism of fatty acids by mitochondria in the mother, caused by deficiency in the LCHAD (long-chain 3-hydroxyacyl-coenzyme A dehydrogenase) enzyme
- Intravenous fluids, blood products and an early delivery has improved prognosis
- Understanding the disease:
  - Deficiency of LCHAD (3-hydroxyacyl-CoA dehydrogenase) enzyme in fetus → accumulation of unmetabolized medium and long chain fatty acids in fetus → these will re-enter the maternal circulation through the placenta → overwhelm the beta-oxidation enzymes of the mother → triglycerides accumulates within maternal hepatocytes → impaired function → liver failure in mother
- Understanding LCHAD:
  - Mutations in the HADHA gene → inadequate levels of enzyme "long-chain 3-hydroxyacyl-coenzyme A (CoA) dehydrogenase" (which is part of a protein complex known as mitochondrial trifunctional protein) → Long-chain fatty acids from food and body fat will not be metabolized and processed → these fatty acids are not converted to energy → this leads to characteristic features of this disorder, such as lethargy and hypoglycemia → Long-chain fatty acids or partially metabolized fatty acids may build up in tissues → damage the liver, heart, retina, and muscles, causing more serious complications
- The gene responsible for LCHAD has been isolated, and the most common mutation found in acute fatty liver of pregnancy is the E474Q missense mutation
- LCHAD deficiency is autosomal recessive in inheritance and mothers are often found to be heterozygous and the fetus, homozygous for the mutation.

Clinical Signs and Symptoms

Usually manifests in the 3rd trimester (34th -36th) of pregnancy, but may occur any time in the second half of pregnancy, or in the puerperium.

Symptoms are usually non specific:
- Nausea
- Vomiting
- Anorexia
- Abdominal pain
- Jaundice and fever may occur in as many as 70% of patients
- Preeclampsia occurs in more severe disease
- Other systems may get involved and manifest as:
  - Acute renal failure
  - Hepatic encephalopathy
  - Pancreatitis
  - Diabetes insipidus (though uncommon).

Lab Abnormalities

- AST/ALT up to 1000 IU/L (usually 300-500)
- Bilirubin ↑↑
- Alkaline phosphatase ↑↑
- ↑ WBCs
- Hypoglycemia
- ↑ INR
- ↓ fibrinogen
- Frank DIC may occur in as many as 70% of patients.

Other Findings

- Fat deposition in the liver
- Microvesicular steatosis
- Rarely, rupture or necrosis of the liver.

Diagnosis

- Very important to differentiate it from other conditions (mentioned earlier)
- Diagnosis is usually made on clinical grounds
- Definitive diagnosis: Liver biopsy (but not done in pregnancy owing to ↑ chances of bleeding in pregnancy).

Treatment

- Admission to ICU
- Intravenous fluids, intravenous glucose and blood products, including fresh frozen plasma and cryoprecipitate to correct DIC
- Fetus → NST
- Delivery anticipated after stabilizing the mother, often vaginal but in cases of severe hemorrhage → cesarean section
- Mortality is reduced to 18%.

8. **Other uncommon conditions occurring during pregnancy, mimicking HELLP**
   Uncommon conditions mimicking HELLP in pregnancy are as follows:

Thrombotic Thrombocytopenic Purpura (TTP)

- Disorder of vessel wall
- Lesions in arteriolar walls in various organs
- Formation of localized platelet thrombi and fibrin deposits at various sites.

Clinical PENTAD of TTP + Normal Coagulation Tests → Pathognomonic of TTP

   I. Microangiopathic hemolytic anemia (Coombs negative)
      - Hemolysis
      - Fragmentation of RBCs
      - ↑ LDH
  II. Thrombocytopenia
 III. Decreased renal function → deposits in renal vasculature
  IV. Disturbed neurological function
      Diffuse and non-focal
      - Headache to visual disturbances
      - Confusion
      - Aphasia
      - Transient paresis
      - Alteration in consciousness
      - Seizures
   V. Fever.

Hemolytic Uremic Syndrome (HUS)

- Vessel wall disorder
- Deposition of localized platelets and thrombi within renal vasculature
- Strongly suspected when:
  - Anemia (Microangiopathic hemolytic anemia)
  - Bleeding (↓ platelets)
  - Renal failure:
    - ↓ Urine output
    - Hyperkalemia
    - Hypertension
- Develops usually in the post-partum period
- Etiology (in children and adolescents): Diarrheal disease
  - E.coli
  - Shigella or
  - Salmonella.

Idiopathic Thrombocytopenic Purpura (ITP)

- A clinical syndrome with thrombocytopenia (which may be manifested as a bleeding disorder with purpura and petechiae)
- Pregnancy has no effect on it (neither does it increases the incidence nor exacerbates a preexisting disease)
- No maternal or fetal morbidity noted, even in cases of very low platelet count.

Systemic Lupus Erythematosus (SLE)

- Autoimmune disorder
- Characterized by deposits of antigen-antibody complexes in capillaries
- SLE may affect multiple organ systems (kidneys, lungs, heart, liver and brain)
- Antiphospholipid antibodies → present in 30-40% of the cases
- Thrombocytopenia occurs in 40-50%
- Hemolytic anemia in 14-23%
- Cerebral lesions and symptoms may develop because of vasculitis and/or cerebro-vascular occlusion that might lead to seizures.

Folate Deficiency

- Common in pregnancy
- Its progression to megaloblastosis is rare
- Hemolytic anemia, thrombocytopenia, and coagulopathy due to folate deficiency may mimic the incomplete HELLP syndrome.

If occurs earlier → Anti phospholipid antibody syndrome has to be excluded.

SUGGESTED READING

1. Ashok Kumar, K Aparna Sharma, RK Gupta, et al. Prevalence and risk factors for hepatitis C virus among pregnant women, Indian J Med Res. 126, September 2007, pp. 211-5.
2. Kjell Haram, Einar Svendsen, Ulrich Abildgaard3: The HELLP syndrome: Clinical issues and management. A Review, BMC Pregnancy and Childbirth. 2009;9:8.
3. Kumaresan Yogeswaran, Scott K Fung. Chronic hepatitis B in pregnancy: unique challenges and opportunities, The Korean Journal of Hepatology. 2011;17:1-8.
4. McIntyre PG, Tosh K, McGuire W. Cesarean section versus vaginal delivery for preventing mother to infant hepatitis C virus transmission (Review), Issue 6, The Cochrane Library, 2010.
5. Neha Gami, Seema Singhal, Manju Puri, et al. An approach to diagnosis and management of acute fatty liver of pregnancy. Int J Reprod Contracept Obstet Gynecol. 2013 Mar;2(1):104-8.
6. Nguyet cam vu lam, Patricia B gotsch, Robert C langan. Caring for Pregnant Women and Newborns with Hepatitis B or C, American Family Physician, November 15, 2010;82(10).
7. Rajendra Kumar Jain. Management of Jaundice in Pregnancy, Medicine Update. 2010, Vol. 20.

CHAPTER 22

HIV in Pregnancy

Tania G Singh, Earl Jaspal

HISTORY

Worldwide
1981 AIDS 1st described in USA
1983 HIV 1 discovered
1984 HIV demonstrated to be cause of AIDS
1985 ELISA developed
1986 HIV 2 discovered (Luc Montagnier and Barresinoussi)
1987 Zidovudine found effective in AIDS

India
1986 HIV was 1st described in Chennai (Dr Sunita Solomon)
1992 First National AIDS control programme launched
1992 NACO was established.

Indian Scenario (NACO Annual Report 2010-2011)

- India has the 3rd largest number of people living with HIV/AIDS (≈ 23.9 lakh people)
  - Children < 15 years account for 3.5% of all infections
  - 83 % are in the age group 15-49 years, out of which 39% cases are among women
- Main route of transmission – heterosexual
- Number of new HIV cases has declined by 50% during the last decade
- Estimated adult prevalence was 0.31% in 2009 (Manipur having the highest)
- Number of pregnant women detected HIV positive (2010) – 0.27%.

Routes of Transmission in India (2010-2011)

- Heterosexual 87.4%
- Parent to child 5.4%
- Injecting drug use 1.6%
- Homosexual/bisexual 1.3%
- Blood and blood products 1.0%
- Unknown causes 3.3%.

Perinatal Transmission

- Vertical transmission accounts for most pediatric HIV infections
- Intrapartum transmission can occur:
  - During labor → through maternofetal exchange of blood
  - Delivery → by contact of infant's skin or mucous membrane with infected blood or other maternal secretions.

"At risk" women

- Exchanging sex for money or drugs
- With a history of STD
- A new or multiple sex partners during pregnancy
- Use of illicit drugs
- Sex partners known to be HIV positive or at high risk
- With signs and symptoms of seroconversion
- Injection drug users
- High prevalence geographic areas or healthcare facilities.

Factors which Increase risk of Mother-to-child Transmission

Clinical factors

1. Immunologically or clinically advanced HIV disease in mother
2. High plasma viral load
3. Maternal injectable drug use during pregnancy
4. Preterm delivery
5. Failure to receive antiretroviral therapy
6. Breastfeeding (risk increases if breast abscesses, nipple fissures, mastitis, oral disease in infant e.g. thrush/sores).

Obstetric factors

1. Increases with every hour after membrane rupture → delivery > 4 hours after rupture of membranes can double the risk of HIV transmission
2. Maternal infection with another STD during pregnancy and certain obstetric procedures like:
   - CVS
   - Amniocentesis
   - Invasive fetal intrapartum monitoring
3. Chorioamnionitis.

Progression of Disease and its Clinical Manifestation

There are 4 stages:

Clinical Stage I

- Patient asymptomatic
- Persistent generalized lymphadenopathy.

Clinical Stage II

- Moderate unexplained weight loss (< 10% of presumed or measured body weight)
- Recurrent respiratory tract infections (sinusitis, tonsillitis, otitis media, pharyngitis)
- Herpes zoster
- Angular cheilitis
- Recurrent oral ulceration
- Papular pruritic eruption
- Fungal nail infections
- Seborrheic dermatitis.

Clinical Stage III

- Unexplained severe weight loss (>10% of presumed or measured body weight)
- Unexplained chronic diarrhea for longer than 1 month
- Unexplained persistent fever (intermittent or constant for longer than 1 month)
- Persistent oral candidiasis
- Oral hairy leukoplakia
- Pulmonary tuberculosis
- Severe bacterial infections (such as pneumonia, empyema, pyomyositis, bone or joint infection, meningitis, bacteremia)
- Acute necrotizing ulcerative stomatitis, gingivitis or periodontitis
- Unexplained anemia (< 8 g/dL), neutropenia (< 0.5×10^9/L) and/or chronic thrombocytopenia (< 50×10^9/L).

Clinical Stage IV

- HIV wasting syndrome
- Pneumocystis (jirovecii) pneumonia
- Recurrent severe bacterial pneumonia
- Chronic herpes simplex infection (orolabial, genital or anorectal of > 1 month's duration or visceral at any site)
- Esophageal candidiasis (or candidiasis of trachea, bronchi or lungs)
- Extrapulmonary tuberculosis
- Kaposi sarcoma
- Cytomegalovirus infection (retinitis or infection of other organs)
- Central nervous system toxoplasmosis
- HIV encephalopathy
- Extrapulmonary cryptococcosis, including meningitis
- Disseminated nontuberculous mycobacterial infection
- Progressive multifocal leukoencephalopathy
- Chronic cryptosporidiosis
- Chronic isosporiasis
- Disseminated mycosis (extrapulmonary histoplasmosis, coccidioidomycosis)
- Lymphoma (cerebral or B-cell non-Hodgkin)
- Symptomatic HIV-associated nephropathy or cardiomyopathy
- Recurrent septicemia (including nontyphoidal Salmonella)
- Invasive cervical carcinoma
- Atypical disseminated leishmaniasis.

HIV Testing

There are mainly 3 types of tests available:

Screening Tests
- ELISA
- Rapid tests
- Chemiluminescent immunoassays (CIA).

Confirmatory Tests
- Western blot
- Immunofluorescence assay
- NAAT (PCR)
- Antigen detection.

Monitoring Tests
- Lymphocyte analysis (CD4 count)
- Viral load assays
- Drug resistance tests
- Human leucocyte antigen assays.

Screening Tests

ELISA (the first generation test)
- Most commonly used, simple, relatively inexpensive
- Sensitivity > 99.5%
- Not very specific
- EIA kit contains antigens from both HIV 1 and HIV 2
- False positive results are seen in:
  - Antibodies to class II antigens
  - Autoantibodies
  - Hepatic disease
  - Recent influenza vaccination
  - Acute viral infections
  - In women taking OCPs
  - From laboratory errors of procedure and specimen handling
- Antibodies can be detected 4-12 weeks after infection
- Results available after 2-3 hours
- Becomes positive 3 months post viral transmission
- May be based on different principles:
  - Indirect
  - Competitive
  - Sandwich
  - Ag/Ab capture.

Rapid tests
- Total reaction time < 20 – 25 min
- Sensitivity 100%
- Specificity >99%
- Commonly used rapid test – TRIDOT. Others – OraQuick Advance Rapid HIV1/2; Reveal G-2 Rapid HIV-1 Antibody; Uni-Gold Recombigen HIV etc.

- Useful in situations where immediate results are required, as testing of a source patient after a needle stick injury and for all women with unknown HIV status in labor
- These tests can be carried out with minimal training and do not require expensive laboratory equipment for testing or biohazardous reagent disposal
- *Test Results after Rapid tests*
    - If Rapid test is negative – result is declared
    - If Rapid test is positive – it must be reconfirmed by either ELISA or Western Blot
        - If that is also negative, result is declared
        - If that is positive, either retest to confirm or result is declared
    - If test is discordant, retest after 6 weeks (referral lab.).

Confirmatory Tests

Western Blot (WB)
- 'Gold standard' for confirmation
- Specificity > 99.9%
- Expensive
- Technically more difficult
- Visual interpretation
    - The virus is disrupted and the individual proteins are separated by molecular weight via differential migration on a polyacrylamide gel and blotted onto a membrane support
    - HIV serum antibodies from the patient are allowed to bind to the proteins in the membrane support and patterns of reactivity can be visibly read
    - The three major viral bands for HIV are the core protein p24 and the two envelope proteins gp41 and gp120/160
- Position of band on the strip indicates antigen with which antibody has reacted
- *Test Results after Western Blot* : *can be Positive/Negative/Indeterminate*
    - A positive or reactive WB demonstrates antibody to two of the three major bands
    - If no viral bands are detected, the test is negative
    - A WB in which serum antibodies bind to any other combination of viral bands is considered indeterminate and a follow-up blood specimen should be obtained 1 month later for repeat HIV antibody testing
    - Almost all persons with HIV infection with indeterminate results will develop a positive result when retested one month later
    - Individuals with repeatedly indeterminate results may undergo further testing using NAAT, to help resolve infection status, as the results may be due to cross reaction with other antibodies and may not represent true HIV infection.

Nucleic acid amplification test (NAAT)
- NAAT is used to detect the presence of genetic material (DNA/RNA) of the HIV virus (amplification of nucleic acid)
- Most sensitive and specific test
- It shortens the window period to 12-15 days
- Gold standard for diagnosis in all stages of infection
- Has two forms – DNA PCR and RNA PCR
- DNA and RNA tests for HIV may function as qualitative diagnostic assays that demonstrate infection or quantitative detection systems that measure the level of circulating copies of HIV nucleic acid for prognostic or therapeutic monitoring (viral load tests)
- All initial positive DNA PCR results require confirmation with a second PCR test on a separate specimen.

- Uses:
    1. To detect HIV infection in newborn. HIV antibody tests are not helpful in infants due to the persistence of maternal antibodies for up to the first 15 months of life. Most newborns with HIV infection are identified from birth within a 4-6 week post-partum period using HIV DNA PCR. Some newborns with the infection may not be detected at the time of birth reflecting the different times of their transmission. In utero infection is suspected when a newborn has a detectable DNA PCR result at 48 hours after birth, whereas transmission during labor and delivery or breastfeeding is detected 2-12 weeks later. Because of the importance of initiating therapy as early as possible, DNA PCR testing is recommended within the first 3 months to identify infants who would greatly benefit from treatment
    2. To screen donated blood
    3. Where serological tests are inconclusive (indeterminate)
- Complex and costly.

Detection of HIV specific core antigen (p24)
- Earliest virus marker
- Detected during window period (the time it takes for a person who has acquired HIV infection to react to the virus by creating HIV antibodies) and in late disease when patient is symptomatic
- Can appear as early as 1-3 weeks after exposure
- Positive in 30-50% of cases.

Monitoring Tests

Lymphocyte analysis (CD4 count)
- CD4 count should be measured at the time of diagnosis of HIV infection and then every 3-4 months
- Treatment decisions should be made only after two successive measurements have been obtained
- Factors influencing test results include:
    - Sex
    - Age
    - Race
    - Drugs (zidovudine, cephalosporins, cancer chemotherapy, nicotine and corticosteroids)
    - Anti-lymphocyte antibodies
    - Splenectomy
    - Differences in reagents and equipment both within a laboratory and between laboratories
- CD4 cell counts should not be used for *diagnosis* of HIV infection as it may be found in a number of other diseases
- CD4 percentage is a direct measurement and is more reliable
- Counted as – (Total white blood cell counts (in thousands) x % of total lymphocytes) x % of CD4 lymphocytes
- If the absolute CD4 count fluctuates but the CD4 count percentage is stable, it indicates that the patient is immunologically stable.

Viral load assays
- Uses
    - Quantifies the amount of HIV-1 RNA circulating in the blood of an infected individual
    - Monitors the effects of ARV therapy
    - Track the viral suppression
    - Detects treatment failure

- Total quantification includes:
  - Cell-free virus (easiest measurement of viral load in an individual's plasma)
  - Virus in infected cells in all compartments of the body
  - Integrated provirus
- Because differences exist in the absolute copy number generated by different viral load assays, the same assay should be used to follow an individual's viral load
- Different assays:
  - *Standard* assays have a lower limit of detection of 400 copies/mL
  - *Ultrasensitive* assays may detect viral loads as low as 5 - 50 copies/mL
  - *Newer* assays have a greater dynamic range when compared to either the standard or the ultrasensitive assay (e.g., 40 - 10,000,000 copies/mL).

Drug resistance tests
- Types:
  - Genotyping
  - Phenotyping
  - Co-Receptor Tropism assays
  - Replicative capacity
- Performed:
  - At baseline, regardless of whether ARV therapy is being initiated (genotypic testing)
  - In patients experiencing treatment failure or incomplete viral suppression while receiving ARV therapy (genotypic and/or phenotypic testing).

HLA testing
- Individuals with (HLA)-B 5701, HLA-DR7, and HLA-DQ3 have an apparent genetic predisposition to development of abacavir hypersensitivity
- Unlike virus-specific tests (HIV genotype, phenotype, co-receptor tropism assays), HLA genotyping is necessary *only once during an individual's lifetime* because it will not change over time.

HIV Testing in Pregnancy (WHO 2013)

1. Counseling and Testing is recommended for women as a routine component of the package of care in all antenatal, childbirth, postpartum and pediatric care settings
2. Testing should be done at the booking antenatal visit
3. Re-testing is *recommended in all mothers* in the 3rd trimester, or during labor, or shortly after delivery because of the high risk of acquiring HIV infection during pregnancy
4. Testing is usually done by HIV serology and if confirmed by other tests, clinical assessment, viral load and CD4 count should be done
5. If feasible, other tests to be done are:
   a. HBV serology
   b. HCV serology
   c. Screening for STDs
   d. Assessment for major noncommunicable chronic diseases and comorbidities
   e. Cryptococcus antigen if CD4 count is ≤100 cells/mm^3 [only in settings with a high prevalence of cryptococcal antigenemia (>3%)]
6. Viral load is recommended as the preferred monitoring approach to diagnose and confirm ARV treatment failure in comparison to CD4 count or clinical staging. Why?
   - It provides an early and more accurate indication of treatment failure and the need to switch to second-line drugs, reducing the accumulation of drug-resistance mutations and improving clinical outcomes

- Measuring viral load can also help to discriminate between treatment failure and non-adherence
    - Many people who are identified with immunological failure (decreasing CD4 count inspite of ARV therapy) in fact have adequate virological suppression and they are misclassified as having treatment failure and are switched, unnecessarily to second-line therapy
7. Treatment failure is defined by a persistently detectable viral load of > 1000 copies/mL after at least six months of using ARV drugs
8. Viral load
    ≤ 1000copies/mL → maintain 1st line Preferred therapy
    > 1000 copies/mL → switch to 1st line Alternative therapy OR 2nd line therapy
9. If viral load is not routinely available, CD4 count and clinical monitoring should be used to diagnose treatment failure
10. If a woman declines an HIV test, this should be clearly documented in her antenatal card, her reasons should be sensitively explored and screening offered again in the 3rd trimester
11. Rapid HIV testing at the time of labor is recommended if HIV infection status has not previously been documented during the index pregnancy.

MANAGEMENT OF HIV INFECTED WOMAN

Can be subdivided into:
1. Medical management
2. Obstetric management

MEDICAL MANAGEMENT[1]

I. General Overview

Nucleoside Reverse-Transcriptase Inhibitors (NRTIs)

- Emtricitabine (FTC) 200 mg once daily
- Lamivudine (3TC) 150 mg twice daily or 300 mg once daily
- Zidovudine (AZT) 250–300 mg twice daily.

Nucleotide Reverse-Transcriptase Inhibitors (NtRTIs)

- Tenofovir (TDF) 300 mg once daily.

Non-Nucleoside Reverse-Transcriptase Inhibitors (NNRTIs)

- Efavirenz (EFV) 600 mg once daily
- Nevirapine (NVP) 200 mg once daily for 14 days, followed by 200 mg twice daily.

Protease Inhibitors (PIs)

- Atazanavir + ritonavir (ATV/r) 300 mg + 100 mg once daily
- Lopinavir/ritonavir (LPV/r) 400 mg/100 mg twice daily.

Integrase Strand Transfer Inhibitors (INSTIs)

- Raltegravir (RAL) 400 mg twice daily.

---

[1] Though there are many other drugs but only those required in pregnancy are mentioned

II. Revised WHO 2013 Guidelines

Antepartum and Intrapartum

The 2013 guidelines no longer recommend Option A, given in 2010 guidelines.

First Line ART

Preferred Regimen

- A once-daily fixed-dose combination of TDF + 3TC (or FTC) + EFV (Tenofovir disoproxil fumarate + Lamivudine/Emtricitabine + Efavirenz)
- Recommended as first-line ART in pregnant and breastfeeding women, including pregnant women in the 1st trimester of pregnancy and women of childbearing age, irrespective of viral load, CD4 count or WHO clinical staging
- The recommendation applies both to lifelong treatment for the own health of the mother and to ART initiated only for PMTCT which is then eventually stopped
- TDF is the preferred NRTI and EFV is the preferred NNRTI
- 3TC and FTC are pharmacologically comparable.

Alternative Regimens

- If the above regimen is contraindicated or is unavailable, use:
    - AZT + 3TC + EFV (or NVP) (Zidovudine + Lamivudine + Efavirenz/Nevirapine)
    - TDF + 3TC (or FTC) + NVP (Tenofovir disoproxil fumarate + Lamivudine /Emtricitabine + Nevirapine).

What are the benefits of this once daily fixed dose?

1. It is easy to implement: Administered to all pregnant women (regardless of "eligibility" for treatment) and continued during pregnancy, labor and postpartum
2. Increased coverage: Immunocompromised women who do not have access to CD4 testing receive appropriate ART without delay
3. Decrease in the rate of vertical transmission
4. Disease progression in mother will be delayed
5. ART will reduce sexual transmission of HIV to sexual partners
6. With the new treatment eligibility threshold of CD4 ≤500 cells/mm^3 (earlier ≤ 350 cells/mm^3), approximately 60% of HIV-infected pregnant women will meet treatment eligibility criteria for their own health
7. Other benefits:
    - Has low cost
    - Is available as a fixed-dose combination
    - Is safe for both pregnant and breastfeeding women and their infants
    - Is well tolerated
    - Severe side effects are rare
    - Has low monitoring requirements
    - A low drug-resistance profile
    - Has a better virological and treatment response
    - Is compatible with other drugs used in clinical care.

Safety of EFV in pregnancy

- Earlier some isolated case reports and retrospective clinical data on neural tube defects among humans have led to concern about using EFV in the 1st trimester of pregnancy

- Of late, the British HIV Association has changed its recommendation and has now allowed EFV to be used in the 1st trimester
- Because the risk of neural tube defects is limited to the first 5-6 weeks of pregnancy and because pregnancy is rarely recognized this early, especially in resource-limited settings, any potential risk of neural tube defects with the use of EFV would be primarily in women who become pregnant while already receiving EFV
- Evaluation of prospectively collected data in humans is reassuring; an updated systematic review and meta-analysis, including the Antiretroviral Pregnancy Registry, reported outcomes for 1502 live births to women receiving EFV in the 1st trimester and found no increase in overall birth defects and no elevated signal for EFV compared with other ARV exposure in pregnancy
- An additional systematic review showed, people receiving NVP are twice as likely as those receiving EFV to discontinue treatment because of adverse events
- A published meta-analysis and a further updated analysis was reviewed, that showed no increased risk of birth defects with EFV compared with other ARV drugs used during the 1st trimester of pregnancy.

Safety of TDF in pregnancy
- Prevalence of overall birth defects in pregnancy – 2.4%
- There is no difference in fetal growth between fetuses who are exposed to and those who are not exposed to TDF
- Limited penetration in breast milk.

Safety of NVP in pregnancy
- ART (triple ARV drugs) is now recommended for pregnant and breastfeeding women regardless of CD4 cell count, concerns remain regarding the use of NVP in women with higher CD4 counts
- A recent systematic review of the risk of NVP-associated toxicity in pregnant women suggests that the frequency of adverse events is no higher than that in the general adult population.

Second Line ART

Preferred regimens
- AZT + 3TC + LPV/r (Zidovudine + Lamivudine + lopinavir /ritonavir)
- AZT + 3TC + ATV/r (Zidovudine + Lamivudine + Atazanavir /ritonavir).

Alternative regimens
- TDF + 3TC (or FTC) + ATV/r (Tenofovir disoproxil fumarate + Lamivudine/ Emtricitabine + Atazanavir /ritonavir)
- TDF + 3TC (or FTC) + LPV/r (Tenofovir disoproxil fumarate + Lamivudine/ Emtricitabine + Lopinavir/ritonavir).

Major Blood Toxicities

EFV
1. CNS side effects:
   - Depression
   - Mental confusion
   - Abnormal dreams
2. Hepatotoxicity

3. Convulsions
4. Hypersensitivity reaction, Stevens-Johnson syndrome
5. Potential risk of neural tube birth defects (very low risk in humans)
6. Male gynecomastia.

AZT

1. Anemia
2. Neutropenia
3. Myopathy
4. Lipoatrophy or Lipodystrophy
5. Lactic acidosis or severe hepatomegaly with steatosis.

NVP

1. Hepatotoxicity
2. Severe skin rash and hypersensitivity reaction (Stevens-Johnson syndrome).

TDF

1. Tubular renal dysfunction
2. Fanconi syndrome
3. Decrease in bone mineral density
4. Lactic acidosis or severe hepatomegaly with steatosis
5. Exacerbation of hepatitis B (hepatic flares).

ATVr

1. Electrocardiographic abnormalities (PR interval prolongation)
2. Indirect hyperbilirubinemia (clinical jaundice)
3. Nephrolithiasis and risk of prematurity.

LPVr

- Electrocardiographic abnormalities (PR and QT interval prolongation, torsades de pointes)
- QT interval prolongation
- Hepatotoxicity
- Pancreatitis
- Risk of prematurity, lipoatrophy or metabolic syndrome, dyslipidemia or severe diarrhea.

Co-trimoxazole Therapy

- For prevention of pneumocystis pneumonia, toxoplasmosis and bacterial infections
- When to start?
    - Any WHO stage and CD4 count <350 cells/mm^3 OR
    - WHO stage 3 or 4 irrespective of CD4 level OR
    - In all, regardless of CD4 percentage or clinical stage, in settings with high HIV prevalence, high infant mortality due to infectious diseases and limited health infrastructure.

What to expect in the first months of ART?

- First six months of therapy are especially important
- Clinical and immunological improvement and viral suppression are expected when individuals adhere to ART
- But opportunistic infections and/or immune reconstitution inflammatory syndrome (IRIS) may develop, as well as early adverse drug reactions, such as drug hypersensitivity, especially in the first three months of ART
- ART significantly decreases mortality overall, but death rates are also highest in the first three months of ART
- These complications are commonest when people starting ART, already have advanced HIV disease with severe immunodeficiency and existing co infections and/or comorbidities, severely low hemoglobin, low BMI and very low CD4 counts or are severely malnourished.

CD4 recovery
- CD4 cell counts rise when ART is initiated during the first year of treatment → plateaus, and then continues to rise further during the second year
- But in few, with very low previous counts, this may not happen
- In such cases, continue prophylaxis for opportunistic infections such as co-trimoxazole preventive therapy.

OBSTETRIC MANAGEMENT

Prepregnancy Management

- Assess viral load
- If not possible → clinical staging and CD4 count
- Start 1st line Preferred therapy (triple line regimen) to all women of childbearing age, IRRESPECTIVE of CD4 count and clinical staging and this therapy is to be continued throughout pregnancy starting from the 1st day
- Adequate and balanced diet with folic acid should be started
- Screening for:
  - Syphilis
  - Rubella
  - Hepatitis B and C
  - Opportunistic infections (P. carinii pneumonia)
- Other routine blood tests:
  - Hemogram
  - Urine analysis
  - Blood group and type
  - FBS/PPBS
- HIV testing of sex partners is to be encouraged
- Counseling for cessation of smoking and illicit drug use is necessary
- Explain the effects of pregnancy on the disease and vice-versa
  - There is a decline in the CD4 cell count, owing to hemodilution of pregnancy which reverts back in the postpartum period
  - Studies have shown a positive correlation between ART and preterm labor
  - Also increased risk of gestational diabetes and preeclampsia have been proposed in these patients

- Counseling regarding risk of vertical transmission, measures available to decrease it and infant feeding options, the benefits to infants of early diagnosis of HIV
- Advice barrier contraceptives to those who choose to continue sexual contact (condoms reduce the risk of HIV transmission by 80%)
- For the HIV-negative person in serodiscordant couples, offer re-testing every 6–12 months
- Where the female partner is HIV negative but husband is positive, assisted reproduction with either donor insemination or sperm washing should be advised
- It is advisable to delay conception until plasma viral load comes down and simultaneously treat if any opportunistic infections are present
- All women who are HIV positive are recommended to have annual cervical cytology.

Counseling

Plays a very vital role in a disease like HIV/AIDS

Pretest counseling
1. Informed consent
2. Emphasize confidentiality
3. Explore high risk behavior
    - Unsafe sex practices
    - IV drug use
    - Blood/blood products received
4. Explore HIV/AIDS knowledge
    - Explain
    - Clarify misconceptions
5. Explore test implication
    - Meaning of negative or positive test result
6. Reason for testing
    - Removes uncertainty
7. Arousing hope: advice and empowerment
    - Focus on quality of life
    - No cure yet but let us hope
    - Express your availability when needed
8. Right to decline testing as it is a voluntary test
9. Causative agent, modes of transmission, methods of testing should be explained to the patient
10. Done on one to one basis or as lectures with slide shows, posters, charts and video clips
11. HIV testing should NOT be imposed as a precondition for employment or providing health care facilities.

Post-test: Test negative
1. Renew relationship
2. Explain negative results
3. Explain about window period
4. Clarify doubts/misconceptions
5. Evaluate need for retest
6. Repeat preventive education.

Post-test: Test positive
1. Renew relationship
2. Follow patients lead when to disclose

3. State result clearly
4. Wait, give time, listen
5. Make adaptive change in lifestyle and plan for future
6. Assess strategies for coping:
   - Evaluate past handling to stressful situations
   - Evaluate patient's social support network
7. Preventive education.

Pregnancy Management

- All pregnant women should be offered HIV counseling and testing (mentioned above)
  - At booking visit
  - Re test in 3rd trimester or peripartum
  - Offer partner testing
- If a woman declines an HIV test,
  - Document this in her ANC card
  - Explore the reasons for decline
  - Try screening again at around 28 weeks
- If testing shows HIV positive results,
  - Team approach [Obstetrician, Pediatrician, Counselor and a Physician (preferably)]
  - The result should be highly confidential
  - Testing of the partner is extremely important
  - If patient desires termination and is < 20 weeks pregnancy, offer safe MTP services
  - Offer effective/dual contraception (condoms, OCPs containing 50 μg estrogen, Depot MPA injections)
  - If patient desires pregnancy- Triple line therapy is started in the 1st trimester and continues throughout pregnancy
- If patient is already on ART:
  Tolerating the drugs well
  - She should not discontinue the drugs, provided, prior information and discussion regarding issues of teratogenicity (almost minimal) and side effects is done
  Not tolerating ART well and/or virological failure
  - Can start 1st line Alternative therapy
- General advice during pregnancy:
  - Regular ANCs once in 15 days
  - Good nutrition and exercise
  - Maintenance of good personal hygiene
  - Safe sex (use of condoms) even if both partners are HIV positive
  - Stop smoking/drug abuse/alcohol
  - Care of breast in preparation for lactation, if woman is desirous of breast feeding
- Multivitamin, folic acid, iron and calcium supplementation is given
- Hepatitis B and pneumococcal vaccination, though purely optional, can be offered in pregnancy
- Nutritional support, infant feeding and family planning counseling should be considered
- Bed nests should be used for prevention of malaria.

Investigations

- CBC, absolute lymphocyte count, blood sugar, urine analysis, blood group and type, LFT, RFT
- Viral load (HIV RNA copies)

- Screen for:
  - Vaginitis and treat at 1st visit, 28 weeks and again at 36 weeks (chlamydia T., N. gonorrhea, bacterial vaginosis)
  - Pap smear for cervical cytology
  - Syphilis, hepatitis B and C and rubella
- Dating and anamoly scans as and when required.

Mode of Delivery

Vaginal versus Cesarean section
- Whichever mode of delivery is followed, special efforts should be made to ensure that delivery care is provided in a non-stigmatizing and supportive manner
- Although cesarean section has been shown to protect against HIV transmission, especially in the absence of ARV drugs or in the case of high viral load, WHO does not recommend it in resource-limited settings specifically for HIV infection
- In these settings, cesarean section is recommended for obstetric and other medical indications only
- LSCS is of doubtful benefit over vaginal delivery, if:
  - Patient is already in labor or
  - Has ruptured her membranes or
  - Viral load is < 1000 copies/mL
- But if cesarean section is taken electively at 38 weeks, it reduces the MTCT risk by 50% (especially when viral load is > 1000 copies/mL). This must be weighed against the risk of infection and complications of surgery
- Factors that increase the risk of complications:
  - Genital infection
  - Obesity or malnutrition
  - Low socioeconomic status
  - Smoking.

General measures to be taken in case of vaginal delivery to minimize chances of transmission during labor and delivery

- Reinforcing recommended antenatal visits and care, especially high-risk management in the late 3rd trimester
- Promoting facility-based delivery by trained skilled birth attendants
- Continue ARV drugs intrapartum
- Use prophylactic antibiotics
- Use standard precautions (for both patient and health care providers) → hand/eye protection from sharp instruments
- Avoiding unnecessary instrumentation and premature rupture of membranes (indicated only at ≥ 7 cm dilatation)
- Use of a partograph to monitor stages of labor
- Pelvic examination to be done with full asepsis and only when essential (risk of infection)
- If there is prolonged rupture of membranes
  - Augment with oxytocin if delay is anticipated and there are no obstetric contraindications to it (increased risk of exposure of fetus to maternal blood and infected secretions)
  - Give broad spectrum antibiotics

- Avoid invasive procedures (fetal scalp electrodes, blood sampling), avoid routine episiotomy and forceps/vacuum delivery
- If instrumental delivery is indicated, outlet forceps are preferable to ventouse
- Pediatrician should be present for newborn resuscitation
- Noninvasive suction of nasogastric secretions
- Washing away blood in the newborn
- Clamp the cord early, do not milk the cord
- AMTSL.

Postpartum

- Support her in her feeding choice
- Proper care of episiotomy wound to prevent infection
- Watch for puerperal sepsis, mastitis and UTI
- Persistence of lochia >15 days, heavy bleeding, foul smelling lochia are abnormal and should be watched for
- Safe disposal of soiled napkins
- Effective contraception should be started early as those on replacement feeds start ovulating and menstruating earlier than those on exclusive breast feeding.

Medical management

Mother

Assess eligibility (WHO clinical stage 3 or 4 or CD4 ≤500 cells/mm^3) for treatment for her own health

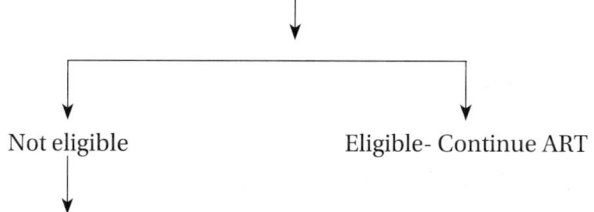

If breastfeeding
- Stop ART after 1 week of complete cessation of breastfeeding and refer to care for reassessment

If not breastfeeding
- Stop ART after delivery.

Infant

Testing

I. HIV exposed infant (in utero or during breastfeeding)
- Virological testing at 4–6 weeks of age
- Aim: To diagnose HIV
- Start ART immediately if HIV infected and simultaneously a second specimen be collected to confirm the initial positive virological test result
- Do not wait for the results of confirmatory tests to start ART.

II. Infant –unknown HIV exposure
- Maternal HIV serological test
  or
- Infant HIV serological test at birth or at the first postnatal visit (at 4-6 weeks)
- Aim: To identify or confirm HIV exposure
- Need virological test if HIV-exposed
- Start ART immediately, if infected.

Follow up
- HIV exposed infants should have a serological test repeated again at 9 months (or at the time of the last immunization visit)
- If results are positive, a virological test is to be done, to identify infants requiring ART.

Treatment
- Infant prophylaxis should begin at birth or when HIV exposure is recognized postpartum.

If Breastfeeding
- Daily NVP (Nevirapine) for 6 weeks.

Replacement feeding
- 4-6 weeks of NVP (Nevirapine) or twice-daily AZT (Zidovudine).

Infant prophylaxis dosing recommendations: NVP

Infant age	Daily dosing
Birth to 6 weeks	
• Birthweight 2000–2499 g	10 mg once daily
• Birthweight ≥ 2500 g	15 mg once daily
> 6 weeks to 6 months	20 mg once daily
> 6 months to 9 months	30 mg once daily
> 9 months until breastfeeding ends	40 mg once daily

Infants weighing < 2000 g should receive mg/kg dosing; the suggested starting dose is 2 mg/kg once daily.

Infant prophylaxis dosing recommendations: AZT (only recommended with replacement feeding)

Infant age	Daily dosing
Birth to 6 weeks	
• Birthweight 2000–2499 g	10 mg twice daily
• Birthweight ≥ 2500 g	15 mg twice daily

Other recommendations:
- Infants weighing < 2000 g should receive mg/kg dosing; the suggested starting dose is 2 mg/kg once daily
- Toxicity from infant NVP requires discontinuing the drug or if infant NVP is not available, infant 3TC can be substituted
- When a breastfeeding mother initiates ART very late in pregnancy (such as < 4 weeks prior to delivery), during labor or postpartum, increasing the duration of infant NVP prophylaxis to 12 weeks can be considered
- Interruption of ART by mother during breastfeeding, places her infant at increased risk of postnatal transmission
- In such situations, providing daily infant NVP during the period of maternal ART interruption should be considered, and this can be stopped six weeks after maternal ART is restarted (or one week after breastfeeding ends, whichever comes first).

WHO recommendations for breastfeeding in HIV mothers

Mothers known to be HIV-infected

- Should receive lifelong antiretroviral therapy or antiretroviral prophylaxis interventions to reduce HIV transmission through breastfeeding.

If infant is uninfected or of unknown HIV status

- Exclusive breastfeeding for the first 6 months of life
- Complementary foods thereafter
- Continue breastfeeding till 1 year of age (This recommendation is based on evidence that the maximum benefit of breastfeeding in preventing mortality from diarrhea, pneumonia and malnutrition is in the first 12 months of life and that the risk of transmitting HIV to infants through breastfeeding is low in the presence of ARV drugs)
- Breastfeeding should only be stopped once a nutritionally adequate and safe diet without breast milk can be provided
- If mothers decide to stop breastfeeding, it should not be abrupt → taper and then stop within a month,
  - Continue ARV prophylaxis for one week after breastfeeding is fully stopped
  - Infants are provided with safe and adequate replacement feeds without hampering their normal growth and development
- Alternatives to breastfeeding include:

For infants < 6 months of age:
  - Commercial infant formula milk, when the following can be met:
    - Safe water and sanitation
    - Sufficient, cleanly prepared, assuring safety, infant formula milk can be provided consistently
    - Family support and affordability to provide infant formula milk exclusively for 6 months OR
  - Expressed, heat-treated breast milk,
    - When the infant has low birth weight or is otherwise ill in the neonatal period and unable to breastfeed OR
    - When the mother is unwell and temporarily unable to breastfeed or has a temporary breast health problem such as mastitis; OR
    - When mothers are planning to stop breastfeeding; OR
    - If antiretroviral drugs are temporarily not available

Note: Home-modified animal milk is not recommended as a replacement food in the first six months of life

For children >6 months of age
  - Commercial infant formula milk (if conditions mentioned above are met) OR
  - Animal milk (boiled for infants under 12 months), as part of a diet providing adequate micronutrient intake
  - Meals, including milk-only feeds, other foods and combination of milk feeds and other foods, should be provided 4-5 times/day.

When the infant is HIV-infected

- Exclusive breastfeed for the first 6 months of life and continue breastfeeding as per the recommendations for the general population, that is up to two years or beyond.

Measures taken by Indian government in reducing HIV and AIDS in the country

The National AIDS Control Programme (NACP), launched in 1992, is being implemented as a comprehensive programme for prevention and control of HIV/AIDS in India.

NACP – Phase III (2007-2012)

Main goal- halting and reversing HIV epidemic in India. Emphasis is mainly laid on preventive measures

1. Targeted intervention programme
   - Target population:
     - *High Risk Groups (HRGs)*
       - Female Sex Workers (FSWs)
       - Men who have Sex with Men (MSM) and
       - Transgenders (TGs)
       - Injecting Drug Users (IDUs)
     - *Bridge populations*
       - Truckers
       - Migrants
   - Measures taken:
     - Treatment for Sexually Transmitted Infections
     - Condom provision → male and female condoms
     - Provision of clean needles and syringes
     - Behavior change communication
     - Creating an enabling environment with community involvement and participation
     - Linkages to testing, care and support services
     - Opioid Substitution Therapy
2. Link worker scheme (LWS)
   - The services provided through this scheme are linked to local health governance system at three levels, which ensures mainstreaming of the HIV response and thus project sustainability
3. Management of STIs and reproductive tract infections
4. Changed strategy of NACP-III → The focus is on moving to behavior change communication from only awareness creation
5. Condom promotion
6. Blood safety
   - Objective → to ensure provision of safe and quality blood even to far-flung remote areas of the country in the shortest possible time, through a well-coordinated National Blood Transfusion Service
7. Standard quality of HIV testing [through "National External Quality Assessment Scheme" (NEQAS) launched in year 2000]
8. ICTC (Integrated counseling and testing center) services → proper pretest and post-test counseling and that the test results provided are reliable and meet the quality standards
9. Care, support and treatment.

SUGGESTED READING

1. Antiretroviral therapy of HIV infection in infants and children: towards universal access: recommendations for a public health approach. World Health Organization. 2010 revision.

2. Consolidated guidelines on the use of antiretroviral drugs for treating and preventing HIV infection: recommendations for a public health approach. World Health Organization 2013.
3. Guideline: vitamin A supplementation in pregnancy for reducing the risk of mother-to-child transmission of HIV. World Health Organization 2011.
4. HIV infection and women's health: AOGD bulletin. Dec 2012; Vol 12 Issue 8.
5. Management of HIV in pregnancy. RCOG Green-top Guideline No. 39. June 2010.
6. NACO Annual Report 2010-11: Department of AIDS Control, Ministry of Health & Family Welfare. Government of India.
7. Rapid advice: revised WHO principles and recommendations on infant feeding in the context of HIV. World Health Organization. November 2009.
8. Rapid Advice: use of antiretroviral drugs for treating pregnant women and preventing HIV infection in infants. World Health Organization. June 2010.
9. Use of antiretroviral drugs for treating pregnant women and preventing HIV infection in infants. World Health Organization. April 2012.

CHAPTER 23

Thyroid Disorders in Pregnancy

Tania G Singh, Earl Jaspal

RELEVANT HISTORY PERTAINING TO THE CASE WITH EXPLANATIONS

Age

Why Important?

- Simple goiter → Occurs in girls approaching puberty and in pregnancy
- Multinodular (solitary and colloid) → occurs in 20s and 30s
- Primary toxic goiter → occurs in young
- Hashimoto's disease → occurs in middle aged women
- Anaplastic carcinoma → Only thyroid pathology occurring in old age.

Sex

- Females > males.

Occupation

- ↑ stress and strain → Thyrotoxicosis.

Residence

- Iodine deficient areas (near rocky mountains)
- Calcium is goitrogenic (areas producing chalk or lime stone).

Swelling

- Onset
- Duration
- Rate of growth
- Is the sleep affected (sleepless nights associated with primary thyrotoxicosis)?

Pain

- Painless – Goiter
- Pain – on inflammation.

Pressure Effects

- Enlarged thyroid → pressure
  - On trachea → dyspnea
  - On esophagus (rare) → dyspnea → esophagus is a muscular tube that can be easily stretched
  - On recurrent laryngeal nerve → hoarseness of voice.

Symptoms

Primary Thyrotoxicosis

- Not much enlargement
- Loss of weight (inspite of good appetite)
- Heat intolerance
- Increased sweating
- Excitability
- Irritability
- Insomnia } CNS involvement
- Tremor of hands
- Weakness of muscles
- Tachycardia (rise in sleeping pulse)
- Exophthalmus
- Staring or protruding eyes
- Difficulty in closing eyelids
- Double vision/diplopia (because of muscle weakness - ophthalmoplegia)
- Edema or swelling of conjunctiva (chemosis) – but is a very late symptom
- Pain in eye → corneal ulceration
- Menstrual cycle - amenorrhea.

Secondary Thyrotoxicosis

When solitary nodule or multinodular or colloid goiter shows manifestation of thyrotoxicosis
- Palpitation
- Ectopic beats
- Arrhythmia } Cardiac involvement
- Dyspnea on exertion
- Chest pain

Hypothyroidism

- Increase in weight despite poor appetite
- Fat, particularly at back of neck and shoulders
- Cold intolerance
- Minimal swelling
- Dry skin
- Puffiness of face with pouting lips and dull expression (mask - like face)
- Loss of hair
- Muscle fatigue/lethargy
- Failing memory
- Constipation/oligomenorrhea.

Past History

- Diet is important (vegetables of brassica family – cabbage, kale, rape) are goitrogens
- Sea fish with low iodine content.

Family History

- In other family members it is usually present.

Physical Examination

Weight

- Thin and reduced weight → hyperthyroidism
- Obese and increased weight → hypothyroidism.

Face

- Excitement ⎫
- Tension   ⎬ hyperthyroidism
- Nervousness ⎭
- Puffy face without expression (mask like face) – hypothyroidism.

Skin (Especially Hands)

- Moist and hot – hyperthyroidism
- Dry and inelastic - myxedema.

Edema

- Non pitting in hypothyroidism.

Vitals

- Sleeping PR to determine degree of thyrotoxicosis:
  - Mild <90/min
  - Moderate 90-110/min
  - Severe >110/min
- Hyperthyroidism: pulse – rapid, irregular
- Hypothyroidism: ↑ BP, bradycardia.

Intelligence

- Low and dull in hypothyroidism.

Local Examination

Inspection

If normal – not obvious on inspection
I. Pizzillo's method
   - Hands placed behind head (clasped hands on occiput)
   - Patient asked to push her head backwards against her clasped hands
   - Swelling may be uniform or isolated nodules present

II. Ask patient to swallow
- A thyroid swelling moves upwards on deglutition (due to the fact that thyroid gland is fixed to larynx)

Other swellings which move:
- Thyroglossal cyst
- Subhyoid bursitis
- Prelaryngeal or pretracheal lymph nodes.

Palpation (Both from Back and Front)

How?
- Patient sits on stool
- Neck always slightly flexed
- Stand behind the patient
- Bilaterally thumbs placed behind neck
- Bilaterally the 4 fingers are placed on each lobe and isthmus

Additional information of 1 lobe:
- By relaxing sternomastoid muscle of that side by flexing and rotating face to the same side

Palpation of each lobe:
- Best by Lahey's method
    - Examiner in front of patient
    - To palpate left lobe → gland pushed to left from right side by left hand of examiner.

Auscultation

- Systolic bruit → primary toxic goiter (↑ vascularity of gland).

Measurement

- Measure circumference of neck at most prominent part of swelling → ↑ or ↓ in size.

General Examination

Eye Signs

1. Lid retraction
    - Over activity of m. levator palpebrae superioris
    - When upper eyelid is higher than normal and lower eyelid is normal in position

Note: (Lid lag – upper eyelid cannot keep pace with eyeball when it looks down following examiner's finger moving downwards from above)

2. Exophthalmus
    - Eyeball pushed forwards due to increase in fat/edema/cellular infiltration in retroorbital space
    - Tests:
        a. Von Graefe's sign: Upper eyelid lags behind eyeball
        b. Joffroy's sign: Absence of wrinkling on forehead when patient looks upwards with face downwards
        c. Stellwag's sign: Staring look and infrequent blinking
        d. Moebius' sign: Inability to converge eyeballs

3. Ophthalmoplegia
4. Chemosis: edema of conjunctiva.

Tremor

- Fine tremor: Exhibits at fingers
  - Straight out arm in front and spread fingers → hyperthyroidism
- Put out tongue straight → keep like this for ≈ 30 seconds → fibrillary twitching → hyperthyroidism.

1. **Anatomy and physiology of thyroid gland**

   Anatomy
   - Is an endocrine gland because its secretion is poured directly into the blood stream
   - Lies against C_5, C_6, C_7 and T_1
   - Embraces upper part of trachea
   - Consists of 2 lobes – right and left, joined by isthmus (typically forming an "H" or "U" shape)
   - Single Lobe (5 × 2.5 × 2.5 cm) has:
     - Apex and base,
     - 3 surfaces-lateral, medial, postero lateral,
     - 2 borders–anterior and posterior
   - Isthmus (1.2 × 1.2 cm) has
     - 2 surfaces-anterior and posterior
     - 2 borders-superior and inferior
   - Weight – 25gm
     - Females > males
     - Increases in menses and pregnancy
   - Thyroid means – 'SHIELD LIKE'
   - 1st endocrine gland to develop in embryo (24 days after fertilization)
   - Has 2 capsules → true and false capsule
   - Blood supply:
     - Arteries – superior and inferior thyroid artery
     - Veins – superior, middle and inferior thyroid vein
   - Lymphatics:
     - Periglandular, prelaryngeal, pretracheal and paratracheal lymph nodes
   - Nerves:
     - Sympathetic: Superior middle and inferior sympathetic gamglia
     - Parasympathetic: Vagus nerves.

   Physiology

   Diet (adequate supply) → iodine is absorbed in small intestine and is released as iodide into blood stream

   ↓

   It is trapped by follicular cells of thyroid gland under the influence of TSH → iodide in thyroid is oxidized to iodine

   ↓

   Iodine iodinates tyrosyl residues like tyrosine present in TBG to form monoiodotyrosine (MIT)

   ↓

   MIT + MIT → DIT
   DIT + MIT → triiodotyrosine (TIT) (T_3)

DIT + DIT → tetraiodotyrosine (T_4; Thyroxine)
↓
Thyroid hormone formed is joined to TBG and stored in colloid of the follicle
↓
Lysosomes cause release of T_4, T_3, MIT and DIT
↓
MIT and DIT are deiodinated. Iodide released is stored in thyroid for reuse → some passes into blood.

Facts
- T_3 more potent than T_4
- T_4 and T_3 are secreted in the ratio of 5:1
- Of T_4 ≈ 30-40% is deiodinated peripherally to form T_3
- Thyroid hormones:
  - 85% are bound to TBG
  - Remaining, bound to T_4 binding pre - albumin or to albumin itself
- 0.05% of T_4 is in free, unbound form
- T_3 → bound to TBG to a lesser extent, 0.5% circulates in free state.

2. **Functions of thyroid hormones**
   1. Increases basal metabolic rate
   2. Protein synthesis → accelerated by
      - Increasing translation of RNA
      - Increasing transcription of DNA to RNA
      - Increasing activity of cellular enzymes
      - Increasing mitochondrial activity
      - Increases absorption of glucose from GIT
   3. Stimulates carbohydrate metabolism
      - Accelerates transport of glucose through cell membrane
      - Increase breakdown of glycogen to glucose
      - Accelerates gluconeogenesis
   4. Increases free fatty acid level in blood due to mobilization of fat from adipose tissues and fat depots
   5. Thyroxine specifically ↓ cholesterol, phospholipids and triglyceride levels in plasma
   6. ↓ in vitamin levels as it is utilized by thyroxine in formation of enzymes
   7. Promotes growth and development of brain during fetal life and during 1st few years of postnatal life (deficiency leads to abnormal development of synapses, defective myelination and mental retardation)
   8. Thyroxine is essential for maintaining body weight,
      - ↑ in thyroxine →↓ body weight
      - ↓ in thyroxine →↑ body weight
   9. Thyroxine ↑ process of erythropoiesis and ↑ blood volume
   10. Thyroxine ↑ circulation of blood by acting mainly on heart
   11. ↑ rate of respiration
   12. Effect on GIT:
       - ↑ appetite and food intake
       - ↑ secretions and moves of GIT

- Therefore, ↓ thyroxine → constipation
- ↑ thyroxine → diarrhea
13. Thyroxine
    - Slight ↑ → work with more vigor
14. Effect on skeletal muscle
    - ↑ secretion → causes weakness in muscle due to catabolism of proteins
15. Effect on sleep
    - ↑T_4 → ↑ stimulation of muscle and CNS → exhaustion and feels to sleep
    - ↓T_4 → excessive sleep (somnolence)
16. T_4 ↑ secretion of other endocrine glands
17. Effect on sexual function
    - Its lack → menorrhagia; polymenorrhea
    - Occasionally, amenorrhea also
    - Hyperthyroidism → oligomenorrhea/amenorrhea.

3. **Thyroid changes in pregnancy**

   Maternal changes
   - Pregnancy-related hyperestrogenism induces a 100% rise in serum thyroxine-binding globulin (TBG) as a result of changes in TBG half-life secondary to altered glycosylation
   - As a consequence, by week 10 of gestation, total T_4 and T_3 serum concentrations are increased and plateau at this level until delivery
   - ↑circulating hCG level in the 1st trimester leads to cross-reactivity with the TSH receptor as they share a common alpha subunit; their beta subunits also have significant homology → temporary ↑in free T_4, T_3 levels and partial suppression of TSH
   - Placental deiodination of maternal T_4, increasing T_4 turnover
   - There is an increase in urinary iodine excretion
   - TSH does not cross the placenta
   - In normal pregnant women, the thyroid gland maintains euthyroidism with only minor fluctuations in serum T_4 and TSH
   - But in women with limited thyroid reserve, due to thyroid autoimmunity or iodine deficiency, hypothyroidism can develop.

   Fetal adaptations
   - Thyroid hormone and specific nuclear receptors are found in fetal brain at 8 week after conception. Therefore, fetus is dependent on mother for thyroxine during this period
   - Fetal thyroid ontogeny begins at 10–12 weeks gestation and is NOT complete until delivery
   - T_4 is not secreted until 18–20 weeks
   - T_4 is critical for many aspects of brain development
   - Although these requirements evolve over months, an especially critical time is the 2nd trimester
   - Maternal T_4 crosses the placenta. Is found in,
     - Human coelomic fluid as early as 4 weeks gestation
     - In amniotic fluid
     - Is detectable in cord blood of newborns with even thyroid dysgenesis
   - Maternal T_3 does not cross the placenta and appears to have little, if any, role in development
   - Deiodination of maternal T_4 by the fetus results in local fetal production of liothyronine (most potent form of thyroid hormone; chemically, it is nearly identical to T_3), which is particularly important for neurological development

- There is presence of increasing concentrations of T_4 and T_3 by 11–18 weeks after conception
- Later in gestation: dependent for iodine
- Normal maternal thyroid function is, therefore, critical in order to provide adequate thyroid hormones for early fetal development and, in particular, early CNS development.

Screening for Thyroid Dysfunction during Pregnancy

Following women are at high risk for thyroid disease, so should be screened definitely:
1. History of hyperthyroid or hypothyroid disease, postpartum thyroiditis, or thyroid lobectomy
2. Family history of thyroid disease
3. Women with a goiter
4. Presence of thyroid antibodies (when known)
5. When symptoms or clinical signs suggestive of thyroid underfunction or overfunction, including anemia, elevated cholesterol and hyponatremia are present
6. Type I diabetes and other autoimmune disorders
7. Infertile women with TSH screening as part of their infertility work-up
8. Previous therapeutic head or neck irradiation
9. History of miscarriage or preterm delivery.

Case 1
A 26yr old primigravida, with 30 weeks POG has come to OPD for regular checkup. She complains of swelling in neck, occasional vomitings and palpitations. On examination: diffuse swelling in neck area which moves with deglutition is present. Weight -54kg, since previous 2 visits → no gain in weight. BP 146/80mmHg, rapid pulse. Per abdomen: uterus ≈ 26-28 weeks size, relaxed, FHS 150/min.
What is your provisional diagnosis?

Hyperthyroidism

Incidence of hyperthyroidism in pregnancy
- 0.4% of all pregnant women.

4. **Why hyperthyroidism is relatively uncommon in pregnancy?**
   Because of:
   1. Low fertility state
   2. Increased pregnancy loss
   3. Gestation related immunological changes suppressing autoimmune disease.

5. **How will you investigate this case?**

   Clinically

   History
   - Weight loss despite ↑ appetite
   - Heat intolerance
   - Palpitations
   - Irritability
   - Tremulousness
   - Vomiting
   - Diarrhea
   - Enlarged neck (noted by patient or family members).

Physical exam
- Rapid pulse
- ↑ systolic but NOT diastolic BP
- Warm moist skin
- Oncholysis
- Sweating
- Tremor of tongue or outstretched hands
- Staring appearance
- Lid lag
- Proximal muscle weakness.

Out of the above symptoms, those normally found in pregnancy are:
- Palpitations
- Tachycardia
- Irritability
- Heat intolerance
- Fatigue

Therefore, can be easily overlooked.

Specific findings in Graves' disease
- Classic thyroid ophthalmopathy
- A significant goiter
- Pretibial myxedema (though rare).

Laboratory findings

While interpreting laboratory values, it is very important to remember certain normal things:
- There is hCG-mediated ↓ in serum TSH levels (which typically fall in the mid to late 1st trimester coincident with rising hCG levels)
  - TSH in first half of pregnancy ranges from 0.03 µU/mL to 0.8 µU/mL
  - Therefore, this should not be interpreted as diagnostic of hyperthyroidism
- Low TSH plasma levels (< 0.1mIU/L) in the presence of elevated free T_4 concentrations → investigations of choice for hyperthyroidism
- Then investigate further with:
  - TSH receptor antibodies (TRAb) → If present, points towards Graves' disease as the etiological factor and differentiates it from gestational thyrotoxicosis in the 1st trimester
  - Thyroid stimulating antibodies (TSA)
  - Thyroid peroxidase antibodies (TPO Ab)
- When TSH is very low, a trend in the serum T_4 and T_3 levels may help in differentiating transient GTT from a truly thyrotoxic state.

6. **Which signs and symptoms can help you differentiate between thyrotoxicosis and characteristic hyper metabolic state of pregnancy?**

   Following signs and symptoms are particularly seen in thyrotoxicosis:
   - Deficient weight gain for gestational age
   - Oncholysis
   - Eye signs including lid lag
   - Muscle weakness
   - Heart rate 100 beats/min (which does not decrease with valsalva manoeuvre).

Causes of Hyperthyroidism in Pregnancy

Most common cause – Graves' disease (85-90%)

Prenatal Counseling
- Women can undergo definitive treatment before pregnancy, which can be either a thyroidectomy or ^{131}I therapy
- Advantage:
  - Risk of maternal thyrotoxicosis during pregnancy is reduced, if not eliminated
  - Fertility is not affected by ^{131}I therapy for thyrotoxicosis
- Pregnancy should be deferred for 4-6 months after ^{131}I therapy
- Women should be made aware that the risk of fetal and neonatal thyrotoxicosis is not eliminated by previous thyroidectomy or ^{131}I therapy
- Most important is to ensure that thyroid function tests are normal at the time of conception and throughout pregnancy
- If patient is on methimazole, she can switch over to propylthiouracil either before conception or early in 1st trimester with frequent check on TFT.

Effect of pregnancy on Graves' disease
- Tends to get worse during the 1st trimester (due to ↑ in hCG, which is structurally similar to TSH)
- Improves later in pregnancy – therefore, lower doses required
- Near term - can even discontinue treatment in euthyroid women
- Get worse again after delivery (postpartum exacerbation, therefore, close monitoring required).

Features
- Production of TSH receptor antibodies
- Stimulate thyroid → overactivity
- Unique features → proptosis and infiltrative dermopathy
- Goiter → common (not always present).

Other causes
Remaining causes
- Multinodular toxic goiter
- Simple toxic adenoma
- Thyroiditis
- Increase intake of thyroxine
- Carcinoma
- Drug induced (amiadarone).

Rare causes
- Gestation transient thyrotoxicosis (GTT)
  - Defined as biochemical thyrotoxicosis in women with an otherwise normal pregnancy
  - Is secondary to the thyrotropic effects of hCG
  - Incidence → 2-3% of all pregnancies especially where hCG levels are much higher such as in multiple pregnancies
  - Present in the mid to late 1st trimester, often with hyperemesis (may lead to weight loss)
  - Usually asymptomatic
  - Resolves spontaneously by 20 weeks gestation and does not require treatment
  - Mild ↑ fT_4 and mild ↓ TSH → in 1st trimester
  - Gestational thyrotoxicosis can be differentiated from Graves' disease owing to presence of the following in the latter:
    - Autoimmunity
    - A goiter
    - Presence of TSH receptor antibodies (TRAb)

- Factitious thyrotoxicosis
- Conditions associated with significant rise in hCG:
  - Hyperemesis gravidarum
  - Twin gestation
  - Hydatidiform mole or Choriocarcinoma.

7. **How does hyperthyroidism in mother affecte fetal thyroid function?**

   Causes of hyperthyroidism secondary to maternal disease:
   - Low maternal transfer of T_4
   - Serum T_4 level in fetus is about 1/3rd of the maternal level
   - Maternal TSH receptor antibodies (TRAb) in Graves' disease are IgG antibodies, which can readily cross the placenta
   - Because the antireceptor antibodies have three different actions on the TSH receptor, these TRAbs can stimulate or inhibit the fetal thyroid
   - Can cause fetal hyperthyroidism after 20 weeks or transient neonatal hypothyroidism
   - Risk factors for neonatal thyroid dysfunction include:
     - History of a previously affected baby,
     - Prior ablative treatment with ^{131}I
     - Elevated maternal TRAb at the time of delivery.

8. **What are the maternal and fetal risks?**

   Following risks are associated:

   Maternal

   If uncontrolled or untreated or inadequately treated
   - Miscarriage
   - Hypertensive disorder of pregnancy
   - Preterm labor
   - Placental abruption
   - Heart failure because of dysfunction of heart muscles with ↑ in blood volume
   - Thyroid storm
   - Congestive heart failure
   - Death (rare).

   Overtreatment of the mother
   - Can result in iatrogenic fetal hypothyroidism.

   Fetal
   - LBW
   - IUGR
   - Still birth
   - Goiter
   - Congenital malformations (ventricular septal defect, cleft lip and palate, polydactyly, diastasis recti abdominis, imperforate anus, anencephaly, ear lobe malformation and omphalocele)
   - Neonatal mortality and morbidity → thyrotoxicosis (thyroid stimulating antibody crosses placenta).

9. **How will you manage the case?**

   General overview of management
   - Main aim of treatment is to set such a dose which can solve 2 purposes:
     1. Keep maternal fT_4 in the upper normal range
     2. Should not cause fetal hypothyroidism

   } Over treatment should be avoided as thyroid hormones are very important for fetal brain

Subclinical hyperthyroidism
- TSH below normal limits
- Free T_4 and total T_4 in the normal pregnancy range
- Disease clinically not evident
- Seen in hyperemesis gravidarum syndrome
- Treatment does not improve pregnancy outcome and may risk unnecessary exposure of the fetus to antithyroid drugs
- Only close monitoring required.

Pregnancy occurs in active Graves' disease
Maternal
- Monitor TSH and free T_4 monthly
- Titrate dose of propylthiouracil accordingly
- Assess TSH Receptor-Ab titers in 3rd trimester to evaluate if fetus is at risk → if elevated → investigate neonatal thyroid function after delivery
- Maternal TFT after delivery

Fetal
Fetus can be monitored by the following parameters ultrasonographically:
- Fetal heart rate (should not be > 160 beats/min)
- Fetal thyroid gland
  - By doppler (associated with fetal hyperthyroidism or hypothyroidism)
  - Goiter can be detected (when present) after 32nd week of pregnancy
- Fetal growth (usually IUGR is observed)
- Hydropic variations
- Fetal cardiac failure

Definitive diagnosis (if needed)
- Requires umbilical cord blood sampling for fetal thyroid function and carries a 1-2% risk of fetal loss

Treatment
- Can be treated satisfactorily by adjusting the dose of antithyroid drug in the mother and by following the fetal response clinically and by ultrasound
- If hyperthyroidism is present in neonate at birth (due to transplacental passage of TRAb), it should be considered as an emergency and managed accordingly.

Newly diagnosed Graves' disease
- Start antithyroid drug as soon as diagnosis is made
- Monitor as above.

Graves' disease relapse during 1st trimester
- ATD therapy should be restarted.

Pregnancy after previous ablative therapy (surgery or radioiodine) for Graves' disease
- Maternal hyperthyroidism is not possible
- Reassess TSH Receptor-Ab levels at beginning of pregnancy (in order to evaluate possibility of fetal or postnatal hyperthyroidism)
- If FSH >160bpm and there is positive maternal TSH Receptor-Ab, it is advisable to initiate treatment with PTU 100–200mg/8 h and also continue LT_4 supplementation to mother to maintain maternal euthyroidism
- The block and replacement method with ATDs (LT_4 plus ATD) should be avoided in pregnancy or used with great caution because of the difficulty in monitoring fetal thyroid function and the increased risk of producing goiter and hypothyroidism.

Principal Drugs

During pregnancy
- Propylthiouracil, Methimazole, Carbimazole
- They inhibit thyroid hormone synthesis via reduction in iodine organification and iodotyrosine coupling.

Propylthiouracil
- Drug of choice because:
  - Less placental transfer
  - ↓T_3 quickly by blocking peripheral conversion of T_4 to T_3
- Dose: 100mg every 8 hourly (200-450 mg/day) → then ↓ accordingly
- Maintenance dose: 50-300 mg/day
- Give the lowest possible dose
- Expect fT_4 to improve first
- TFT (TSH and fT_4) every 4 weeks (2-8weeks)
- Aim of Rx:
  - ↓fT_4 to upper normal or slightly above normal range
  - TSH should remain suppressed - why?
    - Because if mother is fully treated to normal levels of fT4 and TSH, fetus is at high risk for developing hypothyroidism from placental transfer of antithyroid medication
    - fT_4 is preferred to TSH (for dose adjustment) because a change in TSH takes much longer to manifest as compared to fT_4
    - As thyroid function improves, the dose of PTU may be gradually tapered, and when it is in the range of 50–100 mg daily, it is often possible to discontinue the drug altogether (usually in the 3rd trimester)
    - However, relapse of maternal thyrotoxicosis in the postpartum period is common.

Monitoring during pregnancy *on monthly basis:*
- Clinical monitoring of mother and fetus
- Ultrasound → fetus
- Biochemical: TSH and free T_4
- Maternal hormone target levels
  - TT_4: 12–18 μg/dL; FT_4: 2–2.5 ng/dL
  - TSH: 0.1–0.4mIU/L (in late gestation)
  - The median time to normalization of maternal T_4 is around 7–8 weeks.

Methimazole (10-40 mg daily)
- *Methimazole embryopathy*
  - Aplasia cutis
    - A congenital localized absence of skin, typically present as a 0.5–3 cm isolated, punched out, midline lesion at the vertex or occipital area of the scalp
    - The lesions may close spontaneously or skin grafting may be required in more severe cases
    - It occurs spontaneously in approximately 1 in 2000 births,
    - Is often familial
    - Can occur alone or in association with other anomalies
  - Esophageal atresia
  - Choanal atresia
  - Facial abnormalities
  - Hypoplastic nipples

- Tracheoesophageal (TE) fistula
- Developmental delay
- Only used in those cases where PTU cannot be tolerated.

Carbimazole (10-40 mg)

Minor side effects of these drugs
- Urticaria ⎫
- Arthralgia ⎪
- Nausea ⎬ resolve spontaneously
- Metallic taste ⎪
- Pruritis ⎭
- Agranulocytosis – rare → causes fever, sore throat, neutropenia → discontinue drug immediately
- Hepatotoxicity.

During lactation
- Doses not affecting the infant's thyroid hormone levels significantly:
  - PTU – is the drug of choice (< 300 mg/day) ⎫
  - Methimazole up to 20 mg/day can be used ⎬ For a period of 3 weeks to 8 months
  - Carbimazole → 5-15 mg/day ⎭
- Mother should take the drug just after breastfeeding, providing a 3–4 h interval before she lactates again
- From a pharmacokinetic view, there is higher passage of methimazole or carbimazole as compared to PTU into breast milk
  - Methimazole is minimally bound to serum proteins, whereas PTU is more extensively protein-bound in serum, mostly to albumin
  - Methimazole is not ionized in serum whereas PTU, a weak acid, is more ionized in serum (pH 7.4) than in the acidic breast milk (pH 6.8), inhibiting its transfer from serum into the lipid-rich breast milk
- Adverse reactions of ATD therapy (rash, agranulocytosis, hepatic dysfunction, autoimmune sequelae) while mother being on treatment, are not observed in infants with the above mentioned doses.

10. **If medical treatment is unsuccessful, what is the next option?**

    Next option is surgery:
    - Total thyroidectomy
      - Indications: Uncontrolled maternal hyperthyroidism even with high doses of ATD (>300 mg of propylthiouracil or 40 mg/day methimazole)
      - Recommended in 2nd trimester
    - Subtotal thyroidectomy suggested by few → though there is↑ risk of recurrence.

11. **Which investigation you would not like to do in pregnancy and why?**

    Radioactive iodine (^{131}I) uptake and scans: exposes the fetus to >5-10 rads
    - Crosses the placenta
    - Damage fetal thyroid gland permanently
    - Pregnancy avoided at least for 4 months (up to 1yr) after this
    - If pregnancy occurs → termination
    - OCPs → withheld because of ↑ metabolism and disturbed liver function, therefore abstinence advised by few
    - If inadvertently treated in pregnancy, patient should be informed of the possible teratogenic effects and that fetal thyroid uptake of RAI is generally after 12 weeks, exposure to maternal

^{131}I before the 12th week of pregnancy may or may not be associated with fetal thyroid dysfunction
- Exposure after 12 weeks → thyroid ablation, requiring intrauterine thyroid hormone replacement and lifelong therapy for hypothyroidism.

Lactation
- Breastfeeding is contraindicated with it.

12. What is the role of β adrenergic drugs?
- Beta-blockers can be used temporarily for not more than 4 weeks in cases of acute hyperthyroidism or as preparation for surgery
- When used in 3rd trimester-mild and transitory neonatal hypoglycemia, apnea, and bradycardia may be noted, which generally resolves in 1-2 days.

13. Summary of management during pregnancy and postpartum.
During pregnancy
- Tab. PTU 200-450 mg/day (initially)
- Maintenance: 50-300 mg/day
- Repeat TSH and fT_4 every 4 weeks (2-8 weeks)
- Periodic USG (for fetal thyroid size) from 20th week onwards
- ↓dose in 2nd and 3rd trimester
- Investigations:
  - TSH and fT_4
    - If hyperfunction → TSH receptor antibodies
                         Thyroid stimulating antibodies
                         TPO antibodies
    - If euthyroid → stop treatment near term
  - If on USG:
    - Fetal goiter
    - IUGR or Hydrops
    - Mother has ↑ A/b levels
    - Previous child with newborn thyrotoxicosis
    } Cordocentesis and check fetal thyroid hormones and antibody levels
- On checking levels:
  - Hypothyroidism →↓ drugs
  - Hyperthyroidism: ↑ maternal medication
  - If marked tachycardia and arrhythmias → propranolol (β blocking agent)
  - Cord blood → for TSH and fT_4 at delivery.

Characteristics of hyperthyroidism in fetus:
- Goiter
- FHR>160bpm
- Advanced bone age
- Poor growth
- Craniosynostosis
- Hydrops.

Management after delivery

Mother
- Antithyroid drugs → restarted or ↑ after delivery (worsening of Graves' disease not uncommon)
- TFT (TSH and fT_4) → monitored up to 1 year
- Breastfeeding allowed

- Best drug → PTU (minimally excreted)
- Methimazole and carbimazole → also safe
- If ↑ doses of these drugs are given → thyroid function monitored in infant.

Infant
- Neonatal assessment: close monitoring (if hyperthyroid mother)
- TFT → at 5-10 days of age
- Transient thyrotoxicosis – may occur after 7-10 days once antithyroid drugs have cleared from fetal plasma due to presence of circulating maternal autoantibodies
  Symptoms:
    - Vomiting
    - Diarrhea
    - Dehydration
    - Weight loss
    - Irritability
    - Poor feeding
    - Self-limiting
- Supportive treatment required up to 4-6 weeks till antibody clears from fetal system
- If untreated → mortality 15%.

THYROID NODULES AND CARCINOMA

14. Which is the most common thyroid cancer in pregnancy?
Differentiated thyroid carcinoma in young woman

15. How will you treat?
Surgery → treatment of choice
Detection in early pregnancy → surgery in 2nd trimester
Detection in late pregnancy → after delivery

Pregnancy with thyroid nodules
↓
Fine needle aspiration (FNA), if >1 cm (ultrasound guided)
↓
Send for cytopathologic analysis
↓
If found to be malignant or are rapidly growing (in the first or early 2nd trimester)
↓
Pregnancy continued and surgery should be offered in the 2nd trimester, before fetal viability
↓
If cytology shows papillary cancer or follicular neoplasm in their early stages
↓
Wait till delivery for definitive surgery (these well-differentiated cancers are slow growing)
↓
It is prudent to keep TSH suppressed to just minimal levels in these patients by administering thyroid hormone
↓
Simultaneously keep a check on free T_4 or total T_4 levels.

POSTPARTUM THYROIDITIS (PPT)

- "Silent or Postpartum Thyroid Dysfunction"
- A common thyroid disorder that presents during the 1st postpartum year
- It is an exacerbation of an underlying autoimmune thyroiditis, aggravated by the immunological rebound that follows the end of pregnancy, which before pregnancy was clinically silent (Hence called *'silent dysfunction'*).

Incidence

- 1-16%.

Manifestation

It can present as:
- Isolated transient hypothyroidism in 43-48% (onset is usually between 6-12 months postpartum) OR
- Biphasic presentation i.e. hyperthyroidism followed by hypothyroidism OR
- Isolated transient hyperthyroidism in 30% (occurs between 2-10 months postpartum, most commonly at 3 months)

Thyroid antibody positive women are at highest risk (33–50%) of developing PPT.

Best Screening Tool for PPT

- Antithyroid peroxidase antibody
- All high risk women (mentioned above) should be screened for PPT at 3 months postpartum
- TSH and anti TPO antibody should be measured
- Women who are euthyroid and anti TPO antibody-negative require no further follow-up
- Anti TPO antibody-positive women should have a serum TSH performed at 6-9 months postpartum.

Hyperthyroid Postpartum Thyroiditis

- Most common symptoms:
  - Palpitations
  - Fatigue
  - Heat intolerance
  - Irritability/nervousness
- Asymptomatic in 33% of cases
- Untreated, the hyperthyroidism resolves spontaneously within 2–3 months
- This phase is diagnosed by:
  - Low serum TSH and presence of thyroid peroxidase antibodies, in women who are TSH receptor antibody- negative
  - Free T_4 levels are typically elevated but may be normal.

Now this needs to be differentiated from Graves' disease:

1. New onset postpartum Graves' disease is 20 times less common than postpartum thyroiditis
2. Either exophthalmos or a thyroid bruit confirms Graves' disease
3. The goiter of Graves' disease is typically more pronounced than that seen in postpartum thyroiditis

4. A radionuclide uptake may be required to confirm the diagnosis,
    - In the hyperthyroid phase of postpartum thyroiditis, there is minimal uptake, whereas an enhanced uptake is present in Graves' disease.

Hypothyroid Postpartum Thyroiditis

- Painless
- Occurs between 2-12 months postpartum
- Is most commonly diagnosed at 6 months
- Most frequently experienced symptoms:
    - Impaired concentration
    - Carelessness
    - Dry skin
    - Poor memory
    - Decreased energy
- ↑TSH + anti TPO A/b
- Permanent hypothyroidism develops in 20-40% of women following PPT.

Management

- Hyperthyroidism → β blockers (just to alleviate the existing symptoms)
    - Propranolol - drug of choice owing to its easy titration
    - For a maximum of 3 months
- Hypothyroidism
    - Start thyroxine for those who are symptomatic or trying to conceive, keeping in view the risk of subclinical hypothyroidism in 1st trimester on fetal psychomotor development and ↑ miscarriages
    - Continue thyroxine in all subsequent pregnancies for up to 1 year after they have completed family
    - Long term follow up with annual TFT recommended
    - Hypothyroidism being a reversible cause of depression, women with postpartum depression should be screened for hypothyroidism and appropriately treated.

Future Prognosis

- Most women are euthyroid by 1 year
- Risk of recurrence in subsequent pregnancy → ≈ 70%
- Risk of developing hypothyroidism → 2-5% per year.

Case 2. A 27 year old woman attends ANC at 22 wks' gestation in her first ongoing pregnancy, having had 1 previous abortion at the age of 23 yrs. Booked case since 8 weeks of gestation. Vitals, all investigations including USG are normal. She experienced nausea and vomiting until 14 weeks gestation. This has now settled but she remains very tired and feels that she is gaining excessive weight in pregnancy. She also feels cold for much of the time, which surprises her as she understood that pregnant female tends to feel hot. On exam: appears lethargic and of low mood. BP 115/68 mmHg and HR 58/min. Per abdomen: unremarkable and fundus palpable at umbilicus

16. **What can be the provisional diagnosis and which other features will you look for examination?**

    Provisional diagnosis can be
    a. Hypothyroidism
    b. Anemia
    c. Pregnancy itself can have the following:
       - Fatigue and emotional changes
       - Tiredness/lethargy
       - Excessive weight gain
       - Bradycardia

    Other features to be looked at
    - Cold intolerance
    - Constipation
    - Weight gain
    - Dry skin
    - Fatigue
    - Asthenia
    - Drowsiness

    Physical examination
    - Increased Diastolic BP/bradycardia
    - Dry skin
    - Goiter (may or may not be)
    - Delayed reflex – relaxation phase
    - Hair loss
    - Non pitting edema
    - Indentation or pitting:
        - Cardinal sign of subcutaneous edema
        - Pressure maintained for few seconds by examiner's fingers or thumb
        - May persist for several minutes followed by slow reaccumulation of displaced fluid
    - Edema
        - Generalized → disorder of heart, kidneys, liver, gut or due to diet
        - Local → due to:
            - Venous or lymphatic obstruction
            - Allergy
            - Inflammation
            - Myxedema - pretibial (in front of tibia) edema
            - Exophthalmos.

17. **Why in pregnancy female tends to feel hot?**
    - Increase blood flow in skin → dissipate excess heat generated by increased metabolism.

Causes of Hypothyroidism in Pregnancy

- Chronic autoimmune thyroiditis (Hashimoto's disease) – main cause of hypothyroidism in pregnancy (in the absence of iodine deficiency)
- Prior ablation with radioactive iodine or surgery
- ↑↑ doses of antithyroid drugs
- Iodine insufficiency (most important cause of thyroid insufficiency)

- TSH receptor blocking antibodies
- A hypothalamic-hypophyseal origin of hypothyroidism (rare) and can include lymphocytic hypophysitis occurring during pregnancy or postpartum (lack of TSH stimulation causing hypothyroidism → CENTRAL HYPOTHYROIDISM).

Prevalence

- Overt hypothyroidism → 0.3–0.5%
- Subclinical hypothyroidism → 2–3%
- Thyroid autoantibodies are found in 5–15% of women in the childbearing age.

Autoimmune Thyroid Disease

- Most common immune disorder in human
- Most common cause of thyroid hypofunction both subclinical and overt
- Includes:
  - Hashimoto's disease
  - Graves' disease
  - Postpartum thyroiditis
- Measure:
  - Thyroperoxidase (TPO) antibody → Major autoantigen
  - Thyroglobulin (Tg) antibody
- Associated with an 3/4th ↑ risk of spontaneous miscarriage and risk of preterm birth is doubled
- Also a risk factor for perinatal death.

Complications of Hypothyroidism in Pregnancy

- There is a known association between overt hypothyroidism and reduced fertility, but still there is a possibility for them to conceive
- Myxedema rarely presents in pregnancy because these women are INFERTILE
- If controlled → uneventful
- If uncontrolled or remain undetected → there is an ↑ risk of following complications:

Maternal
  - Preeclampsia/Gestational hypertension
  - Eclampsia
  - Anemia
  - Abruptio
  - Preterm delivery
  - Antepartum depression
  - ↑ risk of cesarean section (Indication – fetal distress)
  - PPH
  - Postpartum hypertension
  - Lactation problems.

Fetal
  - Miscarriage
  - IUGR/Low birth weight
  - Increased perinatal mortality
  - Lower IQ and poorer cognitive function in infants.

Laboratory Tests

General overview
TSH and Total T_4 → currently accepted as best. Why?

Total T_4
- Change of TT_4 in pregnancy is much more predictable
- Methods of testing are much more reliable
- TT_4: rises early in pregnancy to 1.5 times its nonpregnant levels [under the influence of a rapid increase in T_4-binding globulin (TBG) levels] and remain stable thereafter
- Therefore, nonpregnant value x1.5 → normal value in 2nd and 3rd trimester
- Target levels in pregnancy → 12–18 µg/dL.

Why not Free T_4?
- There is no absolute value of FT_4 that defines hypothyroxinemia
- Free hormone measurements by automated methodology may perform differently during pregnancy because of the known alterations in two thyroid hormone binding proteins, increased serum TBG levels and decreased serum albumin concentrations
- Measurement of free T_4 hormone concentration by equilibrium dialysis is costly and not universally available
- Target levels in pregnancy → 2–2.5 ng/dL.

TSH
- "Trimester specific" reference ranges for serum TSH
- Lower normal limit:
  - 0.03 mIU/liter in the 1st and 2nd trimesters
  - 0.13 mIU/liter in the 3rd trimester
- Upper normal limit:
  - < 2.5 mIU/liter 1st trimester
  - 3.0 mIU/liter 2nd and 3rd trimesters
- TSH level descends 60–80% by week 10 and recovers slowly thereafter, but it may not reach the preconception normal range until gestation ends.

Thyroid antibodies
- Anti TPO antibodies
- Anti Thyroglobulin antibodies
- If these are increased → Autoimmune thyroid disease (AITD)
- Thyroid antibodies are found in approximately 10% of women
- Therefore, not routinely measured
- Screening advised in cases of recurrent miscarriage.

Therefore, to summarize, **normal recommendations** in pregnancy are as follows:

Screening
- Thyroid function → TSH and Total T_4
- Presence of autoimmune thyroid disease (AITD) → Anti TPO – Ab and Anti Tg – Ab
- Ultrasound → Only when nodular disease is suggested by examination.

Iodine supplementation
- 150 µg/day → non pregnant females
- 250 µg/day (range 200–300 µg/day) in pregnancy and lactation (WHO) but should not exceed 500 µg iodine/day

- Urinary iodine concentration (UIC) to be checked for iodine adequacy in diet (should be 150-250 µg/L)
- Demand increased in pregnancy due to increased thyroid hormone production to maintain maternal euthyroidism and increased urinary iodine excretion.

Effects of Iodine Deficiency on Mother

In pregnancy
- Hypothyroxinemia
- Elevated serum TSH
- Enlargement of the thyroid (by 10–50%)
- Goiter
- There can be overt hypothyroidism (and all complications related to it).

During Lactation
- Increased demands continue during lactation, an iodine-deficient woman may face several years of increased iodine loss leading to goiter
- Even after she stops lactation and the iodine demand decreases, her thyroid may not return to its previous size and there is a risk of multinodular goiter and hyperthyroidism later
- This all can be prevented by adequate iodine supplementation.

On Neonates
- Increases neonate and infant mortality
- Lower birth weight and development is less advanced
- Significantly decreases immunity
- Particularly important for myelination in CNS
- T_4 is very essential for cerebral cortex, cochlea and basal ganglia in 2nd trimester and for brain differentiation and growth in 3rd trimester. In iodine deficiency, maternal T_4 is low, hence brain development is seriously hampered
- The most serious complication of iodine deficiency is cretinism (severe mental retardation, deaf-mutism, spasticity, and stunted growth).

Assessment before Conception

- If known hypothyroid on treatment → achieve TSH levels < 2.5 mU/L (adjust dose)
- If known autoimmune thyroid disease → do TSH prior to or in early pregnancy
- If known other autoimmune disease (Type1 DM): do TSH prior to or in early pregnancy.

Antenatal Management

If hypothyroid (known case)

- Levothyroxine is the treatment of choice for maternal hypothyroidism, if the iodine nutrition status is adequate
- Better to achieve a target TSH level of < 2.5 mIU/liter before pregnancy
- Adjust the dose as early as 4-6 weeks of gestation →↑ it by 30 -50%, then titrate according to TSH levels
- Why should dose be increased?
  - There is a rapid rise in TBG levels resulting from the physiological rise in estrogen
  - There is increased distribution volume of thyroid hormones (vascular, hepatic, fetal-placental unit)
  - There is increased placental transport and metabolism of maternal T_4

- The magnitude of thyroxine increment during pregnancy depends primarily on the etiology of hypothyroidism, namely the presence or absence of residual functional thyroid tissue
- Women without residual functional thyroid tissue (after radioiodine ablation, total thyroidectomy, or due to congenital agenesis of the gland) require a greater increment in thyroxine dosage than women with Hashimoto's thyroiditis, who usually have some residual thyroid tissue
- ↓ to prepregnancy dose immediately after delivery.

Detected for 1st time

- Start levothyroxine
  - 1.8-2.0 µg/kg/day (T_4 → synthetic) in cases of overt disease
  - 100 µg thyroxine daily in mild cases (TSH <10 mIU/liter)
- Increment in thyroxine dose can be based on the initial degree of TSH elevation:
  - Serum TSH between 5–10 mIU/liter → average increment in thyroxine dosage is 25–50 µg/d
  - Serum TSH between 10 and 20 mIU/liter → increase up to 50–75 µg/d
  - Serum TSH >20 mIU/liter → 75–100 µg/d
  - Serum TSH and TT_4 should always be evaluated 3–4 weeks after every change of dosage
  - There should be a 4 hour delay between LT_4 and iron and calcium supplements usually prescribed in pregnancy as these interfere with levothyroxine absorption
- Do TSH after 4 weeks and titrate
- Then do every 6-8 weeks throughout pregnancy
- If patient is non-compliant → check TSH and TT_4 minimum 3 times (once in each trimester)
- Check TFT immediately after delivery and decrease the dose accordingly
- Recheck TSH 4-6 wks postpartum.

Women with Thyroid Autoimmunity (TAI)

- Euthyroid antibody positive women → check TFT every 4 weeks (they are at risk of developing hypothyroidism)
- In the case of recurrent miscarriage → treat with low dose thyroxine with judicious monitoring of thyroid function.

If previous thyroidectomy or ^{131}I ablation done (no native thyroid function)

- ↑↑ dosage required.

Subclinical Hypothyroidism

- TSH ↑ but normal free T_4
- Even mild form (delayed mental and motor function) has:
  - Long term neurodevelopment of offspring → adversely affected
  - ↑ risk of abruptio
  - ↑ cases of preterm birth (< 34 wks)
  - Central congenital hypothyroidism in newborns (requiring thyroxine) → in infants of female with undiagnosed or inadequately treated Graves' disease during pregnancy
- Thyroxine treatment improves obstetrical outcome but does not modify long-term neurological development in the offspring
- Still, prudent to give thyroxine.

Central Hypothyroidism

- Free T_4 ↓ and TSH normal or ↓.

Overt Hypothyroidism

- ↑ serum TSH concentration and ↓ free T_4 concentration.

Author's opinion:
Routinely, if Thyroid function tests are not done, at least it should be checked in the above mentioned women as the symptoms of thyroid disease are so non specific
Studies have proved that targeted thyroid function testing of only high-risk patients would miss about one third of pregnant women with overt or subclinical hypothyroidism
As normal maternal thyroid function is extremely important for normal intellectual development of the child, it should be screened in all women, ideally before conception or in the 1st trimester.

SUGGESTED READING

1. Alex Stagnaro-Green. Postpartum thyroiditis. The journal of clinical endocrinology and metabolism. 2002;87(9):4042-47.
2. Chevy Chase. Management of thyroid dysfunction during pregnancy and postpartum: an Endocrine Society clinical practice guideline. The Endocrine Society. 2007. p 79.
3. Diagnosing thyroid dysfunction in pregnant women. Is case finding enough? The journal of clinical endocrinology and metabolism. 2007;92(1):39-41.
4. Gabriella morreale de Escobar, Maria Jesus Obregon, et al. Is neuropsychological development related to maternal hypothyroidism or to maternal hypothyroxinemia? The journal of clinical endocrinology and metabolism. 2000;85(11).
5. Hypothyroidism in pregnancy. Consequences to neonatal health. The journal of clinical endocrinology and metabolism. 2001;86(6).
6. John T Dunn, Francois Delange. Damaged reproduction: The most important consequence of iodine deficiency. The journal of clinical endocrinology and metabolism. 2001;86(6).
7. Juan C Galofre, Terry F Davies. Autoimmune Thyroid Disease in Pregnancy: A Review. Journal of women's health 2009;18(11).
8. Marcos Abalovich, Nobuyuki Amino, Linda A Barbour, et al. Management of thyroid dysfunction during pregnancy and postpartum: an endocrine society clinical practice guideline. Journal of clinical endocrinology and metabolism. August 2007;92(8) (Supplement):S1-S47.
9. Miho Inoue, Naoko Arata, Gideon Koren, et al. Hyperthyroidism during pregnancy. Canadian Family Physician. Jul 2009;55.
10. Perros P Thyrotoxicosis and pregnancy. PLoS Med. 2005;2(12):e370.
11. Simon Forehan. Thyroid disease in the perinatal period. Australian Family Physician. August 2012;41(8).
12. Susan J Mandel, David S Cooper. The use of antithyroid drugs in pregnancy and lactation. The journal of clinical endocrinology and metabolism. 2001;86(6).
13. Takao Ando, Terry F Davies. Postpartum autoimmune thyroid disease: The potential role of fetal microchimerism. The journal of clinical endocrinology and metabolism. 2003;88(7):2965-71.

Index

A

Abdominal
  circumference (AC) 256
Aberrant cord insertion 255
Abnormal
  trophoblastic hyperplasia 177
Abortion 60, 123, 161, 437
  1st trimester 123
  2nd trimester 124
  complete 161, 164
  ectopic 359
  incomplete 140, 141, 161, 364
  inevitable 140, 159, 161, 163, 359, 364
  missed 140, 161, 169
  spontaneous 8, 10, 12, 126, 144, 167, 225, 245, 381, 624
  threatened 140, 141, 146, 161, 162, 359, 364
Abruptio placenta 184, 186-192, 225, 529
  classification 189
  clinical features 191
  management 192
  pathophysiology 188
  risk factors 187
  sonography 191
Acarbose 293
ACE inhibitors 320, 321, 322, 436, 453
  in pregnany 307
Acetaminophen 515
Achondroplasia 248
Acidosis 91, 477, 607, 670
  fetal 333
  lactic 650
Activated charcoal 681
Active phase 335
  protracted 334
Acute appendicitis 147
Acute chest syndrome 91, 95
Acute fatty liver of
  pregnancy 360, 694
Acute papillary necrosis 90

Acute respiratory distress
  syndrome 204, 476
Acute tubular necrosis 204
Acyanotic heart defects 466
Adenomyosis 105
Adenovirus 111, 248
ADH 348
Adnexal masses 377
Adnexal torsion 363, 369, 380
Adrenal insufficiency 113
Adult polycystic kidney
  disease 319
AED, pharmacokinetics during
  pregnancy 625
Albendazole 67
Albumin 672
Albuminuric retinopathy 319
Alcoholic cirrhosis 80
Aldosterone 348
Alkaline
  phosphatase 674, 675, 678
Allis clamp test 340
Alopecia, reversible 156
Alpha fetoprotein 9
Alpha glucosidase inhibitors 293
ALT 317, 675, 678, 682, 686, 687, 691
Amenorrhea 119, 132, 142, 161, 162, 163, 164
American Academy of
  Pediatrics 572
Amiodarone 451
Amlodipine 322
Amniocenteses 225, 245, 658
Amnioinfusion
  antepartum 260
  intrapartum 260
Amnion 527
Amnionicity 217, 230, 239
Amnioreduction 245
Amniotic fluid 22, 25
  embolism 194, 196, 459, 520, 529
  functions 26
  in 1st trimester 26

  in 2nd trimester 26
  index 243
  measurement 244
Amniotic sacs 218
Ampicillin 372, 438, 589
Amylophagia 49
Anaplastic carcinoma 718
Anembryonic gestation 165
Anemia megaloblastic 63
Anemia microangiopathic
  hemolytic 691
Anemia 29, 45, 52, 63, 170, 237, 261, 330, 351, 436, 439, 527, 633, 708
  acute 96
  causes of 81
  chronic hemolytic 52, 80
  classification of 57
  consequences of 91
  Cooley's 85
  deficiency 73
  dimorphic 51
  effect on fetus 61
  effect on mother 60
  folate deficiency 50, 52
  frank iron deficiency 62
  hemolytic 63, 84, 292, 658
  iron deficiency 50, 51, 52, 55, 59, 61, 62, 63, 80, 86, 92, 519
    blood transfusion 77
    manangement of 64
    role of erythropoietin 77
  leading factors 58
  macrocytic 97
  megaloblastic 96, 99
    causes of 98
    incidence 98
    mechanism 97
  in late pregnancy and labor 76
  microcytic hypochromic 80
  national rural health mission
    recommendations 79
  noniron deficiency
    microcytic 77

pernicious 63
short gun therapy of 73
sickle cell 44, 50, 59, 63, 88, 89
   acute manifestation 90
   antepartum
      management 93
   blood transfusion 94
   care of the fetus 94
   care of the mother 93
   chronic manifestation 89
   intrapartum care 94
   management 91
   preconceptional
      counseling 91
   sideroblastic 51, 80, 81
   vitamin B_{12} deficiency 52
Anencephaly 10, 17, 45, 157, 255, 404
Anesthesia
   epidural 339
   general 339
   spinal 338
Aneuploidies 217, 230, 242, 258
Angina 454
Angiotensin receptor
   blockers 92, 320, 453, 461
Angiotensin-converting enzyme
   (ACE) inhibitor 92, 461
Angular cheilitis 64
Angular stomatitis 64
Anhydramnios 224, 257
Anisocytosis 62
Annexin V 111
Annular pancreas 243
Antenatal care 3
Antepartum asphyxia 261
Antepartum coagulation 446
Antepartum fetal surveillance
   (APFS) 267
Antepartum hemorrhage 10, 57, 93, 184, 382, 392, 524, 655
   in early pregnancy 140-181
   in late gestation 183-213
      complications
         associated 186
      fetal and neonatal
         complications 185
      massive hemorrhage 185
      maternal
         complications 185
      mild bleeding 185
      mode of delivery 186
      steroid usage 186

Antibodies
   anticardiolipin (ACL) 111, 127
   anti-HEV 690
   anti-phospholipid 104, 110, 129
   anti-prothrombin 129
   antisperm 105
   antithyroid 105
   antitrophoblast 105
   anti-β_2
      glycoprotein 1 111, 128
   fluorescent treponemal 22
   IgG 499, 505
   IgG anti-HAV 682
   IgM 499
   IgM anti-HAV 682
   phosphatidylinositol 111
   phosphatidylserine 111
   phosphotidylcholine 111
   phosphotidylethalomine 111
   phosphotidylglycerol 111
   thyroglobulin (TGAB) 125, 131, 737
   thyroid 738
   thyroperoxidase (TPO) 131, 732, 737
   TSH receptor (TRAB) 727-729, 732
Anticoagulants, naturally
   occurring 193
Anti-D immunoglobulin 172, 198, 207, 550, 563, 653-656, 662
Antiepileptic drugs 624
Anti-hypertensive drugs 312
   atenolol 309
   compatible with
      breastfeeding 309
   diazoxide 309
   hydralazine 308
   hydrochlorthiazide 309
   labetalol 308
   methyldopa 308
   nitro-prusside 309
   prazosin 309
Antiphospholipid antibody
   syndrome 105, 110, 113, 128, 129, 301, 314, 697
   classification 128
   complications of 112
   treatment 135
Antiplasminogen 194
Antithrombin 3 104, 193, 194, 370
   deficiency 107, 314

Antitubercular drugs
   first line 488
   non-compliance 490
   second line 488
   third line 488
Anuria 307
Aortic aneurysm 423, 427, 428
Aortic annular dilation 455
Aortic diseases 468
Aortic dissection 431
Aortic regurgitation 423-425, 428, 429, 432, 455
   auscultation 456
   management 456
Aortic stenosis 429, 432, 453
   calcific 428
   compensated state 454
   congenital 466
   decompensated state 454
   management 454
Apex beat 426
Apex impulse 422
APGAR scores 10, 61, 329, 411, 609
APLA 111, 137, 263
Aplasia cutis 10
Appendectomy 376
Appendicitis 367, 376
   acute 361, 367
aPTT 127
Aqueductal stenosis 505
Arcuate uteri 123
AROM 212, 324, 336
Arrhythmia 243, 439, 454
   management of 464
ART
   first line 706
   second line 707
Arterial thrombosis 107
Arteriovenous fistula 425
Artesunate 480
Arthrogryposis 248
Artificial mechanical valve
   prosthesis 439
Ascites 245, 246, 506
Asherman syndrome 119, 204
Asphyxia 10, 213, 250
Aspirin 184
Assessment, sacral curve 32
AST 317, 675, 678, 691
Asthma 36, 570
Astomia 243
Asymptomatic hypercholanemia
   of pregnancy 678

Atazanavir 705
ATDs 729
Atenolol 320, 322
Atherosclerosis 112
Atovaquone 483
Atrial arrhythmias 451
Atrial dilatation 449
Atrial fibrillation 424, 439, 441, 447, 449, 464
Atrial flutter 439
Atrial septal defect (ASD) 429, 434, 466, 625
Atrial tachyarrythmias 424
Attitude 28
Atypical cyst 160
Autism 571
Autosplenectomy 88
Autoimmune disorders 110
Autoimmune thyroid disease 737
Azithromycin 483
AZT 714
Azygous artery of vagina
 anterior 543
 posterior 543

B

B lymphocytes 484
Baby-friendly initiative (BFI), benefits 570
Bacillus Calmette–Guérin (BCG) 491
Bacteriuria 371, 585
Bacteroides 512
Bagel sign 144
Ballantyne syndrome 246, 608
Balloon valvuloplasty 442, 456
Ballotment 215
Bart's hydrops fetalis syndrome 84
Basal artery 543
Baum's curette 546
Behavioral disorder 494
Benign vaginal adenosis 122
Benzodiazepines 630
Beta 2-glycoprotein 128
Beta blockers 308, 421, 440, 461, 462, 463
Beta HCG 142, 143, 144, 148, 150, 152, 153, 155, 158, 159, 171, 173, 231, 249
Betamethasone 237, 693
Biguanides 292

Bile acids 677
 in ICP 678
 in normal pregnancy 678
Biliary colic 361
Bilirubin 54, 86, 311, 314, 317, 678
 conjugated 674, 678
 metabolism 672
 total 674
 unconjugated 674, 691
Biliverdin 672
Bimanual compression 532, 537
Bimanual examination 40
Binding proteins 111
Bipolar cord coagulation 227
Birth asphyxia 296
Birth trauma 284
Bishop's score 297, 328, 469, 613
 modified 34
Blastocysts 109, 218
Blind cervical pouch 122
Blob sign 144
Blumberg's sign 368
Bone marrow depression 156
Brachial plexus
 injury 250, 284, 296
Brachiocephalic circulation 268
Bradycardia 424
Brain defects 231
Braxton-Hicks
 contractions 21, 336
Breast abscess 590
 treatment 597
Breast cancer 571
Breast engorgement 589, 594
Breast feeding frequency 582
Breast milk
 comparison 573, 574
 contents 572
 of diabetic mother 575
 production 572
 qualities of 574
 storage 576
 tips for using 580
Breast pumps 579
 types of 579
Breast signs 4
Breast-sucking patterns 583
 nonnutritive sucking 583
 nutritive sucking 583
Breast, weaning 577
Breastfeeding 154
 contraindications to 575
 factors influencing 580
  negative impact 581
  positive impact 580

Breech delivery 405
 assisted 407
 complications associated with cesarean section 406
 fetal complications 411
 maneuvers for cesarean delivery 405
 spontaneous 406
 vaginal 406
Breech presentation 123
Broad ligament 546
 abscess 586
 hematoma 529
Bronchiectasis 255
Bronchitis 586, 592
 chronic 592
Brudzinski's sign 632
Budd Chiari syndrome 113
Burns-Marshall technique 409
Burr cells 691

C

C. difficile 593
Cabergolin 579
Calcium channel antagonist 308
Calcium channel blockers 421, 463
Calcium supplementation 310
Campylobacter 593
Candesartan 461
Candida albicans 565
Captopril 307, 321, 322, 461
Carbamazepine 625, 628, 630
 associated malformations 631
Carbetocin 532
Carbimazole 730, 731
Cardiac abnormalities 231, 624
Cardiac activity 142, 147, 150, 153, 161, 162
Cardiac arrest, in pregnancy 470
Cardiac asthma 450
Cardiac failure 29
Cardiac malformation 631
Cardiomegaly 84
Cardiomyopathies 247, 284, 433, 435, 449
 dilated 433
 hypertrophic 433
 restrictive 433
Cardiopulmonary circulation 449
Cardiopulmonary overload 317
Cardiovascular collapse 476

Cardiovascular system
    auscultation 427
        aortic area 427
        Erb's area 427
        mitral area 427
        pulmonary area 427
        tricuspid area 427
    inspection 422
    palpation 426
    percussion 426
Carey Coombs murmur 429
Carvallo's sign 450
Carvedilol 461
Casein 569
Cataracts 496
CD4 701, 706, 707, 709
Cefazolin 372
Ceftriaxone 632
Celiac disease 59
Cell salvage 550
Cerclage
    cervical 208, 398
    high transvaginal 118, 389
    history-indicated 117, 389
    occlusion 118, 389
    rescue 118, 389
    transabdominal 118, 389
    transvaginal 118, 389
    ultrasound-indicated 117, 389
Cerebral calcification 501
Cerebral edema 638
Cerebral hemorrhage 90, 638, 641, 643
Cerebral infarction 90
Cerebral ischemia 113, 638
Cerebral microthrombi 113
Cerebral palsy 397, 514, 654
Cerebral sinus thrombosis 623
Cerebral white matter damage 514
Cerebrovascular accident 623
Cervical abnormalities 141
Cervical assessment 613
Cervical atresia 119, 122
Cervical cervix 326
Cervical hematoma 529
Cervical incompetence 105, 114, 120
Cervical insufficiency 382, 388
Cervical lacerations 635
Cervical length 115–118, 217, 386
Cervical polyp 213
Cervical softening 383
Cervical spine injury 412
Cervical swab 104

Cervical tears 134, 529
Cervicovaginal fistula 326
Cervix
    mechanical dilatation 344
    ripening of 383
Cesarean section 336, 339
    Cherney procedure 341
    complications 345, 353
        adhesion formation 354
        bowel obstruction 354
        dehiscence 353
        infection 353
        operative 345
        paralytic ileus 354
        postoperative 346
        superficial wound separation 353
    extraperitoneal cesarean section 343
    indications for 338
    Joel-Cohen technique 341, 342
    lower segment 326
    methods of removal of placenta 344
        cord traction 344
        manual removal 344
        placental drainage with spontaneous delivery 344
    Misgav-Ladach technique 342
    modified Misgav-Ladach technique 342
    Mouchel incision 341
    Pelosi-type 340
    Pfannenstiel incision 341
    Porro operation 343
    Porro Veit operation 344
    Porro's Müller operation 343
    postoperative
        care 346
        infections 349
    preoperative preparation 339
    prevention of adhesions 355
    traditional vertical 342
    trial of labor informed consent 330
    types of 337
        classical CS 337
        elective 337
        emergency 337
        LSCS 337
        primary cesarean section 337
        repeat cesarean section 337

upper segment 326, 343
    uterine incision
        extra-abdominal 345
        intra-abdominal repair 345
    wound drainage 344
Chadwick's sign 4
Chenodeoxycholic acid 677
Chest infection 346
Chest pain, causes 431
Chlamydia 126, 587
Chloasma gravidarum 23
Chloasma uterinum 38
Chloroquine 478, 483
Chlorpromazine 112, 292, 649
Chlorthiazides 320
Chocolate cyst 147
Cholecystectomy, laparoscopic 373
Cholecystitis 90
    acute 361, 367, 372
Cholelithiasis 90, 367, 372, 374
Cholestasis 292
    extrahepatic 674
    intrahepatic 674
Cholestyramine 681
Cholic acid 677
Chorea gravidarum 112
Chorioamnionitis 118, 126, 337, 382, 389, 392, 395, 510, 524, 540, 587, 621
Chorioangioma 248, 360
Choriocarcinoma 167, 177, 178, 728
Chorion 217, 527
Chorionic villi 148, 160, 169, 172, 177
Chorionicity 217, 220, 222, 230
    complications related to 221
Chorioretinitis 500
Chromosome abnormalities 258
Chronic anovulation 86
Chronic hepatitis 85
Chronic kidney disease 319
Chronic leg ulcers 91
Chronic liver disease 80, 193
Chronic renal disease 29
Circular artery of cervix 543
Circulatory collapse/shock 480
Circumvallate placenta 184
Cirrhosis 193, 674
Cisplatin 178
Cleft lip 45, 157, 631
Cleft palate 45, 157, 242, 625, 631
Clifford's syndrome 608, 609
Clindamycin 478

Clostridium tetani 587
Clostridium welchii 587
Cloxacillin 590
Clubbing 431
Clubfoot 157
CMV 261
COA 435
Coarctation of aorta 319, 423, 429, 467
Collapsing pulse 455
Colloids 197
Colostrum 43, 560, 572
Common iliac artery 545
Complete heart block 247
Complete mole 141
Congenital adrenal hypoplasia 12
Congenital glaucoma 496
Congenital heart disease (CHD) 44, 45, 431, 446, 465, 496
   ASD 433
   antenatal measures 465
   intrapartum and postpartum measures 465
   Eisenmenger's syndrome 433
   Fallot's tetralogy 433
   PDA 433
   preconception counseling 465
   VSD 433
Congenital myotonic dystrophy 248
Congenital nephrosis 247
Congenital rubella syndrome 492, 493
Congestive cardiac failure 241, 428, 431
Conjunctivitis 156
Constipation 49
Contraception
   estrogen-progestin contraceptives 575
   for breastfeeding women 564
   for nonbreastfeeding women 564
   progestin only contraceptives 575
Controlled cord traction (CCT) 526
Convulsions
   pseudo 622
   recurrent management of 645
   true 622
Coombs test 658
   amniotic fluid analysis 659
   direct 658
   indirect 22, 658, 659

Cor pulmonale 436
Cord clamping
   delayed 525
   early 525
Cord embolization 227
Cord entanglement 230
Cord ligation 227
Cord prolapse 338, 403, 412
Cordocentesis 655
Corneal resection 151
Coronary artery disease 571
Coronary sinus 268
Corpus luteal cyst 141, 143, 147
   hemorrhagic 359
Corrigan's neck sign 456
Corrigan's pulse 455
Corticosteroids 208, 222, 485
Cortisol 279, 580
Co-trimoxazole therapy 708
Couvelaire uterus 185
Cracked nipple 589
Craniosynostosis 625
C-reactive protein 571
Criggler-Najjar syndrome 673
Critical stenosis 453
Crohn's disease 59
Cryoprecipitate 198
Cryptosporidium 498
Crystalloids 197
CTG monitoring 238
Culdocentesis 149
Cushing's syndrome 319
Cyanosis
   central 432
   peripheral 432
Cyanotic heart defects 255, 467
Cyclophosphamide 175
Cystadenoma 378
Cystic fibrosis 8, 44
Cystic periventricular leukomalacia (PVL) 396
Cystitis 368
   acute 361, 371, 372
Cytokines 188
   anti-inflammatory 110
   proinflammatory 110
   role of 110
Cytomegalovirus 503
   clinical manifestations 504
   congenital 504
   IgG avidity assay 505
   intrauterine transmission 504
   modes of transmission 504
   prenatal diagnosis 505
   prevention 506

   screening 506
   serious complications 504
Cytotrophoblast 111, 168

D

D dimer 196, 691
Dactinomycin 174, 175, 178
DCDA 220
Deep vein thrombosis 29, 45, 128, 439, 449, 591
Degenerating myoma 362, 369, 380
Delivery, vaginal 327, 328
Denominator 28
Deoxycholic acid 677
Depot medroxyprogesterone acetate 299
Dermatitis herpetiformis 63
Descent
   arrest 335
   failure 335
   protracted 335
Desferrioxamine 87
Dexamethasone 680, 693
Dextrans 197
Dextrocardia 157, 427
DHEAS 11
Diabetes 36, 37, 45, 72, 86, 103, 105, 126, 248, 255, 261, 266, 283, 313, 328, 485, 494, 612
   classification of 283
   in pregnancy 279
Diabetic vasculopathy 296
Diaphragmatic hernia 243, 247
Diarrhea 49
Diastolic dysfunction 459
Diastolic shock 426
Diazepam 628, 648
Dichorionic diamniotic pregnancy 218, 220, 221
Dichorionic pregnancy 218
Dicrotic pulse 425
Didelphys 130
Diffuse trophoblastic hyperplasia 168
Digitalis 440
Digoxin 453, 461, 463
Diltiazem 440, 441
Dilute Russell's viper venom test 127
Dinoprostone 525
Discriminatory zone (DZ) 148
Disseminated intravascular coagulopathy 173, 185, 193–199

clinical features of 195
conditions associated
　with 194
diagnosis 195
in antepartum hemorrhage 199
management 197
profile 196
Diuretics 310, 320, 455
　pregnancy, 307
Dizziness 430
Dobutamine 441
Domperidone 584
Dopamine 441
DOTS 489
Double decidual sac 142
Down's syndrome 8, 11, 12, 16,
　22, 230, 231, 247, 274, 404
Dravet syndrome 628
Drepanocytosis 88
Dubin-Johnson syndrome 674
Ductus venosus (DV) 273
Duke's criteria 456, 457
Duodenal stenosis 243
Dwarfism 44
Dysmenorrhea 123
Dyspareunia 123
Dysphagia 63
Dyspnea 430, 450, 452, 455, 459
　exertional 454
　paroxysmal nocturnal 430
Dysuria 361, 362, 590

E

E. coli 262, 350, 696
Early pregnancy factor 7
Ebstein's anomaly 243, 247
Ecchymosis 63
Eclampsia 194, 196, 303, 315, 318,
　338, 392, 395, 459, 631, 637,
　693, 737
　atypical 639
　clinical features 640
　effects on
　　fetus 647
　　mother 647
　fluid management 639
　impending 316, 365, 639
　　symptoms 316
　management 641
　　emergency care 641, 642
　　magnesium infusion 644
　　obstetric
　　　management 641, 646

indications of cesarean
　section 646
postpartum 646
organ system
　derangements in 638
Eclamptic fit 640, 647
Ectopic pregnancies 7, 655
　intrauterine 145
　unruptured 153
Ectopic unruptured 140
Edema 29
　physiological 29
Eden's criteria 648
Efavirenz (EFV) 705–707
　in pregnancy 706
Ehlers-Danlos
　syndrome 437, 467, 468
Eisenmenger's syndrome 436
Ejection click 430
Electrolyte imbalance 636
Elisa 6, 7, 22, 62, 128
EMA-CO regimen 174, 175, 178
EMA-EP regimen 175
Embryo 142
Embryonic pole 161, 165
Emtricitabine 705, 706
Enalapril 307, 321, 322, 461
Encephalitis 508, 623
Encephalocele 10, 242
Endocannabinoids 574
Endocarditis 445, 455, 457
　definite 457
Endocrine disorders 319
Endometrial biopsy 131
Endometrial cancer 571
Endometrial sclerosis 119
Endometriosis 120
Endometritis 200, 610
　postoperative 345
Endometrium 142, 143, 187,
　331, 565
Endomyometritis 514
Endovascular
　cytotrophoblasts 109
Entecavir 686
Epidermal growth factor 573
Epignathus 274
Epilepsy 36, 45, 623
　management
　　antepartum 629
　　contraception 630
　　intrapartum 629
　　postpartum 630
　pregnancy
　　and fetus 624
　　effects on 624

Epithelioid trophoblastic
　tumour 167, 179
Eplerenone 462
Ergometrine 186, 443, 525,
　530, 531
Ergonovine 594
Ernest page's classification 189
Erythroblast
　basophil 55
　orthochromatic 55
　polychromatophilic 55
Erythroblastopenia 50
Erythroblastosis fetalis 249
Erythrocyte zinc protoporphyrin
　concentration 62
Erythrocytes 53, 55
Erythromycin 590
Erythropoiesis 55
　ineffective 673
Erythropoietin 55
Escherichia coli 512, 587
Eslicarbazepine 627
Esophageal atresia 243, 730
Esophageal reflux 393
Estradiol 86, 298
Estrogen 279, 384, 580
Etoposide 174, 175, 178
Exchange transfusion 667, 669
　complications 670
　continuous exchange 669
　post exchange care 670
　prerequisites for 668
　push-pull method 669
　types of 668
External ballottement 40
External cephalic version 413
External iliac artery 544
External iliac vein injury 546
Extrinsic hemolysis 247

F

Facial clefts 231
Factor V Leiden 104, 314
Fallopian tube 151, 158
Famciclovir 509
Fanconi syndrome 708
Fatty liver 194
FDP titer 196
Femoral artery 544
Ferritin 54, 61, 65, 80
Ferroportin 55
Ferrous fumarate 70
Fetal akinesia 243
Fetal anasarca 245

Fetal anemia 213
Fetal anomalies 17, 186
Fetal asphyxia 199
Fetal biometry 216
Fetal bradycardia 336
Fetal cerebral circulation 272
Fetal circulation 522
    normal 268
Fetal distress 260, 337, 524
Fetal growth 134
Fetal growth restriction 211
Fetal head entrapment 403, 411
Fetal heart failure 653
Fetal hydantoin syndrome 631
Fetal hypoxia 185
    transient 336
Fetal malformations 284, 624
Fetal malpresentation 124, 201, 338
Fetal renal hamartoma 243
Fetal soufflé 22
Fetal venous circulation 273
Fetomaternal hemorrhage 10, 656, 657
FHR monitoring 94, 192, 193, 239, 259
FHS 22, 201, 207, 215, 217, 253, 308, 340
Fibrin 108, 195
Fibrinogen 108, 192, 193, 196, 198
Fibrinolysis 108, 194, 195
Fibroblasts 352, 355, 484
Fibroid polyp 549
Fibroid uterus 519
FIGO anatomical staging 173, 178
First pelvic grip 31
First trimester 3–20
    laboratory tests 5
    signs 4
    symptoms 3
    ultrasound features 13
Flank pain 362
Flow cytometry 664
Focal trophoblastic hyperplasia 169
Focused antenatal care (FANC) 69
Folate deficiency 49, 697
Folate supplements 82
Folic acid 56, 67, 72, 92, 97, 234, 236, 483
Folinic acid 175, 178
    antagonist 153

Fortification 68
    biofortification 68
    conventional 68
    home 68
Fragile X syndrome 44
Fresh frozen plasma (FFP) 198
Fritsch syndrome 119
Frusemide 440
FT_4 131, 730, 732
Fundal grip 30
Fundal height 23, 40, 103, 265, 561

G

Gabapentin 627, 630
Galactogogue 584
Galactosemia 575
Gardnerella vaginalis 512
Gastric delivery systems 72
Gastroenteritis 593
Gastroschisis 10, 242
GDM 35, 138, 280
    antenatal management 295
        first trimester 295
        labor 296
        postpartum 297
        second trimester 295
        third trimester 296
    insulin therapy 286
    medical nutrition therapy 285
    nutritional therapy 285
    treatment 285
Gentamycin 372, 438, 589
Geophagia 49
Gestation
    multiple 519
    nonmolar 176
    transient thyrotoxicosis (GTT) 727
Gestational age 318
    determination of 35, 230
    prediction of 251
Gestational diabetes
    recurrence of 291
    risk
        factors 280
        in newborn 284
        to fetus 284
        to mother 284
    screening and diagnosis 281
        Carpenter and Coustan 281
        DIPSI 282
        IADPSG 281
        WHO/NICE 281

Gestational prediabetes 280
Gestational sacs 13, 144, 154, 159, 160, 165, 217
Gestational trophoblastic disease 153, 167, 314
    quiescent 180
Gestational trophoblastic neoplasia 176
    chemoresistant 179
Gestational trophoblastic tumours 167
GI atresia 255
Gilbert's syndrome 673
Glipizide 292
Globin 56
Globin chain
    alpha 82
    beta 82, 84, 89
Glomerular thrombosis 113
Glomerulonephritis 319
Glossitis 52, 63
Glucocorticoids 138, 346
Gluconeogenesis 287
Glucose challenge test 281
Glucose monitoring 290
Glucose-6-phosphate dehydrogenase deficiency 50, 90, 247, 673
Glutathione S-transferase alpha 678
Gluteal claudication 546
Glyburide 292
Glycemic control 296
Glycogenolysis 287
Glycoprotein 108
Goiter 728
    primary toxic 718, 721
    simple 718
Gonadotropins 216
Gonococci 587
Gonorrhea 46
Goodell's sign 4
Gosling index 270
Graham Steell murmur 450
Grandmal seizures 640
Grannum B. Hobin's grading 604
Granulocytosis 91
Graves' disease 726, 729, 737
    effect of pregnancy on 727
    relapse 729
Gravid uterus 379
Group B streptococcus 512
GTN
    follow-up after treatment 179

high-risk metastatic 174
invasive, mole 173
low-risk metastatic (stage II, III and score 0–6) 174
postmolar 176
GTT 103
Guar gum 681

H

H. pylori infection 59, 60
Haptoglobin 691
Hartman's sign 4
Hashimoto's disease 718, 737
Hb electrophoresis 82, 92
HbA 89
HbA$_1$C 103, 126, 263, 298
HbA$_2$ 89
HbcAg 8
HbF 89
HbH disease 87
HbS 89, 96
HbsAg 8, 94
HBV 689
    CDC vaccination schedule 687
    DNA 687
HCG 11, 168, 169, 180, 727
    false-positive
        causes of 149
        characteristics of 149
    maternal serum 11
    phantom 149
HCV RNA 689
HDL 298
Heart disease 45
Heart failure 728
    decompensated 462
Heart sounds 427
Hegar's sign 5
Hellin's rule 232
HELLP
    clinical symptoms 692
    diagnostic criteria 692
HELLP syndrome 12, 235, 314, 316,
        318, 338, 360, 647, 690, 691, 697
    guidelines in treatment of 693
    platelet therapy for 693
Hematemesis 49
Hematoma 324
    intrauterine 187
    rectus sheath 327
    retroplacental 191

Hematopoiesis,
    extramedullary 85
Hematuria 6, 49, 59, 63, 90, 205, 213, 362, 371, 377, 431
Heme 65, 83
Hemiplegia 176, 431
Hemochromatosis 80, 82, 85
    hereditary 81
Hemocytoblast 55
Hemoglobin 53, 56, 88, 237
    Bart's 84
    electrophoresis 212
    haptoglobin complex 691
    synthesis 56
Hemoglobinopathies 21, 45, 50, 82, 83
Hemoglobinuria 59, 477, 480
Hemolysis 80
Hemolytic disease of the newborn (HDN) 665
Hemolytic malignancy 63
Hemolytic uremic syndrome (HUS) 493, 696
Hemopericardium 150, 471
Hemophilia 44, 550
Hemophilia A 519
Hemoptysis 450
Hemorrhage 49
    catastrophic 160
    intracystic 378
    stages of 520
Hemorrhoids 49, 54, 98, 184, 216
Hemosiderosis 85
Hemothorax 471
Heparin 135, 137, 446, 447
    induced thrombocytopenia (HIT) 136
        HIT type I 136
        HIT type II 136
    low molecular weight 136, 184, 310, 461
    unfractionated 136
Hepatic dysfunction 731
Hepatic veins 268
Hepatitis 50, 372, 504, 586, 681
    toxic 674
    viral 674
Hepatitis A 248, 682
Hepatitis B 45, 86, 532, 683, 708, 709, 712
    immunoglobulin (HBIG) 687
    viral markers 683
        anti HbcAg 684
        anti HbeAg 684

        anti HbsAg 684
        HbcAg 683
        HbeAg 683
        HbsAg 683
    management 686
    risk of transmission 685
    vaccine HBV
        in combination with DTAP 685
        in combination with HAV 685
        in combination with HIB vaccine 685
        recombinant 685
Hepatitis C 45, 80, 86, 687, 709, 712
    management 688
    risk of transmission 688
    screening 688
Hepatitis D 689
Hepatitis E 689
Hepatocytes 672
Hepatomegaly 85, 91
Hepatosplenomegaly 63, 84, 86, 496, 505
Hepatotoxicity 708, 731
Hepcidin 55, 56
Hereditary spherocytosis 50
Hernia
    femoral 375
    incisional 328, 343, 346
    inguinal 375
Herniorrhaphy 545
Herpes esophagitis 507
Herpes genitalis 507
Herpes gladiatorum 507
Herpes labialis 507
Herpes simplex virus 507
    diagnosis 509
    disease manifestations 508
    management 509
    modes of delivery 510
    modes of transmission 508
    neonatal infection 510
    prevention of neonatal herpes 510
    risk of transmission to the neonate 508
Herpes viral encephalitis 507
Herpes viral meningitis 507
Herpetic gingivostomatitis 507
Herpetic whitlow 507
HEV-RNA 690
HI encephalopathy 250

HILL's sign 456
Hingorani sign 379
HIV 86, 112, 255, 484, 571, 688
  at risk women 699
  CD4 count 703
  clinical manifestation 699
    clinical stage I 699
    clinical stage II 700
    clinical stage III 700
    clinical stage IV 700
  medical management
    infant 713
    mother 713
  mode of delivery 712
  mother-to-child
    transmission 699
  perinatal transmission 699
  postpartum 713
  pregnancy
    management 705, 711
  prepregnancy
    management 709
  routes of transmission 698
  specific core antigen 703
  testing 701
    in pregnancy 704
  viral load assays 703
  WHO recommendations for
    breastfeeding in 715
HLA testing 704
HLA-A 109
HLA-B 109
HLA-E 109
HLA-G 109
Hoffman criteria 160
Holosystolic murmur 452
Home pregnancy tests 7
Homocysteine 104
Hookworms 98
Howell-Jolly bodies 99
HSG 130
Hughes syndrome 110
Human chorionic
  somatomammotropin 279
Humoral immune
  mechanisms 110
Hyaline membrane disease 186
Hyaluronic acid 383
Hydralazine 309, 441, 453,
  461, 462
Hydramnios 217, 224, 230,
  244, 255
Hydrocephalus 17, 157, 231, 242,
  404, 501, 505

Hydronephrosis 377
  acute 362, 368, 377
Hydrops fetalis 216, 224, 301, 506,
  663, 732
  classification 245
  immune hydrops 245
    cause 246
  nonimmune hydrops
    (NIFH) 245, 246, 261
    causes 247
Hydroxychloroquine 138
Hydroxyurea 92
Hyperandrogenism 125
Hyperbilirubinemia 186, 284, 329,
  505, 667, 673, 678
Hyperemesis 168, 173
Hyperemesis gravidarum 728
Hyperhomocysteinemia 129
Hyperinsulinemia 125, 134, 284
Hyperkalemia 670, 696
Hyperlactatemia 477
Hypermetabolic state of
  pregnancy 726
Hyperparasitemia 477
Hyperparathyroidism 374
Hyperprolactinemia 124, 135
Hyperpyrexia 261
Hyper-reflexia with sustained
  clonus 313
Hypertelorism 446
Hypertension 36, 45, 75, 90, 113,
  216, 241, 246, 258, 266, 353,
  612, 640
  accelerated 459
  chronic 187, 301, 303, 307,
    313, 319, 320
    management of 320
  essential 303, 319
  gestational 10, 112, 235, 284,
    301, 303, 310, 311, 320, 458
  in pregnancy 303
    classification 303
  mild 311, 313
  moderate 311, 313
  pulmonary 466
  secondary 303, 319
  severe 311, 313, 321
  transient 303
  white coat 303, 320
Hypertensive disorders
  fetal monitoring 312
  fundus changes 305
  labor management in 318
  maternal monitoring 311

  postpartum
    management of 321
Hypertensive
  encephalopathy 623, 638
Hyperthyroidism 168, 173, 392,
  720, 724, 725, 732
  features in fetus 732
  fetal thyroid function 728
  in pregnancy causes of 726
  maternal and fetal risks 728
  subclinical 729
Hypertrophic obstructive
  cardiomyopathy
  (HOCM) 425
Hyperventilation 433
Hyperventilation syndrome 622
Hypoadrenalism 50
Hypocalcemia 392, 636, 670
Hypocalvaria 307
Hypocortisolism 12
Hypofibrinogenemia 190, 195, 228
Hypogastric artery
  ligation 541, 543
Hypoglycemia 392, 631, 633,
  636, 670
Hypogonadotrophic
  hypogonadism 86
Hypokalemia 349, 391
Hypomagnesemia 284
Hypomenorrhea 119
Hyponatremia 292, 349, 636
  euvolemic 636
  hypervolemic 636
  hypovolemic 636
Hypopituitarism 50, 572
Hypoproteinemia 29, 246, 353
Hypospadias 45, 625
Hyposplenism 88, 90
Hypotension 75, 307, 308,
  391, 556
  postural 308
Hypothyroidism 50, 86, 135, 719,
  720, 730, 732
  central 737
  in pregnancy
    causes of 736
    complications of 737
  subclinical 125
Hypoxic cytotrophoblasts 11
Hypoxic ischemic
  encephalopathy 260, 329
Hysterectomy 185, 204, 208, 326,
  330, 544, 546
  abdominal 537
  in placental invasion 210

Hysteria 622, 623
Hysterotomy 537

I

Idiopathic thrombocytopenic
 purpura (ITP) 696
Ileocolic veins 376
Immunoglobulins,
 intravenous 138
Immunological tests, for
 pregnancy diagnosis 5
Impaired fasting glucose 297
Implantation bleeding 141
Incompetent cervix 134
Increta 544
Indomethacin 245, 258, 380
Induction of labor (IOL) 610
 contraindications 612
 definition 612
 methods of induction 614
 pharmacological methods 615
  mifepristone 615
  oxytocin 615
  prostaglandins 615
  relaxin 615
 prerequisites 613
 risks 613
Infective endocarditis 431, 432,
 440, 453, 456
Inferior mesenteric artery 544
Infertility 120, 123, 132, 146,
 253, 327
Infliximab 485
Inhibin A 12
Insulin extended insulin zinc
 suspension 289
Insulin resistance 279
Insulin ultra short-acting 289
Insulin 293, 580
 allergy 288
 efficiency 291
 exogenous 287
 glargine 289
 human 287
 intermediate acting 288
 protamine zinc insulin 289
 regimens for
  administration of 289
 resistance 288
 secretagogues 294
 sensitizers 292, 294
 short-acting 288
 ultra long acting 289

Intercurrent fits 639
Internal iliac artery 542
Internal iliac vein laceration 546
Interstitial pneumonitis 504
Intertuberous diameter 325
Intestinal atresia 231
Intestinal obstruction 362, 368,
 374, 375
Intestinal perforation 374
Intra-amniotic infection 519
Intracerebral hemorrhage 176
Intrahepatic cholestasis of
 pregnancy
 clinical features 676
 effects on fetus 677
 effects on mother 676
 investigations 677
 management of 680
 prognosis 681
Intrapartum asphyxia 284
Intrauterine
 adhesions 114, 119, 133
Intrauterine device 146
Intrauterine fetal demise 12, 61,
 112, 118, 185, 227, 261, 281,
 296, 372, 392, 524, 612
 cause 263
  antepartum 263
  postpartum 263
 investigations 266
 management 264
 treatment proper 267
Intrauterine infections 335
Intrauterine synechiae 119
Intraventricular hemorrhage 395,
 396, 446, 514
Intrinsic hemolysis 247
Intuberculous meningitis 486
Iodine deficiency 739
Iodine supplementation 738
Iron 56, 82
 carbonyl 72
 deficient erythropoiesis 61
 demand in pregnancy 64
 dextran 73, 74
 distribution in the body 53
 III hydroxide polymaltose
  complex 71
 parenteral administration
  contraindications 73
  indications 73
  intramuscular 74
  intravenous 74
 preparations 73

 poisoning 73
 requirements
  in lactation 60
  in pregnancy 60
 preparations oral 71
 sorbitol 73
 sorbitol citric acid complex 74
 sucrose 73, 75, 78
Ischial spines 325
Isorbide dinitrate 462
IUCD 49, 145
IUGR
 asymmetrical 254, 255, 266
 clinical examination 264
 doppler in 270
 symmetrical 254, 255, 266
IVC 273, 274
 thrombosis 247
IVF 142

J

Janeway lesions 432
Jaundice in pregnancy 675
 causes
  acute hepatitis 675
  AFLP 675
  HELLP 675
  hyperemesis
   gravidarum 675
  ICP 675
Jaundice 52, 63, 85, 90, 673
 causes 673, 675
 forms of 674
 physiological 581
Jauniaux and Campbell
 classification 199
Joffroy's sign 721
JVP 433, 438
 abnormal 424
 normal 423

K

Kallman syndrome 12
Kaolin clotting time 127
Kaposi sarcoma 700
Kegel's exercises 562
Kernicterus 654
Kernig's sign 632
Klebsiella 350
Kleihauer acid elusion screening
 test 664
Kleihauer Betke tests 185, 207,
 212, 263, 657

Koilonychia 63, 64
Korotkoff sounds 302, 425
Kuppuswamy scale 37

L

Labetalol 309, 320, 322
Labor/Labor 318
  1st stage 333
  2nd stage 333
    expulsive phase 333
    propulsive phase 333
  3rd stage 333
  4th stage 333
  pains
    false 360, 365
    true 360
  induction 469
  obstructed 94, 123, 524
  preterm 360, 677, 728
  prolonged 334, 405, 524, 588, 609, 635
    dangers of 335
    management 336
  spontaneous 324, 328, 330
  threatened preterm 359
Lacosamide 628
Lactalbumin, alpha 569
Lactation 58
Lactic acidosis 293
Lactoferrin 572
Lactoglobulin beta 569
Ladin's sign 4
Lambda sign 218
Lamivudine 686, 705, 706
Lamotrigine 625
Laparotomy 150, 152, 160
Laser photocoagulation 227
Lateral grip 30
LCHAD (long-chain 3-hydroxyacyl-coenzyme A dehydrogenase) enzyme 694
LDH 99, 298, 317
LDL cholesterol 293
Leg cramps 43
Leiomyoma 105, 114, 120, 130
  submucous 134
Lennox–Gastaut syndrome 628
Letzke's classification 196
Leucovorin 155
Leukocytosis 372
Level II scan 24
Levetiracetam 624, 626

Lie 27
Liley's curve 660
Linea nigra 40
Lipogenesis 279
Lisinopril 307, 461
Listeria monocytogenes 261, 512
Lithocholic acid 677
Livedo reticularis 112
Liver function tests 490
  etiology of complications 679
    fetal 679
    maternal 679
  in ICP 678
  in normal pregnancy 678
Liver laceration 471
Liver transaminases 490
Lochia 562, 589
Lochia alba 566
Lochia rubra 566
Loeys-Dietz syndrome 469
Lopinavir 705
Low-birth weight 186
Lower uterine segment 342
LPD 134
LPVR 708
Lumbar artery 544
Lumbosacral plexus 598
Lump in axilla 596
Lung maturity 296
Lupus anticoagulant 111
Luteinizing hormone 124
LV dysfunction 435
Lytic cocktail 649

M

M. tuberculosis 484
M. tuberculosis complex 485
Macrocytosis 99
Macrolides 593
Macrophages 109, 484
Macrosomia 10, 249, 296, 330, 338, 609–611
Magnesium sulfate 317, 396, 641
Malaria 57, 66, 98, 255, 266, 473, 586
  algid 477
  artemisinin combination therapy 479
  clinical features 479, 632
  complicated 476, 479, 623
  falciparum 632
  diagnosis 477
  obstetric management 481

  prevention 475, 482
  prophylaxis in pregnancy 483
  recurrence in 482
  transmission 474
  treatment 480, 633
  uncomplicated 475, 478
Malformations 403
Malignant trophoblastic tumours 170
Malnutrition 48
Malpresentation 330, 378, 612
Management of cardiac patient in labor 443
Maneuvers, Leopold's 30, 40, 335
Maneuvre 409
  Bracht 407
  Erich Franz bracht 410
  Johnson 549
  Løvset and Bickenbach 408
  original ritgen 408
  zavanelli 411
Mantoux test 487
Maple syrup urine disease 575
Marfan's syndrome 433, 435, 436, 469
Mastitis 589, 596
Maternal circulation 522, 657
Maternal infections 338
Matrix metalloproteinases 188
McDonald's rule 23, 265
Mean arterial pressure 304
Meckel-Gruber syndrome 258
Meconium 563, 606, 611, 679
  aspiration 250
  cause of 608
  syndrome (MAS) 607, 608
  injury, mechanisms of 608
  peritonitis 247
Meconium-stained amniotic fluid (MSAF), causes of 607
Megaloblastic erythropoiesis 99
Megaloblasts 99
Meglitinides 294
Melena 49
Mendelson's syndrome 345, 370
Meningitis 586, 623, 631
Meningoencephalitis 494, 504
Menorrhagia 122, 724
Menstrual age, methods for determining 250
Menthol 681
Metabolic acidosis 135, 480
Metabolic syndrome 571
Metformin 134, 292

Methergin 530
Methimazole 730
Methotrexate therapy
   fixed multiple dose 155
   in placental invasion 210
   single dose 155
Methotrexate 150, 153, 159, 174, 178
   congenital anomalies associated 157
   contraindications 154
   indications 154
Methyldopa 309, 311, 320, 646
Methylergonovine 594
Metoclopramide 584
Metoprolol 322
Metritis 586
Metronidazole 589, 594
MHC antigen 105
MHC molecules 109
Microcephaly 231, 242, 446, 494, 496, 506
Micrognathia 157
Micronutrient deficiencies
   calcium 67
   folate 66
   iron 66
   vitamin B_{12} 66
   vitamin D 67
   essential 68
Middle cerebral artery 272
   pulsatility index 273
Middle sacral artery 543, 544
Mifepristone 165, 166
Miglitol 294
Milk ejection reflex 582
Milk secretion 572
Mirror syndrome 246
Miscarriages 35, 104, 110, 120, 466, 728
Misoprostol 165-167, 330, 400, 524, 525, 530, 531
   oral tablets 618
Mitral regurgitation 424, 428, 429, 432, 451, 452
   management 453
Mitral stenosis 424, 428, 429, 432, 449, 450
   β blockers 451
   calcium channel blockers 451
   diuretics 451
   management during pregnancy 450

   obstetric management 451
   percutaneous balloon mitral valvuloplasty (PBMV) 451
Mitral valve prolapse 452
Mitral valve reconstruction 453
Moebius' sign 721
Molar mass 173
Molar pregnancy 11
Mole
   carneous 161
   chorioadenoma destruens invasive 176
   hydatidiform 167, 168, 265, 728
      complete 168, 180
      partial 169
   invasive 167, 171
Monocytogenes 126
Montgomery's tubercles 22
MRSA 587
MTHFR gene defect 107
Müllerian anomalies 114
Müllerian ducts 120, 121, 130
Mullerian fusion 105
Multicystic encephalomalacia 222
Multigravida 335
Multiparity 58, 249
Multiple birth deliveries 337
Multiple gestation 216
   average duration of pregnancy 233
Multiple pregnancies 23, 37, 338
Murmurs 429
Murphy sign 373
Muscular dystrophy 8, 44
Mycobacterium tuberculosis 485
Mycoplasma hominis 512
Myocardial infarction 112, 457
Myocarditis 247, 458, 460, 500, 504
Myocardium 268
Myoma 248
Myomectomy 119, 134, 204, 327
Myometrium 133, 142, 159, 177, 205, 331, 542, 679
Myotonic dystrophy 243, 404
Myxedema 720

N

N. meningitides 631
Nasal bone 15, 16
Nateglinide 294
National Anemia Prophylaxis Program 67

Necrotizing enterocolitis 571
Necrotizing fasciitis 590
Neonatal academia 609
Neonatal lacerations 329
Neonatal resuscitation 327
Neonatal thrombosis 112
Neoplasm 319
Nephrolithiasis 362, 377, 708
Nephrotoxicity 210
Neural tube 14, 231
   defects 10, 11, 17, 44
Neurogenic collapse 549
Neurohormonal blockade 464
Neutropenia, severe 156
Nevirapine 705, 714
   in pregnancy 707
New Ballard scoring system
   neuromuscular maturity 399
   physical maturity 399
Nifedipine 309, 311, 320, 322, 391
Nipple infection 597
Nipple pain 595
Nipples
   flat 595
   hypoplastic 730
   inverted 595
Nitabuch's layer 605
Nitroglycerine 441
Nonalcoholic steatohepatitis 80
Noonan's syndrome 248
NSAIDs 321
Nuchal arms 403
Nuchal cord 261
Nuchal translucency 15, 16, 230, 236
Nucleic acid amplification test (NAAT) 702

O

O'Sullivan's hydrostatic method 549
Obesity 351
Obstetrical paralysis 598
Obturator sign 368
OGTT 23, 126, 237, 281, 282, 295, 297
Oligohydramnios 12, 224, 232, 244, 253, 256-258, 307, 380, 404, 405, 436, 506, 607, 610, 624
   bilateral renal agenesis 257
   causes 257
   complications 260

management 259
Potter's facies 257
role of maternal hydration 259
urinary tract obstruction 258
Oligomenorrhea 251, 254
Oliguria 308, 313, 349
Omentum 326
Omphalocele 10, 242
Onycholysis 726
Oophorectomy 379
Open heart surgery 442
Opening snap 430
Ophthalmoplegia 722
Opitz-Frias syndrome 248
Oral contraceptives 234
Oral hypoglycemic agents (OHAs) 291
  sulfonylureas 291, 293
Orthopnea 430, 433, 439, 450, 452, 454, 455, 459
Osiander's sign 4
Osler nodes 432
Osteogenesis imperfecta type II 248
Osteomyelitis 486
Osteoporosis 138
Ovarian artery 541, 543
Ovarian cancer 379, 571
Ovarian cysts 130, 150, 168, 170, 215, 377
  hemorrhagic 363
  rupture of 362, 369, 377, 379
Ovarian tumours 216, 378
Overt diabetes 280, 282
Oxcarbazepine 627
Oxytocin 186, 239, 240, 324, 333, 336, 384, 524, 525, 530, 531, 534, 561, 594, 603, 613, 616, 620
  side effects 620

P

P. falciparum 473, 478, 479, 481
P. knowlesi 473
P. malariae 473
P. ovale 473
P. vivax 473, 477, 478, 481
Pagophagia 49
Pain abdomen 358-380
  gynecological causes 362
  medical/surgical causes 361, 366, 371

obstetric causes 359, 364
  trimester I 359
  trimester II 359
  trimester III 360
Painful myoma syndrome 380
Palmer's sign 5
Palpitations 433
Pancreatic β-cells 291
Pancreatitis 373, 708
  acute 361, 367, 374
Panencephalitis 494
Papilloedema 316
Paralytic ileus 346
Parametritis 586, 588
Parasitic infections 64
  prevention of 69
Parasternal heave 426
Parathyroid hormone 306
Paratubal cysts 122
Paroxysmal nocturnal dyspnea 450, 452, 459
Partial mole 141
Partial thromboplastin time 196
Parvovirus 111, 126
Patent ductus arteriosus (PDA) 307, 434, 466
Pawlick's grip 31
PCOS 103, 104, 105, 125, 281, 293
Pedal edema 622
Pedersen hypothesis 283
Pelvic assessment 32, 40, 330
  intertuberous diameter 33
  ischial spines 33
  pelvic side walls 32
  pubic arch 33
  sacral promontory 32
  sacrosciatic notch 33
  subpubic angle 33
  symphysis pubis 33
Pelvic infections 587
Pelvic irradiation 119
Pelvic side walls 325
Pelvic sonogram 143
Pelvis
  adequate 328
  arterial supply of 541
  contracted 324
Pena-Shokeir syndrome 243
Penicillins 453, 584, 590
Peptic ulcer disease 50, 98, 154
Percutaneous nephrostomy 377
Pericardial effusion 245, 422, 427, 451
Pericardial rub 430
Pericarditis 431

Perineal care 562
Peripartum cardiomyopathy (PPCM) 457
  compensated management 460
Peripheral edema 308
Peripheral neuropathy 113
Peritoneum 337, 340
Peritonitis 588
  generalized 586
Periventricular calcification 506
Periventricular leukomalacia 231
Persistent cord presentation 405
Persistent trophoblastic neoplasia 181
Petechiae 432
Pethidine 650
Pharyngitis 586
Phenformin 293
Phenobarbitone 628, 630, 631, 633
  associated malformations 631
Phenyl ketonuria 44, 575
Phenytoin 628, 630, 649
  associated malformations 631
Pheochromocytoma 319
Phlebitis 350
Phospholipids 111
Phosphotidylserine 111
Physiological anemia in pregnancy 57
PICA 49
PID 146, 147
Pigmentary retinopathy 493, 496
Pioglitazone 294
Pipingas technique 535
Piskaçek's sign 4
Placenta accreta 204, 205, 338, 346, 544
Placenta increta 204
Placenta percreta 204
Placenta previa 145, 184, 185, 199-204, 235, 238, 326, 327, 330, 338, 346, 395, 404, 405, 519, 525
  definitive diagnosis 201
  etiopathogenesis 200
  risk factors 199
  TAS 201
    role in 203
  USG terminology 203
Placenta
  at term 523
  bilobed 211

grading system 26
manual removal 130
retained 524, 528
    management 534
Placental abnormalities 10, 120
Placental abruption 185, 235, 313, 322, 346, 360, 366, 728
Placental anastomoses 231
Placental enlargement 246
Placental insufficiency 111, 258, 271, 273, 605, 609
Placental invasion 204
    2D color doppler 205
    3D power doppler 206
    antenatal management 206
    grayscale ultrasound 205
    massive treatment of 209
    mode of delivery 208
    time of delivery 208
Placental lactogen 580
Placental lacunae 205
Placental mosaicism 11
Placental perfusion 111, 336, 653
Placental polyp 594
Placental separation, signs of 522
Placental sign 4
Placental site trophoblastic tumour (PSTT) 181, 167, 177
Placentomegaly 245
Plasma inflammatory cytokines 458
Plasma protein-A 12
Plasmin 108
Plasminogen activators 194
Plasminogen inhibitors 194
Plasmodium 498
Platelets 196, 198
Pleural effusion 245, 246
Pleurisy 592
Plugged duct 596
Plummer-Vinson syndrome 63
Pneumococcal meningitis 631
Pneumocystis pneumonia 700
Pneumonitis 156, 339, 500, 546, 586, 592, 609
Polychromasia 62
Polycythemia 284, 667, 670
Polydactyly 625
Polyhydramnios 10, 187, 216, 232, 235, 244-246, 281, 296, 301, 382, 404, 519, 653
    acute 360, 366
    causes 241
    chief complaints 241
    classification 241
    GPE 242
    investigations 242
    signs 242
Polykinetic tendon reflexes 316
Polymenorrhea 724
Polymorphism 59
Ponderal index 254, 255
Porphyria 50, 81
Porphyria cutanea tarda 80
Portal hypertension 52, 653
Portal vein 376
Position 28
    trendelenburg 379
Post-term pregnancy 603-611
    amniotic fluid changes 606
    calculation of gestational age in 604
    cord 607
    cord problems 604
    fetal risks 609
    intrapartum 611
    maternal risks 610
    meconium 604, 607
    placental changes 604
Postinfectious encephalitis 493
Postmaturity dysmaturity syndrome 604, 608
Postnatal visit, examinations and assessments 564
Postpartum blues 598
Postpartum care 559
Postpartum depression 598
Postpartum endometritis 126
Postpartum
    hemorrhage 60, 84, 518, 635
Postpartum hemorrhage 186, 336, 527, 588
    acute 518
    antifibrinolytic agents 550
    atonic 525
    blood transfusion 551
    consequences of 527
    diagnose 520
    etiology 519
    major 518
    management of 527
    minor 518
    oxytocin in uniject 532
    precautions 524
    recombinant factor VIIa 550
    secondary 518, 565, 594
Postpartum hypertension 737
Postpartum psychosis 598
Postpartum thyroid disease 125
Postportocaval shunting 80
Post-term pregnancy
    management of 610
    risk factors 603
Postural hypotension 430, 459
Pott's disease 486
Pouch of douglas 342, 379, 586
Pourcelot index 269
PPCM
    clinical presentation and diagnosis 459
    differential diagnosis 459
PPROM 34, 102, 118, 187, 225, 235, 260, 381, 389, 390, 395, 614
Precipitous delivery 519
Preconception counseling 44
Precordium 422
Prediabetes 282
Preeclampsia
    acetyl salicylic acid role in 306
    management 314
    postnatal management 315
    risk factors for 313
    severe 365
    women at high risk 322
Preeclamptic angina 316
Pregabaline 624, 627
Pregestational diabetes 280
Pregnancy loss
    biochemical 104
    early 104
    recurrent 102-138
Pregnancy 147
    abdominal 360, 366
        examination 363
    anemia in 48
    anticoagulation in 447
    associated plasma protein-A 231
    blood changes 521
    blood pressure recording in 39
    cervical 159
    cornual 159
    dichorionic 219, 227
    DIET in 17
    ectopic 35, 143, 146, 364
        extrauterine 144
        tubal 145
    effects of fibroid 381
    extrauterine 153
    general history in 35
    heart disease in 432

heterotopic 150, 158
hydronephrosis of 371
interstitial 158
intra-abdominal 160
laparoscopy during 370
management of common
   symptoms of 42
medical termination of 165
molar 140, 143, 194, 301,
   359, 365
   anti-D prophylaxis 172
   contraception 172
   evacuation of 170
   hysterectomy 171
   management 170
   ultrasound features of 180
monoamniotic 219, 223
monochorionic 218, 219, 227
   diamniotic 218, 220, 221,
      223
   monoamniotic 218, 220,
      221, 229
multiple 261, 265, 314, 330
nausea and vomiting in
   early 42
of unknown location 143
ovarian 160
physical examination 38
physiological changes in 369
prolonged 612
RH negative 36, 652
   antepartum
      management of 666
scar (cesarean) 160
sickle cell disease 92
surgical termination of 166
systemic examination 38
twin 220
   role of ultrasound in 217
weight gain in 20
Prelabor scoring 34
Prelaryngeal/pretracheal lymph
   nodes 721
Premature birth 120
Prenatal genetic screening tests
   1st trimester 9
   2nd trimester 9
Preplacental abruption 191
Presentation 27, 28
breech 27, 28, 123, 343, 403, 613
   diagnosis 404
   flexed or complete
      breech 404
   footling 405

footling or incomplete 404
frank or extended
   breech 404
kneeling breech 404, 405
cephalic 27, 343
shoulder 27
vertex 32
Presenting part 27, 333
Preterm babies
   characteristics 398
Preterm birth 93
   rate 124
   risk factors for 382
Preterm delivery 12, 110, 138,
   185, 186, 737
Preterm infants
   complications of 396
Preterm labor 10, 11, 35, 60, 76,
   118, 123, 222, 225, 235, 237,
   284, 381-401, 388, 405, 442,
   466, 468
   cervical length 385
   corticosteroids in 395
   pathophysiology 383
   progesterone 397
   tocolysis 390
Preterm neonates, complications
   associated 400
Previous cesarean section
   pelvic assessment 324
   placental location 328
Previous cesarean
   scar integrity assessment 331
   trial of labor 330
Primaquine 478
Primary hyperaldosteronism 319
Primidone 630
Primigravida 253, 333
Probenecid 673
Procainamide 112
Proerythroblasts 55
Progesterone 7, 124, 131, 134,
   279, 310, 321, 384, 580,
   598, 679
   vaginal 398
Progestin 298
Proguanil 483
Prolactin 279, 580
   deficiency 572
   disorders 105
Prolonged latent phase 334
PROM 258, 613
Promethazine 650
Propylthiouracil 730

Prostaglandins 111, 189, 594
   contraindications 615
   dinoprostone (PGE$_2$) 616
      dinoprostone vaginal
         inserts 617
      intracervical gel 616
      intravaginal tablets 617
   misoprostol (PGE1) 617
      oral misoprostol
         solution 617
      vaginal misoprostol 617
         benefits of 619
         pharmacodynamics 619
   receptors 384
Protein C 104, 111, 193
   deficiency 107, 314
Protein S 104, 193
   deficiency 107, 314
Proteinuria 6, 90, 246, 301, 304,
   305, 311, 313-315, 623,
   640, 675
   testing for 304
Prothrombin 108
Prothrombin gene 104, 107
   mutation 187
Prothrombin time 196, 198
Prune belly syndrome 258
Pseudosac 143
Pseudotumour cerebri 63
Psoas sign 368
Psoriasis 153
Pubic arch 325
Puerperal sepsis 60, 336, 346, 381,
   527, 585, 635
   infectious causes 586
   management 589
   noninfectious causes 586
   signs and symptoms 588, 635
   sites of infection 588
   tests 635
   treatment 635
Puerperal tubal ligation 321
Puerperal venous thrombosis 61
Puerperium 378, 559-600
   abnormal 585-600
   normal 559-585
   physiological changes
      abdominal wall 567
      afterpains 568
      body weight 569
      cardiovascular system 568
      cervix 566
      endometrium 565
      gastrointestinal tract 568
      hematologic changes 569

lactation 569
lochia 566
nursing 569
perineum 567
placental site involution 566
skin 569
temperature 567
urinary tract 568
uterine vessels 566
uterus 565
vagina 567
vulva 567
Pulmonary atresia 274
Pulmonary crepitations 459
Pulmonary edema 87, 313, 316, 317, 450, 454, 476, 477, 480, 633
acute 441
Pulmonary embolism 61, 112, 321, 346, 439, 440, 457
Pulmonary embolus 113, 459
Pulmonary hypertension 92, 113, 224, 257, 258, 260, 392, 427, 428, 433, 435, 436, 449, 466
primary 436, 437
Pulmonary regurgitation 429
Pulmonary stenosis 274
Pulmonary surfactant 400
Pulmonary valve stenosis 468
Pulmonary venous hypertension 449
Pulmonic stenosis 424, 435, 456, 467
management 456
Pulsatility index (PI) 270
Pulse alternans 425
Pulse bigeminus 425
Pulse paradox 425
Pulsus bisferiens 455
Pulsus parvus et tardus 424, 454
Punctate basophilia 80
Pyelitis 368
Pyelonephritis 50, 58, 319, 590
acute 361, 372, 515
investigations 515
management 515
presentation 515
signs and symptoms 515
Pyrimethamine 502, 503
Pyruvate kinase deficiency 247
Pyuria 371

Q

Quantiferon-TB gold (QFT-G) 487
Queenan's curve 660, 667
Quickening 22
Quinine 480, 481, 633
Quintero staging system 224

R

Radial artery 543
Radiofrequency ablation 227
Radioreceptor assay 6
Radiolucent bone disease 496
Raltegravir (RAL) 705
Ramipril 461
Recti muscles 341, 567
Rectus sheath 340, 341, 342
Recurrent pregnancy loss
anatomic causes 105, 129
anatomical factors 114
causes 105
diagnosis of 127
diagnostic criteria 128
endocrine abnormalities 124, 131
endocrine and metabolic causes 105
genetic causes 104
genetic factors
monosomy X 106
tetraploidy 106
triploidy 106
trisomy 16 106
trisomy 21 106
trisomy 22 106
immunological causes 105, 109
infectious disorders 105
placental abnormalities 105
role of infection in 126
secondary 104
thrombotic factors 105
RPL
tertiary 104
treatment of 132
unexplained 138
Reflux nephropathy 319
Renal artery stenosis 319
Renal disease 50, 266, 313
Renal dysfunction 260
Renal dysplasia 257

Renal failure 307
chronic 59
Renal insufficiency 113
Renal tubular dysplasia 436
Renal tubular necrosis 185
Renal vein thrombosis 247
Renin-angiotensin-aldosterone 307
Repaglinide 294
Respiratory distress syndrome 186
Reticulocyte 55
Retigabine 628
Retinal edema 316
Retinal vasospasm 313
Retroplacental abruption 191
Return of menstruation and ovulation 566
Reversal of end diastolic flow (REDF) 272
Revised National TB Control Programme (RNTCP) 490
Rhabdomyoma 247
Rheumatic carditis 439
Rheumatic heart disease 431, 449, 455
Rheumatoid arthritis 110
Rheumatoid factor 149
RH-isoimmunization 612
Rifampicin 673, 680
Right atrial enlargement 427
Right ventricular hypertrophy 468
Ritonavir 705
Robert's sign 262
Rosetting technique 664
Rosiglitazone 294
Rotor's syndrome 674
Round ligament 359
Rubella 126, 248, 492
clinical presentation 492
diagnosis 495
fetal infection 494
infant evidence 496
maternal evidence 495
mode of transmission 492
prevention 494
risks 493
treatment 496
vaccine 497
vertical transmission 494
Rufinamide 628

S

Runge syndrome 608
Rupture uterus 336, 529
Ruptured ectopic 140

Saccharomyces cerevisiae 685
Sacral curve 325
Sacral promontory 324
Sacrococcygeal teratoma 10, 274
Sacrosciatic notch 325
Sacrum 325
S-adenosyl—L-methionine 681
Salmonella 593, 696
Salmonella choleraesuis 90
Salmonella enteritidis 90
Salmonella paratyphi 90
Salmonella typhimurium 90
Salpingectomy 151, 158
Salpingitis 586
Salpingitis isthmica nodosa 145
Salpingo-oophorectomy 380
Salpingotomy 151, 152
Salu's sign 305
Sarcoplasmic reticulum 384
Scar endometriosis 328
Scar
   unknown 329
   uterine 329
Schamrott's sign 432
Schistosomiasis 119
Sclerotic endometrium 119
Second trimester
   signs 21
   symptoms 21
   ultrasound features 25
   vaginal examination 21
Secondary amenorrhea 86
Seizure disorders 45
Selective feticide 226
Selenium 458
Sengstaken Blakemore tube 533
Septate uterus 123
Septate vagina 130
Septated cystic hygroma 16
Septic shock 586
Septicemia 372, 586, 588, 623
Septostomy 226
Serum alkaline phosphatase
   levels 372
Serum amylase 374

Serum bilirubin 668
Serum ferritin 62, 86
Serum pregnancy tests 6
Serum progesterone 149
Serum transferrin receptor 62
Serum unconjugated estriol 11
Serum α fetoproteins 204
Severe hemorrhages 316
Sheehan's syndrome 527, 572
Sher's classification 190
Shigella 696
Short limbs 157
Short rib-polydactyly
   syndrome 248
Shoulder dystocia 250, 609
Sibai regimen 645
Sickle cell disease
   (SCD) 83, 88, 98
   effect of pregnancy on 92
Sickle cell nephropathy 90
Sickle-hemoglobin C 89
Silent stroke 90
Sinus bradycardia 247
Skeletal dysplasia 243
Skull bossing 91
Small bowel obstruction 362
Small fetus 254
Smith lemli opitz
   syndrome 12, 258
Society for hysteroscopy 119
Sodium valproate 112
Somatic fetopathy 283
Sperm
   abnormal 110
   DNA decondensation test 135
   DNA fragmentation assay 135
Spherocytosis 673
Sphincter hemorrhages 112
Sphincter of Oddi 373
Spina bifida 10, 17, 45, 157, 625
Spinal abscess 587, 593
Spinal cord injury 346
Spiramycin 502
Spironolactone 462
Stallworthy's sign 201
Staphylococci aureus 90, 587, 593
Star gaze 405
Status epilepticus
   causes 631
   management 631
Stellwag's sign 721

Stercobilin 673
Stevens-Johnson
   syndrome 626, 708
Stillbirths 8, 10, 11, 186, 728
Stiripentol 628
Stomatitis 156
Streptococcus pneumonia 631
Streptococcus spp. 593
Streptococcus pyogenes 587
Strychnine poisoning 650
Subchorionic abruption 191
Subchorionic hemorrhage 141
Subhyoid bursitis 721
Subpubic angle 325
Sudden infant death
   syndrome (SIDS) 571
Superfecundation 234
Superfetation 234
Superficial thrombophlebitis 591
Superior vena cava 268
Sutures
   B lynch 537, 538
   hayman 539
   pereira 539
   U type 540
Symphysis pubis 24, 324, 325
Syncope 430, 454, 622
Syncytiotrophoblasts 11
Syndactyly 157
Synechiae 105
Syphilis 46, 103, 110, 111, 248,
   709, 712
Systemic hypertension 428
Systemic lupus erythematosus
   (SLE) 45, 103, 110, 113,
   255, 261, 697
Systolic thrill 454

T

T lymphocytes 484
T. Gondii 502
T_3 722, 724, 725
T_4 723, 724, 725, 729, 730
   free 738
   total 738
Tachyarrhythmia 439
Tachycardia 424
Tay-Sachs disease 44
T-cells 109, 135
Tears 536

Telbivudine 686
Tenderness
    extrauterine 363
    uterine 363
Tenofovir 706
Tenofovir (TDF) 705
    in pregnancy 707
Tenosynovitis 493
Tetanospasmin 633
Tetanus toxoid immunization
        schedule 21
Tetanus 623
    neonatal 634
    symptoms and signs 633
    treatment 634
    vaccines 634
Tetralogy of Fallot (TOF) 468
Thalassemia 8, 59, 62, 63, 80, 82, 83
    alpha 83, 84, 87, 247
        management of 87
    beta 83, 85
        management of 86
    intermedia 86
    major 80, 82
    minor 86
    sickle beta
        plus 89
        zero 89
    syndromes 82
T-helper 2 cells 135
Thiazide diuretic 461
Thiazolidinediones 294
Third trimester
    examination 27
    signs 27
    symptoms 27
    ultrasound features 35
Thrill 426
    continuous 426
    presystolic 426
    systolic 426
Thrombin 108, 136
Thrombocytopenia 63, 112, 292,
        307, 313, 476, 477, 493, 494,
        504, 505, 670, 691, 697
    heparin-induced 136
    neonatal 272, 308
    with preeclampsia 519
Thromboembolic disorders 591
Thromboembolism 208, 445,
        451, 447
    venous 370
Thrombophilia 107, 184, 187, 255,
        261, 314

inherited 105, 107, 129
    testing 104
Thrombophlebitis 112, 527, 585
    septic 586
    superficial 586
Thromboplastin 162
Thrombosis 108, 110, 112, 128,
        346, 546
    arterial 129
    deep vein 112
    renal arterial 113
    venous 112
Thrombotic thrombocytopenic
        purpura (TTP) 696
Thromboxane A2 111, 193
Thyroglossal cyst 721
Thyroid autoimmunity 125
Thyroid cancer in pregnancy 733
Thyroid changes in
        pregnancy 724
Thyroid disorders 45, 103, 105, 131
Thyroid dysfunction 125
    in pregnancy 725
Thyroid function tests 103
Thyroid gland 14, 722
Thyroid hormones,
        functions of 723
Thyroid nodules 733
Thyroid peroxidise autoantibodies
        (TPOAB) 125
Thyroid profile 263
Thyroid storm 728
Thyroidectomy
    subtotal 731
    total 731
Thyroiditis 494, 727
    hyperthyroid
        postpartum 734, 735
    postpartum 734, 737
Thyroid-stimulating hormone 131
Thyrotoxicosis 6, 170, 248, 429,
        439, 720, 726, 728, 732
    primary 719
    secondary 719
Thyroxine 723, 727
Tinnitus 316
Tissue plasminogen activator
        (TPA) 355
Tocolysis 192, 208
    drugs 391
        atosiban 393
        beta agonists 391
        calcium channel
            blockers 391

        contraindications 395
        indomethacin 393
        isoxsuprine 392
        magnesium sulfate 394
        nitroglycerin 394
        rofecoxib 394
        terbutaline 394
Topiramate 627, 630
TORCH 126, 263, 266
Total breech extraction 407
Toxoplasma 498
    amniocentesis 500
    diagnosis 499
    gondii 498
    prenatal screening 499
    primary prevention 499
    transmission to fetus 501
    vertical transmission 501
Toxoplasmosis 126, 248
    congenital 499, 501
    treatment 502
Tracheoesophageal (TE)
        fistula 731
Transferrin 53, 61, 80
Transverse myelopathy 113
Traumatic vaginal delivery 284
Trendelenburg position 215, 216
Treponema pallidum
        hemagglutin assay 22
Trichophagia 49
Tricuspid regurgitation 223, 224,
        428, 429, 432, 449, 450, 459
Tricuspid stenosis 424, 428, 429
Triploidy 10, 12
Trisomy 11, 16, 21
Troglitazone 294
Trophoblast 109, 111, 152, 210
Trophoblastic diseases 6
Trophoblastic
        embolization 169, 173
Tryptophan 105
TSH 168, 727, 730, 732, 738
T-sign 218
Tubal ectopic pregnancy
    diagnosis
        transabdominal (TAS) 147
        transvaginal (TVS) 147
    etiology 145
    physical examination 146
    presentation 146
    risk factors 145
    treatment 150
        surgical route 150

Tubal ectopic
   unruptured 155
Tubal ligation 145
   failure 146
Tubal rupture 150
Tubal surgery 146
Tuberculin reaction 487
Tuberculosis 36, 45, 48, 50, 57, 103, 111, 319, 483
   active 486
   causative agent 485
   diagnosis 486
   extrapulmonary 485, 486
   genital 119
   latent 487, 492
   osseous 486
   pathogenesis 484
   pregnancy management 491
   prevention 490
   pulmonary 485, 486, 586, 592, 700
   risk factors 485
   signs and symptoms 485
   transmission 484
   urogenital 486
Tuberculous pleurisy 486
Tubo-ovarian
   abscess 147, 377, 586
Tumour necrosis factor 188
TVS 150
Twins 230
   conjoined 215, 229
   dichorionic 220
   dizygotic 219
   dizygous 216
   monoamniotic 219, 220, 222, 238
   monochorionic 238
   monozygotic 218
   uniovular 360
   with previous scar 240
Twin entrapment 240
Twin gestation 187, 728
   amniotic fluid assessment 232
   cervical length
      measurement 232
   contributing factors 233
   fetal
      complications 235
      surveillance 231
   management 236–240
      first trimester 236
      indications for cesarean section 238

   optimal time of
      delivery 237
   prepregnancy 236
   second trimester 237
   third trimester 237
   maternal complications 234
   screening for anomalies 230
      first trimester 230
      second trimester 231
Twin reversed arterial perfusion
syndrome (TRAP) 228
   diagnosis 229
   differential diagnosis 228
   treatment 229
Twin-to-twin transfusion
   syndrome (TTTS) 230, 232, 238, 243, 248
   anastomosis 223
   antenatal criteria 223
   features of donor twin 224
   features of recipient twin 224
   laser ablation 225
   management 225
   serial amnioreduction 225
Typhoid 586
Tyrosine kinase 287

U

Umbilical artery 22, 223, 224, 254–256, 270, 271
   doppler 312
Umbilical cord 69
   compression 610
   short 548
Umbilical vein 273, 274
Umbilical venous dilatation 245
Umbilical venous flow 275
Unicornuate uterus 123
Ureaplasma urealyticum 512
Ureteral stent placement 377
Ureteric artery 543
Ureteroscopic retrieval 377
Ureterovesical reflux 371
Urinary calculi 147
Urinary fistula 546
Urinary tract infections 92, 590
Urine culture/sensitivity 266
Urine pregnancy tests
   (UPT) 5, 145, 164, 169
Urobilin 673
Urobilinogen 672
Urolithiasis 362, 368, 377

Ursodeoxycholic acid
   (UDCA) 677, 680
Uterine anomalies 105
   agenesis 121
   arcuate uterus 122, 123, 124
   bicornuate uterus 122, 123
      treatment 133
   canalization defects 124
   classification of 121
   congenital 145
   DES related 122, 130
   didelphys 122, 123
   embolization of 210
   septate uterus 122
      treatment 133
   subseptate 123
   unicornuate uterus 121, 123
      treatment 133
Uterine artery 225, 270, 541, 542
   branches 543
   doppler 271, 304, 314
   ligation 540
Uterine atony 523, 549
Uterine contractions 336
Uterine development 121
Uterine hyperstimulation 619
Uterine incarceration 381
Uterine incision 340, 343
   J-shaped 327
   T-shaped 327
Uterine inversion 519, 528, 547
   causes and risk factors 548
   classification 548
   diagnosis 548
   management 549
   pathophysiology 548
Uterine leiomyoma 215
Uterine malformations 404
Uterine massage 526, 532
Uterine natural killer cells 109
Uterine perforation 176
Uterine rupture 120, 184, 330, 338, 360, 365, 519, 544, 549, 613
Uterine scar 200
Uterine synechiae 133
Uterine tamponade 533, 551
Uterine torsion 381
Uteroplacental blood flow
   assessment 269
Uteroplacental
   circulation 269, 335
Uteroplacental
   insufficiency 112, 611

Uteroplacental sinuses 201
Uterotonic agent 525
Uterovaginal prolapse 549
Uterus
  agenesis treatment 132
  atonic 546
  didelphys 130
  hypoplasia 132
  septate 159
  subinvolution of 588, 593
UTI 377
UTI in pregnancy 371

V

Vaginal anastomosis 122
Vaginal artery 543
Vaginal birth after cesarean (VBAC) 327, 337
  contraindications to 327
  induction of labor in 329
  risks
    for infant 329
    of failed 329
Vaginal discharge 161
Valcyclovir 509
Valproic acid 630
  associated malformations 631
  malformations associated 625
Valsartan 461
Valvuloplasty 453

Vancomycin 590, 632
Vancomycin 1 438
Varicose veins 43, 216
Vasa previa 184, 525
  diagnosis 212
  differential diagnosis 211
  management 213
  risk factors 211
Vasculopathy 255
Vasoconstriction, thromboxane-mediated 306
Vasodilators 461, 463
Venous thrombosis 107, 440
Ventricular aneurysm 422
Ventricular bigemini 424
Ventricular hypertrophy 449
Ventricular septal defect 424, 429, 434, 466, 468
Vesicoamniotic shunt 260
Vesicouterine pouch 337
Vesicovaginal fistula 326
Vesicular mole 249
Vigabatrin 628, 630
Vincristine 175
Virilization 379
Vitamin
  B_{12} 65, 72, 97
    deficiency 49, 50, 98
  C 66, 87, 97
    deficiency 98

  D 236
  K 680
Voglibose 294
Volvulus 375
Von Braun-Fernwald's sign 4
Von Graefe's sign 721
Von Willebrand's disease 519
Vulvovaginal trauma 213

W

Warfarin 137, 255, 446, 448
Water hammer pulse 425, 455
West syndrome 628
Western blot (WB) 702
Wharton's jelly 607
White matter injury 396
Wilson's disease 674

Y

Yolk sacs 142, 218

Z

Zidovudine (AZT) 705
Zonisamide 624, 627
Zuspan regimen 645
Zygosity 219, 230